AF183172

FOETUS AND PLACENTA

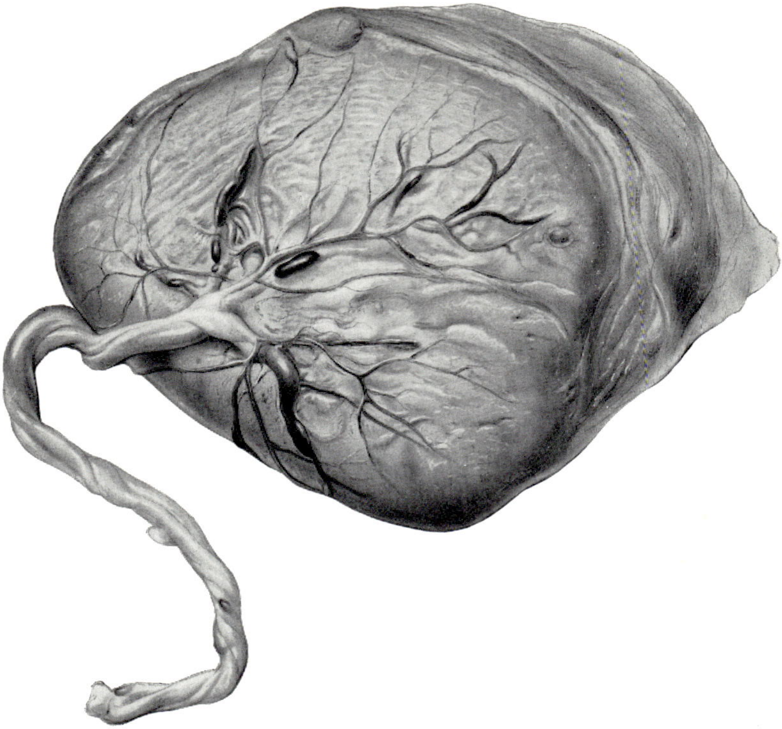

FRONTISPIECE. The human placenta – an incomplete endocrine gland. From a drawing by D. P. Hammersley.

FOETUS AND PLACENTA

EDITED BY

ARNOLD KLOPPER
M.D. Ph.D. F.R.C.O.G.

Department of Obstetrics and Gynaecology
University of Aberdeen, Scotland

AND

EGON DICZFALUSY
M.D.

Reproductive Endocrinology Research Unit
Karolinska Sjukhuset, Stockholm, Sweden

BLACKWELL SCIENTIFIC PUBLICATIONS
OXFORD AND EDINBURGH

© BLACKWELL SCIENTIFIC PUBLICATIONS 1969

All rights reserved. No part of this publication may be reproduced, stored in a retrieval system, or transmitted, in any form or by any means, electronic, mechanical, photocopying, recording or otherwise, without the prior permission of the copyright owner.

SBN 632 05140 X

FIRST PUBLISHED 1969

Printed in Great Britain by
ADLARD AND SON LTD
DORKING, SURREY
and bound by
THE KEMP HALL BINDERY

Contents

Contributors

SAM BRODY, M.D., Department of Obstetrics & Gynaecology, University of Gothenburg, Sweden.

EGON DICZFALUSY, M.D., Swedish Medical Research Council, Reproductive Endocrinology Research Unit, Karolinska Sjukhuset, Stockholm, Sweden.

H.G. DIXON, PH.D., M.B., B.S., F.R.C.P.(Ed.), F.R.C.O.G., Department of Obstetrics and Gynaecology, University of Bristol, Bristol, England.

DWAIN D. HAGERMAN, M.D., Department of Biochemistry and Department of Obstetrics & Gynecology, University of Colorado School of Medicine, Denver, U.S.A.

DR. MED. H.-D. HIERSCHE, Univ.-Frauenklinik, Mainz, Germany.

ARNOLD KLOPPER, M.D., PH.D., F.R.C.O.G., Department of Obstetrics & Gynaecology, University of Aberdeen, Aberdeen, Scotland.

SALVATORE MANCUSO, M.D., Universita Cattolica del Sacro Cuore, Istituto di Clinica Ostetrica e Ginecologica, Roma, Italy.

M.C. MACNAUGHTON, M.B., F.R.C.O.G., Department of Obstetrics & Gynaecology, University of Dundee, Dundee, Scotland.

W.B. ROBERTSON, B.SC., M.D., M.C.PATH., Department of Pathology, St. George's Hospital Medical School, London, S.W.1.

SAMUEL SOLOMON, PH.D., Department of Biochemistry and Experimental Medicine, McGill University and The University Clinic, Royal Victoria Hospital, Montreal, Canada.

Dr. med. K. THOMSEN, Department of Obstetrics and Gynaecology, University of Hamburg, Hamburg, Western Germany.

MAUREEN YOUNG, Ph.D., Department of Gynaecology, St. Thomas's Hospital Medical School, London, S.E.1.

E. V. YOUNGLAI, Ph.D., Department of Biochemistry and Experimental Medicine, McGill University and The University Clinic, Royal Victoria Hospital, Montreal, Canada.

Preface

When Mr Per Saugman of Blackwell Scientific Publications first suggested the idea of a book on the placenta to us, the thought was to produce a compendium somewhat on the lines of Snoeck's classic *Le placenta humain*, bringing together some of the experience gained since its publication. When, however, we came to examine our capabilities in this respect we found them short and decided, perhaps defensively, that there was no great need for a general survey covering all aspects of recent work on the placenta. We were aware that all over the world there were men whose scientific interests centred on the placenta; we have gambled that there is still a sufficient commonality among placentologists for there to be a place for a book which is not devoted to one interest, nor pretends to survey anything more than a haphazard selection of aspects. We have been concerned with the divisive trend in placentology as in other scientific fields and often felt the need to know more of the developments in related disciplines to our own also concerned with placental function. Endocrinologists, pathologists, anatomists, biochemists, paediatricians and obstetricians have a common interest in the placenta. Our object has been to make a contribution to the means by which they might look over the barriers between disciplines and see the green pastures next door.

This book has in its genesis undergone many sea changes. Not the least of these has been the change of emphasis from the concept of the placenta as a single functional entity to that of the foeto-placental unit. In fact we have had to extend this unity to cover not only the contents of the uterus, but in some respects to include the uterus itself. This is a generalization which we have found useful in endocrinology; from our other contributors it appears that it is applicable to other disciplines also.

It had been our intention to examine all those areas of foeto-placental physiology where the content of knowledge was changing most rapidly and to seek a contribution from one of those immediately concerned with research on a particular aspect. In the event, this too, proved too ambitious a project for we would have required several volumes for adequate coverage. The outcome has been that the selection of material for this volume represents largely the interests and contacts of its editors. Our only justification is that it is a segment of experience common to many placentologists.

We are aware of the strong endocrinological bias engendered by our common interest in this subject. There has been an explosion of information about placental endocrinology in the last decade and this is an appropriate moment to attempt to integrate the data into a coherent description of placental function. Although each chapter is complete in itself, we hope the sections on anatomy, enzymology, placental transfer and the like will be accepted as complementary to the central theme of endocrinology. Perhaps the most notable of the many aspects in which this volume is deficient is pathology. Happily, the handbook on the placenta by Strauss, Benirschke and Driscoll which has appeared since our work began has been largely devoted to this aspect and considers placental pathology with a great deal more expertise and detail than we could hope to attain.

A word of explanation about the format and style of this book. The other contributors are all recognized authorities in their field and we have not considered it wise to impose too rigid a conformity of language and layout on them. The reader may find himself disconcerted by abrupt transitions from British to American usage and spelling. We consider individuality of expression more precious than the convenience of uniformity although in such mundane matters as usage in references we have laid some bonds on the freer European spirits and on all we have imposed the limitation of confining their remarks to the human animal.

This book has been longer in production than we care to own. None of the fault lies with our publishers who have treated our own shortcomings with exemplary patience and fulfilled their part with speed and efficiency. As usual in reviews our contributors have drawn their material from many publications. It would be tedious and an empty ceremony to list them all. We hope that the private thanks of the authors and public acknowledgement of our indebtedness will satisfy. Our wives, Mary and Anne, have helped us across barriers of language and rearranged their lives to make the production of this book possible.

Arnold Klopper
Egon Diczfalusy

Aberdeen and Stockholm 1969.

1
The Growth of the Conceptus and its Blood Supply

H. G. DIXON & W. B. ROBERTSON

Although much of the available information on the interrelationship of the growth patterns of uterus, placenta and foetus is based upon animal evidence, it is obvious that, in the human, differential growth patterns of these three elements exist.

Reynolds (1947) has shown that in the rabbit the conceptus possesses a spherical shape up to the 22nd day. The growth of this conceptus in a spherical or ovoid shape leads to a marked increase in tension of the uterine wall which rises geometrically in proportion to the increase in radii of the conceptus. Reynolds considers that the high tissue tension is a direct stimulus to uterine growth. During this phase the maternal blood flow through the uterus falls progressively until at the 22nd day a critically low level of flow is reached, being relieved in a dramatic fashion by a physiological mechanism which Reynolds has called 'conversion'. It consists of a sudden change in shape of the conceptus and its enclosing uterus from ovoid to cylindrical. Any further increase in size of the conceptus now evokes local tissue tension increase in a linear rather than a geometric proportion. The rapid conversion into a cylindrical shape reduces intra-uterine tension in accordance with established hydrostatic principles. Because of the lowered tissue tension there is a remarkable improvement in uterine blood flow, restoring it to the amount flowing in early pregnancy, but after the 24th day of gestation the flow again begins to fall. Reynolds provides experimental evidence to show that the high tissue tension in the preconversion stage is a stimulus to direct growth and hyperplasia of the uterine tissue, but that after conversion, owing to the lowered tension no further growth occurs, the hyperplastic elements of the uterine wall simply being 'paid out'.

Although there are obvious anatomical differences between the uterus of the rabbit and that of the primate, an essentially similar state of affairs has been shown to occur in the rhesus monkey by Gillespie *et al.* (1949) and in the human by Gillespie (1950). Gillespie has shown that, although the human uterus is pear-shaped, at the onset of pregnancy it gradually becomes spherical and is certainly so by the 20th week. From then on it elongates rapidly. Additional evidence that the primate uterus behaves in much the same way as that of the rabbit has been provided by Ramsey (1949), who has shown that in the preconversion stage in the monkey the endomyometrial arteries proliferate and become very closely coiled. Following the conversion phenomenon, which in the monkey occurs at or shortly after the 100th day, these arteries are very rapidly uncoiled along their whole length. From personal observation of human term placentae *in situ* and placental bed biopsies, the authors feel that this uncoiling of the spiral arteries, although it undoubtedly occurs to some extent in the human, is not nearly such a remarkable phenomenon as it is in the monkey.

Bearing in mind this basic information on the growth of the uterus during pregnancy we must now turn to the pattern of both foetal and placental growth in the human. The measurement of both these parameters is far more difficult than the simple assessment of uterine growth. Not only is the size of the foetus determined to some extent by genetic factors but its rate of growth is also considerably affected by alterations in the utero-placental environment. The situation with regard to growth of the placenta is perhaps even more difficult, as, in the villous period, the placenta undergoes a stage of active proliferation from about the 13th day to the end of the 4th month, and then a period of slow enlargement, *pari passu* with that of the uterus from the 5th month to term (Wilkin 1965).

From an obstetrical point of view it is the growth of the foetus during the second half of pregnancy which offers the greater interest and this has recently been studied by Hendricks (1964). He showed that during the second half of pregnancy the foetal growth is relatively rapid when measured in terms of daily percentage weight increments, being in the range of 1·6 to 1·8 per cent from week 20 to week 34. After week 34 the rate begins slowly to drop, being approximately 1·4 per cent at week 36. Thereafter the decrease in daily percentage increments is sharp, reaching 0·6 per cent at term and 0·2 per cent at week 43. There is, of course, a considerable variation in weights from foetus to foetus at the same stage of gestation and in the large numbers studied by Hendricks the standard deviation ranged between 11·4 and 15·3 per cent of the mean value. He adopted a figure of approximately 13 per cent and considered that no matter how large a group is studied the standard deviation will never depart very far from this percentage. These findings are of considerable interest when reviewed in the light of the finding of Dixon *et al.* (1963). They found a gradual diminution in the clearance of radioactive Na from 34 weeks to term, continuing past term. Whilst Hendricks considers that the birth weight is probably the most useful overall index of the stage of development reached by any foetus he is careful to point out the fallacies of such a belief and indeed much present work in neonatal paediatrics appears to show that the neurological development of the child is a far better index of its gestational age than its birth weight.

The weight of the placenta at various stages of gestation has been studied, amongst others, by Kloosterman & Huidekoper (1954) who have calculated what they call a 'placental coefficient', which is simply the ratio of placental weight to foetal weight. At 8 weeks this ratio is 2·0 whereas at term it varies between 0·13 and 0·19. In other words, in early pregnancy the growth of the placenta is rapid as compared to that of the child, but in later pregnancy, whilst the child is growing relatively rapidly the placenta increases only slightly in size. The explanation of this phenomenon lies in the method of development of the placenta. Between the 13th day and the end of the 4th month, during what Wilkin terms the stage of elaboration, the primary villi are developing into secondary and tertiary villi and a foetal placental circulation is being established. Later the foetal cotyledons and placental septa are formed. The details of this process will be considered later. After the 4th month, placental development is achieved both by an increase in area of placental surface and by an increase in thickness. The thickness in particular increases rapidly between the 4th and 7th months. All placental growth after the 4th month is achieved entirely by enlargement of the formed foetal cotyledons, which Crawford (1962) estimates increase their volume some 500 times between the 12th and the 40th week. There is no evidence that the number of cotyledons increases during this final stage of placental growth. Placental weights were also studied by Hendricks (1964) and his findings were in broad agreement with those of Kloosterman & Huidekoper. He showed that the initial growth of the placenta is much more rapid than that of the foetus as it achieves 50 per cent of its final weight in the same time that the foetus takes to achieve 30 per cent. Similarly he found the slowing of placental growth at the end of pregnancy to be more marked than that of the foetus although the percentage standard deviation of the mean among the placentas was somewhat larger than that for the foetuses, being approximately 21 per cent. These simple mechanistic criteria of placental growth are not very helpful from the functional point of view. In terms of the latter it is important to distinguish between useful tissue, (the placental parenchyma and gas-exchanging area), and supporting structures.

The problem of the early embedding of the fertilized ovum and the development of a maternal blood supply to the placenta is a subject which has attracted the attention of many workers over a long period of time. Here it is possible only to give the briefest review of the generally accepted sequence of events. For further information the interested reader should refer to Hamilton & Boyd (1960) and these authors' several other masterly contributions to the subject, as well as to the work of Wilkin (1965). The mechanics of early nidation and trophoblastic invasion do not concern us here excepting, perhaps, the observation of Böving (1962) who, from a study of early implantation in the rabbit, concluded that invasion was specifically aimed for the subepithelial vessels of the endometrium. The invasion only spreads after the penetration has reached the vessels for which it is 'aiming'.

The blastocystic trophoblast of the early ovum in the process of implantation differentiates into primitive cytotrophoblast and primitive syncytiotrophoblast and soon after differentiation the syncytiotrophoblast begins to show marked vacuolation. These vacuoles appear about the 9th day and the 12th to 13th day there is a well developed system of lacunae throughout the syncytiotrophoblast. The process of invasion into the endometrium by the cytotrophoblast has opened maternal blood vessels, although whether these are specific targets in the human, as they are in the rabbit, is, as yet, not known. Hamilton & Boyd (1960) note that there appears to be no disordered destruction of maternal tissue nor haemorrhage into the decidua. In contrast the endothelium of the maternal vessels at the points of communication is in neat apposition to the peripheral syncytium. These authors also point out that the erythrocytes which pass from the opened vessels into the lacunar spaces of the syncytiotrophoblast show abnormal histological staining reactions, taking up eosin poorly when compared with maternal erythrocytes in blood vessels away from the implantation site. They suggest that the erythrocytes in the lacunar spaces are, at this stage, in a special physiological state, but their basis for this suggestion is difficult to follow if any sort of maternal placental circulation exists.

As development progresses between the 13th and the 18th day, the lacunae run together and the strands of syncytiotrophoblast, losing their irregular pattern tend to become more and more radially orientated around the chorion. Thus there is formed a single cavity lined almost throughout by syncytiotrophoblast and crossed by strands of the same tissue. The strands are converted into primary villi by the proliferation of cytotrophoblastic tissue in their centre. The blood filled cavity surrounding them is the intervillous space.

Between the 18th and 21st day the primary villi are further transformed by the development of a central axis of mesoblastic tissue which is in continuity with the primary extraembryonic mesoblast. These secondary villi are then converted into tertiary villi by the formation of haemopoietic tissue and vascular buds (Wilkin 1965). Where these tertiary villi are in contact with the syncytiotrophoblast covering decidua their cytotrophoblast extends outwards so that it begins to form a complete, although irregular, cytotrophoblastic layer around the conceptus, the so-called trophoblastic shell. In this way the original primitive syncytiotrophoblast is split into two parts. The superficial one lines the intervillous space and is persistent whereas the deeper part, in contact with maternal tissue, persists only in part, possibly giving rise to the giant cells so characteristic of the placental bed.

Thus we have the definitive syncytium lining the whole intervillous space whilst the tertiary villi are for the most part attached to the cytotrophoblastic shell, a characteristic which gives them the name of anchoring villi. The syncytium covering these villi begins to give off buds, most of which are later penetrated by cytotrophoblast cells and then by mesodermal tissue to give rise to daughtervilli. Sometimes, however, the syncytial buds become pedunculated and cut off so that they find their way into the maternal circulation.

Although it is not until the 14th or 15th day that the spiral arteries proper are opened by cytotrophoblastic invasion and the maternal placental circulation through the intervillous space becomes established, it seems highly probable that the suggestion of Hamilton & Boyd (1960) that a sluggish circulation exists as soon as the capillaries of the superficial endometrium and venous sinusoids are invaded, is correct.

At this stage of placental development there are some 20 to 40 main stem villi. Each of these, by a process of budding, now gives rise to between 25 and 50 daughter villi and, according to Wilkin (1958), most of these daughter villi run down towards the basal plate to which they become attached by their trophoblastic investment and then run for a short distance back up into the intervillous space. With increasing growth of the uterus, the area of the placenta increases and thus the anchoring points of these daughter villi are carried further apart. Wilkin believes that during this process they become arranged into symmetrical structures of anchoring stems around a median axis to which he has given the name 'Systemes Tambours'. Whether Wilkin's explanation of the method of their formation is correct or not, there seems very little doubt that in its final form the foetal cotyledon consists of one or more such structures arising from a main stem villus.

The problem as to how these foetal structures are related to the maternal blood supply of the intervillous space is complex and, as yet, unsolved. There is no agreement even on the simple question as to how many maternal blood vessels open into the intervillous space. Spanner (1936), working with a corrosion preparation from a pregnancy of some six months gestational age, found 94 arteries with a total of 488 openings into the intervillous space. Boyd (1956) on the basis of partial counts arrived at figures of 180, 310 and 320 arterial openings in three different term placentae. Brosens (1964a) in a serial section examination of one half of a placenta found only 36 arteries with even fewer veins. In a step serial section examination of some 2/5ths of an *in situ* term placenta Brosens & Dixon (1966) found one arterial opening to every two square centimetres of basal plate. Boyd is quoted by Wilkin (1965) as now feeling that there are approximately 100 arterial openings into the intervillous space of the term placenta and this figure would be in reasonable agreement with that of Brosens and Dixon. The explanation for the discrepancy in the figures which have been given probably depends upon three factors. Firstly, Ramsey (1959) has shown, in the rhesus monkey, the uneven distribution of arterial communications with the intervillous space. If in the human there exists a similar uneven distribution as Brosens & Dixon suggested, then the partial counts are probably in error. Secondly, not all the counting has been done on term *in situ* placentae and it is possible that in early pregnancy each spiral artery opens through a number of orifices which disappear in later pregnancy. Finally, counting vessel openings in the scattered remnants of decidua attached to a delivered placenta is likely to be fallacious.

Wilkin is attracted to the idea that there are in the region of 100 arterial openings into the intervillous space as this allows him to speculate on the possibility, which he emphasizes is by no means proven, that each of the 100 or so 'Systemes Tambours' has its own spiral artery opening at the centre of its ring of attachment. Attractive though this concept may be, it is difficult to correlate with personal observations. If it were so it would imply that the spiral arteries opened more or less uniformly along the basal plate. This is manifestly not true. Furthermore, it implies that the arteries open along the decidual plate but away from the septa which form later in pregnancy.

Bumm (1893) stated his belief that 'the arteries are mainly lying in the decidual projections and septa and eject their blood from the side of the cotyledon inwards to the intervillous space'. Unfortunately his work has been repeatedly misquoted by some authors who were apparently under the impression that the septa extended from the basal plate to reach the chorionic plate and the belief arose that Bumm thought the spiral arteries opened into the intervillous space near the chorionic plate. Reference to Bumm's original work is, however, sufficient to dispel this misconception. The septal opening of the spiral arteries was confirmed by Hinselman (1958), and Stieve (1941) amended Bumm's observations only slightly in that he specified that he had found the openings of the spiral arteries predominantly at the base of septa. However, Wieloch (1923) and Ramsey (1956) have criticized Bumm's findings and speculated that the structures that he considered to be septal arteries were, in fact, artifacts or tissue fissures. Hamilton & Boyd (1960) found the arteries opening at variable situations in the basal plate, and Spanner (1936) described them as opening in the area underlying the central part of the foetal cotyledon. Brosens & Dixon (1966) found that almost all the maternal arteries opened into the intervillous space a little above the general level of the decidual plate; usually at the base of, or a short way up, a septum (Fig. 1.1a, b and c). The nature of the material used by Brosens & Dixon allowed them to follow maternal vessels from their openings into the intervillous space down to levels in the myometrium where recognition of the nature of the vessels was easy. Occasionally a small artery was found opening into the intervillous space having no relationship to a septum but they noted that every sizable septum had at least one spiral artery opening at its base. If this anatomical work is correct then it follows that one must postulate some method of formation of the septa which allows them to develop at the sites of arterial entry.

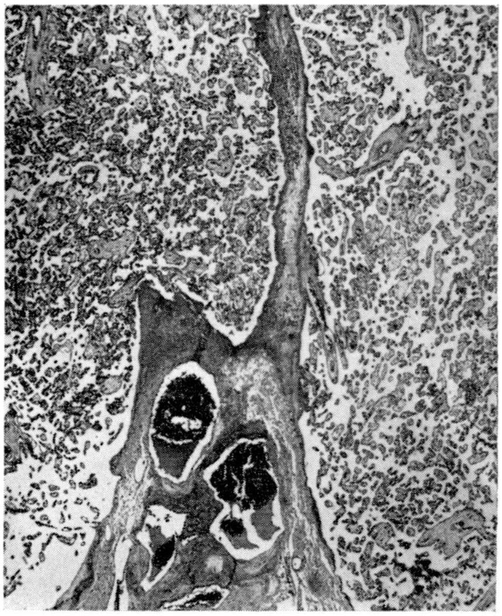

(a)

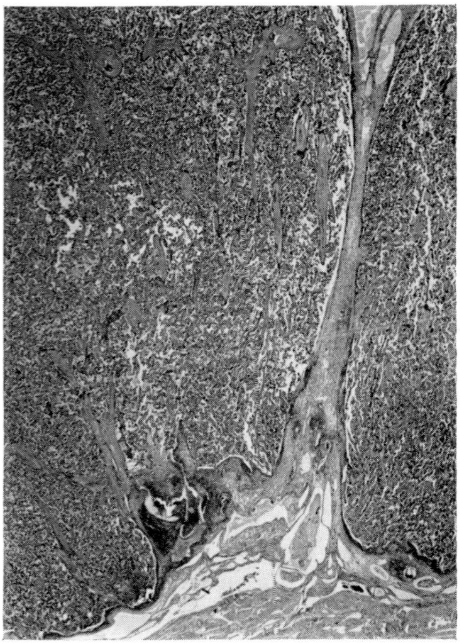

(b)

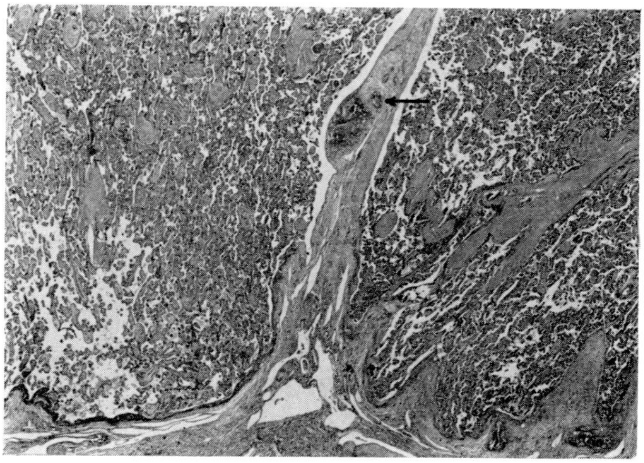

(c)

FIG. 1.1a, b and c. Maternal arteries at various levels in the placental septa. By courtesy of the Editor, *J. Obstet. Gynaec. Brit. Cwlth.* (a) = H. and E. × 12·6. (b) = H. and E. × 4·5. (c) = H. and E. × 7.

At one time the septa were regarded as being simply folds of the basal decidua and undoubtedly maternal tissue is incorporated into the base of the septum. Examination of early placentae from about the 14th week, however, leaves equally little doubt that apart from its juxta basal portion the septum at that stage consists of cytotrophoblast (Fig. 1.2). Wilkin (1965) has proposed that the septa develop from the formation at the periphery of the cotyledonary 'Systemes Tambours' of islands of cytotrophoblastic tissue containing strands of sclerosed avascular villous connective tissue, frequently surrounded by fibrinoid. By progressive

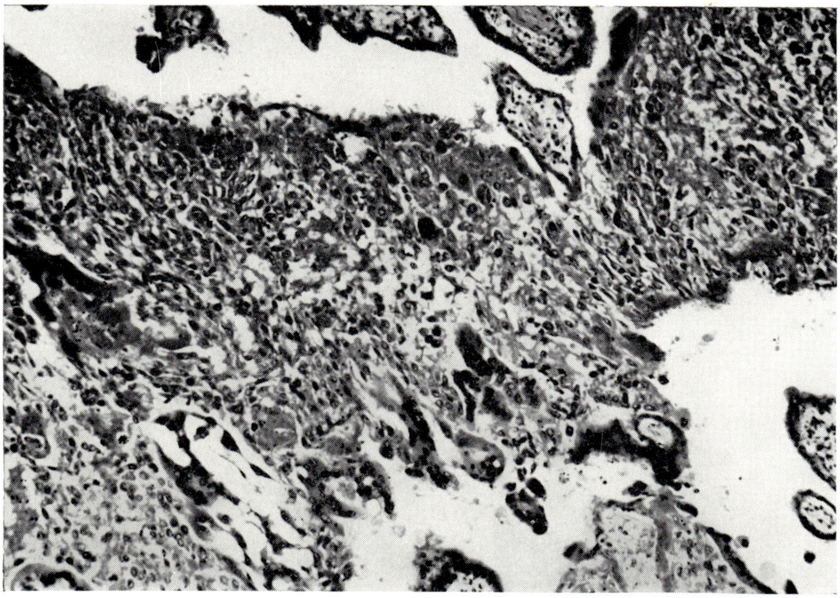

FIG. 1.2. High power view of transverse septum at 14 weeks gestation (see Fig. 1.4); composed mostly of cytotrophoblast with some syncytiotrophoblast proliferating from villi. H. and E. ×56.

fusion these cytotrophoblastic islands form incomplete cellular septa around the foetal cotyledon. These septa then fuse with the cytotrophoblast of the basal plate at the moment that the definitive syncytium of the floor of the intervillous space disappears. Later on in pregnancy, when the marked thickening of the placenta is occurring, a part of the basal plate consisting of both its cytotrophoblastic layer and the maternal decidual layer, becomes incorporated in the base of the septum. Wilkin himself tends to the view that the vessels found at the base of the septa are veins. The present authors' own observations lead them to believe that the veins drain through much larger orifices which are always found on the flat basal plate (Fig. 1.3). These venous openings usually join together just beneath the basal plate to form the so-called 'venous lakes'

(Ramsey 1956). Not only do the vessels in the base of the septa show throughout their length the physiological changes which occur specifically in spiral arteries during pregnancy and to which reference will be made later in this chapter, but as has been said, it is possible on serial sectioning to follow any vessel down to a level at which its nature can no

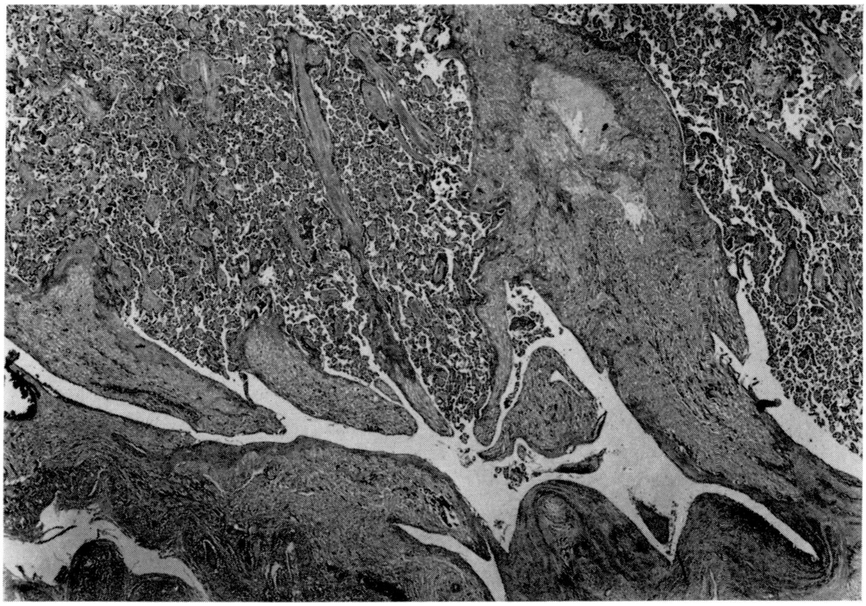

FIG. 1.3. Venous drainage at basal plate. By courtesy of the Editor, *J. Obstet. Gynaec. Brit. Cwlth.* H. and E. × 12.

longer be in doubt. How then can one explain the formation of the septa at sites where previously opened arteries are situated?

It is permissible to speculate that during the process of thickening of the placenta that occurs between the 4th and 7th month, arteries that were previously situated on a flat area of decidual plate are pulled into the base of a septum. This, however, does not explain the fact that for the most part, even in early pregnancy, arteries are found in decidual hummocks, nor the fact that it is only relatively small arteries that are found at term opening elsewhere than at the base of a septum. Furthermore, on serial sectioning of early placentae not all the villi reach the basal plate (Fig. 1.4) and in mature placentae very strong anchoring villi are found attached to the septa at all heights (Fig. 1.5). The villus which has anchored to the basal plate displays a remarkable propensity to proliferate cytotrophoblast at its tip and it is probable that even those villi which do not reach the basal plate retain this property. It could, therefore, be that the masses of cytotrophoblast which are seen from the 14th week onwards in the intervillous space are not so much proliferations from the periphery of attached villi but proliferations from the tips of unattached villi. Because of the peculiar behaviour of invading tropho-

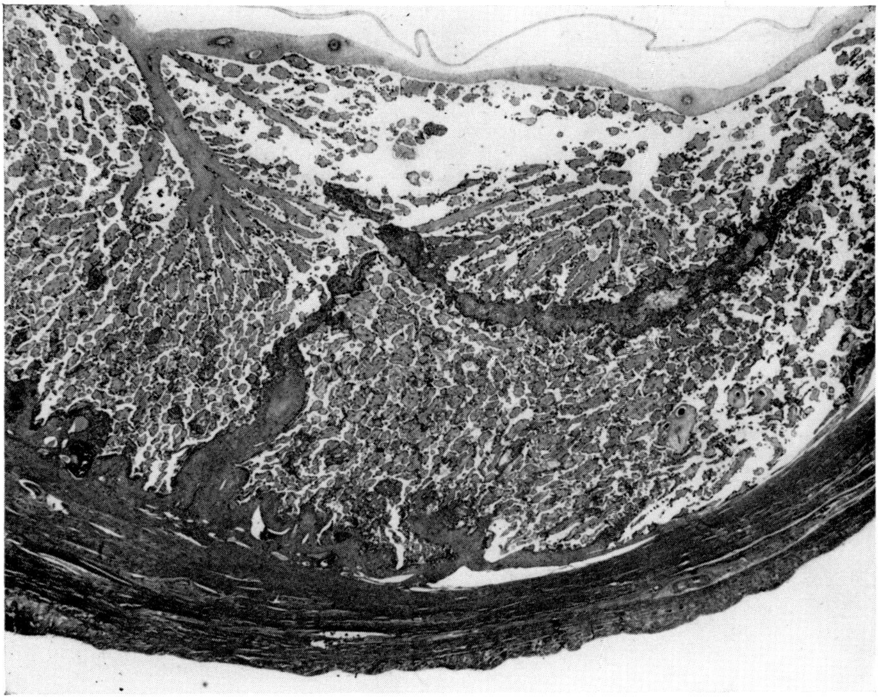

FIG. 1.4. Section of 14 weeks placenta *in situ* showing villous attachment to transverse primitive septum. By courtesy of the Editor, *J. Obstet. Gynaec. Brit. Cwlth.* H. and E. ×2·4.

blast in their vicinity, the vessel mouths at this stage of pregnancy are found in small decidual hummocks and it seems reasonable to suppose that the sheets of cytotrophoblast proliferated at the end of unattached villi will eventually fuse with these hummocks giving rise to a septum, with strong villous attachments that persist to term. Later on in the development of a septum the histological picture becomes somewhat confused because of the deposition of fibrinoid but the writers are in agreement with Wilkin that trophoblast can sometimes be found in the heart of a septum at term (Fig. 1.6).

As part of their studies of the *in situ* placenta by serial section techniques Brosens and Dixon constructed a model of the maternal side of the placenta (Fig. 1.7). In addition to demonstrating their views that most spiral arteries open just above the general level of the decidual plate,

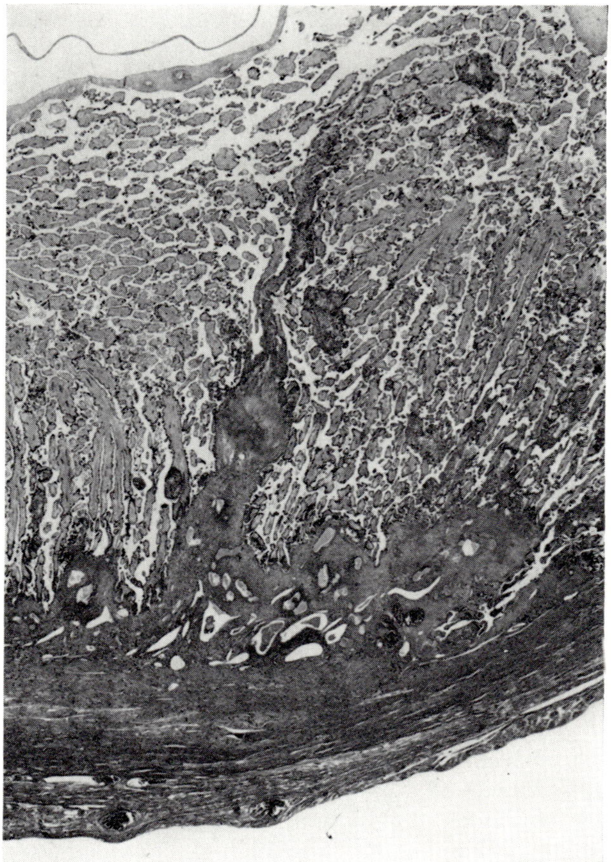

FIG. 1.5. Term Placenta *in situ* showing anchoring villi attached to septum at all levels. By courtesy of the Editor, *J. Obstet. Gynaec. Brit. Cwlth.* H. and E. ×3.

whether in the lower part of a septum or in a small protrusion of basal plate, this model also showed that the septa varied a great deal in height and length. They are frequently perforate and appear to be quite haphazardly distributed, allowing a free intercommunication between every part of the intervillous space. In many instances a septum appeared to separate a group of arterial openings from a group of venous drainage channels. Although they could find no evidence to support Bumm's original suggestion that the spiral artery openings were orientated to direct the blood flow laterally towards the foetal cotyledons, Brosens &

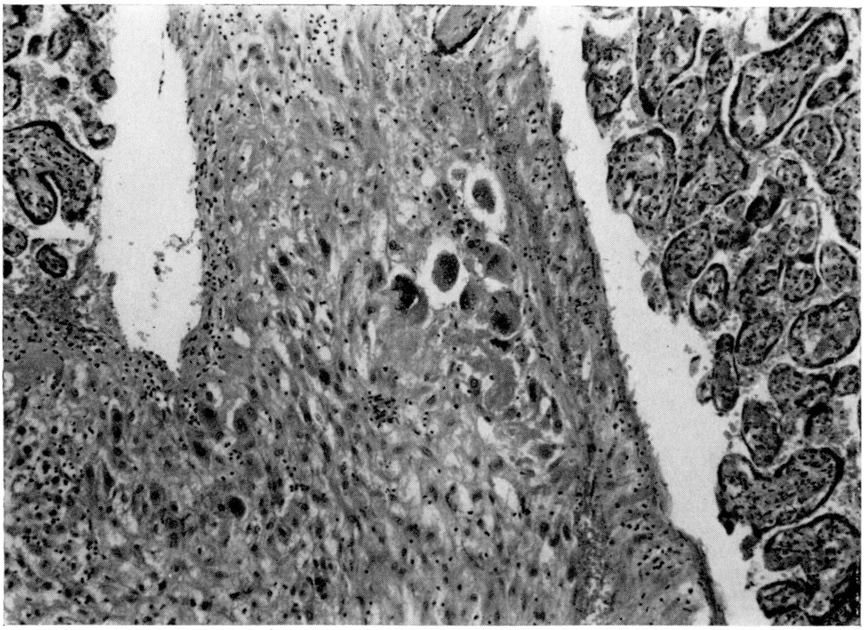

FIG. 1.6. Trophoblast in septum of term placenta. H. and E. × 100.

Dixon suggested that the septa may well play a more important part in directing blood flow through the intervillous space than that usually attributed to them.

Although there was much discussion before the present concept of random openings of arteries and veins throughout the entire basal plate came to be accepted, most workers on the placenta appear to have accepted, almost without question, the concept that there is a coinciding functional and anatomical compartmentation of both foetal and maternal components of the placenta. The finding of the great irregularity of both distribution and size of the septa makes it doubtful whether each foetal cotyledon, that is each major stem villus, lies separated from its neighbours within a neat surrounding ring of maternal septa complete with arterial supply and venous drainage.

Whilst we do not know the precise functional anatomy of the intervillous space, there is some information available on the behaviour of the intervillous space flow during the phases of uterine activity and rather less about its alteration during some of the complications of pregnancy.

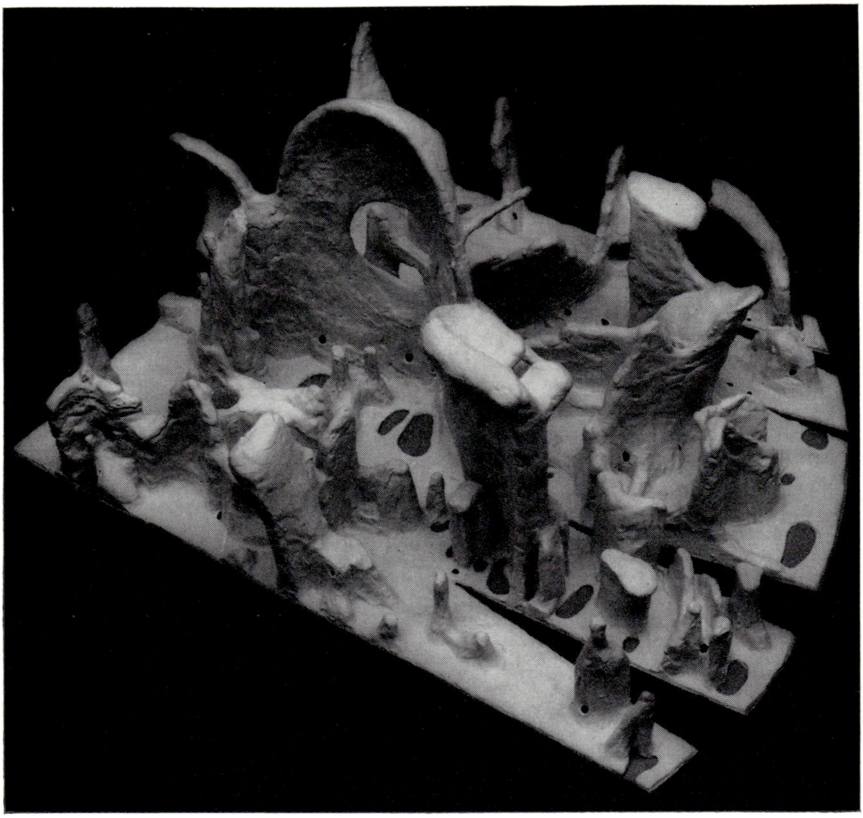

FIG. 1.7. Model of maternal surface of 2/5th of term placenta. By courtesy of the Editor, *J. Obstet. Gynaec. Brit. Cwlth.*

Since the work of Ramsey (1956 and 1963) on the monkey and Borell, Fernstrom & Westman (1958) on the human placenta, it is now generally accepted that blood flows through the intervillous space as a more or less constant stream, fed from the irregularly scattered orifices of the spiral vessels by funnel shaped jets of blood at a relatively high pressure. These jets not only bathe the villi with oxygenated blood but force out the blood already in the space through the venous drainage openings which lie scattered in the basal plate. There seems little doubt that this picture approximates at any rate to the true one and it is thus scarcely surprising that Fuchs, Spackman & Assali (1963) found that the pO_2 and pCO_2 of intervillous space blood varied widely from site to site.

The recent observations of Martin and his colleagues (1964) suggest that the haemodynamics of the intervillous space are more complicated than this simple picture would imply. These workers carried out in the rhesus monkey repeated radioarteriographic placentograms during uterine relaxation and were able to show alterations in the pattern of the arterial entries that were seen. They noted that the arterial spurts appeared or disappeared quite independently of any recorded myometrial activity or change in the maternal blood pressure. They suggest that these changes are due to some inherent vasomotor capacity of the arteries supplying the intervillous space but are obviously quite uncertain as to the mechanism and significance of the phenomenon they have demonstrated. There is some evidence that a similar phenomenon occurs in the human, but as yet we know remarkably little about the mechanism of regulation of intervillous space flow. The two prime variants that have to be considered are the changes in maternal systemic blood pressure and changes in intra-uterine pressure. Rather more is known about the latter than the former.

As might be expected, uterine contraction causes closure of the venous channels and then the arterioles and the pressure in the intervillous space rises (Hendricks 1958, Corner *et al.* 1963). Caldeyro-Barcia (1957) has shown that the maternal flow is slowed under these circumstances. These findings have been confirmed by Borrell *et al.* (1964) in the human during therapeutic abortions between the 18th and 20th week of gestation. They found that uterine contractions prevented the introduction of contrast medium into the intervillous space in three-quarters of the patients they investigated and that in the remainder the space was poorly or only partially visible. The uterine veins were generally not visible and there was a marked prolongation of the period of time during which the main branches of the uterine artery and its myometrial divisions could be seen, showing that there was retardation of the arterial blood flow. They could, however, find no definite correlation between the intensity of the contraction and the degree of circulatory retardation. All these authors suggest that the sequence of events affecting the intervillous space during uterine activity is governed by entirely mechanical phenomena related to myometrial contraction and a rise of intrauterine pressure.

The fact that the intervillous space pressure follows, as would be expected from simple hydraulic principles, the pressure of the intra-amniotic cavity has been demonstrated by Hendricks *et al.* (1959) and Ramsey *et al.* (1959). This relationship between the intervillous space pressure and the amniotic fluid pressure must remain the same despite alterations in maternal blood pressure. Quite how this is effected is obscure. It is not possible to demonstrate a rise in intra-amniotic pressure in even the most severe essential hypertensive in spite of the claims that have been made that this pressure is raised in pre-eclampsia. We must, therefore, assume that there is some mechanism which succeeds in holding a delicate balance between the maternal blood pressure and the pressure in the intervillous space which in turn is dictated by the general intrauterine pressure. The nature of this mechanism is unknown but it is presumably related to the vasomotor activity of the spiral arteries which results in their intermittent closure. As will be seen later, histological study of the spiral arteries in the human between the myometrio-decidual junction and their opening into the intervillous space, suggests that far from being the muscular type of vessel that one would associate with a brisk, yet delicate vasomotor action, these vessels have lost almost all their musculo-elastic tissue. Before considering these histological changes we must outline what little is known on the changing rate of intervillous space flow during normal pregnancy.

The problem of the estimation of this flow rate in the human female is one of considerable complexity. Assali and his co-workers (1953) and Metcalfe *et al.* (1955) adapted the nitrous oxide technique of measuring blood flow to the pregnant uterus and obtained flow rates in early pregnancy in women who were undergoing therapeutic abortion and from some women near term at the time of Caesarean Section. The complexity of this method as well as the more simple practical difficulty of obtaining venous blood samples truly representative of the venous outflow from the entire uterus, apparently accounts for the fact that no observations were made in abnormal pregnancies. Assali has himself shown that the dye-dilution technique is useless in the measurement of uterine blood flow and has more recently been using the electro-magnetic flowmeter to measure uterine blood flow at the time of therapeutic abortion between 10 and 28 weeks gestation. The results he has obtained correspond very roughly to those obtained by the nitrous oxide technique but he considers them more uniform. Whilst these methods are of theoretical interest and importance, they are not suitable for the investigation of a large number of healthy pregnant women. In two articles (Browne & Veall 1953 and Dixon *et al.* 1963) workers at Hammersmith have reported their results on the rate of intervillous space flow by a relatively simple technique of direct injection of ^{24}Na into the intervillous space and measurement of its half dispersal time. They have been able to show that in the normal pregnancy there is apparently a slight, but progressive slowing of intervillous space flow rate from 34 weeks to term. Simple though the method is, when compared with others, it is not without its difficulties both practical and theoretical.

Fuchs *et al.* (1963) have pointed out that, with a sufficient amount of ingenuity, blood can be aspirated from any part of the uterus. Browne and his co-workers agree with this statement but hold that previous localization of the placenta to the anterior aspect of the uterus is an essential pre-requisite for this type of investigation. A danger does exist that blood and even chorionic villi may be aspirated from a venous lake immediately beneath the decidual plate and the ^{24}Na injected, but in these instances Browne noted that the half dispersal time of the ^{24}Na is extremely short and, in fact, corresponds to that obtained when the substance is injected into a vein in the antecubital fossa.

One obvious objection to the injection of ^{24}Na into the intervillous space is that a needle has to be passed through the myometrium. The mere trauma of this manoeuvre could induce uterine contraction with resultant disturbance in the flow rate in the intervillous space. In fact, the results obtained have been sufficiently consistent to lead to the belief that such contraction either does not occur or that its effects are the same in every patient. Although Ramsey (1964) has experienced no difficulty in injecting radio opaque substances into the intervillous space of the monkey, there is nonetheless a very real need for a more refined yet simple method of estimating intervillous blood flow in the human.

Because of the lack of such a technique there is, therefore, no direct confirmation of the findings of Dixon *et al.* (1963) of a progressive fall in the intervillous space flow rate between 34 weeks and term. Equally there is no evidence to refute it. If the finding be substantiated it fits in very well with the suggestion made by Assali *et al.* (1960). Quoting previous work in the pregnant sheep and assuming that the pattern of flow is the same in the human, they suggested that the blood flow to the uterus increases rapidly at the height of placental growth but levels off after the placenta reaches full maturity at 33 or 34 weeks. Equally it would provide an explanation for the observations which have been made on foetal growth rates during pregnancy and for the findings of Flexner *et al.* (1948) that the rate of transfer of sodium across the placenta increases up to 35 weeks and then falls progressively to term. Finally it fits closely with the suggestion of Cope (1958) that the fall in plasma volume and rise in packed cell volume which occur in late pregnancy are evidence of diminution in size of the arterio-venous shunt at the placental site causing the associated changes in the circulation to begin to revert to normal.

Whatever the precise mechanism governing the alterations in intervillous flow rate during pregnancy, a major part must be played by the spiral arteries in the placental bed which are the sole source of the blood supply to the intervillous space. It is tempting to think of these as vessels capable of responding very quickly to vasomotor influences and in this way adjusting the flow rate. But the profound structural alterations which occur in the distal segments of the spiral arteries in pregnancy make it unlikely that these vessels are capable of any response to such influences. In view of the obvious importance of the function of the spiral arteries during pregnancy it is regrettable that we know so little about their adaptive changes during the course of pregnancy and how these changes are brought about.

Hamilton & Boyd (1960) have described in some detail the changes which occur in the maternal vessels of the endometrium during implantation and during the early stages of placental development. From our own limited observations in early pregnancy we agree with these authors that the proliferating cytotrophoblast is responsible for the breaching of the arteries and veins which establishes the intervillous circulation. Just how this is achieved in unknown as no lytic properties have so far been demonstrated in trophoblastic cells and if cytotrophoblast does elaborate lytic enzymes, then they are remarkably specific for maternal vascular tissue. Be that as it may, the characteristic picture that is seen in the decidual portion of the spiral artery in early pregnancy is of a vessel whose normal musculo-elastic wall has been almost totally destroyed and replaced by fibrinoid material. The endothelial lining has disappeared and is frequently replaced by a layer or even layers of cells which by morphological criteria must be cytotrophoblast (Fig. 1.8). In fact plugs of cytotrophoblast can be found almost occluding the lumen. Hamilton & Boyd have argued that these masses of cytotrophoblast have an important part to play in damping down the effects of the maternal blood pressure which might dislodge the conceptus. Though this argument may be correct we feel that these cytotrophoblast cells are also responsible for the changes that occur in the spiral vessels in early pregnancy and possibly have a continuing function to perform as pregnancy progresses to term. The structural alterations are so extensive that in a single random section it is well nigh impossible to tell which are arteries and which are veins.

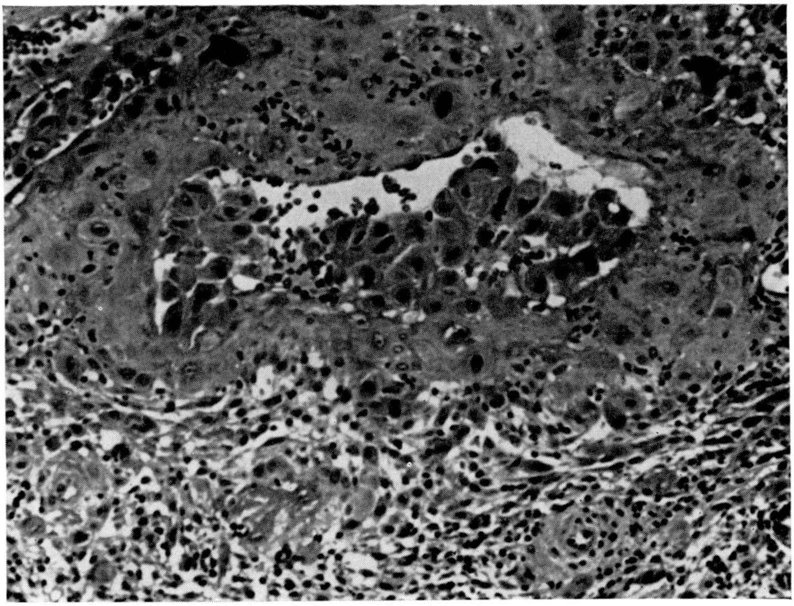

FIG. 1.8. Mass of cytotrophoblast in lumen of spiral artery in early pregnancy. H. and E. × 135. By courtesy of the Editor of *J. Path. & Bact.*

Only by serial sectioning of placentae *in situ* can the vessels be traced to their origin from the deeper myometrial vessels at a level where their true identity is easily established.

It is obvious that adaptive changes in the spiral arteries must continue throughout pregnancy to allow these vessels, which in the non-pregnant uterus supply only a small area of endometrium, to become capable of carrying the 600 ml of blood that are required every minute by the term placenta (Browne & Veall 1953). Unfortunately for the research worker, mid pregnancy specimens are not readily obtained and the changes that occur in the spiral vessels throughout pregnancy can only be inferred from studies in early pregnancy and in placental bed biopsies and uterine specimens at or near term (Dixon & Robertson 1958 and 1961, Brosens *et al.* 1967). The complexity of the vessel changes and the small portions of maternal tissue that adhere to the delivered placenta make it of limited value in morphological studies of maternal vessels. One must be able to trace the spiral vessels from their origin in the myometrium to their termination in the intervillous space to make meaningful interpretation.

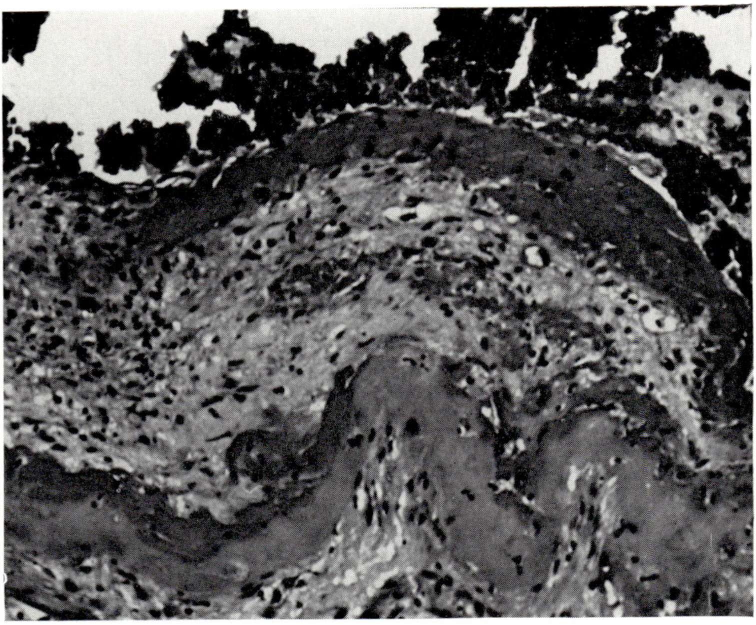

FIG. 1.9. Wall of spiral artery as it opens into intervillous space at term showing layered mural thrombi. H. and E. × 175. By courtesy of the Editor of *J. Path. & Bact.*

In late pregnancy the spiral arteries show a remarkable transformation from their normal appearance in the non-pregnant uterus. In their decidual portions, particularly where they open into the intervillous space, they bear little resemblance to any normal vascular structure. Here the wall of the vessel is widely dilated and tortuous and in every instance all muscular and elastic tissue has disappeared, being replaced by a mixture of layered fibrinoid and fibrous tissue. Mural thrombi of different ages are found, some relatively fresh, others partially or completely organized (Fig. 1.9). The frequency of mural thrombus formation is presumably due to the fact that at this level most vessels have lost their continuous endothelial lining. As it is this segment of the vessel which is found when the delivered placenta is examined, and because it frequently shows intimal thickening due to recurrent mural thrombosis, it is understandable that certain investigators (Marais 1962, Brosens 1964b) have considered that arterio-sclerosis of the spiral arteries occurs in normal pregnancy. While the use of this term may be justifiable in a

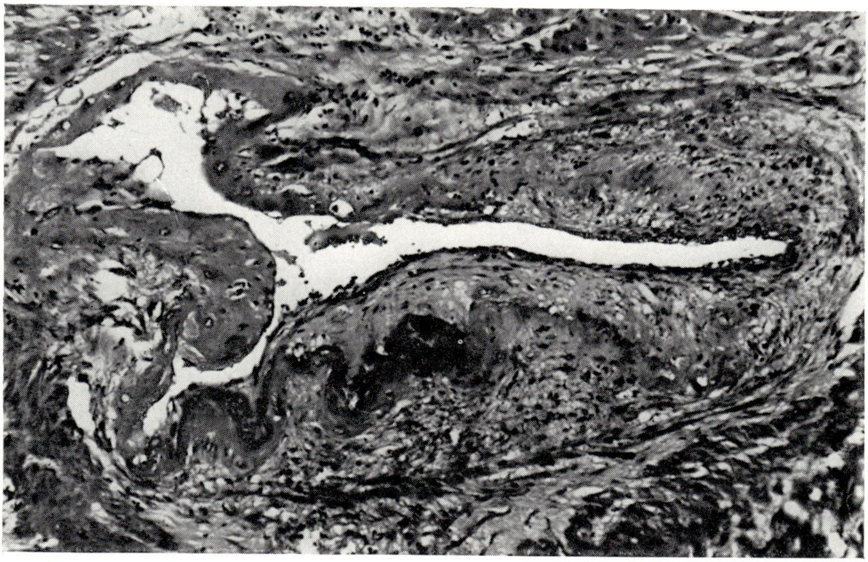

FIG. 1.10. Myometrial segment of spiral artery showing extensive physiological changes at term. H. and E. ×80. By courtesy of the Editor of *J. Path. & Bact.*

purely descriptive sense, it has pathological implications that cannot be so readily accepted. Occlusive thrombosis of occasional spiral arteries occurs in apparently normal pregnancy. This could explain areas of true placental infarction and degeneration but significant disease of the spiral arteries, as opposed to structural alteration, is not a feature of normal pregnancy. The finding of fresh thrombi in, and evidence of haemorrhage from, terminal decidual fragments of these vessels attached to the delivered foetal placenta should occasion no surprise when the trauma to the placenta during the second and third stages of labour is considered.

Examination of placental bed biopsies and even better of intact pregnant uteri, provides a clear picture of these physiological changes in the spiral arteries throughout their course from their origin in the radial arteries to their termination in the intervillous space. At the level of the

they are the remnants of the original trophoblastic invasion or indicate a renewed invasion, is problematical.

We have called those vessels which communicate with the intervillous space 'spiral arteries', but it must be emphasized there are other branches

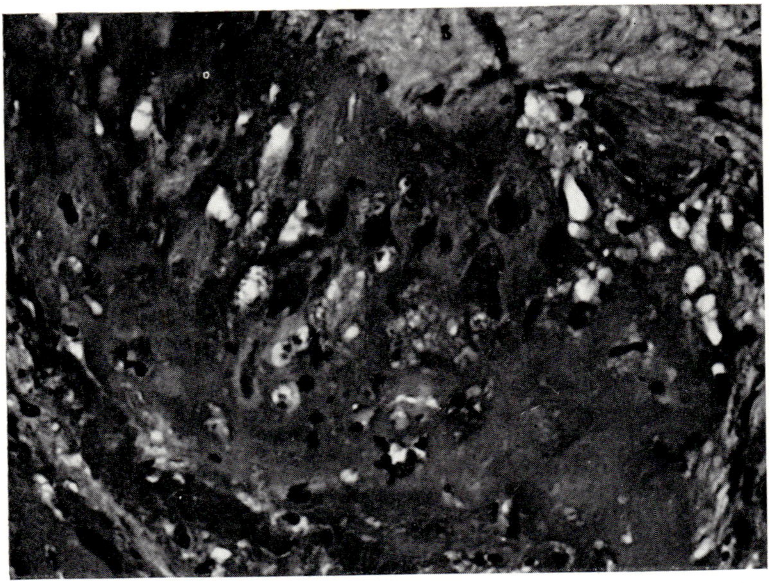

FIG. 1.13. Degenerate cytotrophoblastic cells in fibrinoid layer of spiral artery at term. H. and E. × 280. By courtesy of the Editor of *J. Path. & Bact.*

of the radial arteries which supply only the superficial myometrium and the other tissues of the placental bed. They have no communication with the intervillous space. There is no difference between the two types of vessel in the non-pregnant uterus as both are the spiral arteries of the endometrium. During implantation and early placentation the cytotrophoblast breaches only a random selection of the maternal vessels in the decidua and it is these we have chosen to term spiral arteries. The others we designate basal arteries. This distinction is both valid and useful, as the different functions of the two types of artery in pregnancy have a bearing upon their physiological changes and pathological lesions.

The basal arteries, as could be anticipated, show none of the changes described in the spiral arteries except for an apparent loss of elastic tissue which may either be real or due to a change in elastic staining reaction. There is also a hyperplasia of the smooth muscle of the media giving, in fixed tissue, a false appearance of a thick walled vessel with a narrow lumen (Fig. 1.14). The muscular hyperplasia and loss, or alteration, in the elastica, are presumably necessary to accommodate the increase in blood flow in the pregnant uterus although, as the basal arteries do not

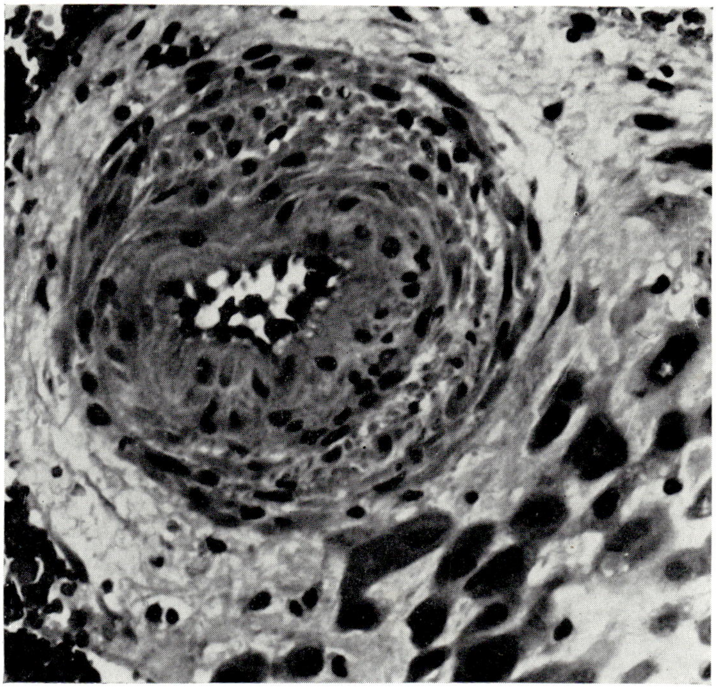

FIG. 1.14. Muscular basal artery with artifactual 'stenosis'. (Note placental bed giant cells at bottom right and absence of physiological change in vessel wall.) H. and E. × 350. By courtesy of the Editor of *J. Path. & Bact.*

supply the intervillous space, the requirements will be considerably less than for the spiral arteries.

The veins after leaving the intervillous space run more or less parallel to the basal plate. It is only the proximal portions, lying in Nitabuch's layer that show some of the features of the physiological changes that affect the spiral arteries. The lumen is widely dilated and the tips of normal villi can often be seen in it. The walls have lost their normal architecture and show extensive fibrinoid necrosis in the midst of which cytotrophoblast cells can be identified (Fig. 1.15).

More proximally, beneath the basal plate and in the myometrium the veins, apart from enlargement and loss of elastic tissue, appear to be little affected structurally by pregnancy. Some multi and mono-nucleate giant cells are found around the veins, even immediately beneath the endothelium (Fig. 1.16), but the vein wall shows no apparent response to their presence. As in the spiral arteries fresh thrombi are not a feature

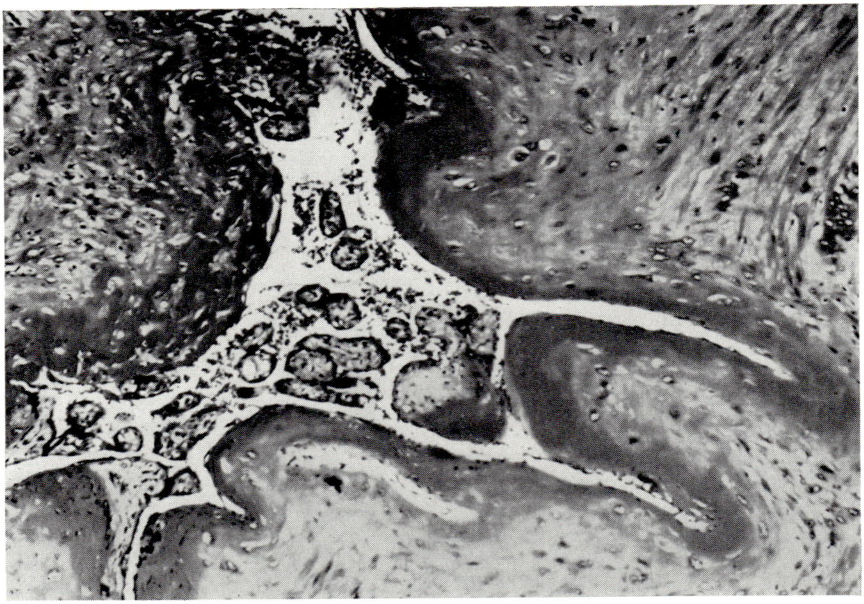

FIG. 1.15. Venous opening from intervillous space. Term normal pregnancy. H. and E. ×80. By courtesy of the Editor of *J. Path. & Bact.*

of the veins in normal pregnancy but the frequent presence of intimal cushions of fibrous tissue and smooth muscle suggests mural thrombi are formed in early pregnancy. As with the basal arteries the histological appearances of the veins in pregnancy is not greatly influenced by their position in the placental bed.

The exact mechanism by which these physiological changes in the spiral arteries are brought about is unknown. The morphological evidence points to an interaction between cytotrophoblast and the maternal arteries in the early stages of pregnancy. Some authorities (Park 1959, Ober & Grady 1961) have suggested that decidual cells are involved, but the absence of these changes in the basal arteries surrounded by decidua and their absence from vessels in the decidua vera would seem to negate this suggestion. The contention of Marais (1962) that the cell responsible is some unspecified intimal cell raises similar objections. Furthermore, we have noted in our studies that the physiological changes are maximal in the centre of the placental bed which is presumably the site of implantation and minimal towards the periphery. These changes are found not only in the decidual segments of the spiral arteries but also in the superficial myometrial segments. This anatomical distribution favours a foetal rather than a maternal origin for the cells in the arterial walls.

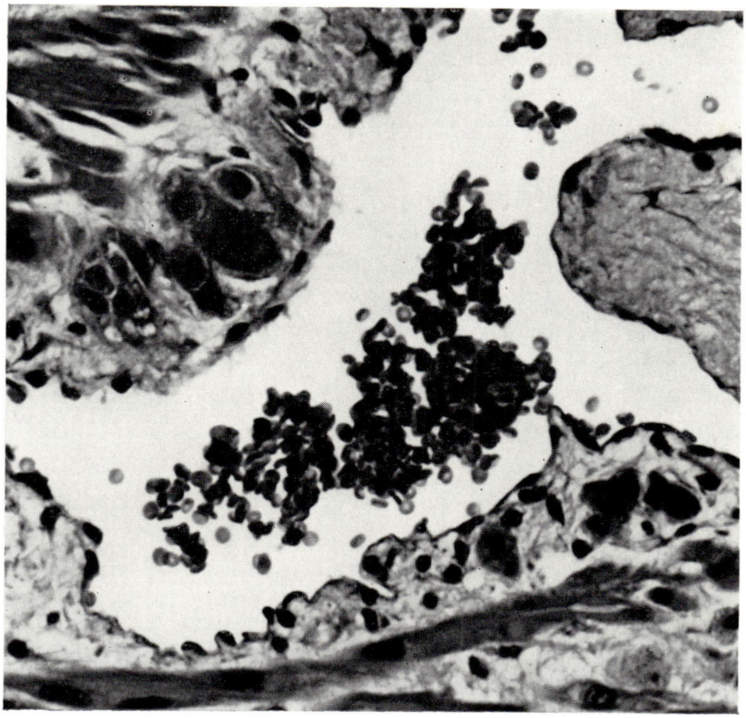

FIG. 1.16. Myometrial segment of vein draining intervillous space with intimal giant cells. (Note absence of reaction in vein wall.) H. and E. × 350. By courtesy of the Editor of *J. Path. & Bact.*

Assuming that cytotrophoblast is responsible for the initial change and admitting ignorance of the exact means by which it penetrates the vessel wall, how do the changes develop? It is tempting to think of a purely mechanistic sequence. The cytotrophoblast partly destroys the vessel wall allowing insudation of plasma to produce the fibrinoid material in the manner described by Lendrum (1963) for various diseases affecting arteries. He called this process 'plasmatic vasculosis'. When the musculo-elastic wall of a blood vessel is damaged the normal intraluminal pressure could cause progressive dilatation and it is possible that this simple mechanism is all that is required for the utero-placental circulation. Thus, initial damage to the maternal vessels and the necessity for an increased blood flow to the growing uterus and conceptus might force the damaged vessels to accommodate. Such a mechanism seems unlikely when it is remembered that the changes in the vessels are progressive and gradually extend proximally to reach even the distal portions of the radial arteries. It seems more probable that some control system is operative to regulate the supply and demand situation created by the growth of the placenta and foetus. An obvious, but purely speculative answer, is that the cytotrophoblast, securely established in the walls of the spiral arteries, continues to exert, by some means whether it be lytic, hormonal or immunological, an effect throughout pregnancy.

Whilst there seems little doubt that the purpose of the structural alteration in the spiral arteries in pregnancy is to allow the transport of a considerably larger volume of blood to the growing placenta and foetus, the very nature and extent of the changes would make these blood vessels incapable of normal vascular responses which are dependent on intact smooth muscle for their operation. As there must be a fairly delicate control system for the blood supply, its site of action must be more proximal than the level of the spiral arteries and is probably in the radial arteries. Martin and his colleagues (1964) from their observations during *in vivo* experiments with pregnant rhesus monkeys, suggested that vasoconstriction occurs near the radial spiral artery junction. On morphological grounds it is thus difficult to explain the findings of Dixon and his colleagues (1963) of progressive diminution in intervillous blood flow in the human from 34 weeks, to term and even beyond, unless it be that the mural thrombi and intimal proliferation play a more significant part in the reduction of blood flow through the affected vessels than seems likely. This reduction in blood flow is probably achieved by some purely physiological mechanism operative on the radial vessels. There is, however, at the moment no morphological evidence for any such suggestion and the precise way in which the progressive diminution in blood flow through the intervillous space towards the end of pregnancy is brought about, must remain a matter for conjecture.

The alterations that occur in intervillous space flow towards the end of pregnancy are only a facet of the whole problem of maternal blood supply to the uterus and conceptus. It is widely believed to-day that much of the pathology of the foetus and the foetal placenta is due to alterations in the maternal blood supply, caused either by a failure to increase normally for reasons that we do not understand, or by maternal hypertension and associated pathological lesions of the spiral vessels. The solution to many problems of clinical obstetrics must lie in a better understanding of the maternal-foetal junction. We are still ignorant of the precise anatomy. We know little of its haemodynamics, less of changes in the maternal blood flow that occur during health and disease in pregnancy and virtually nothing of the mechanisms by which such changes are brought about. Very few fields of medical research can offer better prospects of successful co-operation between anatomist, physiologist, pathologist and clinician.

NOTE ADDED IN PROOF

In the time that has elapsed between the preparation of this text and its appearance in print there have appeared amongst others the following articles which are of great importance to the topics discussed.

BOYD J.D. & HAMILTON W.J. (1967) Development and structure of the human placenta from the end of the third month of gestation. *J. Obstet. Gynaec. Brit. Cwlth.* **74**, 161.

FREESE U.E. (1968) The utero-placental vascular relationship in the human. *Amer. J. Obstet. Gynec.* **101**, 8.

REFERENCES

ASSALI N.S., DOUGLASS R.A., BAIRD W.W., NICHOLSON D.B. & SUYEMOTO R. (1953) Measurement of uterine blood flow and uterine metabolism. IV. Results in normal pregnancy. *Amer. J. Obstet. Gynec.* **66**, 248.

ASSALI N.S., RAURAMO L. & PELTONEN T. (1960) Measurement of uterine blood flow and uterine metabolism. VIII. Uterine and fetal blood flow and oxygen consumption in early human pregnancy. *Amer. J. Obstet. Gynec.* **79**, 86.

BORELL U., FERNSTROM I., OHLSON L. & WIQVIST N. (1964) Effect of uterine contractions on the human utero-placental blood circulation. *Amer. J. Obstet. Gynec.* **89**, 881.

BORELL U., FERNSTROM I. & WESTMAN A. (1958) Eine Arteriographische Studie Des Plazentarkreislaufs. *Geburtsh. u. Frauenh.* **18**, 1.

BOVING B.G. (1962) *Contrib. Embryol. Carnegie. Inst. Washington*, **37**, 35.

BOYD J.D. (1956) In *Gestation. The Transactions of the Second Conference*, p. 132, C.A.Villee, ed. The Josiah Macey Foundation, New York.

BROSENS I. (1964a) Personal communication.

BROSENS I. (1964b) A Study of the spiral arteries of the decidua basalis in normotensive and hypertensive pregnancies. *J. Obstet. Gynaec. Brit. Cwlth.* **71**, 222.

BROSENS I. & DIXON H.G. (1966) The anatomy of the maternal side of the placenta. *J. Obstet. Gynaec. Brit. Cwlth.* **73**, 357.

BROSENS I., ROBERTSON W.B. & DIXON H.G. (1967) The physiological response of the vessels of the placental bed to normal pregnancy. *J. Path. & Bact.* **93**, 569.

BROWNE J.C.M. & VEALL N. (1953) The maternal placental blood flow in normotensive and hypertensive women. *J. Obstet. Gynaec. Brit. Emp.* **60**, 141.

BUMM E. (1893) Uber die Entwicklung des mutterlichen Blutkrieslaufes in der menschlichen Placenta. *Arch. Gynak.* **43**, 181.

CALDEYRO-BARCIA R. (1957) In *The Physiology of Prematurity*, p. 131. Josiah Macey Foundation, New York.

COPE I. (1958) Plasma and blood volume changes in late and prolonged pregnancy. *J. Obstet. Gynaec. Brit. Emp.* **65**, 877.

CORNER G.W. Jnr., RAMSEY E.M. & STRAN H.M. (1963) Patterns of myometrial activity in the Rhesus monkey in pregnancy. *Amer. J. Obstet. Gynec.* **85**, 179.

CRAWFORD J.M. (1962) Vascular anatomy of the human placenta. *Amer. J. Obstet. Gynec.* **84**, 1543.

CROMPTON M.R. & LAYTON D.D. (1961) Delayed radionecrosis of the brain following therapeutic X-radiation of the pituitary. *Brain*, **84**, 85.

DEMPSTER W.J., HARRISON C.V. & SHACKMAN R. (1964) Rejection processes in human homotransplanted kidneys. *Brit. Med. J.* **2**, 969.

DIXON H.G., BROWNE J.C.M. & DAVEY D.A. (1963) Choriodecidual and myometrial blood flow. *Lancet*, **2**, 369.

DIXON H.G. & ROBERTSON W.B. (1958) A study of the vessels of the placental bed in normotensive and hypertensive women. *J. Obstet. Gynaec. Brit. Emp.* **65**, 803.

DIXON H.G. & ROBERTSON W.B. (1961) Vascular changes in the placental bed. *Path. Microbiol.* **24**, 622.

FENNELL R.H., REDDY C.R.R.M. & VAZQUEZ J.J. (1961) Progressive systemic sclerosis and malignant hypertension. Immunohistochemical study of renal lesions. *Arch. Path.* **72**, 209.

FLEXNER L.B., COWIE D.B., HELLMAN L.M., WILDE W.S. & VOSBURGH C.J. (1948) The permeability of the human placenta to sodium in normal and abnormal pregnancies and the supply of sodium to the human fetus as determined with radioactive sodium. *Amer. J. Obstet. Gynec.* **55**, 469.

FUCHS F., SPACKMAN T. & ASSALI N.S. (1963) Complexity and nonhomogeneity of the intervillous space. *Amer. J. Obstet. Gynec.* **86**, 226.

GILLESPIE E.C. (1950) Principles of uterine growth in pregnancy. *Amer. J. Obstet. Gynec.* **59**, 949.

GILLESPIE E.C., RAMSEY E.M. & REYNOLDS S.M.R. (1949) The Pattern of uterine growth during pregnancy in monkeys as shown in an X-ray study. *Amer. J. Obstet. Gynec.* **58**, 758.

HAMILTON W.J. & BOYD J.D. (1960) Development of the human placenta in the first three months of gestation. *J. Anat.* **94**, 297.

HENDRICKS C.H. (1958) The hemodynamics of a uterine contraction. *Amer. J. Obstet. Gynec.* **76**, 969.

HENDRICKS C.H. (1964) Fetal and placental growth: the second half of normal pregnancy. *Obstet. Gynec.* **24**, 357.

HENDRICKS C.H., QUILLIGAN E.J., TYLER C.W. & TUCKER G.J. (1959) Pressure relationships between the intervillous space and the amniotic fluid in human term pregnancy. *Amer. J. Obstet. Gynec.* **77**, 1028.

HINSELMANN H. (1958) In *Biologie und Pathologie des Weibes*, 2nd erz, p. 1. L.Seitz und A.I.Amrich, eds. Urban und Schwarzenberg, Berlin.

KLOOSTERMAN G.J. & HUIDEKOPER B.L. (1954) The significance of the placenta in Obstetrical Mortality. *Gynaecologia*, **138**, 529.

LENDRUM A.C. (1963) The hypertensive diabetic kidney as a model of the so-called collagen diseases. *Canad. Med. Ass. J.* **88**, 442.

MARAIS W.D. (1962) Human decidual spiral arterial studies. Part III. *J. Obstet. Gynaec. Brit. Cwlth.* **69**, 225.

MARTIN C.B. Jr., MCGAUGHEY H.S. Jr., KAISER I.H., DONNER M.W. & RAMSEY E.M. (1964) Intermittent functioning of the utero-placental arteries. *Amer. J. Obstet. Gynec.* **90**, 819.

METCALFE J., ROMNEY S.L., RAMSEY L.H., REID D.E. & BURWELL C.S. (1955) Estimation of uterine blood flow in normal human pregnancy at term. *J. Clin. Invest.* **34**, 1632.

OBER W.B. & GRADY H.G. (1961) Subinvolution of the placental site. *Bull. N.Y. Acad. Med.* **37**, 713.

PARK W.W. (1959) Disorders arising from the human trophoblast. In *Modern Trends in Pathology*, p. 180. D.H.Collins, ed. Butterworth, London.

PARONETTO F. (1965) Immunocytochemical observations on the vascular necrosis and renal glomerular lesions of malignant nephrosclerosis. *Amer. J. Path.* **46**, 901.

RAMSEY E.M. (1949) The vascular pattern of the endometrium of the pregnant Rhesus monkey (Macaca Mulatta). *Contrib. Embryol. Carneg. Instn.* **33**, 113.

RAMSEY E.M. (1956) In *Gestation. The Transactions of the Second Conference*, p. 229. C.A.Villee, ed. The Josiah Macey Foundation, New York.

RAMSEY E.M. (1956) Circulation in the maternal placenta of the rhesus monkey and man, with observations on the Marginal Lakes. *Amer. J. Anat.* **98**, 159.

RAMSEY E.M. (1959) Vascular adaptations of the uterus to pregnancy. *Ann. New York Acad. Sci.* **75**, 726.

RAMSEY E.M., CORNER G.W. Jnr. & DONNER M.W. (1963) Serial and cineradio-angiographic visualization of maternal circulation in the primate (hemochorial) placenta. *Am. J. Obstet. Gynec.* **86**, 213.

RAMSEY E.M. (1964) *Proceedings of the 4th World Congress of the International Federation of Obstetrics and Gynaecology* (in press).

RAMSEY E.M., CORNER G.M. Jnr., LONG W.N. & STRAN H.M. (1959) Studies of amniotic fluid and intervillous space pressures in the rhesus monkey. *Amer. J. Obstet. Gynec.* **77**, 1016.

REYNOLDS S.R.M. (1947) Uterine accommodation of the products of conception: physiological considerations. *Amer. J. Obstet. Gynec.* **53**, 901.

Spanner R. (1936) Mutterlicher und kindlicher Kreislauf der menschlichen Placenta und seine Strombahnen. *Ztch. Anat. Entwickl. Gesh.* **105**, 163.

Stieve H. (1941) Die Entwicklung und der Bau der menschlichen Placenta. *Z. Micr. Anat. Forsch.* **50**, 1.

Wieloch J. (1923) Beitrag zur Kenntnis des Baues der Placenta. *Arch. Gynak.* **118**, 112.

Wilkin P. (1958) In *Le Placenta Humain*, p. 23. J.Snoek, ed. Masson, Paris.

Wilkin P. (1965) *Pathologie du Placenta.* Masson, Paris.

2
Utero-placental Pathology

W.B.ROBERTSON & H.G.DIXON

INTRODUCTION

Pathologists have neglected no field of their subject more than that of abnormal pregnancy. Much has been written on the placenta after delivery, on still-births and neonatal deaths but little on the pregnant uterus and the maternal side of the placenta. Moreover the relationships between the three integral parts of the conceptus–uterus, placenta, and foetus,–are ill understood, especially in abnormal pregnancy. Another section has illustrated how much has yet to be learned about normal placentation, the growth of the foetus, placenta and uterus and it is a sad reflection on morphologists that there is even now incomplete agreement about the normal anatomy of the utero-placental unit. This basic anatomical ignorance hinders the acquisition of knowledge of function and constitutes a poor background for the delineation of pathological lesions.

Delivered foetal placentae, still-births and neonatal deaths provide an abundance of material for morbid anatomical and histological study. Indeed the very bulk and complexity of such material is daunting but this alone is not the answer to the neglect of the subject by the vast majority of pathologists; nor is the fact that study has only been possible when uteri with placentae *in situ* from cases of maternal death were available. These are now rare so that relatively few pathologists have an opportunity of performing detailed examinations on such tissue. Yet the key to the solution of many obstetric problems may lie in the uterus itself and particularly in the maternal side of the placenta. Disease of the foetus may be explained by abnormalities in the delivered placenta but the suspicion must remain that many placental lesions are due to abnormalities on the maternal side of the placenta and the containing uterus.

After all it is the uterus and the maternal placenta which sustain the foetal placenta and the foetus itself throughout pregnancy. It therefore cannot truly be said that the exact cause of a lesion in the foetal placenta and hence the foetus has been found unless the maternal placenta has been examined. This reservation applies particularly whenever it is suspected that inadequacy of maternal blood supply to the placenta is a major factor in foetal morbidity and mortality. The pathologist investigating ischaemic disease of the heart, brain or limbs concentrates his attention on the blood supply to those organs and tissues. He who attempts to investigate ischaemic disease of the placenta and foetus must do likewise, either by investigation of uteri with placentae *in situ*, or by examining the fragments of maternal tissue adherent to the foetal placenta (Zeek & Assali 1950, Marais 1962a), or by using the placental bed biopsy technique (Dixon & Robertson 1958). No doubt other techniques will be evolved as interest in the subject receives its due attention.

The perinatal mortality survey conducted in 1958 by the National Birthday Trust (Butler & Bonham 1963) shows that the commonest cause of stillbirth is intra-uterine anoxia. Obstetricians often talk of placental insufficiency, undoubtedly a very real entity although its clinical diagnosis is fraught with difficulty, but in many cases they have no sound morphological evidence to support their diagnosis. Some clinical causes of this syndrome of placental insufficiency such as severe essential hypertension, pre-eclampsia, cyanotic heart disease and diabetes are well recognized, but all too frequently the mechanisms whereby the precarious symbiosis of foetus and mother becomes frankly dangerous are not understood. Some, such as intra-uterine infection, obviously affect the whole utero-placental unit with ultimate deleterious effects on the foetus. Rhesus iso-immunization and multiple pregnancy are genetically determined foetal factors frequently associated with placental malfunction and increased foetal morbidity and mortality. It seems highly probable that genetic factors will also prove to be operative in many cases of unexplained abortion, intra-uterine death and in placental malfunction where abnormally small babies with correspondingly small placentae are born.

The hypertensive states of pregnancy, abruptio placentae and post-maturity constitute important obstetrical clinical problems. The aetiologies of these conditions are unknown but they all result in clinical placental insufficiency. From a pathological point of view arguments as to whether foetal, placental or maternal factors are paramount only hinder progress. In these conditions, above all others, it is necessary to consider the whole conceptus in relation to the maternal tissues. In morphological studies, the uterus, placenta and foetus must be regarded as a single, although complex unit if correlation of pathological lesions is to be achieved and dynamic interpretations attempted.

Because of all the difficulties inherent in the complete investigation of abnormal pregnancies it is the purpose of this chapter to review the present state of our knowledge of utero-placental pathology with particular emphasis on the placental bed, where foetal and maternal tissues are most intimately related and upon which depends the viability of the conceptus. The extensive work on the delivered foetal placenta and the foetus itself has helped considerably in explaining the cause of many stillbirths and neonatal deaths and so aided preventive measures. Bearing in mind the role played in perinatal mortality by intra-uterine anoxia, pathologists, to be of further assistance to their clinical colleagues, must now help to unravel the pathological changes, affecting particularly the blood supply, that occur on the maternal side of the placenta.

THE UTERUS IN ABNORMAL PREGNANCY

CONNECTIVE TISSUES

The uterus is normally so efficient in responding to pregnancy by hyperplasia that it has come to be taken for granted. There have been few who have suggested that failure on the part of the uterine tissues to respond adequately to the needs of the placenta and foetus is a cause of abnormal pregnancy or abortion. One exception is Sophian (1953) who postulated that increased intra-uterine pressure, due to resistance of the myometrium to stretch, provokes a utero-renal reflex which, he alleges, is the cause of pre-eclampsia. His arguments are largely theoretical and backed by much debatable patho-physiological evidence but there is no support from morphological or other studies of the uterine muscle for his thesis. In fact little is known about the physiological response of the tissues of the uterus to pregnancy and even less about the pathological changes which may occur in abnormal pregnancy.

Recently attempts have been made to start exploring this wilderness of ignorance. Danforth & Buckingham (1964) reviewed connective tissue mechanisms in relation to pregnancy but could do little more than draw attention to recent advances in our knowledge of connective tissues in general biological terms. Amongst other things they noted that elastase inhibitor was increased during pregnancy and suggested that this could affect not only the matrix and blood vessels of the uterus but also vessels and connective tissues in other sites. Laguens & Lagrutta (1964) studied the ultramicroscopy of the smooth muscle of the uterus in pregnancy and in the non-pregnant state. Not surprisingly they concluded that in pregnancy the smooth muscle cells undergo hyperplasia with active synthesis of protein. The collagen content of the uterus increases rapidly with advancing pregnancy and returns to normal proportions even more rapidly in the puerperium (Harkness 1956). Morrione & Seifter (1962) calculated that, in the human, the collagen content of the uterus at term is eight times that of the non-pregnant uterus but the uterus loses nearly three-quarters of this increase by the 8th day *post partum*. The mechanism by which the involuting uterus disposes of its collagen is unknown and there is no information available on collagen metabolism in abnormal pregnancy. Fainstat (1964) studied the collagen of the pregnant uterus in rats and showed that in advancing pregnancy there was a dispersion of collagen fibres with a progressive accumulation of ground substance. In noting that trophoblast did not appear to destroy or digest tissue but simply infiltrated by pushing cells and tissue aside, he stressed the importance of the extra-cellular constituents in the mechanism of placentation.

The reaction of a uterus to pregnancy does not merely depend on whether the pregnancy is normal or abnormal, but also on other factors such as parity. Little modern work appears to have been done on this question. Using single blocks from 163 pregnant or immediately post-partum uteri from their files, Dilts & Greene (1964) showed that, contrary to previous belief, there is a gradual increase in the amount of elastica in and around vessels with increasing parity but this increase is not influenced by age.

BLOOD VESSELS

While we still have much to learn about the effect of normal pregnancy, and even more of abnormal pregnancy, on the connective tissues of the uterus the situation is more encouraging when we consider the vasculature of the pregnant uterus. It has been appreciated for a long time that the recurrent hyperplasia and involution of the uterus in successive pregnancies has an effect upon the larger blood vessels such as the uterine and ovarian arteries. Gillman (1964) makes a plea for the intensive study of these arteries, pointing out that the alterations they are required to undergo in pregnancy provide a background for the development of true arterial disease later in life. Multiparous humans and animals eventually develop more pathological lesions in their uterine arteries than their nulliparous sisters. Whether abnormal, particularly hypertensive, pregnancy has an effect upon, or is affected by, these changes in the main

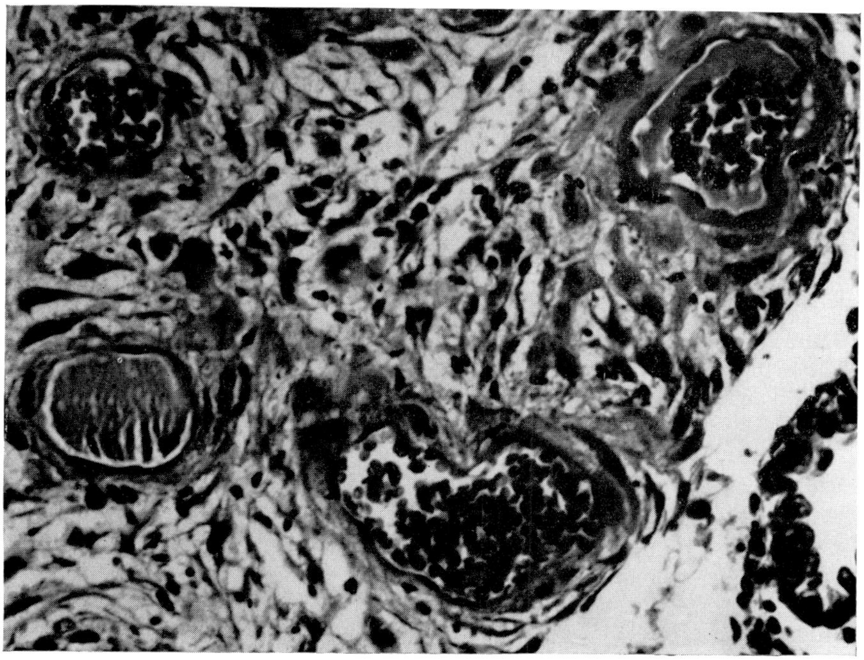

FIG. 2.1. Early hyalinization of decidual arterioles: essential hypertension. H. and E. × 275.

blood vessels of the reproductive system has still to be determined. Of more immediate concern is the effect of abnormal pregnancy upon the smaller parenchymal arteries of the uterus and in particular those of the placental bed which supply the intervillous space. In another chapter we have discussed the physiological response of the placental bed vessels to normal pregnancy and we wish now to describe some pathological responses of these same vessels to abnormal pregnancy.

In 1953 Browne & Veall showed that the intervillous space blood flow is reduced in maternal hypertension whatever its cause. This observation was confirmed by Dixon and his colleagues (1963). Knowing that long-standing and severe acute, hypertension are associated with organic changes in systemic blood vessels it seems reasonable to search for such lesions in the vessels feeding the intervillous space. Occasional reference to vascular lesions are found in the literature of the late 19th and early 20th century but it was not until Hertig (1945) described what he called

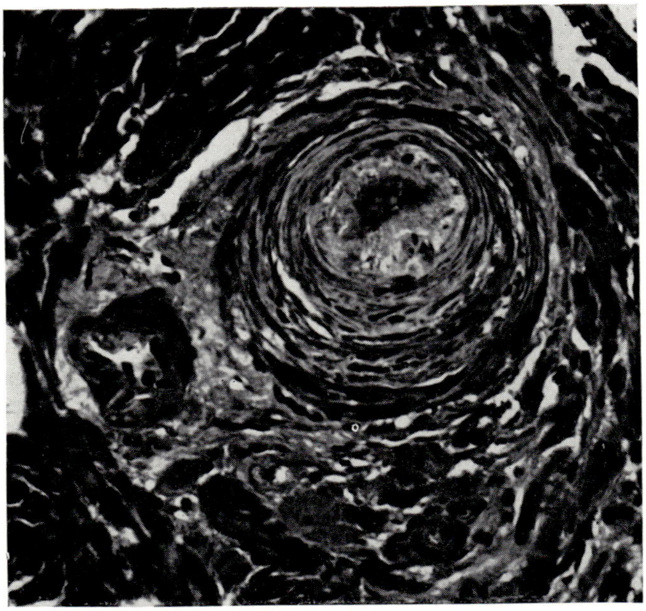

FIG. 2.2. Severe degree of arteriosclerosis in myometrial basal artery: severe essential hypertension. Picro-Mallory. ×275.

'acute degenerative arteriolitis', occurring in the spiral vessels associated with 'hypertensive albuminuric toxaemia of pregnancy' that interest was aroused. Investigating hypertensive pregnancy, Zeek & Assali (1950) studied many delivered placentae and a number of Caesarean hysterectomy and post-mortem specimens. In cases of pre-eclampsia they described a vascular lesion of both the spiral and basal arteries which they termed 'acute atherosis'. Essential hypertension was associated with hyperplastic arteriosclerosis of the same vessels. Since they found these lesions only in the decidual portions of the vessels, they suggested that placental tissue must be involved in their aetiology. Burstein and his colleagues (1957) doubted the interpretation of the morphological findings of Zeek & Assali and called into question their use of the term 'acute atherosis', pointing out that the development of an acute inflammatory vasculitis in general pathology is not accompanied by an atheromatous element. It is obvious that much of the earlier work was handicapped by the lack of suitable material for detailed histological examination. We, (Dixon & Robertson 1958, 1961), have described a simple technique by which such material can be obtained at the time of Caesarean section

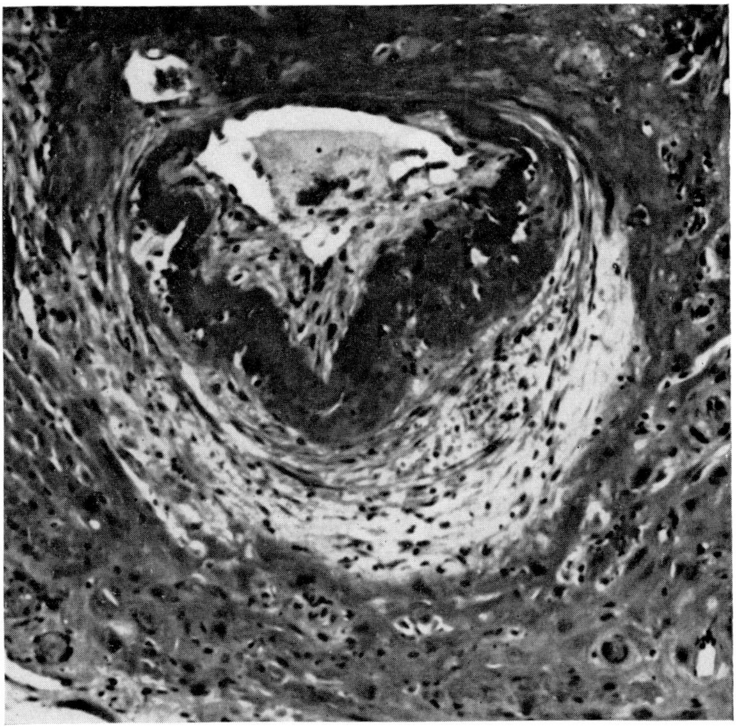

FIG. 2.3. Spiral artery showing hyperplastic changes with luminal stenosis, superimposed upon physiological changes: essential hypertension. H. and E. ×70.

when quite large biopsies of the maternal tissue underlying the foetal placenta can be taken with suitable forceps. The specimens can be fixed or processed in any desired fashion. Working with this material we showed that vascular lesions are found in both spiral and basal arteries of the placental bed when pregnancy is complicated by maternal hypertension. Using placental bed biopsy and other methods for obtaining maternal placental tissue various authors (Duparc 1960, Marais 1962b, Brosens 1964, Maqueo *et al.* 1964, Wilkin 1965) have confirmed the presence of pathological lesions of the maternal blood vessels in pregnancy complicated by hypertension. Recently we (Robertson *et al.* 1967) have given a more detailed account of these lesions and shown how the appearances in the spiral vessels can be modified by concomitant physiological changes. Our findings are summarized in the following paragraphs.

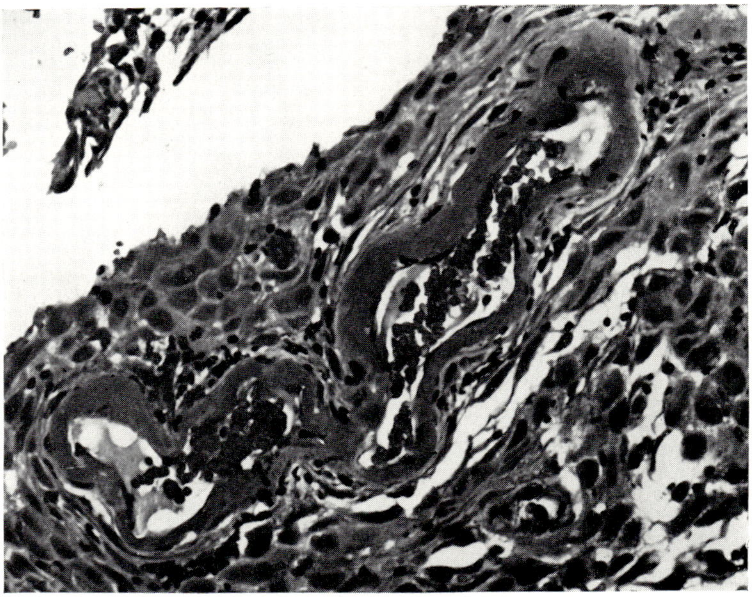

FIG. 2.4. Fibrinoid necrosis of decidual (basal) arteriole: pre-eclampsia. H. and E. × 220.

Essential hypertension

Systemic hypertension is associated with two distinct vessel lesions in the smaller arteries and arterioles. Neither is specific for hypertension but both are more prominent and pronounced in individuals with hypertension than in those without. Arteriolar hyalinization, by which is meant the deposition in the intimal and medial tissues of homogeneous, finely granular material which is strongly eosinophilic, occurs with increasing frequency with advancing age. In essential hypertension this lesion, probably best seen in the glomerular afferent arterioles of the kidney, occurs prematurely and severely but still requires many years of a high level of blood pressure to reach pathological significance. It is therefore not surprising that hyalinization of myometrial and decidual arterioles is seen only rarely in pregnant women with chronic hypertension (Fig. 2.1).

Hyperplastic arteriosclerosis, in which there is a proliferation of fibrous tissue, elastic tissue and smooth muscle in the intima and media leading to thickening of the arterial wall and narrowing of the lumen, is

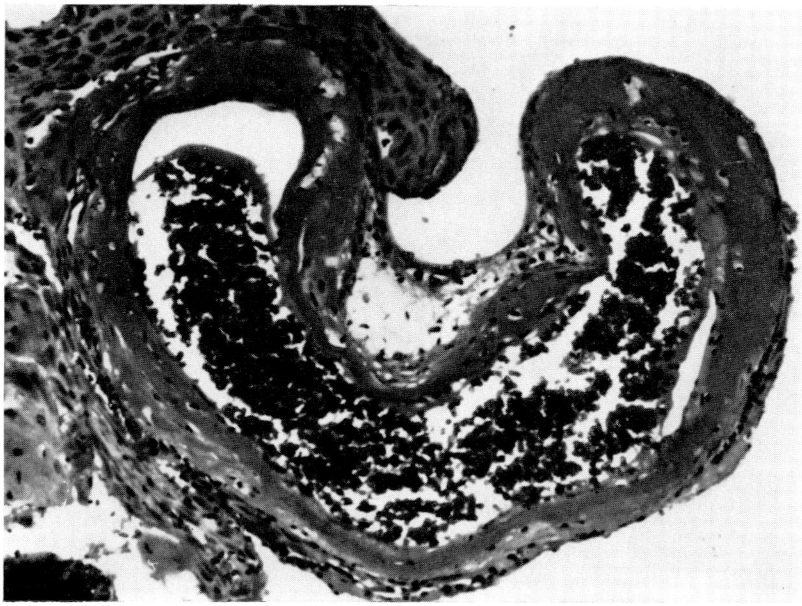

FIG. 2.5. Fibrinoid necrosis with lipophage infiltration in a decidual (basal) arteriole: pre-eclampsia. H. and E. × 140.

associated with severe grades of essential hypertension, usually of long duration. This lesion, unlike hyalinization, is common in the placental bed arteries in essential hypertension and is seen in its purest and easily recognized form in the basal arteries, that is in those arteries which supply only superficial myometrium and decidua and do not communicate with the intervillous space. Figure 2.2 shows an extreme example which had developed in a pregnant woman with chronic hypertension by 32 weeks gestation, in spite of hypotensive therapy which had kept the maternal blood pressure within the range 120/80 to 160/100 mm Hg.

In the spiral arteries the appearances associated with essential hypertension are less clearly defined because of the pre-existing physiological changes described in chapter one. Although there are considerable structural alterations in the vessel wall due simply to pregnancy, essential hypertension produces a marked hyperplasia of fibrous tissue and smooth muscle leading, in some cases, to near occlusion of the lumen (Fig. 2.3).

There can be no doubt that the hyperplastic changes seen in the basal and spiral arteries of the placental bed in essential hypertension are far in

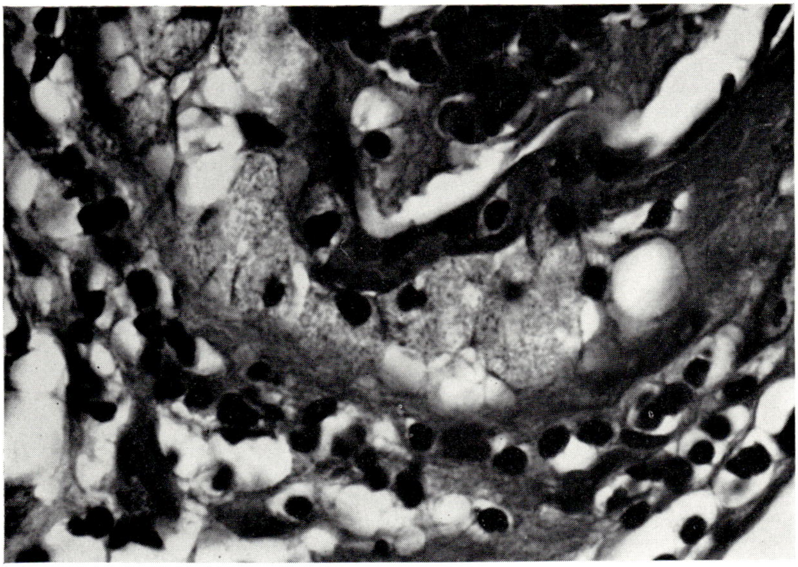

FIG. 2.6. Acute atherosis with lipophages and round cell infiltrate: pre-eclampsia. H. and E. × 704.

excess of those seen in other organs in systemic hypertension of similar degree and duration. Because of the morphological similarities between the physiological changes in the spiral arteries in normal pregnancy and the lesions superadded when pregnancy is complicated by essential hypertension, some authors have regarded hypertensive lesions as being simply an exaggeration of normal changes. Since, however, hyperplastic arteriosclerosis in the basal arteries, which are relatively unaffected by normal pregnancy, can only be attributed to the effects of hypertension we prefer the view that the physiological changes in the spiral arteries are due to the action of cytotrophoblast and that the hyperplastic lesions in those same arteries are associated with the altered haemodynamics of hypertension.

Pre-eclampsia and eclampsia

The acute onset of hypertension in pre-eclampsia resembles in some ways the malignant or accelerated phase of essential hypertension. It is therefore not surprising that the arterial lesions in pre-eclampsia have much in common with the vascular lesions of malignant hypertension but, as there are differences in the clinical manifestations and basic

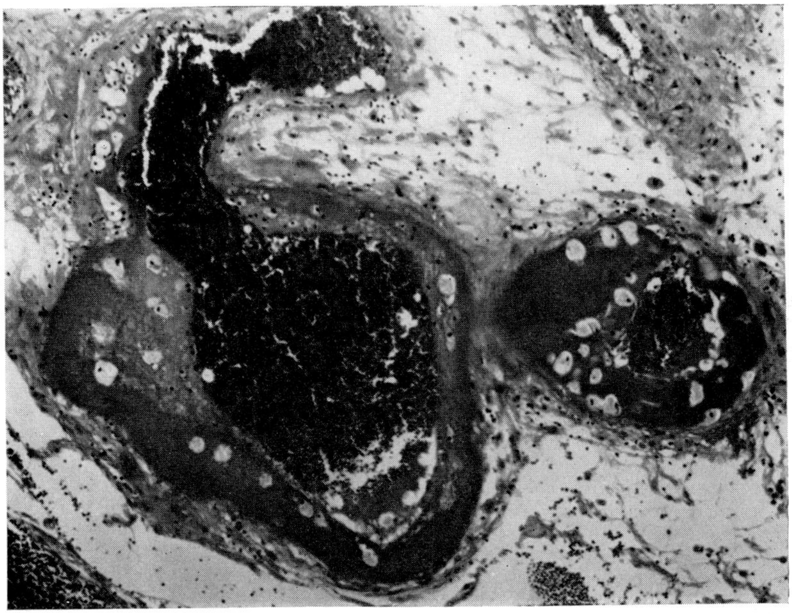

FIG. 2.7. Severe acute atherosis with distension of the damaged decidual vessels: eclampsia. H. and E. ×80.

mechanisms of these two conditions, so there are distinguishing features in their arterial lesions. One of the characteristic, but by no means invariable, features of malignant systemic hypertension is fibrinoid necrosis of the walls of small arteries and arterioles, usually best seen in the afferent arterioles in malignant nephrosclerosis. Lendrum (1963) considers that elements, including fibrinogen, of the plasma infiltrate the damaged vessel wall by a process of 'insudation' so that the arterial tissues stain positively with dyes which have a strong affinity for fibrin. As fibrinogen, or fibrin, is not the sole component of the lesion, he proposed that the term 'fibrinoid necrosis' be replaced by 'plasmatic vasculosis'.

In pre-eclampsia and eclampsia a form of fibrinoid necrosis or plasmatic vasculosis of the placental bed arteries is the characteristic lesion found. Most authors who have investigated this aspect of the subject agree that the vessel lesion is almost pathognomonic but disagree as to its pathogenesis. The elucidation of the pathogenesis of the lesion is best sought in the basal arteries of the placental bed as these vessels show none of the structural alterations due to cytotrophoblast effect on the

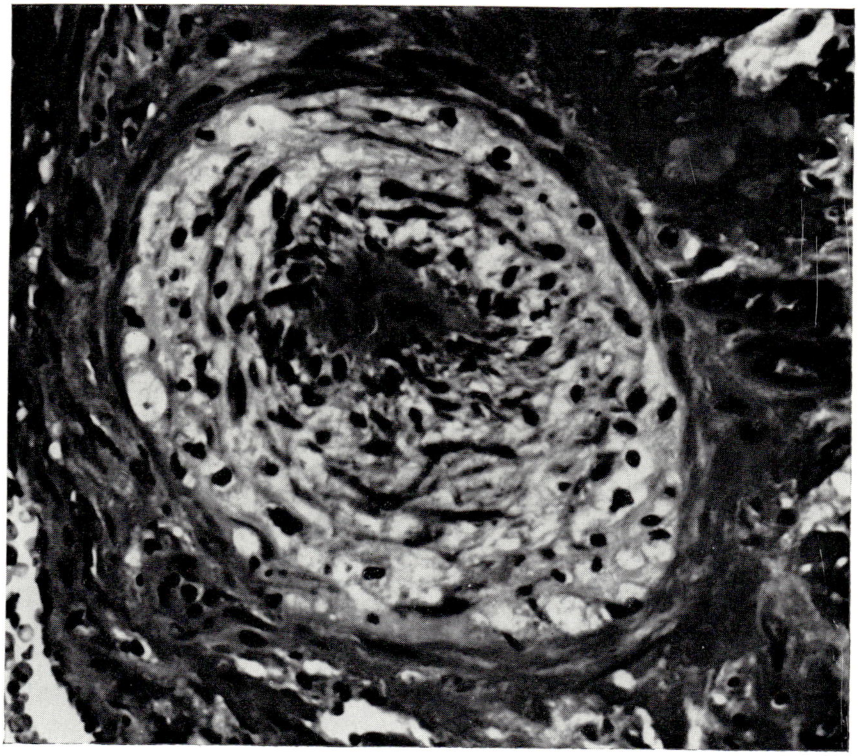

FIG. 2.8. Myometrial basal artery with severe stenosis due to intimal hyperplasia and foam cell infiltration: essential hypertension plus pre-eclampsia. H. and E. × 350.

vessel wall. In the early stages fibrinoid necrosis is the first recognizable lesion. In sections stained with haematoxylin and eosin (Fig. 2.4) the vessel wall takes the eosin avidly and the fibrinoid nature of the change can be confirmed by its intense fuchsinophilia with trichrome stains and the fact that it is periodic acid Schiff (P.A.S.) positive. Somewhat later the fibrinoid material is infiltrated with foam cells (Fig. 2.5), which can be shown to contain lipid by frozen sections and appropriate lipid stains. The origin of the foam cells has been debated but it seems most likely that they are derived from the round cells, i.e. lympohcytes and histiocytes, which are seen in and around the damaged vessel wall (Fig. 2.6). It is this cellular infiltrate and particularly the lipophages that serve to distinguish the arterial lesion of pre-eclampsia from that of malignant hypertension, and to which Zeek & Assali (1950) gave the name 'acute

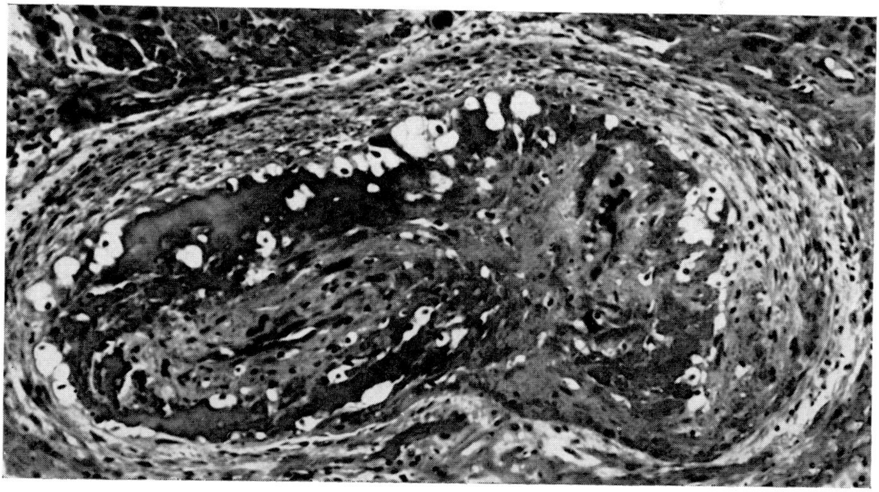

FIG. 2.9. Myometrial segment of spiral artery showing acute atherosis complicating the physiological changes of pregnancy: essential hypertension plus pre-eclampsia. H. and E. × 140.

atherosis'. Since fibrinoid necrosis or plasmatic vasculosis is compounded of substances other than fibrin, it would seem reasonable to suggest that the lipid in the arterial lesion comes, at least in part, from the plasma lipoproteins.

In the decidual segments of the basal arteries, possibly because of the looseness of the surrounding tissues, the damaged arteries and arterioles tend to become progressively distended in severe pre-eclampsia and eclampsia (Fig. 2.7). It is not difficult to visualize rupture of such severely damaged vessels. In the myometrial segments of the basal arteries fibrinoid necrosis is not such a prominent feature and lipophage infiltration, accompanied by a fibroblastic reaction, tends to dominate the picture. Because of this, possibly aided by the support given to the vessels by the surrounding myometrium, apparent stenosis of the lumen is seen at this level (Fig. 2.8).

In the spiral arteries communicating with the intervillous space and already showing considerable morphological alteration due to cytotrophoblast activity, acute atherosis is superimposed upon the physiological changes. This combination produces a complex picture of new fibrinoid

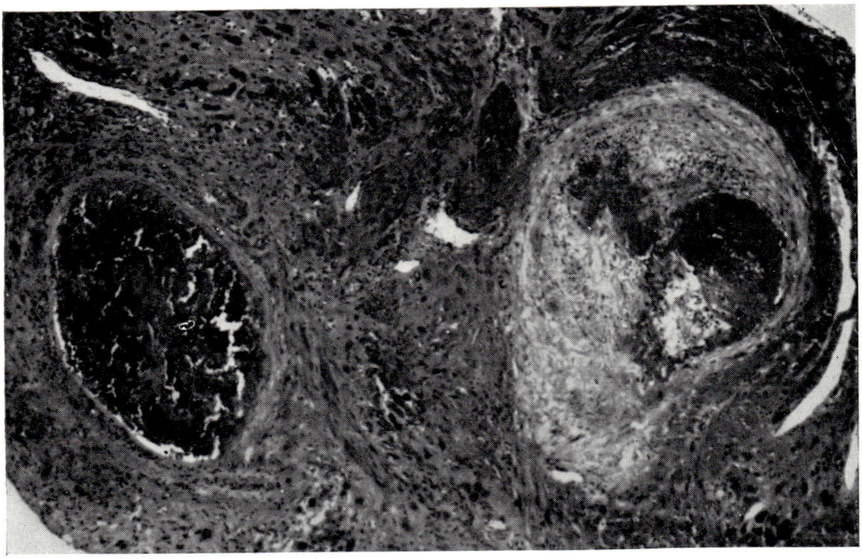

FIG. 2.10. Severe damage to spiral artery (left) with thrombosis of the decidual segment (right) and resultant decidual infarction: essential hypertension plus pre-eclampsia. H. and E. ×56.

necrosis and lipophage infiltration added to the older mixture of fibrinoid and fibrous tissue (Fig. 2.9).

When pre-eclampsia occurs in a chronic hypertensive woman the additive effects of the vessel lesions and, in the case of the spiral arteries, their superimposition on physiological changes, produce the most severe vascular damage seen in the placental bed. Necrotizing and proliferative processes may be accompanied by occlusive thrombosis with infarction of the decidua (Fig. 2.10). Secondary thrombosis in veins and decidual haemorrhage may also be seen.

From their studies of the fragments of decidua and maternal vessels adherent to the delivered placenta some authors (Marais 1962c, Wigglesworth 1964, Wilkin 1965) have stressed the frequent occurrence of recent thrombi in the terminal segments of the spiral arteries. Whilst we accept their morphological findings we feel that caution should be exercised in attributing pathogenetic significance to such thrombi since they may well develop during the physical trauma of labour and the separation of the placenta. Our study of *in situ* placentae and placental bed biopsies leads us to believe that fresh occlusive thrombi are rarely seen in the

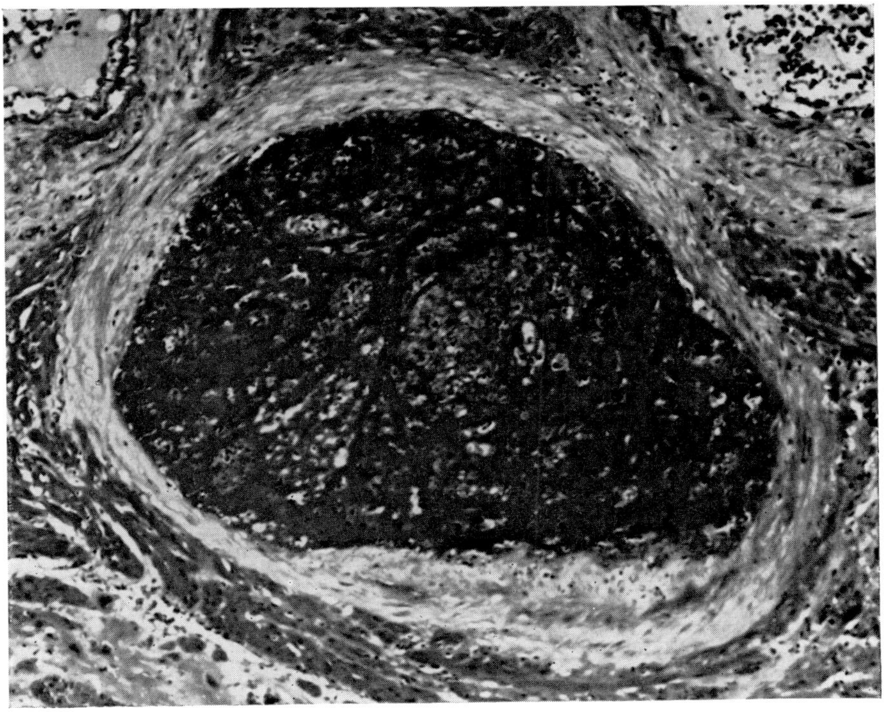

FIG. 2.11. Occlusive thrombosis in the myometrial segment of a spiral artery: essential hypertension plus pre-eclampsia. H. and E. × 100.

retained segments of the spiral arteries before placental separation except when the pregnancy has been accompanied by chronic, and even more by acute, hypertension (Fig. 2.11).

SIGNIFICANCE OF VASCULAR LESIONS IN THE PLACENTAL BED

It would seem that the lesions we have demonstrated in the spiral and basal vessels in hypertensive pregnancy afford an adequate morphological explanation of the finding by Browne & Veall (1953) of a reduction in intervillous blood flow amounting in some instances to 60 per cent.

Similarly the fact that the extent and severity of the lesions is related to the clinical severity of the hypertension would account for the findings of Dixon, Browne & Davey (1963) that the reduction in the intervillous space flow rate is more marked in the more severe instances of hypertension. Although they agreed with the findings of Morris and his colleagues (1955) that there was a slowing of myometrial blood flow in the presence of maternal hypertension, Dixon and his colleagues were unable to find the same correlation between the degree of elevation of blood pressure and the myometrial flow as they did with the intervillous space flows. They suggested that myometrial blood flow is a less sensitive index of variations in maternal blood pressure than intervillous blood flow and that it may be influenced by other factors. Such a suggestion would be in keeping with the morphological findings that have been described. The vessel lesions are, except in the most severe cases, restricted to the vessels of the placental bed and to the more distal segments of these arteries.

There can be no doubt that the vascular lesions, particularly the destructive and occlusive ones, are a more than adequate explanation for much of the pathology found in the foetal placenta in the hypertensive states of pregnancy.

AETIOLOGY AND PATHOGENESIS OF SPIRAL ARTERY DISEASE

While it can therefore be assumed that much placental malfunction and consequent foetal anoxia can be explained in terms of defective utero-placental blood supply, we are still largely ignorant of the immediate cause and pathogenesis of spiral artery disease. The problem of haemodynamic influences on arterial disease extends far beyond hypertension in pregnancy and is one of the most urgent questions in medicine today. Yet the effects of hypertension upon pregnancy provide an almost ideal natural experimental model for the elucidation of the pathogenesis of arterial lesions and their intensive study could provide information of inestimable value to general pathology. In chapter one we have described in detail the remarkable morphological changes which occur in normal pregnancy in the maternal blood vessels of the placental bed. The decidual portions of these vessels are shed with the delivered placenta, but the basal and superficial myometrial segments remain and, despite the profound alterations which they have undergone during pregnancy, return to normal morphology and function within a short space of time following delivery. In any other anatomical situation these vessel changes, which for very good reasons we have called 'physiological', would be regarded as pathological and would certainly not be considered reversible. Yet they are completely reversible, and we have not the least idea of how this reversibility is achieved.

When the vascular lesions encountered in pregnancy complicated by hypertension are considered several other questions arise. The first is why vascular lesions are found at all. The level of the hypertension and its short duration in pregnancy would not be expected to produce lesions in the renal arteries and arterioles even during pregnancy and indeed it does not. Nor would hypertension of similar degree and duration cause vascular disease in non-pregnant young women. These observations suggest either that factors other than the high blood pressure are involved in the production of the vascular lesions in the placental bed or that the vessels of the placental bed are much more sensitive to alterations in haemodynamics than vessels elsewhere.

The latter explanation may be true of the vessel changes found in the placental bed in the presence of essential hypertension. Short (1966) using a technique by which he was able to fix small arteries and arterioles of between 20 and 200 μ diameter in distension has shown that the mean lumen diameter is reduced in hypertension although the wall is of the same thickness as in normotension. It therefore seems possible that in the hypertensive woman the decidual arteries are of smaller calibre than those in the non-hypertensive. We have already discussed the tremendous changes in the haemodynamics of the placental site consequent upon nidation and it seems reasonable to suppose that the effects of such disturbance would be greater in the hypertensive woman with her narrower arteries than in the normotensive. There is no doubt that the lesions found in the placental bed arteries are quite characteristic of essential hypertension although the mechanism by which they occur in these arteries, at levels of blood pressure which would not produce any change in vessels elsewhere in the body, is unknown. Nonetheless these vessel changes develop slowly and progressively throughout the entire term of pregnancy so that both the conceptus and its blood supply may be able to adapt in some way, thus explaining the better prognosis for the foetus in uncomplicated maternal essential hypertension than in uncomplicated pre-eclampsia (Harley 1966).

The situation in pre-eclampsia is different. Here we have a rapid onset of hypertension affecting vessels which have previously undergone only the normal physiological changes. Hypertension is, of course, not the sole manifestation of pre-eclampsia. In its developed form pre-eclamptic patients will show both albuminuria and oedema to greater or lesser degrees. Furthermore the foetal prognosis in pre-eclampsia is, as has been stated, far worse than for uncomplicated essential hypertension. It is therefore not suggested that the placental bed arterial lesions can be attributed to hypertension alone, however acute its onset.

The typical lesion of pre-eclampsia, best seen in the basal arteries of the placental bed where it is unobscured by physiological changes, comprises fibrinoid necrosis of the artery wall with infiltration of the damaged wall by lipophages, lymphocytes, histiocytes and occasional plasma cells. It is now realized that fibrinoid necrosis of arteries and arterioles in socalled malignant hypertension cannot be explained by the acute hypertension alone (Kincaid-Smith *et al.* 1958). Paronetto (1965) using immunofluorescent techniques on kidney tissue from patients with malignant nephrosclerosis, demonstrated complement in the fibrinoid necrosis of the renal arteries. Since complement combines with immunological complexes he suggested that the lesions have an immunological component comparable to the arterial lesions of the collagen group of diseases. Morphologically the placental bed arterial lesions of pre-eclampsia have much in common with the renal arterial lesions in cases of scleroderma complicated by hypertension.

Arterial damage, morphologically almost identical to that of 'acute atherosis' is seen in other situations when hypertension is not a factor. Sheehan (1944) and Crompton & Layton (1961) illustrated such arterial lesions in tissues with delayed irradiation necrosis. The latter authors thought that the irradiation could not have caused the arterial damage directly, because of the long delay, but that some form of allergy or hypersensitivity was involved. They suggested that irradiation produces an alteration in protein, cells or cell constituents which renders them autoantigenic. Perhaps the most remarkable similarity between arterial lesions of this type is encountered when acute atherosis is compared with the arterial lesions of rejected human renal homotransplants. Dempster and his colleagues (1964) described and illustrated arterial pathology which is almost identical, at least in morphology, to acute atherosis. They believe that an immunological reaction of some sort is involved in the pathogenesis of the arterial lesions and suggest that the host plasma cells and plasma cell precursors recognize foreign (i.e. donor) endothelium, attack it and disrupt it to initiate the arterial damage.

We are aware of the dangers inherent in accepting analogies based on morphological appearances alone and of making dynamic interpretations from static pictures. Nonetheless, the similarities of the placental bed arterial lesions of pre-eclampsia to the arterial lesions of malignant hypertension, to the collagen diseases, to irradiation necrosis and to homograft rejection tissue, all of which appear to involve immunological mechanisms to some degree, cannot be ignored and surely demand further investigation. There is nothing new in the idea that pre-eclampsia may have an immunological background. The acceptance by the maternal tissues of the 'foreign' tissues of the foetus without provoking an antigen-antibody reaction is one of the great unsolved physiological mysteries. It is difficult to resist the temptation to assume a breakdown of the normal suppression of antigen-antibody mechanisms in pre-eclampsia, especially as some manifestations of this disease of pregnancy suggest allergy or hypersensitivity. There are, however, formidable objections to such a hypothesis. No circulating antibodies have so far been demonstrated in mother or foetus, but on the other hand the search for such antibodies cannot be regarded as having been exhaustive in view of the many techniques now available for their detection. If one were to accept that the arterial lesions in the placental bed are immunologically determined, then it is difficult to explain why they occur only in the placental bed and not elsewhere in the body. Furthermore, since the lesions occur in the maternal and not the foetal vessels one would have to assume, on the basis of the homograft rejection mechanism, that the foetus 'rejects' the mother. Such an assumption would necessitate proof that the cells in and around the damaged maternal vessel walls are foetal lymphocytes, plasma cells and histiocytes. Alternatively, one could postulate that, in cases of pre-eclampsia, the foetal tissues (trophoblast) act upon the maternal tissues in such a way as to render them auto-antigenic so initiating an auto-immune sequence of events.

OTHER CAUSES OF PLACENTAL INSUFFICIENCY

In view of the similarity, in many respects, of the clinical effects of other varieties of placental insufficiency on the foetus, it is perhaps disappointing that one finds nothing in the way of lesions in the vessels of the placental bed in post maturity, diabetes, or 'small for dates' babies unless these conditions are also complicated by hypertension. On the other hand, investigations of the intervillous blood flow rate in both post maturity and diabetes have yielded unconvincing and uncertain results. Browne (1954) reported his initial experiments in this field and although he thought that a diminished maternal blood supply to the placenta was probably a factor in the foetal wastage due to post maturity, had to

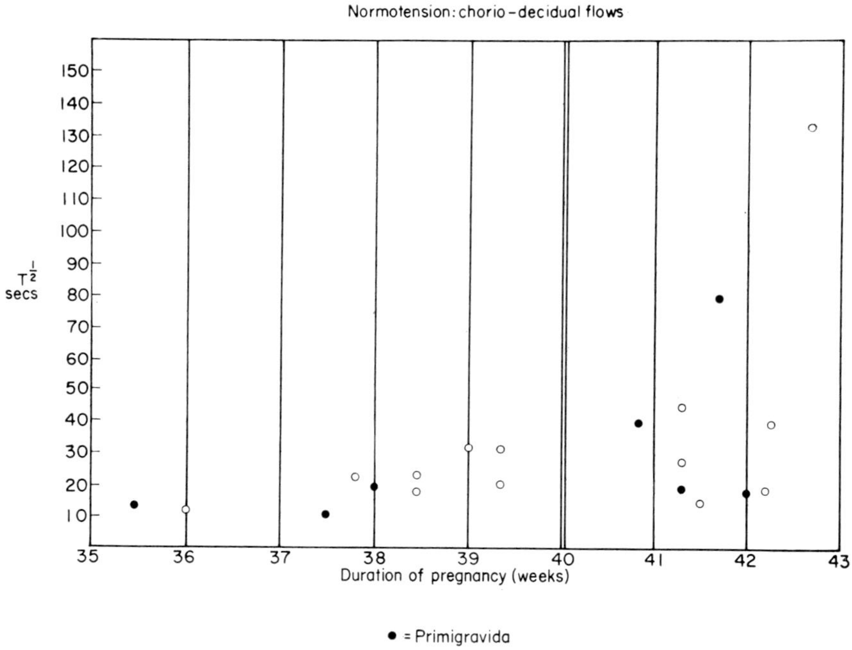

FIG. 2.12. Choriodecidual (intervillous) blood flows in pregnancy before and after term.

admit that he had found no evidence that such a reduction actually occurred. Dixon and his colleagues (1963) showed that in normotensive pregnancy there appeared to be a slight but progressive slowing of the intervillous blood flow between 35 weeks and term but that past term the picture changed (Fig. 2.12). Some patients showed a moderate decrease in flow past term, compatible with a continuation of the progressive reduction in flow shown before term. Subsequent unpublished investigations have shown that, in fact, most postmature patients fall into this group. There are, however, a small number of patients past term who show a marked decrease in the rate of flow, although such a finding has not been correlated with any marked worsening of the foetal prognosis in these individual cases of post maturity. A slightly larger number of patients show an apparent increase in flow rate past term but the possibility remains, as so often in obstetrical practice, that in spite of precautions the estimation of gestational age in these patients was incorrect. Such an error could have led to a recording being made on a patient thought to be past term but whose pregnancy was in fact not mature. If the results of clinical investigations are so indeterminate, it is hardly surprising that morphological findings have so far been largely negative.

Anoxic stillbirths in which there is no clear cut reason for the anoxia form a disturbingly high proportion of perinatal mortality. It is doubtful if a single aetiology will emerge but a number of these cases show true infarcts of the placenta (Wigglesworth 1964, Wilkin 1965) and the histological features of placental ischaemia. From this one is tempted to infer that occlusive disease of the spiral arteries is the cause of these stillbirths. Wigglesworth calculates that survival of the foetus is unlikely if more than 30 per cent of the placenta is infarcted, while Aherne & Dunnhill (1966) consider 5 sq. metres (approximately half the normal) of villous surface is the lowest limit for foetal survival. Before concluding that placental infarcts due to thrombosis in the spiral arteries are the cause of many of the otherwise inexplicable deaths *in utero*, it is well to consider the possibility that the infarcts merely accompany and are not the cause of the stillbirths. Even if placental infarcts were the cause of the foetal death, the aetiology and pathogenesis of the spiral artery lesions which led to thrombosis would still have to be determined.

THE FOETAL PLACENTA

To give an account of the extensive accumulation of literature on the delivered placenta would be a Sisyphean task, beyond the scope of this chapter. The reader is referred to the excellent studies of Benirschke (1962), Gruenwald (1964), Wilkin (1965), Benirschke & Driscoll (1967) and others who have reviewed critically their own work and the literature of the pathology of the placenta. Our concern is to attempt to relate certain lesions found in the delivered placenta to the pathological changes we have described in the maternal vessels of the placental bed.

GROSS PATHOLOGY

The most obvious lesion in the foetal placenta, easily seen with the naked eye, is infarction. It seems strange that a pathological process so well understood by pathologists when encountered in the heart, kidney, spleen or brain should lead to argument when it occurs in the placenta. The confusion and controversy that exists regarding the significance of placental infarcts is due not only to failure to distinguish true from pseudo-infarction but also to lack of appreciation of the parts played by the maternal and foetal blood vessels in their causation. There seems no good reason for departing from accepted pathological principles to explain placental infaction. By far the commonest cause of ischaemic necrosis of tissue is the shutting off of the arterial blood supply to that tissue, usually by thrombus or embolus. The placenta is no exception. If the spiral arteries of the placental bed could be routinely examined in cases showing infarcts of the delivered placenta, thrombosis of the vessels supplying the infarcted area would surely be found. We have demonstrated this in pregnancy complicated by hypertension when placental infarction is common. Zeek & Assali (1950), Benirschke (1962), Marais (1962c), Wigglesworth (1964) and Wilkin (1965) amongst others, agree that true infarction of the placenta is more logically and easily explained by pathological changes in the maternal than in the foetal vessels. It is perhaps understandable that the foetal vessels should be incriminated if the delivered foetal placenta only is examined.

We still do not know the definitive parts played by the maternal and foetal blood supply in the nourishment of the villous tissue of the placenta. Such evidence as we have indicates that the trophoblast, at least, is entirely dependent on the maternal blood supply and only when the maternal supply is deficient does the trophoblast undergo ischaemic degenerative and necrotic changes. In hydatidiform mole where the villi contain no foetal vessels, the trophoblast flourishes. In placentae where the villi are enmeshed in massive fibrin deposits and show stromal fibrosis with endarteritis of the foetal vessels, it is tempting to think that the changes are due to foetal vascular pathology but it is no less likely that the sclerosis of the villi is due to anoxia caused by the encasing fibrin and that the endarteritis of foetal vessels is a secondary phenomenon. There are certainly many examples in general pathology of such involutionary changes in blood vessels in damaged or atrophied organs.

The blood vessels of the atrophied post-menopausal ovaries undergo progressive endarteritis with the cessation of ovarian function.

Wilkin, whilst believing that true infarction of the placenta is due to spastic or organic obliteration of the maternal vessels, considers that focal ischaemic necrosis of villi with deposition of fibrinoid is the result of 'local suppression' of the foetal circulation by thrombosis in the foetal vessels of the villous trunks. The production of fibrinoid he attributes to cytotrophoblast derived from Langhans cell residues in areas of villous damage. These focal lesions 'necrose ischaemique' (N.I.D.F.) as he terms them, may enlarge to quite considerable size and, in ageing, come to resemble old hyalinized infarcts in the gross, and have been interpreted as such by many people. Intervillous thrombosis is another common lesion of the placenta and when it is extensive and old it may also resemble and be mistaken for chronic infarcts. This process, which is entirely comparable to the thrombosis which occurs in aneurysmal sacs in large arteries, is seen particularly in the sub-chorial and marginal zones of the placenta. It is so common that it may be regarded as normal and the topography of the lesions indicates that they are probably due to stasis of maternal blood at points furthest from the spiral artery openings with consequent anoxic degenerative change in the trophoblast of the more remote villi.

Another gross lesion, placental haematoma, has been confused with true, particularly acute, infarction. Classically associated with accidental haemorrhage, placental haematoma is always of serious import, but its aetiology and pathogenesis are far from understood. When accidental haemorrhage complicates the hypertensive diseases of pregnancy it seems reasonable to infer from the morphological evidence available, that damage to the maternal vessels due to altered haemodynamics is the key factor. Nonetheless, the exact mechanism for production of the haemorrhage is not known. Spasm, arterial and venous thrombosis and combinations of these three have been cited. The only satisfactory way to elucidate the morphological aspects of this lesion would be to examine a series of accidental haemorrhages with intact uteri and the placenta *in situ*, a difficult task in modern obstetrical practice. Moreover, the very destructive nature of the lesion renders histological interpretation difficult. When accidental haemorrhage occurs in an apparently healthy pregnant woman, the so-called non-toxaemic variety, the problem is even more baffling. Several theories have been advanced including hormonal imbalance (Moore 1961), trauma, autonomic nerve stimulation

(Wilkin 1965) and folic acid deficiency (Hibbard & Hibbard 1963). Whatever the aetiology may prove to be, we still have to determine the mechanism by which the maternal vessels are ruptured to produce the haemorrhage.

It now seems reasonably certain that among gross placental lesions, excluding placental malformation and the abnormally situated placenta, only true infarction of the placenta and haematoma, both determined by maternal vascular pathology, are of clinical significance. The other gross lesions including intervillous thrombosis, focal necrosis, and fibrin or fibrinoid deposition around and in villi can be regarded as normal phenomena of the maturation and ageing of the placenta. The fact that these features may be exaggerated in abnormal pregnancy should not cloud the issue of what constitutes true pathological lesions in the placenta.

MICROSCOPIC PATHOLOGY

A subject of even greater complexity than gross placental lesions, is the microscopy of the abnormal or presumed abnormal placenta. The problem of sampling error is now well recognized (Benirschke 1962, Gruenwald 1964, Fox 1964a, Wigglesworth 1964). Fox has shown that there are highly significant and consistent variations in the morphology of villi in both the horizontal and vertical planes of the placenta. He considers that the subchorial and marginal regions of the placenta suffer a relative anoxia which causes many of the more subtle alterations in villous morphology seen with the light microscope. In view of this, great caution is necessary in attributing pathogenetic significance to such features as syncytial knots, villus basement membrane thickening, fibrinoid necrosis of villi, stromal fibrosis, and endarteritis of foetal vessels. If anoxia from disturbance of the maternal blood supply is responsible for many, if not all, of these changes then it is hardly surprising that they have been found more frequently in the hypertensive states of pregnancy.

One microscopic feature of the damaged, particularly the anoxic or ischaemic placenta, is proliferation of the Langhans cells to form a large type of cytotrophoblast (the 'Cellules X' of Wilkin). Wigglesworth (1964) regards this differentiation of the Langhans cell into a new form of cytotrophoblast rather than syncytium as the main microscopic finding common to all forms of placental insufficiency, and Fox (1964b) suggests that this Langhans cell proliferation is both a qualitative and quantitative index of placental ischaemia.

The effect of maternal hypertension upon the size of the placenta and hence of the foetus has been illustrated in a novel fashion by Aherne & Dunnhill (1966). Using point counting and mean linear intercept determination methods for quantitation, they showed that the volume of the placenta, the villous surface area (and hence the foetal capillary surface area), and the intervillous space volume are all significantly reduced in hypertensive pregnancy. They found a close correlation between the size of the foetus and the villous surface area of the placenta. These findings can be explained at least in part by the spiral artery pathology of hypertensive pregnancy as the normal growth of the placenta is dependent upon an adequate maternal blood supply.

Their findings of reduced placental volume, villous surface area and intervillous space volume in placentae from 'small for dates' babies are no less interesting but less readily explained. No definitive study of the maternal blood vessels in such cases has been undertaken although it is urgently required. The possibility that a primary hypoplasia, possibly genetically determined, of the placenta is involved, has been mooted but not proven. That the mechanism of production of the small placenta may be different in the hypertensive and 'small for dates' cases is suggested by one finding of Aherne & Dunnhill although they do not comment upon it. They calculated that the mean volume of the placental foetal capillaries at term was 45 ml in normal cases, 56 ml in hypertensive cases and only 38 ml in placentae with 'small for dates' babies. Whether the increased volume of foetal capillaries in the hypertensive cases or the decreased volume in the 'small for dates' cases is the more surprising is a matter for debate, but it does indicate a possible difference in the causation of the two forms of placental insufficiency.

GENERAL CONSIDERATIONS

Of the diverse types of abnormal pregnancy it would seem that we cannot yet offer reasonable pathogenetic mechanisms for many stillbirths, 'small for dates' babies and post-maturity. The utero-placental pathology associated with rhesus isoimmunization, diabetes, heart disease and other maternal disorders can be explained in terms of these diseases but the hypertensive states of pregnancy, particularly pre-eclampsia, present an almost unique problem. It is here that the need for a comprehensive approach is the most apparent. We have tried to show that much of our knowledge of pathology in the foetus and delivered placenta is, as it were, second hand because the primary lesion, though not the aetiology, of many pathological complexes lies in uterine blood supply, especially to the placental bed. In maternal essential hypertension there would appear to be a close correlation of arterial pathology with reduction in intervillous blood flow. In pre-eclampsia there is a similar correlation but the nature of pre-eclampsia and the morphology of its placental bed vascular lesions clearly indicate that factors other than hypertension are involved in the production of the clinical, metabolic and pathological manifestations of the condition. The further investigation of the arterial lesions offers exciting research possibilities that may have a bearing not only on the aetiology of pre-eclampsia but also on the aetiology and pathogenesis of other forms of arterial disease.

So far attempts to explain many instances of placental insufficiency in terms of spiral artery disease have been unsuccessful, probably for the very good reason that all forms of placental insufficiency are not due to, or associated with, organic changes in blood vessels. The terms 'ischaemia' and 'anoxia' have implications far beyond mechanical or functional interference with the blood supply. While disordered morphology may be a good starting point for the investigation of many disease processes it is unrewarding and may even be misleading in others where it is a better end point. In recent years there has been such an increase in tools and methods available to the pathologist and other investigators in the fields of ultramicroscopy, histochemistry, immunology, tissue culture and cytogenetics, to mention but a few, that the scope for further work in the problems of abnormal pregnancy is unlimited.

ACKNOWLEDGMENTS

We are grateful to the Editor of the *Journal of Pathology and Bacteriology* for permission to reproduce figures 2.1, 2.2, 2.4, 2.5, 2.6, 2.7, 2.8, 2.9, 2.10 and 2.11, and to the Editor of the *Lancet* for permission to reproduce figure 2.12.

REFERENCES

AHERNE W. & DUNNILL M.S. (1966) Quantitative aspects of placental structure. *J. Path. Bact.* **91**, 123.

BENIRSCHKE K. (1962) A review of the pathologic anatomy of the human placenta. *Amer. J. Obstet. Gynec.* **84**, 1595.

BENIRSCHKE K. & DRISCOLL S.G. (1967). *The Pathology of the Human Placenta.* Springer-Verlag. New York.

BROSENS I. (1964) A study of the spiral arteries of the decidua basalis in normotensive and hypertensive pregnancies. *J. Obstet. Gynaec. Brit. Cwlth.* **71**, 222.

BROWNE J.C.McC. (1954) Maternal placental blood flow in postmaturity. In *La Prophylaxie en Gynécologie et Obstetrique*, p. 1015. Georg et Cie, Geneva.

BROWNE J.C.McC. & VEALL N. (1953) The maternal placental blood flow in normotensive and hypertensive women. *J. Obstet. Gynaec. Brit. Emp.* **60**, 141.

BURSTEIN R., BLUMENTHAL H.T. & SOULE S.D. (1957) Histogenesis of pathological processes in placentas of metabolic disease in pregnancy. I. Toxemia and hypertension. *Amer. J. Obstet. Gynec.* **74**, 85.

BUTLER N.R. & BONHAM D.G. (1963) *Perinatal Mortality.* E. & S.Livingstone, Edinburgh.

CROMPTON M.R. & LAYTON D.D. (1961) Delayed radionecrosis of the brain following therapeutic X-radiation of the pituitary. *Brain*, **84**, 85.

DANFORTH D.N. & BUCKINGHAM J.C. (1964) Connective tissue mechanisms and their relation to pregnancy. *Obstet. Gynec. Surv.* **19**, 715.

DEMPSTER W.J., HARRISON C.V. & SHACKMAN R. (1964) Rejection processes in human homotransplanted kidneys. *Brit. med. J.* **2**, 969.

DILTS P.V. & GREENE R.R. (1964) Effects of increasing parity on the myometrium. *Amer. J. Obstet. Gynec.* **89**, 1049.

DIXON H.G. & ROBERTSON W.B. (1958) A study of the vessels of the placental bed in normotensive and hypertensive women. *J. Obstet. Gynaec. Brit. Emp.* **65**, 803.

DIXON H.G. & ROBERTSON W.B. (1961) Vascular changes in the placental bed. *Path. et Microbiol.* **24**, 622.

DIXON H.G., BROWNE J.C.McC. & DAVEY D.A. (1963) Choriodecidual and myometrial blood-flow. *Lancet*, **2**, 369.

DUPARC J. (1960) Etude histologique de la caduque dans les grossesses normales et pathologiques. These Med., Lyons.

FAINSTAT T. (1964) The helical collagen fibres in the uterus. IV. Extracellular studies of uterus. *Amer. J. Obst. Gynec.* **89**, 1026.

FOX H. (1964a) The pattern of villous variability in the normal placenta. *J. Obstet. Gynaec. Brit. Cwlth.* **71**, 749.

FOX H. (1964b) The villous cytotrophoblast as an index of placental ischaemia. *J. Obstet. Gynaec. Brit. Cwlth.* **71**, 885.

GILLMAN T. (1964) A plea for arterial biology as a basis for understanding arterial disease. In *Biological Aspects of Occlusive Vascular Disease*, p. 3. D.G.Chalmers & G.A.Gresham, eds. Camb. Univ. Press.

GRUENWALD P. (1964) Examination of the placenta by the pathologist. *Arch. Path.* **77**, 41.

HARKNESS R.D. (1956) Metabolism of collagen. In *Lectures on the Scientific Basis of Medicine*, Vol. V, p. 183. Athlone Press, London.

HARLEY J.M.G. (1966) Pregnancy in the chronic hypertensive woman. *Proc. Roy. Soc. Med.* **59**, 835.

HERTIG A.T. (1945) Vascular pathology in the hypertensive albuminuric toxemias of pregnancy. *Clinics*, **4**, 602.

HIBBARD B.M. & HIBBARD E.D. (1963) Aetiological factors in abruptio placentae. *Brit. Med. J.* **2**, 1430.

KINCAID-SMITH P., MCMICHAEL J. & MURPHY E.A. (1958) The clinical course and pathology of hypertension with papilloedema (malignant hypertension). *Quart. J. Med.* **27**, 117.

LAGUENS R. & LAGRUTTA J. (1964) Fine structure of human uterine muscle in pregnancy. *Amer. J. Obstet. Gynec.* **89**, 1040.

LENDRUM A.C. (1963) The hypertensive diabetic kidney as a model of the so-called collagen diseases. *Canad. Med. Ass. J.* **88**, 442.

MAQUEO M., AZUELA J.C. & VEGA M.D.DE LA (1964) Placental pathology in eclampsia and pre-eclampsia. *Obstet. and Gynec.* **24**, 350.

MARAIS W.D. (1962a) Human decidual spiral arterial studies. Part 1. *J. Obstet. Gynaec. Brit. Cwlth.* **69**, 1.

MARAIS W.D. (1962b) Human decidual spiral arterial studies. Part IV. *J. Obstet. Gynaec. Brit. Cwlth.* **69**, 234.

MARAIS W.D. (1962c) Human decidual spiral arterial studies. Part V. *J. Obstet. Gynaec. Brit. Cwlth.* **69**, 944.

MOORE H.C. (1961) Periplacental haemorrhage, foetal death and lesions of the kidney and other viscera in pregnant rats receiving progesterone. 1. The uterus and placenta. *J. Obstet. Gynaec. Brit. Cwlth.* **68**, 570.

MORRIONE T.G. & SEIFTER S. (1962) Alteration in the collagen content of the human uterus during pregnancy and post-partum involution. *J. Exp. Med.* **115**, 357.

MORRIS N., OSBORN S.B. & WRIGHT H.P. (1955) Effective circulation of the uterine wall in late pregnancy measured with ^{24}NaCl. *Lancet*, **1**, 323.

PARONETTO F. (1965) Immunocytochemical observations on the vascular necrosis and renal glomerular lesions of malignant nephrosclerosis. *Amer. J. Path.* **46**, 901.

ROBERTSON W.B., BROSENS I. & DIXON H.G. (1967) The pathological response of the vessels of the placental bed to hypertensive pregnancy. *J. Path. Bact.* **93**, 581.

SHEEHAN J.F. (1944) Foam cell plaques in the intima of irradiated small arteries (one hundred to five hundred microns in external diameter). *Arch. Path.* **37**, 297.

SHORT D. (1966) Morphology of the intestinal arterioles in chronic human hypertension. *Brit. Heart J.* **28**, 184.

SOPHIAN J. (1953) *Toxaemias of Pregnancy*. Butterworth, London.

WIGGLESWORTH J.S. (1964) Morphological variations in the insufficient placenta. *J. Obstet. Gynaec. Brit. Cwlth.* **71**, 871.

WILKIN P. (1965) *Pathologie du Placenta. Etude Clinique et Anatomo-clinique*. Masson, Paris.

ZEEK P.M. & ASSALI N.S. (1950) Vascular changes in the decidua associated with eclamptogenic toxaemia of pregnancy. *Amer. J. Clin. Path.* **20**, 1099.

3
The Functional Morphology of the Placenta, the Foetus, the Membranes and the Umbilical Cord

K. THOMSEN & H.-D. HIERSCHE

THE PLACENTA

DEFINITION OF THE ORGAN

The association of the endometrium and the chorion is called the placenta (plakous = the cake). The placenta serves as a resorption, excretion and exchange organ, for the respiration and nourishment of the foetus, and provides for the transport of raw materials and waste products. Recent research has shown that the membranes also play a considerable role in the exchange of material between mother and foetus. The placenta, however, is also a screen between maternal and foetal organisms, thus ensuring the separate development of the human foetus.

The relationship of the mucous membrane of the uterus and the trophoblast varies with the species of animal concerned. On the basis of these differing relationships, Grosser (1927), put forward his very useful classification for the morphological and functional description of the placenta, which was subsequently further developed by Mossman (1937, 1959). This purely morphological subdivision does not, however, do justice to what we now know of the functional characteristics of different placentae (Page 1957).

From the evolutionary point of view Grosser's classification (Fig. 3.1) is morphologically correct for man in its general scope. In the haemochorial placenta, the human has a highly specialized organ, yet justifiable doubts have arisen as to whether the human placenta is the most highly specialized form. A further reduction in the number of layers separating maternal and foetal blood is anatomically possible, for instance in the haemoendothelial portions of the placenta of the guinea pig (Mossman 1937). The various types of placentae in Grosser's classification permit only limited conclusions concerning biological evolution.

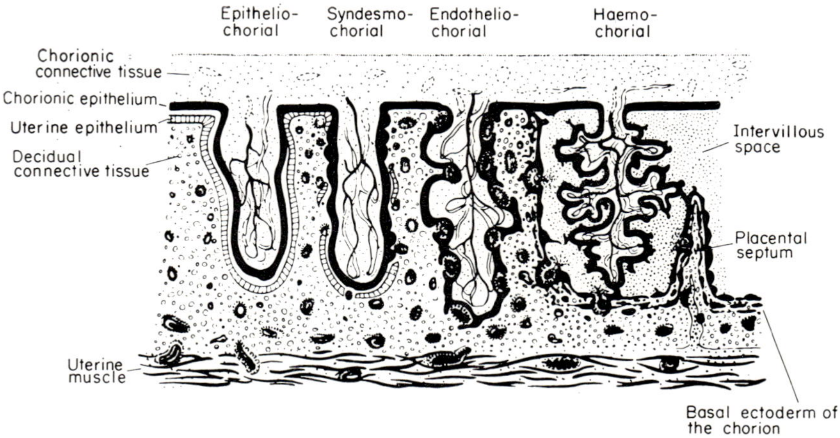

FIG. 3.1. Schematic representation of different types of placentation according to Grosser.

HUMAN PLACENTATION

The placental development of primates is characterized by the reduction of the vitelline sac and allantois and by great depth of implantation with the formation of a haemochorial placenta.

On the 4th day of development the fertilized egg enters the uterus as a blastula in the 5–12 cell stadium, (18th day of a 28 day menstrual cycle). The blastocyst with 58–107 cells still lies free in the cavity of the uterus. Implantation begins on the 20th day of the cycle, and probably takes several days to complete (Hertig 1960). The great majority of implantations in the case of the human take place in the fundus of the uterus and in the posterior wall. The tendency for implantation to occur in this area is surely not due to chance (Hertig *et al.* 1956). The investigations of Schmidt-Mathiessen (1968) show that the dominant prerequisite for implantation is the strict synchronization of the developmental stages of the blastocyst and the endometrium.

Comparable animal experiments suggest that the decidualization and loosening of the endometrium necessary for nidation is engendered by endogenous histamine, i.e. by acetyl choline secretion (Shelesnyak 1959, Marcus *et al.* 1963). The blastocyst itself can also be considered a loosening factor by possibly causing decidualization in an endometrium sensitized by oestrogen and progesterone (Strauss 1967). Mast cells and eosinophil granulocytes might be sources of histamine as is suggested by research done on rats. The implantation itself is facilitated as far as the trophoblast is concerned by proteolytic enzymes, by amoeboid movements and by phagocytosis, and in the endometrium by loosening, by increased fragility of the vessels and decreased protein metabolism in the decidua. On the basis of their observations, Shelesnyak & Kraicher (1963) divide implantation into two phases whereby a sudden surge of oestrogen secretion plays a decisive role: (1) decidualization of the endometrium by the liberated histamine; (2) nidation, for which both trophoblastic and maternal action are important. The position of the nidation pole means that, like the endometrium, the trophoblast plays a part in the specific orientation of the blastocyst (Strauss 1967).

While the maternal mucous membrane is enzymatically destroyed by the now rapidly proliferating trophoblast, the embryo penetrates deeply into the decidua. The latter reacts by extensive hypertrophy and so creates a site for implantation into which the embryo gradually expands.

The breach in the decidua is closed by a 'mucous plug'. Eventually, a largely intact decidua capsularis forms over the embryo, and by the 4–5 lunar month comes to adhere to the decidua parietalis. As it penetrates actively into the decidua and pushes the pars marginalis away, the rapidly growing trophoblast proliferates in the maternal tissues and opens the maternal blood vessels. The latter already show increased fragility and permeability (Capodacqua *et al.* 1961, Wilkin 1960, Schmidt-Mathiessen 1963, 1968). It can therefore be assumed that the opening of the maternal vessels is the result of common maternal and foetal action which is delicately determined by biochemical interaction (Strauss 1967). The maternal blood, and also probably glandular secretions (Strauss 1967) penetrate into the lacunae composed of three-dimensional masses of syncytium in trabecular order, lined with thin cytotrophoblastic layers. The period during which the maternal blood pours into the interstices of the foetal tissues is called the lacunar phase of placental development. In man it takes place in the first or second week (Starck 1955). During this period man has a labyrinthine placenta. A weak circulation begins in the lacunar system, and the lacunae grow wider following a further opening out of the maternal sinus. The surrounding masses of syncytium with their proliferating cytoplasmatic inner layers become flattened into plates. At this time (end of 2nd to beginning of the 3rd week), one cannot yet demonstrate the presence of mesenchyme. At the same time, the action of the trophoblast produces degenerative changes in the endometrium in the neighbourhood of the egg. This area of penetration is composed of necrotic decidua, fibrin and maternal leucocytes.

Whether these leucocytes are the site of production or liberation of the histamine, as mentioned earlier, or a sign of a maternal defence reaction to the invading trophoblast is still an unresolved problem (Schmidt-Mathiessen 1963, 1968, Shettles & Schmidt-Mathiessen 1963). As the trophoblast cannot dissolve any fibrin (Ludwig 1959) the mucous coagulum prevents the egg from returning to the cavity of the uterus and, on the other hand, makes it more difficult for the trophoblast to penetrate too deeply into the maternal tissues.

Between the 3rd and 4th week the formation of crude secondary villi about 150 μ in size takes place. A central layer of mesenchyme appears in the rapidly ramifying and growing primary villi. Whether this derives from mesenchyme outside the embryo and its proliferation into the villus, and should be regarded as a differentiation product of the trophoblast, is still a matter of dispute.

Pictures taken by light microscopy show star shaped mesenchymal cells in the loose embryonic connective tissue, and these with their branches appear to build up a three dimensional syncytium. However, electron microscopical investigations show that the most delicate processes of the cells of the embryonic tissue, some 700–1,000 Å in size, do not communicate. They come into apposition either side to side (Fig. 3.2) or end to end, or come into contact through interdigitation (Fig. 3.3). So the lattice of mesenchymal cells is not a syncytium.

During the period of the rapid proliferation of the cytotrophoblast, primary adhesive villi develop, (the rafters of the cytotrophoblast), which form a cellular connection of chorion villi with the maternal tissue.

Five weeks post menstruum rudimentary blood vessels appear in the chorionic villus. At first they develop near the adhesive stem in the chorionic mesenchyme. Vitelline sac and allantois vessels also develop.

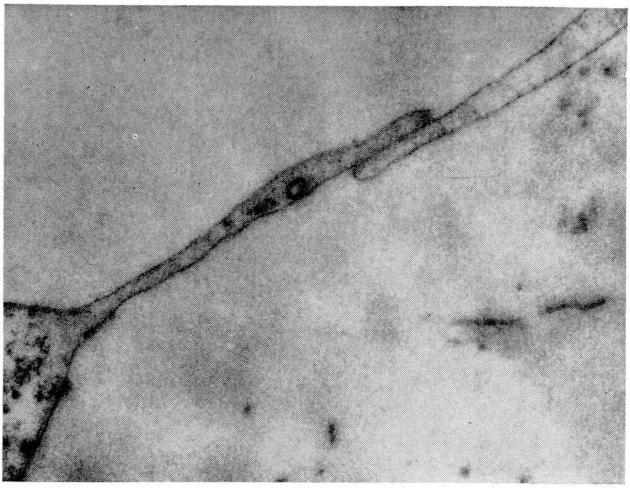

FIG. 3.2. Projections of the mesodermal cells of the chorion in contact with each other. (Magnification 48,000 times.) From Bargmann & Knoop (1959).

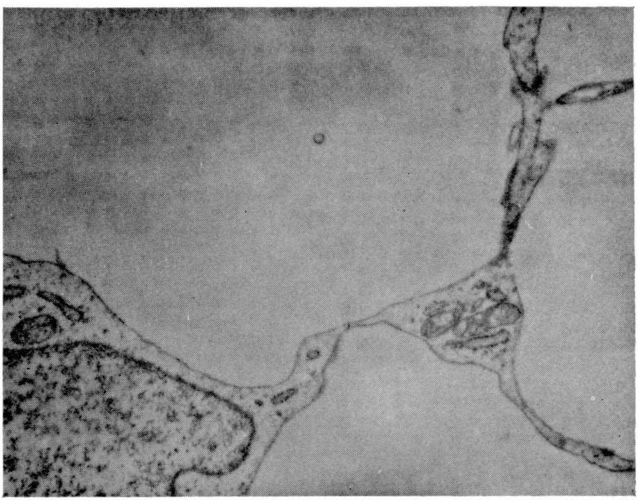

FIG. 3.3. Mesodermal cells of chorion in contact with extensions of other cells. Note the interdigitation of the projections in the upper right of the section. (Magnification 36,000 times.) From Bargmann & Knoop (1959).

In man both these organs have lost their primary significance, and are only mentioned as a matter of evolutionary history. Their system of blood vessels does, however, aid the vascularization of the chorionic villus, and thus its transformation into the tertiary villus of the haemochorial human 'pot' placenta. The main component of the tertiary villus next assumes the form of a loose mesenchyme, poor in cells and fibrillae

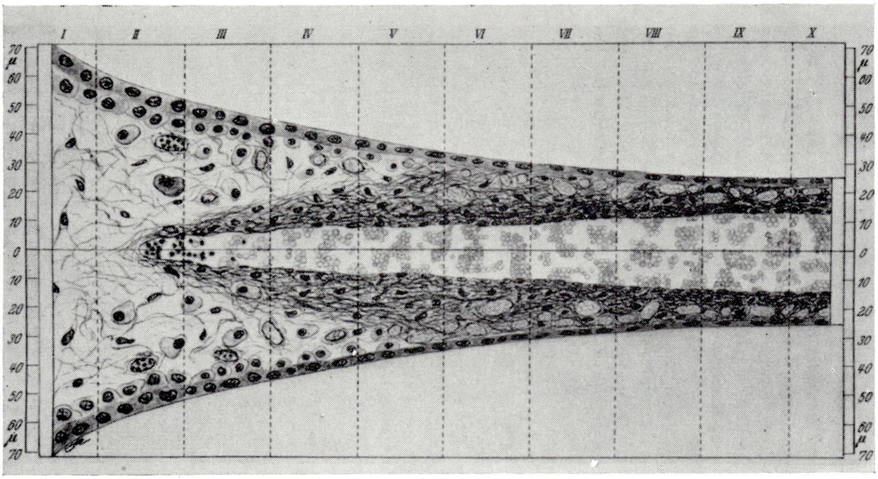

FIG. 3.4. Life cycle of the normal chorionic villus according to Hörmann (1951).

and with capillaries filled with nucleated elements of the red blood series. The villus is covered by a layer of trophoblast without cell divisions which, at its base, is connected with a row of cellular trophoblasts. Electron microscopy has not revealed cell boundaries in the syncytium.

FURTHER DEVELOPMENT OF THE PLACENTA

During the first phase of development, cytotrophoblastic rafters without veins serve as resorption and anchoring systems. After vascularization, and further dichotomous division and proliferation of the large villi, the metabolically active area advances more and more towards a union with the chorion. This leads to the establishment and sub-division of the resorption villus and the main villus.

During the period of its further differentiation that resorption villus decreases in diameter until the 9th month (Fig. 3.4). In the first month of pregnancy the end villus still has an average diameter of 136 μ (up to a maximum of 350 μ). In the 5th lunar month average values, according to Hörmann (1948, 1950, 1951) are only 71 μ (50–150 μ) in the 8th month 50·5 μ (50–100 μ), in the 9th and 10th month 49·8 μ (40–100 μ). The percentage of the larger end villi decreases as pregnancy progresses (Hörmann 1951) leading to an increasing similarity in the diameters of the villi (Fig. 3.5). Diminution of the villous diameter leads to an

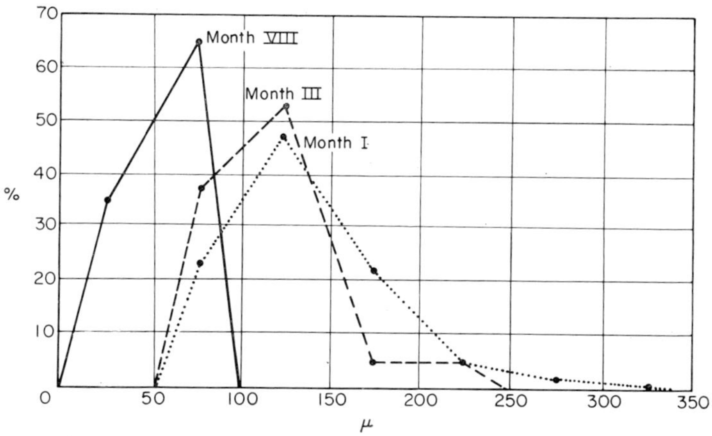

FIG. 3.5. Example of the percentage of villi having diameters between 0 and 350 μ in the 1st, 3rd and 8th month of pregnancy. From Hörmann (1951).

enlargement of the functional surface. This was proved statistically by Knoop (1960).

From about the 11th week *post menstruum*, mature embryocytes are found in the foetal vessels, together with nucleated elements of the red blood series. In normal conditions the nucleated red blood corpuscles have disappeared by about the 12th week *post menstruum*. At this time a rarification of the Langhans' cell layer sets in. It is assumed that it is taken into the syncytium, and there used as replacement material. However, according to earlier research it does not disappear altogether (Thomsen & Blankenburg 1956). After reduction of the Langhans' cells there is a rapid development of the foetal vascular system, with a specific orientation to the periphery of the villus and the growth of sinus-like formations. Where there is close contact between the basal membranes and the foetal vessels, the nuclei of the syncytium pass to one side. Clusters of nuclei come about in the syncytium with thickening of the trophoblast. It is still not clear whether these are active centres of proliferation in the syncytium. Howorka (1956, 1960) has made it seem probable that the syncytium has the power of proliferation. Yet one also finds in diseased villi accumulations of nuclei, with vascular degeneration, and these must surely be of degenerative origin.

During the maturation of the villi, endothelium, basal membranes and the segment of syncytium free of nuclei come together to form metabolic membranes (syncytio-capillary membranes). This nucleus free

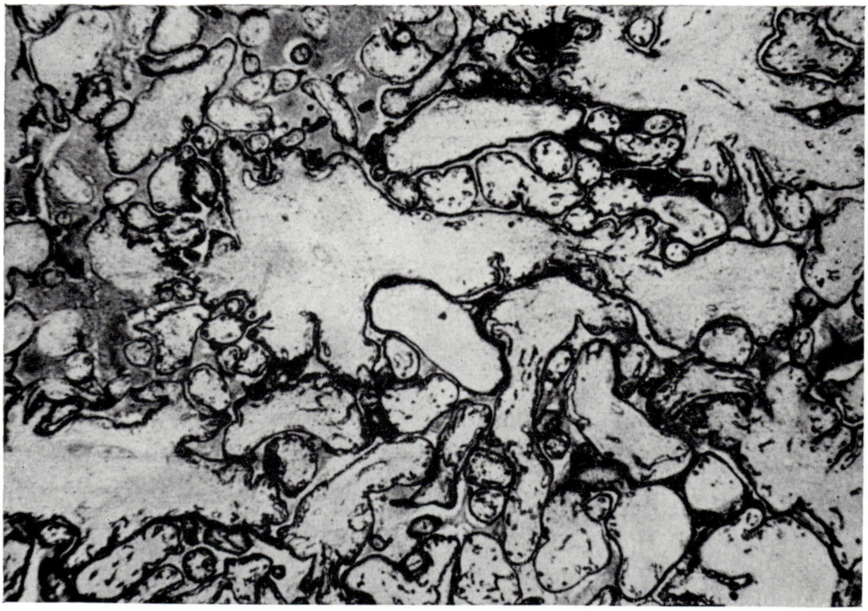

FIG. 3.6. A demonstration of nucleotidase in a 12th week placenta. The villous capillaries show a strong positive reaction but the larger vessels contain no enzyme.

membrane is about 2–5 μ thick, and the component layers (syncytium and endothelium and basal membrane) can only be distinguished by electron microscopy. All earlier research shows that the syncytiovascular membranes are of great importance for the exchange of material between mother and embryo.

During the period of further development, the capillaries not only change into large capillary vessels, (sinusoids), but clearly also change their function. A positive 5′nucleotidase reaction is found between the 15th and 20th week, at first only in the endothelium of the sinusoids

(Fig. 3.6). As the activity of the 5′nucleotidase reaction increases in the vessels of the larger villi, the activity in the capillaries of the resorption villi decreases.

The outer surface of the syncytium shows a brush border which electron-microscopy shows to be a patch of microvilli (Fig. 3.7). This patch is obviously a fluctuating structure. Electron microscopic findings of the surface of the villi will be discussed later.

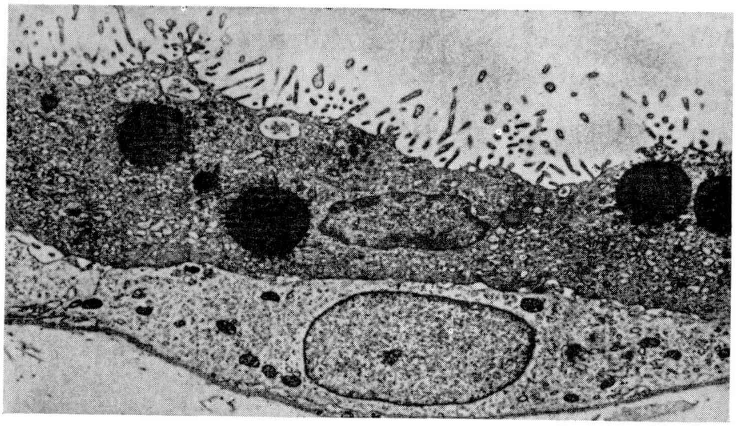

FIG. 3.7. Syncytiotrophoblast with microvilli and lipoid inclusions. There is also a Langhans cell below. (Magnification 12,000 times.) After Bargmann & Knoop (1959).

About the 14th week, the Hofbauer-von-Chaletsky-Neumann cells decrease in numbers. Demonstration is made more difficult, especially by decreased susceptibility to staining and increased pressure of fibroblasts and fibrocytes. They can, however, be shown in the mature normal placenta histochemically (Thomsen & Netz 1955, Thomsen & Blankenburg 1956), and by electron-microscopy (Bargmann & Knoop 1959, Arnold *et al.* 1961). In pathological placentae, on the other hand, they can be clearly recognized as, for example, in the margins of haemorrhagic infarcts.

The cytotrophoblast rafters make a specially important contribution to the formation of the main villi. Once the resorption villus reaches the stage where it is composed almost entirely of huge capillary vessels (sinusoids) they are only foetal support elements, and do not directly serve for the exchange of material. Unlike the resorption villus their diameter increases continuously. At the beginning of the haemotrophic phase of the placental metabolism, the main villus is 100–150 μ. Three to four months later it is 300–400 μ and in the tenth month of pregnancy 150–1500 μ in thickness. During the maturation of the placenta there develops a nodular cell structure of collagen which spreads into the chorion layer and pushes into the main villus. Here one can trace real

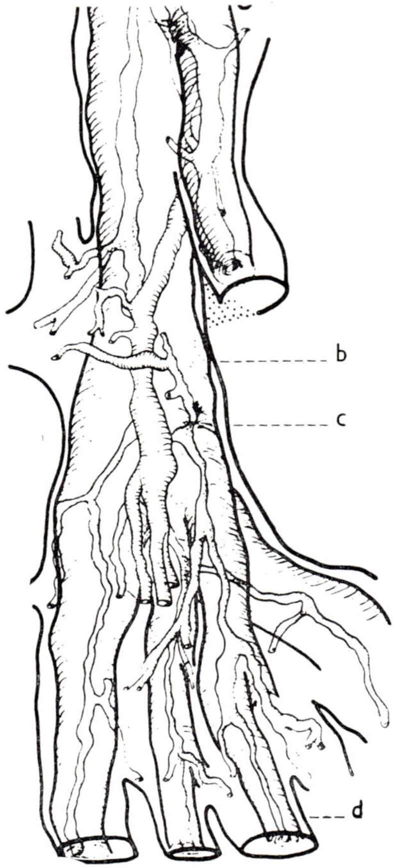

FIG. 3.8. Schematic reconstruction by serial sections of a main villus and the manner in which it subdivides. After Becker (1962).

collagen pillars, while no collagenation takes place in the resorption villus. Tenzer (1962) has made a graphic reconstruction of these pillars, and found a sharply contoured framework of collagen that sometimes comes to a dead end after going through the whole width of the organ, or otherwise attaches itself to the columns of the decidual plate, or even penetrates into the latter (Fig. 3.8). So there arises a real conflict between the pars foetalis and the pars materna placentae. During this conflict between the connective tissues, the vascular system of these villi becomes surrounded by a ring of connective tissue as shown in Fig. 3.9. This is often wrongly described as periarteritis fibrosa. During the de-

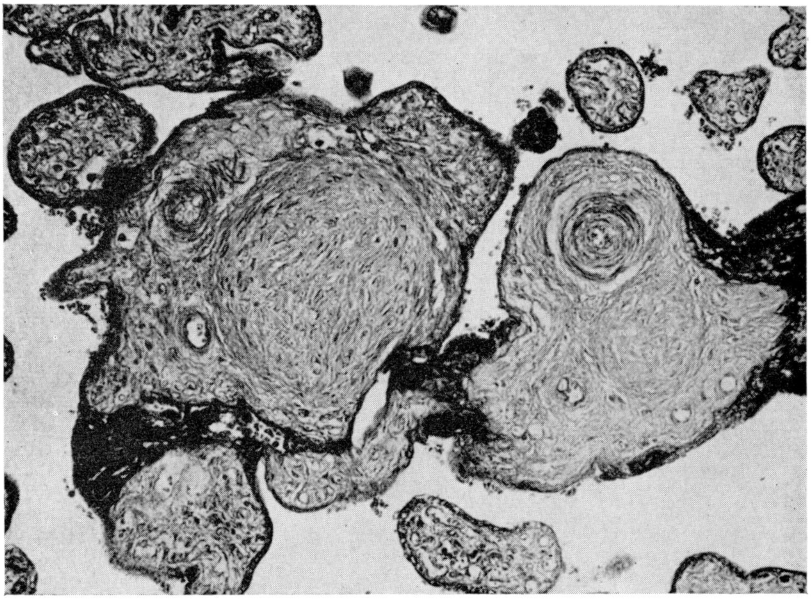

FIG. 3.9. On the left is a main villus with a fibrous ring around the artery. On the right is a clearly demarcated collagenous column. (Magnification 108 times.) After Becker (1962).

velopment of the placenta the arterial walls themselves become disorganized. At first they present muscular elastica-free vessels, but later fibrous permeation of the arteries of the main villus takes place, and the arterial walls become thickened (Becker 1962).

MATURATION OF THE PLACENTA

There is no consensus as to the determinant morphological factors for the definition of the maturation of the placenta. Some writers pay most attention to the vascular system and its differentiation, others to the apparatus of connective tissue, and yet others give the greatest weight to the behaviour of the trophoblast. Becker (1960) compared anatomical findings on five hundred children and their placentae, and on this basis set out the following four signs. (1) Diminution of the diameter of the resorption villus at the right time. (2) Transformation of the capillaries into large capillary vessels (sinusoids) under pressure from the stroma of the villus. (3) Formation of the syncytio-capillary metabolic membranes. (4) The fibrous degeneration of the main villus and the fibrosis of its vessels.

Poor synchronization between the maturation of the placenta and that of the foetus is not uncommon. Becker (1960) found morphologically fully mature placentae in 10 per cent of premature births, whilst the child was still immature in terms of its length, weight and the maturity of its organs. In such cases, further differentiation of the placenta is impossible, and the birth of an immature embryo follows. On the other hand, in cases of postmaturity the placenta has not reached full maturity, whereas the child already shows all the signs of maturity. Thus it is postulated that the maturity of the placenta has greater bearing on the timing of delivery than has that of the child. Both retardation and acceleration of the maturation of the placenta in relation to that of the foetus can be a pathogenic factor for the development of the embryo (Becker 1960, Bleyl 1962). For the development of the placenta which stops at an early stage, degenerative changes and calcification will usually follow, leading, says Becker, to arrested maturation, and the death of the embryo.

THE MATURE PLACENTA

MACROSCOPIC DESCRIPTION

The mature placenta is an almost circular disc shaped organ. According to various authors its diameter may be 15–20 cm. As its disc shape suggests, the placenta grows thinner towards the edge, often with a sudden drop very near to the edge. Inside the placenta the height varies very much. An average weight for a normal single placenta (without the foetal membranes and umbilical cord), is said to be 500 gm (Strauss 1967). This varies, and a normally developed organ can weigh as much as 1,000 gm. A weight below 300 gm indicates a halt in morphological and functional maturation leading to inadequate development of the child.

There is a significant relationship between the weight of the placenta and that of the child (Zschiesche & Gerlach 1963). The placentae of male embryos are heavier than those of female ones. The weight of the placenta increases with parity (Hendricks 1964). Moreover the placentae of mothers living in good social conditions are heavier than those of mothers in bad social circumstances. The final thickness of the placenta is attained by the end of the 4th month. In the 2nd half of pregnancy the placenta grows only by the formation of additional layers (Hamilton & Mossman 1962). The increased size of the placenta is mainly due to the

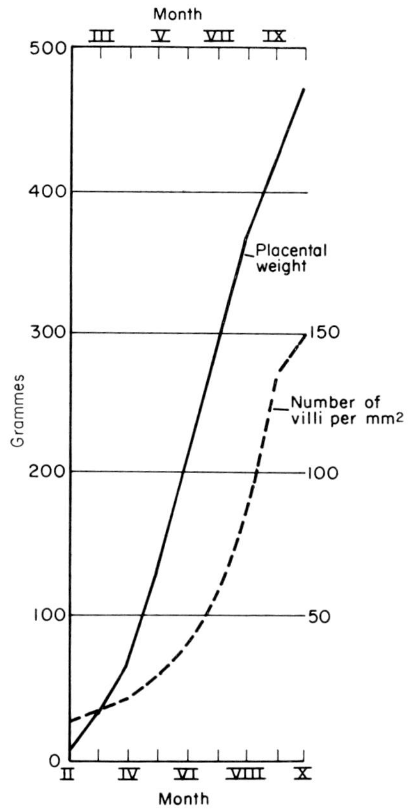

FIG. 3.10. Comparison between the increasing weight of the placenta and the number of villi per sq. mm on cross section. After Knoop (1960).

resorption villi, with large capillary systems which increase five hundred fold during development of the placenta (Crawford 1962). Figure 3.10 shows the relationship between the weight of the placenta and the number of villi. Thin membrane-like forms of placenta known as *placenta membranata* are not uncommon. The trophoblast cells have not penetrated sufficiently into the decidua during the invasion phase, probably due to the absence of an adequate bed for the egg. In such forms one can often find areas where placental tissue is entirely lacking, leaving openings in the tissue: *placenta fenestrata*,

The placenta may consist of a larger or smaller number of lobes of equal size. According to the number of lobes there is present a *placenta bi, tri, or multi lobulata.* The last of these is uncommon. In a sample of 10,000 Aguero (1957) found 326 placenta bi-lobulata, and 15 with three to five lobes. If, however, the organ is composed of more than two parts wholly separated from each other, whose vessels come together in the membranes to enter the umbilical cord, it is described as a *placenta bi, tri, or multi partita.*

A more common form is a main placenta with one or more smaller lobes attached to it: *placenta succenturiata.* In the post-partum period the latter may tear away from the main lobe, be retained in the cavity of the uterus, and cause haemorrhages.

At the edge of the placenta there is often a broad circular yellowish-white band to be found histologically and histochemically. This appears to be fibrin. This form is termed *placenta marginata* or, where the fibrin formation is especially clearly defined, shaped like a glove, inturned and wall-like it is termed *placenta circumvallata.* Both forms can be termed *placenta extrachorialis.* When the placenta is fully formed the point of insertion of the membranes is normally the edge of the placenta. Where the placenta is relatively insufficient and the trophoblast has retained some of its powers of adaptation, the organ spreads up more widely to adapt the exchange area to the demands made on it. This brings into being a partly extrachorioamnial placenta. Scott (1960) again stressed its clinical consequences which consist of bleeding during pregnancy and during delivery, as well as a tendency to abort which can in such cases be considered as a desperate measure of adaptation. According to the literature, extrachorionic placentae occurred in 7–40 per cent of all placentae. This form of placenta is not necessarily connected with increased damage or danger to the child but is often the real cause of bleeding from the sinus marginalis, the significance of which is over-estimated and is only valid in exceptional cases. The *placenta pseudo-zonaria* was observed by Aguero (1957) twice out of 10,000 placentae.

THE MATERNAL BLOOD CIRCULATION OF THE PLACENTA

The human placenta consists of placentomes according to Strauss (1967), which communicate together. A placentome consists of a chamber of the maternal blood compartment composed of septa and the clustered root-like foetal villous system projecting into it. However, further research by Becker & Jipp (1963) into the trophoblastic shell of the human placenta has shown a different picture. These authors, taking large shallow serial sections step-wise horizontally to the basal plate, have never found a reticulated structure. After dissecting the tissues of the villi from the basal plate, narrow sheets and columns rising from the basal plate were found. On the other hand, septa were not seen. These sheets and columns show great variety of form, especially varying heights. Most of them are perforated. The columns are certainly unsuitable for giving direction to the blood stream. The sheets are flat formations growing narrower towards the chorion plate. The base amounts to no more than 2·8 cm. Nor do Becker & Jipp (1963) attribute any decisive haemodynamic role to them on the basis of their structure and position. This was confirmed by Lemtis (1966). Columns and sheets are therefore an essential part of the supporting apparatus of the placenta and protect the organ from compression. These findings show that a placenta limited by septa does not exist. Lemtis (1966) found circulation units independent of the villi. The main stems of the foetal villi with their branches come from the chorion plate and rest on the 'lunar landscape' of the basal plate (Fig. 3.11 and 3.12).

Hörmann (1953) and Freese (1966) have demonstrated that the maternal blood circulates in a three dimensional capillary slit and not in an intervillous 'space' as has been assumed before. X-ray cinematographic, serial angiographs, plastoid injections and histological studies (Freese 1966, Freese *et al.* 1966) attest the presence of an intracotyledonary space. Evidence is accumulating that one spiral arteriole for each cotyledon discharges the maternal blood into the intracotyledonary space; from there it enters the intervillous capillary slits before returning to the maternal circulation (Freese 1966).

More recent research has shown that directly below the chorion plate the main villus divides into many branches (second order branches) and these again divide dichotomously (third order branches). These branches go to the basal plate and anchor themselves there partly as adhesive villi. At the same time, the main villi are formed with their end branches in root-like cluster formations. Only a few end villi finally turn back to the chorion plate. According to Crawford (1956a, 1956b, 1962) the cotyledon can be subdivided into at least four sub-cotyledons and some neighbouring sub-cotyledons become interdigitated. Arteriovenous or

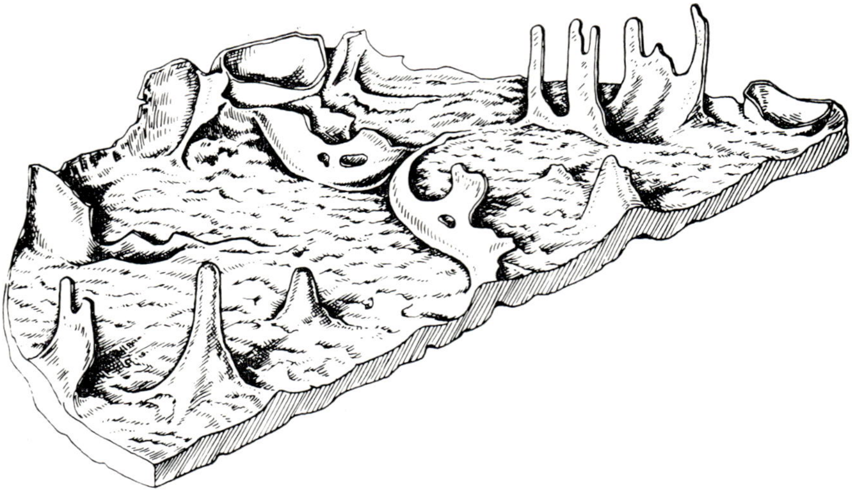

FIG. 3.11. Three dimensional reconstruction of a segment of the basal plate with a baseline of 20 cm.

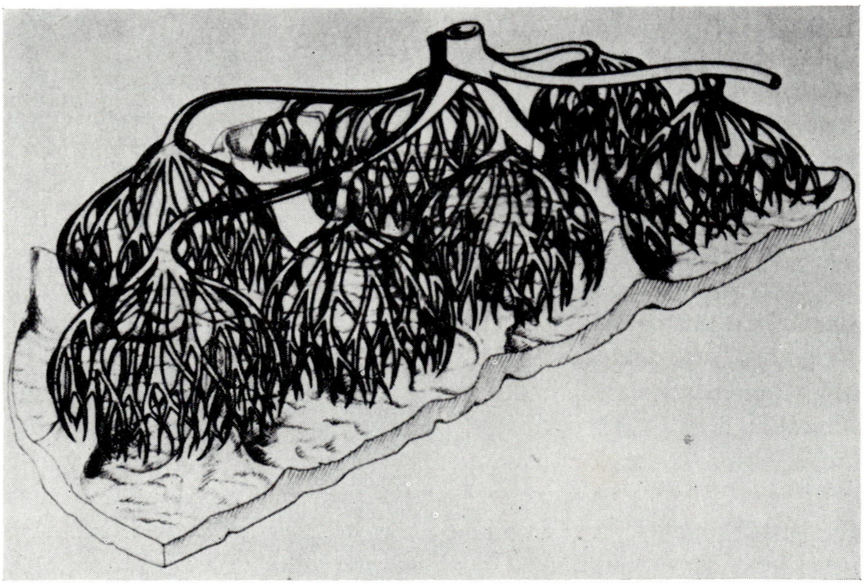

FIG. 3.12. Schematic reconstruction of the basal plate with its sheets and columns. From this is derived the system of foetal cotyledons. the subchoreal web of vessels. After Becker (1962).

interarterial anastomoses do not occur in the area of the circulation of the cotyledon. The vessels of the main villus are thus terminal vessels.

Until now, the conception of the circulation of the maternal blood in the intervillous slit has been as follows: the utero-placental arteries become jet-like, narrowing at their mouths. The pressure gradient of the maternal and intervillous circulation is 75 mm Hg. The maternal blood is sprayed as a Borrell's jet into the sub-chorionic lake. It was then supposed to travel in a stream counter to the foetal blood past the chorion villus into the funnels of the basal veins. The best possibility of exchange between the maternal and foetal blood is created by the sharp difference in the circulation speeds and the concept of the contrary directions of the maternal and foetal circulations.

It can be assumed that the blood stream can be directed through vasomotor regulatory circuits. This would make the circulation in the intervillous space fit in with the earlier conception. The subchorionic space and the marginal sinus prevent overfilling of the intervillous space. The marginal sinus is of minor importance serving as an outflow for the maternal blood.

Recent research by Lemtis (1966) has cast serious doubts on this conception. On grounds of perfusion studies, studies based on x-ray films and corrosion preparations, it is possible to show that the maternal intervillous blood paths involve a capillary cleft in which there are areas with a rapid flow and areas with a slower flow. Since the foetal line of flow also contains areas of rapid flow and areas with a slower flow through them a functionally determined blood supply is suggested. Even when higher pressure injections were used a Borrell's jet reaching to the subchorionic sinus is not shown. The contrasting flow spreads out into the intervillous capillary cleft in circular, oval or ellipsoid form like a smoke ring. The diameter of such a ring is from 1 to 2 cm. Taken together the picture is one of separate circulatory spheres. According to Lemtis, the findings indicate the presence of pre-existing directed blood flow paths in the maternal capillary system of the placenta, composed of 'bundles of capillary pathways'. According to Lemtis (1966) a ring shaped circulation is typical of the blood flow in the maternal system of intermediate villi. It requires little pressure for the blood to flow through the pre-formed and pre-directed circulatory paths. This might be considered a safety device for the foetus in the event of defective maternal circulation. Even if injected under high pressure the contrast solution flows along pre-formed capillary paths and not along the shortest route.

THE VILLUS

The villus of the mature placenta consists mainly of these tissues: The basic stem is formed by a delicate reticular, non-collagenous tissue containing many sinusoidal capillaries. This tissue is limited by two layers of trophoblast, the external syncytium and the internal Langhans layers. The latter does not, however, constitute a continuous layer in the ripe placenta but is composed of scattered observable single cells which are taken up by the syncytium. Special methods e.g. histochemistry (Thomsen & Blankenburg 1956), and electron microscopy (Bargman & Knoop 1959, Hashimoto *et al.* 1960, Wakitani 1961), always show them to be present.

The syncytium (plasmodium)

Howorka (1956, 1960) unlike earlier investigators, was able to observe a real growth of the syncytium in the tissue culture which demonstrates that this layer of tissue is independent of substitute material composed of Langhans cells.

Contrary to some haemochorial animal placentae, the syncytium of the human villus shows under the electron microscope no sub-division into separate cells. It is not clear at present whether the outer trophoblast layer of the villus results from the fusion of separate cells (syncytium) or a continuous nuclear division without subsequent cell division (plasmodium). We are using the term 'syncytium' or 'syncytiotrophoblast', as the case may be, without thereby seeking to take a position on its genesis.

The syncytiotrophoblast consists of a single layer of epithelium which grows increasingly thin as the villus develops. The nuclei also decrease in circumference. In the mature villus one can identify areas free of nuclei and accumulations of nuclei in which adjacent nuclei can build bridges. In the areas free of nuclei the endothelium of the sinusoids of the villus and the basal membranes may be so close to the syncytium that all three layers coalesce into a unit–the so-called syncytio-capillary membrane, the separate parts of which can no longer be identified by electron microscopy and which is often no more than 2 μ in thickness. All chorionic villi, however, continue to show an intact syncytium even where it appears to be extremely thin in a few places over a prominent Langhans cell. In the region of the syncytium of the immature villus, plasmatic projections are to be found (Howorka 1956, 1960, Kanematsu 1961) which are only connected with the underlying epithelium by quite thin processes.

The brush border on the top surface of the syncytium earlier detected by light microscopy consists of an evenly developed patch of cytoplasmatic processes (microvilli) placed at intervals of from 80 to 250 mμ (Boyd & Hughes 1954, Wislocki & Dempsey 1955, Sawazaki and colleagues 1957, Bargmann & Knoop 1959, Hashimoto and colleagues 1960). These microvilli (Fig. 3.7) apparently serve to enlarge the surface area; whether they signify an essential requirement for the exchange of

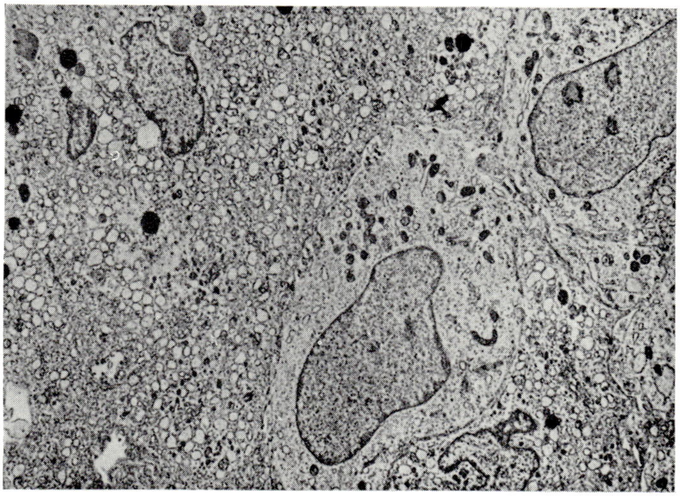

FIG. 3.13. Two Langhans cells surrounded by syncytiotrophoblast. In the syncytium are vesicles and osmophilic inclusions. (Magnification 9,500 times.) After Bargmann & Knoop (1959).

material has recently been questioned (Arnold *et al.* 1961). The lengths of the microvilli vary from 1,000 to 2,000 mμ; their diameters range from 100 mμ to 250 mμ. In the region of the apex the little strands of cytoplasm are often thickened into globules and a few even divided into branches. In them a granular vacuolated protoplasm is to be found. These microvilli are not rigid structures but capable of wavelike motion.

As the differentiation of the villus progresses, these microvilli begin to change their form. Up to the 11th week they increase in length and thickness. From the 15th week on the other hand, they grow smaller and at term are often no more than 500 mμ long. The thickness of the microvilli also decreases after the 31st week and finally is as little as 150 mμ. Thus, there is a shrinkage of the microvilli as the villus matures. By electron microscopy, areas can even be found quite free of microvilli.

More especially, there is a lack of microvilli in the area of the buds. According to the observations of Amstutz (1960) they are scarce in, or absent from, the area of syncytio-vascular membrane (see, however, Figs. 3.16 and 3.17). This implies that the microvilli serve the exchange of material during the growth of the top layer and otherwise are inconstant in appearance. The significance of the so-called 'bald patches' free of microvilli is still unclear. The doubly contoured outer membrane may disappear at points where the micro-villi touch so that the syncytial protoplasm appears to flow together. This is supposed to bring about the stabilization of the system of the villi so that it is possible that the microvilli have a supporting function.

Whilst the light microscope shows a relatively structureless syncytio and karyoplasma, ultra microscopic observation makes it possible to determine the morphological basis for the high metabolic performance of the syncytium. The nuclei of the syncytium often lie together in clusters and are clearly polymorphous and often show an eccentric nucleolus. They are limited by a double membrane which is perforated by so-called nuclear pores. The cytoplasm of the syncytium often has indentations into the nuclei which may extend for 300 mμ.

Some regular structures are found in the syncytial cytoplasm. They may occur singly or in groups, are osmophilic and ovoid or spherical in shape with diameter from 400 to 2,500 mμ (Fig. 3.13). These spheres are identical with the lipoid inclusions of the syncytium described by Wislocki & Dempsey (1948). Their significance as substrates of steroid hormone production was discussed by Thomsen & Lorentzen (1956); Bargmann (1957), Ortmann (1959), Hashimoto and colleagues (1960). Irregularly shaped but often definitely circular vacuoles of various sizes (800–2,000 mμ diameter) can also be distinguished.

By electron microscopic observation, one can find small vesicles, very close together, disposed throughout almost the whole width of the syncytium (Figs. 3.13 and 3.14), and these are one of its essential charac-

---

FIG. 3.14. Electron microscope structure of whole thickness of villous trophoblast. Above are the microvilli (V) and below the basal membrane, (indicated by an arrow). Between them lies the somewhat irregularly disposed nuclei of the syncytium. Thin extensions of the protoplasm of the syncytium between the Langhans cells reach the basal vesicles and inclusions as well as larger canals, (indicated by white arrows). (Magnification 5,360 times.) After Ashley (1965).

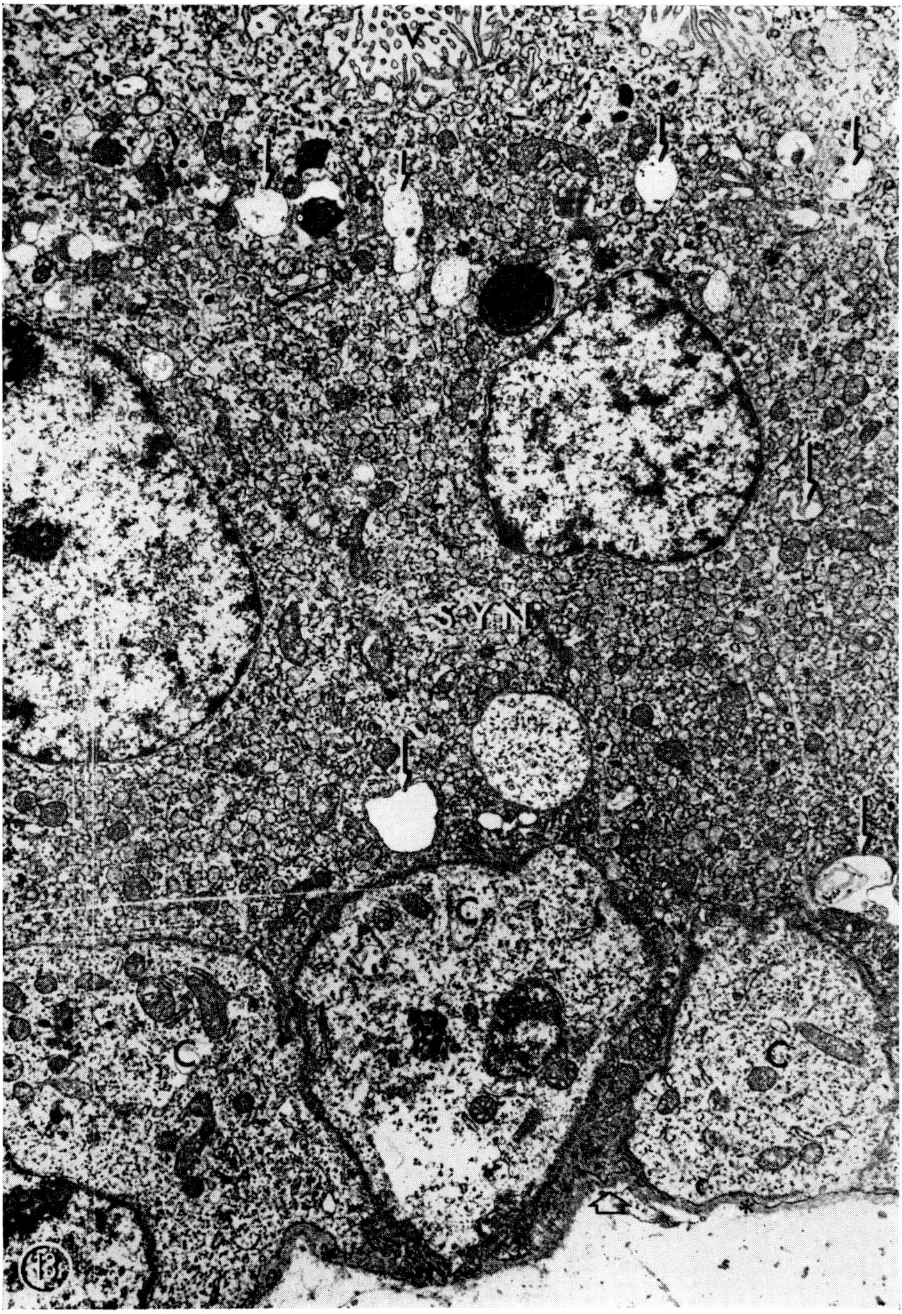
V
SYN
C
C
C
13

teristics. They have diameters ranging from 200 to 500 mμ and are contained in a clearly defined membrane. Some sections of the membrane, often extensive, are osmiophilic. Here tiny granula are found which are often taken to be RNA granules, partly because of their size. Wislocki & Dempsey (1955) thus attribute these structures to the ergastoplasm. There are also small vesicles to be found in the syncytium whose content appears to be homogeneous even under the electron microscope and shows a very low optical density. Moreover here lie RNA granula.

The mitochondria of the syncytium show a stratified structure and are about 600 mμ long and some 80 mμ in width. In this case, electron microscopy has made a contribution to functional morphology: the mitochondria have been found to be most numerous in the neighbourhood of the lipoid inclusions; a localization such as we are familiar with as regards the fat producing cells (Bargmann & Knoop 1959). The Golgi apparatus of the syncytium can be resolved into a complex granular membrane (see Figs. 3.15, 3.16, 3.17 and 3.18).

Kanematsu (1961) describes small vesicles, mostly homogeneous, but some filled with granula, found in the periphery of the syncytium in living villus preparations which sometimes increase and may be concerned with hormone production. Immediately beneath the area of the microvilli, Ikawa (1959) observed numerous vacuoles, some sharply divided off by membranes from the surrounding cytoplasm but others connected with it by openings.

Pinocytosis is put forward as an explanation, not only for the intake of liquid but also for the entry of plasma protein and lipids into the syncytium (Yamaguchi and colleagues 1960).

By electron microscopy, two zones of distinguishable ultrastructure can be differentiated in the syncytium. The alpha zone is thinner than the beta zone (Burgos & Rodriguez 1966). The alpha zone corresponds to the syncytio-capillary metabolic membrane (Fig. 3.15). The ultra structure of the alpha zone shows many microvilli, pinocytosis, vesicles, apical canaliculi, phagocytosis and lysosomes (Figs. 3.16 and 3.17). Electron microscopy of other specially active resorptive tissue suggests that the

---

FIG. 3.15. Electron microscopic enlargement of an endvillus. One can see interdigitations between the syncytium (ST) and the cytotrophoblast (CT). A: Alpha zone. B: Beta zone. IS: Intervillous capillary space. N: Nucleus. S: Stroma of the connective tissue. E: Endothelium. BM: Basal Membrane (indicated by an arrow). FC: Foetal capillary. (Enlarged 13,600 times.) From Burgos & Rodriguez (1966).

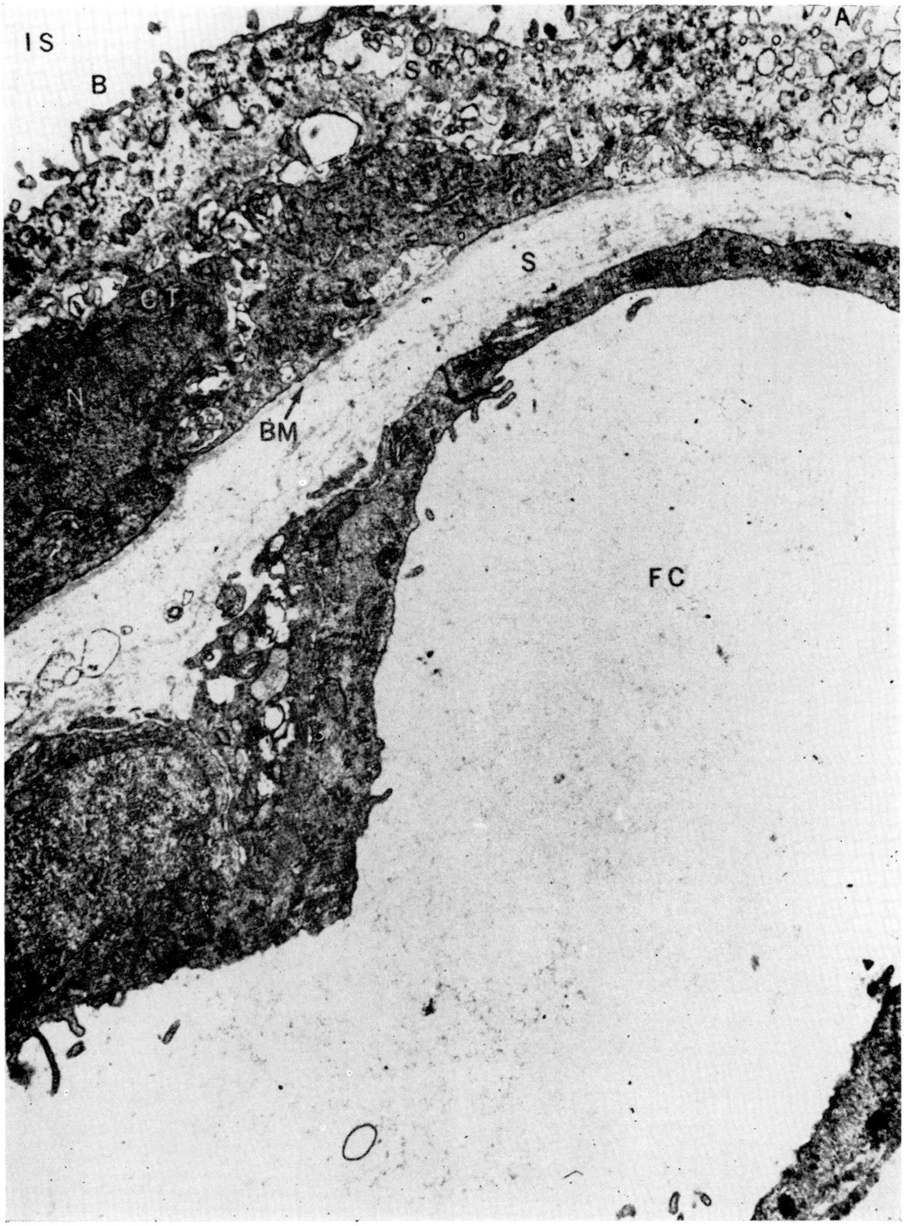
IS
B
S
A
CT
N
S
BM
FC

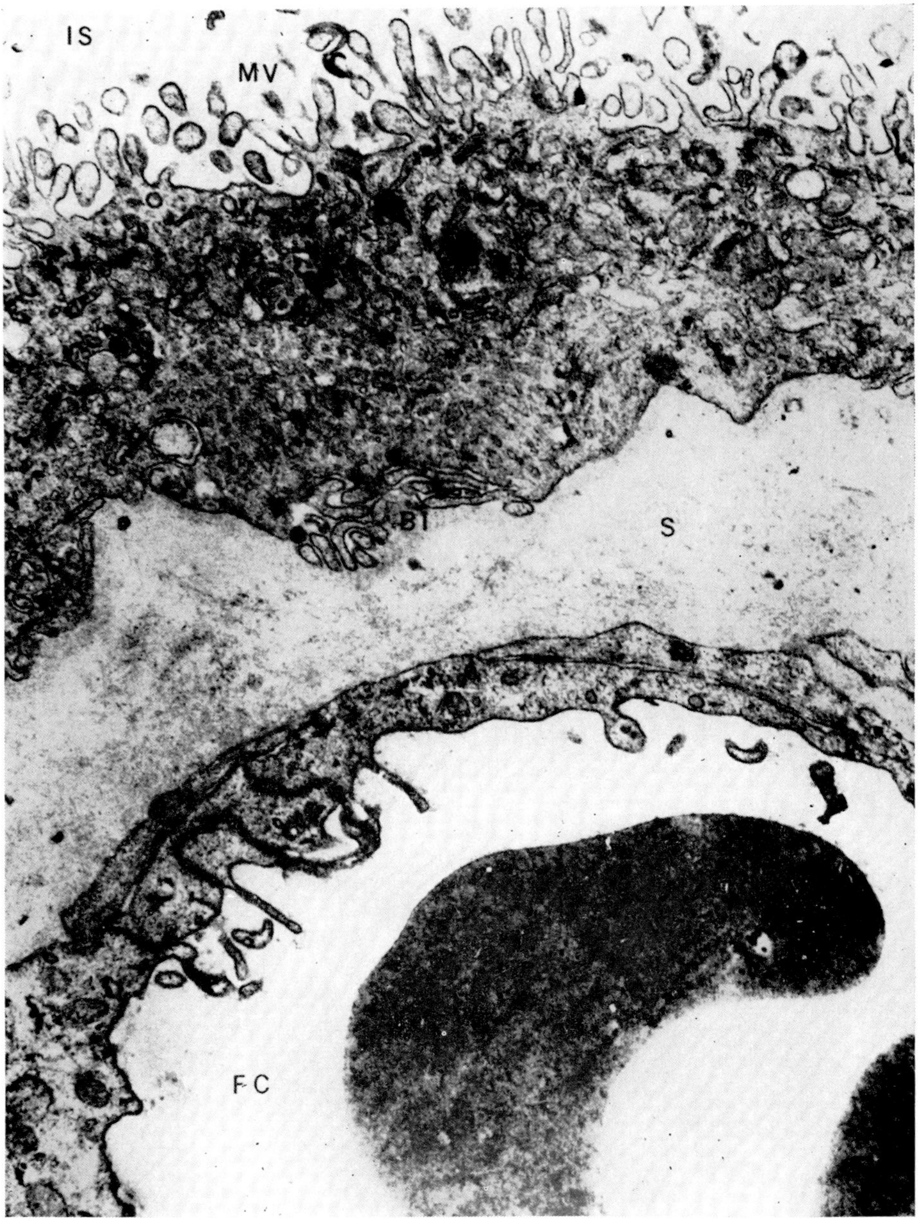

FIG. 3.16. The free end of a villus. The alpha zone with thick microvilli (MV) and basal indentations. IS: Intervillous capillary space. S: Stroma of connective tissue. FC: Foetal capillary. (Enlarged 13,760 times.) After Burgos & Rodriguez (1966).

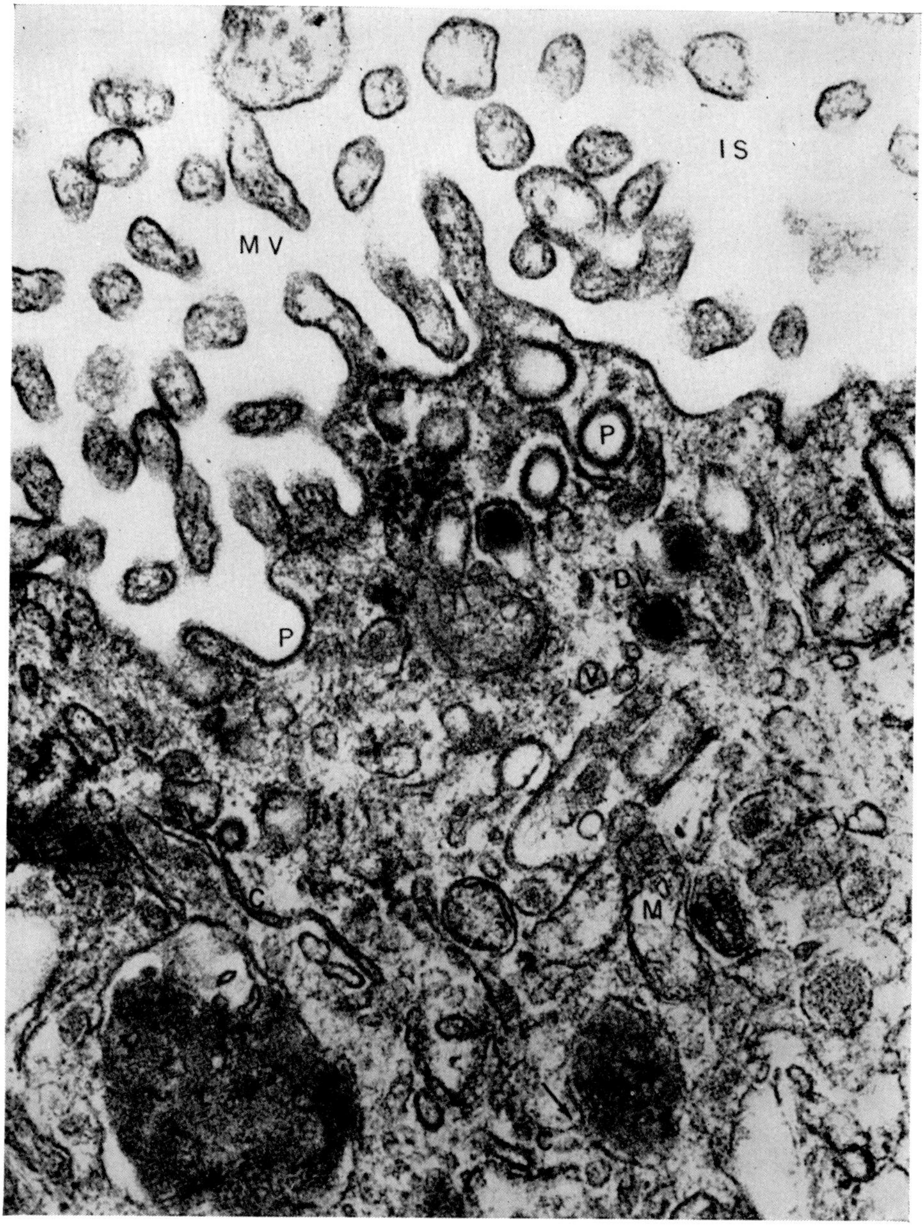

FIG. 3.17. Greatly enlarged syncytial surface in the region of the alpha zone. MV: Microvilli. P: Pinocytes. V: Vesicle. C: Canaliculi. DV: Vacuoles with dense material. L: Lysosomes. M: Mitochondria. The arrow shows a connection between a canaliculus and a vacuole. IS: Intervillous capillary space. (Magnification 42,400 times.) After Burgos & Rodriguez (1966).

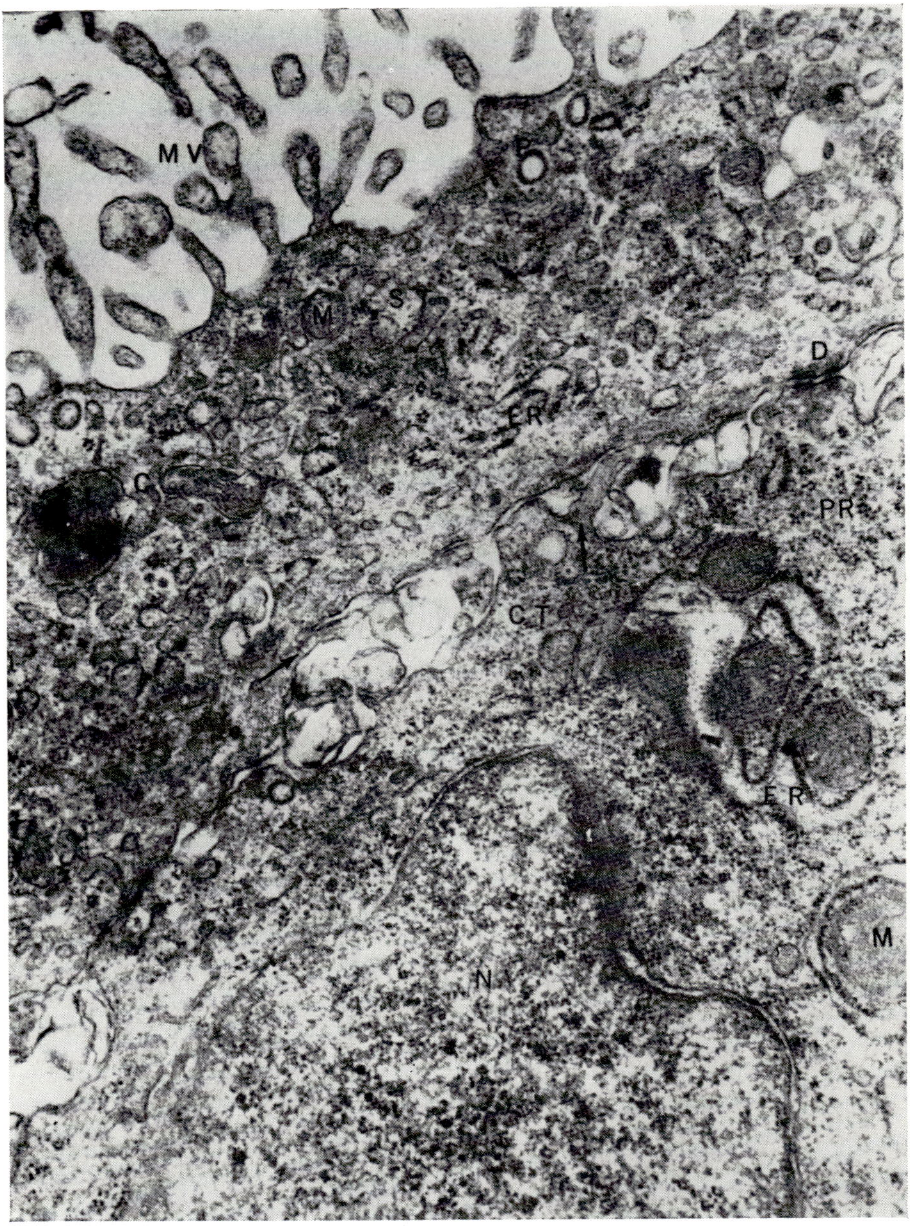

FIG. 3.18. The beta zone of the cytotrophoblast. CT: Cytotrophoblast. M: Mitochondria. ER: Endoplasmic Reticulum. PR: Polyribosomes. ST: Syncytium with endoplasmic reticulum mitochondria and occasional pinocytes. C: Canaliculi. L: Lysosomes. The arrow shows an interdigitation between syncytium and cytotrophoblast. D: Desmosomes. MV: Irregular microvilli. (Magnification 22,400 times.) After Burgos & Rodriguez (1966).

presence of this assortment of organellae is an expression of brisk transport within the cells.

The beta zone has many nuclei and highly developed ergastoplasm, ribosomes and polyribosomes (Fig. 3.18). This finding is a strong indication of a high synthesizing performance by the cells. Burgos & Rodriguez

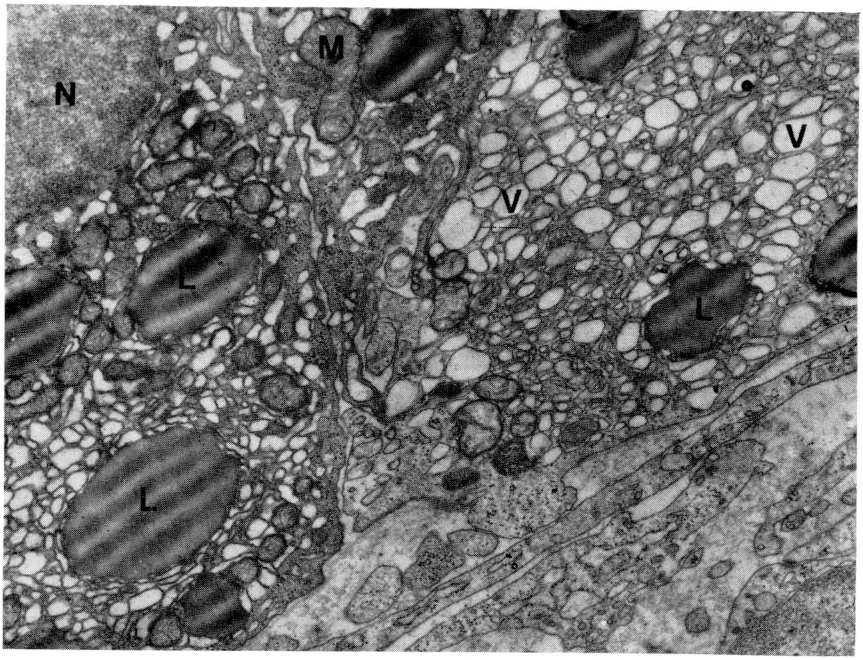

FIG. 3.19. Intermediate cells of the rabbit ovary after stimulation with gonadotrophin. L: Lipoid vesicles. M: Tubular mitochondria. V: Markedly dilated endoplasmic vesicle. N: Nucleus. (Magnification 27,200 times.) Stegner & Beltermann (1967).

(1966) have correlated this finding with the synthesis of peptides, proteins, nucleic acid, glycogen and fatty acid; also with the production of the placental hormones (HCG, progesterone, oestrogens). The wealth of ergastoplasm and RNA is sure evidence of protein synthesis. Both components are present in quantity in the beta zone but are sparse in the alpha zone.

In connection with hormone production, the results of investigations by Beltermann & Stegner (1968) and Stegner & Beltermann (1967) are noteworthy. Following stimulation with human hypophyseal gonadotrophin (HPG), the ovaries of newborn mice showed the following characteristic picture; large tubular mitochondria, a highly developed system of endoplasmatic membranes and plentiful lipoid inclusions. Mature functioning interstitial cells present a similar picture. It is therefore possible that the wealth of organellae described may be determined by the functioning of the cells.

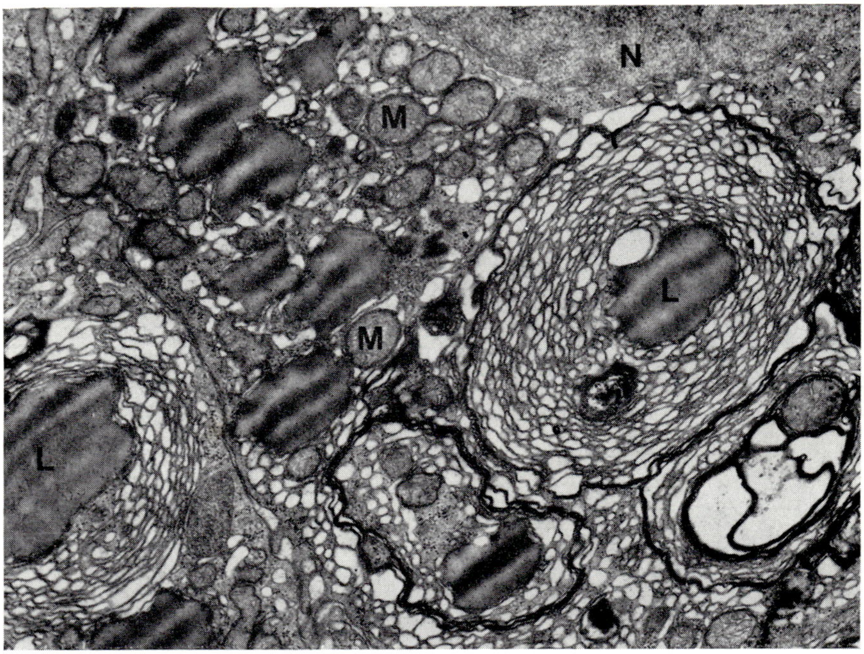

FIG. 3.20. Interstitial cells of the rabbit ovary after overstimulation with gonadotrophin. Clearly demarcated endoplasmic membrane system with a concentric arrangement of lipoid inclusions. It may be that these represent zones where steroid hormones are synthesized or that they are regressive changes. L: Lipoids. M: Tubular mitochondria. V: Concentrically arranged endoplasmic membrane systems. N: Nucleus. (Magnification 27,200 times.) After Stegner & Beltermann (1967).

Comparative studies of the Leydig cells of the testes (Schwartz & Merker 1965) and of the intermediate cells of the rabbit ovary clearly show that the active steroid hormone producing cells have in common the characteristics of a highly developed system of vesicular endoplasmatic membranes and the transformation of the crystalline mitochondria into tubular mitochondria (Figs 3.19 and 3.20).

The experimental observations of Ashley (1965) show that colloid thorium dioxide and ferritin, after incubation with syncytium are fairly rapidly permeated from the maternal top layer through the cytoplasm to the basal membranes. According to Ashley (1965) the basal membrane is

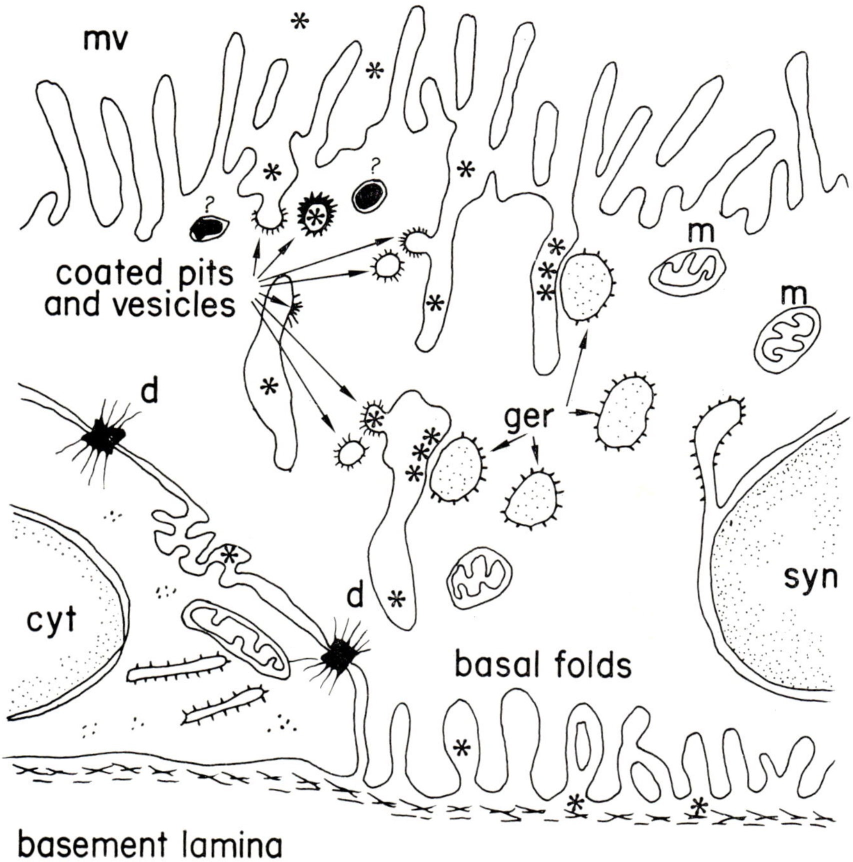

FIG. 3.21. Schematic representation of the passage of thorium and ferritin particles through the trophoblast (*): Ferritin particles. Between the microvilli (MV) one finds absorbing pits and vesicles as well as connecting canals. The particles pass from the microvilli to capillary openings between the syncytiotrophoblast (syn) and the cytotrophoblast (cyt). The cells are connected by desmosomes (d). Ferritin particles are taken along the membranes of the canals in the immediate neighbourhood of the endoplasmic reticulum (ger). The particles reach the extracellular space between the basal folds of the syncytiotrophoblast and the upper surface of the basal membrane. The mitochondria (M) are unevenly distributed. Denser structures of uncertain origin, bound to membranes occur in special vesicles. After Ashley (1965).

the last effective filter and regulator for substances which are to reach the embryo. A schematic presentation of Ashley's experimental results is shown in Fig. 3.21.

Cellular slits are another way of transport through the syncytium (Sawasaki *et al* 1957). Radioactive reinjected maternal erythrocytes can pass to the child with the placenta intact (Suhring, Green, Rochlin & Blakemore 1961). We agree with Page (1960) who stated: 'From time to

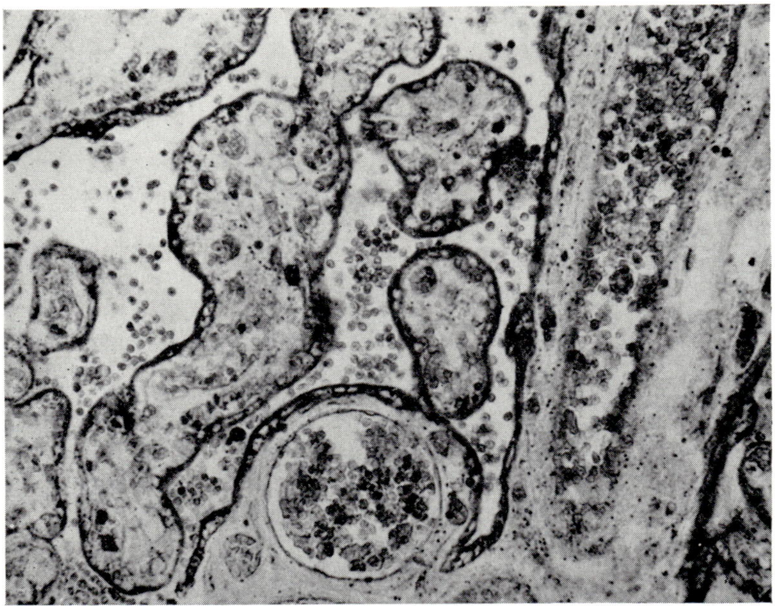

FIG. 3.22. Placenta from the 40th week of pregnancy. Stained with Sudan Black. (Magnification 90 times.) After Thomsen & Lorentzen (1956).

time, possibly in all placentae there may develop variable numbers of cross leaks in the barrier through which intact cells may pass. In this instance, the direction of passage must depend upon the hydrostatic pressure gradient existing at that moment on the two sides of the barrier'.

According to the researches of Windle (1940) glycogen is present only in the maternal placenta. Hertig (1960) found in a 13 day old placenta: 'Relatively little glycogen within the syncytial trophoblast'. Boyd (1960) and Villee (1960) confirmed the findings on placentae 18, 24 and 28 days old. The primordial egg is always free of glycogen (McKay 1960).

Other carbohydrates are the mucopolysaccharides, mucoproteins and glycoproteins. Their histochemical evaluation was critically appreciated by Gedigk (1952). The gonadotrophic hormones of the chorion are also mucoproteins. It is not clear at present whether the outer trophoblast layer of the villus results from the fusion of single cells (syncytium) or a continuous nuclear division without subsequent cell division (plasmodium). In spite of many investigations histochemical methods have so far failed to localize the site of production of the gonadotrophic hormones.

The syncytium is rich in lipids. During placental development the larger droplets are transformed into smaller ones. The lipid granules are found mainly on the periphery and in the basal portion of the syncytium (Fig. 3.22). Some of the smaller lipid droplets appear to be formed by pinocytosis. While the distribution of the fat in the syncytium is mainly in the periphery and in the basal areas (Wislocki & Dempsey 1948, Thomsen & Lorenzen 1956, Thomsen 1959) tiny isolated droplets of fat have been found in the nuclei and in the microvilli.

In the fat content of the placenta 67·7 per cent consists of lipids, among which phospholipids constitute 76·6 per cent, the remainder being composed of neutral fats. Since histochemical methods of differentiating between lipids and neutral fats are not sufficiently specific, it is still usual to limit determinations to the total fat content. Whether lipids are synthesized *de novo* in the placenta or how they pass through it has not been determined. Kleine (1966, 1967a, b, c) has demonstrated in incubation experiments that (1-^{14}C) acetate is incorporated by mature human placental villi into fatty acids, cholesterol and fatty acid free phosphatides. These ^{14}C-labeled fatty acids again are incorporated in mono-, di-triglycerides, cholesterol esters and phosphatides. The mature human placenta has to be considered as an organ of synthesis of lipids which are required in great amount by the foetus.

After critical evaluation of all these results, it can be said that the positive basophilia of the syncytium is an indication that it is rich in RNA as seen in Table 3.1. There is positive metachromasia in the syncytium but the histochemical value of this statement is disputed.

A central role in the metabolism of albumin is played by 5′nucleotidase which catalyzes the splitting of the nucleotide into nucleoside. The nuclei and the top layer of the syncytium in the immature villus react positively for 5′nucleotidase. Enzyme activity in the syncytium does not increase after the 30th week of pregnancy (Fig. 3.23).

Phosphatases appear wherever transphosphorylation takes place They are of importance in numerous metabolic activities such as glycogenesis. The protoplasm of the syncytium is rich in alkaline phosphatase (pH 9·0–9·8), the nuclei are negative (Thomsen 1955a and b). This finding was confirmed by cell fractionation studies (Strauss & Stark 1960), and by unstained preparations (Strauss & Hiersche 1962). There is little alkaline phosphatase activity until the 10th week, thereafter, it increases to the end of pregnancy. Strauss & Hiersche (1962), showed that the localization of the alkaline phosphatase was dependent on the technique used in working up the material (Fig. 3.25). The cellular trophoblast is free of phosphatase (Fig. 3.24). Basophilia is strong in the young villus whereas phosphatase activity is limited, while in the mature placenta, the position is reversed. The greatest concentration of alkaline phosphatase (pH 9·0–9·8) lies in the mitochondria (Stark & Jung 1956, 1959).

TABLE 3.1

	Syncytium	Langhans cells	Columns	Shell	Septal Islands	Decidua
Glycogen	+	+/−	+	+	+	+
Acid mucopolysaccharides	−	−	−	−	−	+
Glycoproteins	+	−	+/−	+/−	+/−	−
Lipids	+	−	−	+	+	+
Phospholipids	+	−		−	−	−
Sulphydryl groups	+/−	+/−	+/−	+	+	+/−
Basophilia	+	+	+	+	+	+/−
Metachromasia	+	+	+	+	+	−
5′-Nucleotidase	+	−	?	+	+	−
Alkaline	+	−	+/−	−	−	−
Acid phosphatase	+	−	+/−	+/−	+/−	−
DPN- and TPN-diaphorase	+	−	?	?	?	+
Succino-dehydrogenase	+	−	?	+	+	+

Acid phosphatase (pH 0·5.5·6) is more labile than alkaline phosphatase. Its histochemical demonstration is more difficult and associated with a greater liability to artefacts. In the syncytium of the immature villi there is a strong reaction to acid phosphatase, quite unlike the position with alkaline phosphatase (Fig. 3.26). In some areas of the syncytium the reaction is weak or entirely absent. In the 2nd half of pregnancy, the activity of acid phosphatase in the syncytium decreases. In unstained

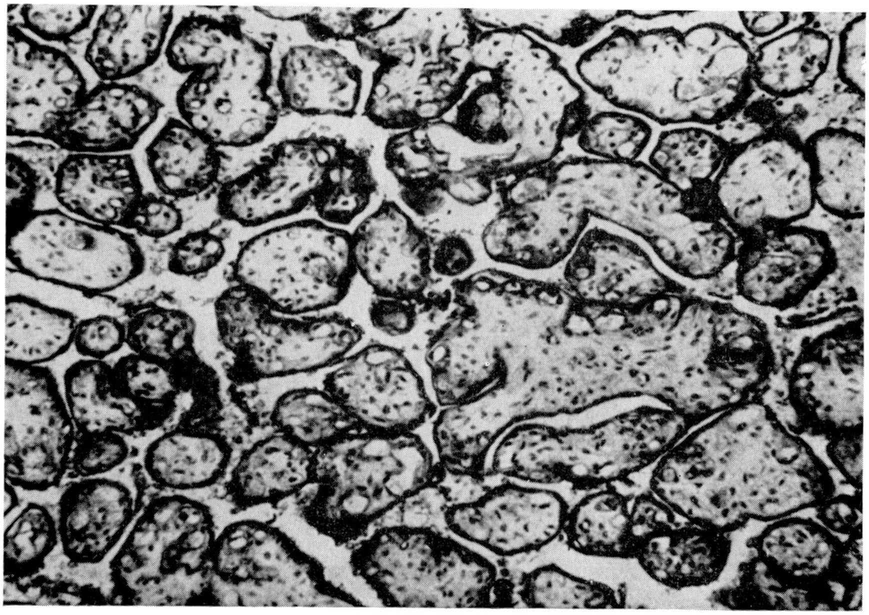

FIG. 3.23. Mature placenta from 37th week of gestation. A demonstration of the distribution of nucleotidase. There is strong activity in the stromal nuclei. (Enlarged 216 times.)

sections alkaline phosphatase is found almost exclusively in the basal areas (near the stroma) while acid phosphatase occurs particularly in the peripheral cell areas near the intervillus space.

Quantitative analysis of the total phosphatase content of the human placenta (Humke 1963) showed that this enzyme increases up to the end of pregnancy. On the 12th to 14th day of a real postmaturity, the phosphatase content decreases again in correlation with the reduction in the function of the placenta.

The yellow respiratory enzymes of the DPN- and TPN-diaphorase group were shown to be present in the human placenta by Strauss & Hiersche (1962). The formazan crystals which appear in a histochemical demonstration are distributed as fine granules throughout the syncytium and unlike alkaline and acid phosphatase are not specially localized. Absorption techniques show them to be in apposition to the outer sur-

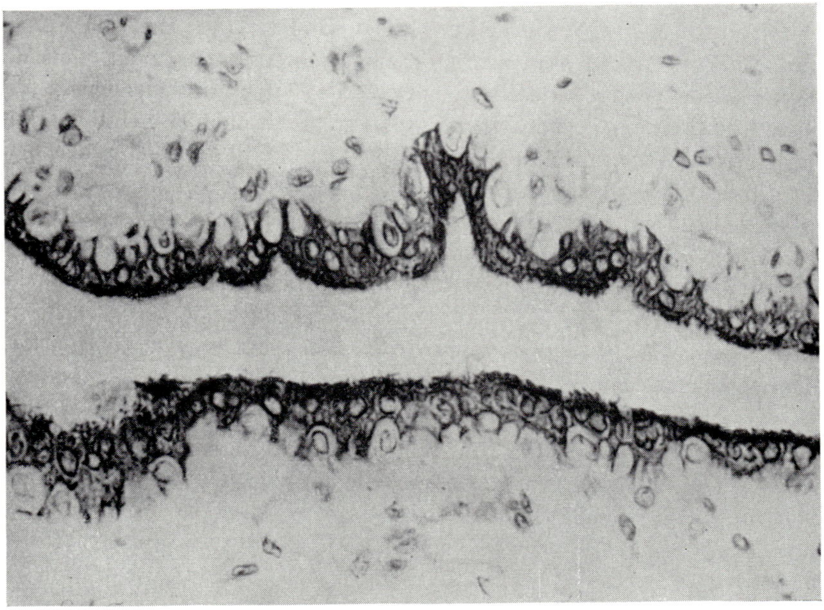

FIG. 3.24. Placenta from the 17th week of pregnancy. A demonstration of alkaline phosphatase. The reaction is negative in the Langhans cells and positive in the syncytium. (Enlarged 260 times.) Thomsen (1955a).

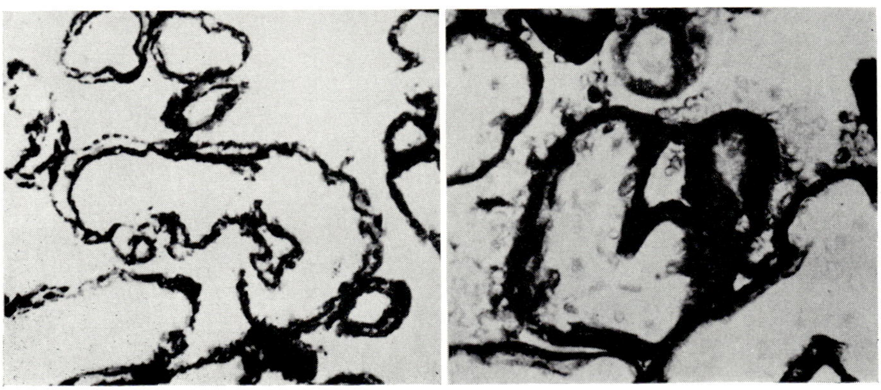

(a) (b)

FIG. 3.25. Demonstration of alkaline phosphatase by the Gomori reaction. (a) After embedding in paraffin wax. (b) Without embedding. After Strauss & Hiersche (1962).

faces of the nuclei but these themselves are free of DPN- and TPN-diaphorase. Sometimes an enzyme-free basic substance separates granula arranged like strings of beads in the syncytium from those in the endothelia of the foetal vessels (Fig. 3.27).

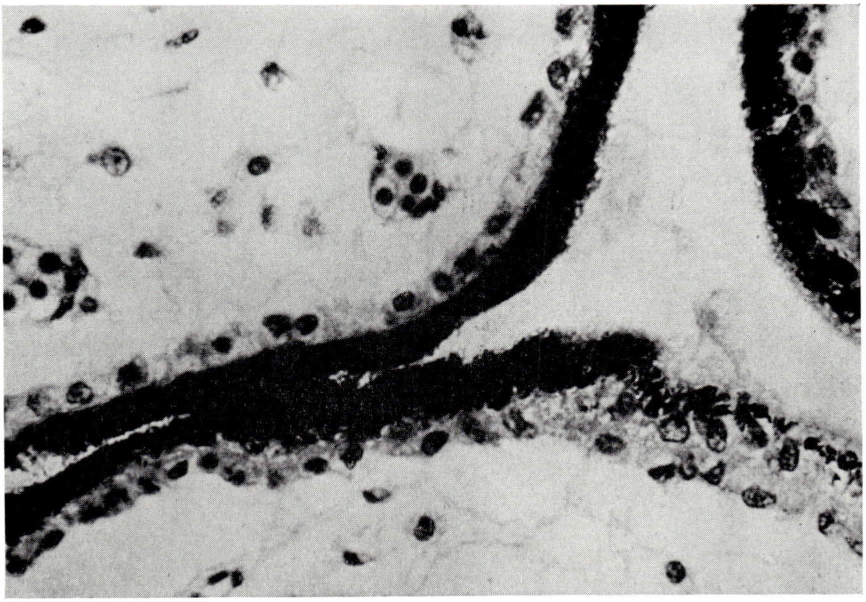

FIG. 3.26. Placenta from the 10th week of pregnancy. A demonstration of acid phosphatase. Counterstained with haematoxylin and eosin. The syncytium is strongly positive, the Langhans layer weakly positive, and the mesenchyme and villous vessels are negative. There are nucleated red cells in the villous vessels. (Enlarged 360 times.) After Thomsen (1955b).

Succinodehydrogenase also occurs in the placenta (Table 3.1). This enzyme is directly connected with the respiratory chain in that it transmits the hydrogen to the cytochrome b.

Langhans cell layer

Cellular Villous Trophoblast

The Langhans cells are cubic with an oval or round nucleus and a strongly eosinophilic cytoplasm. On the average they measure 3 μ and even under the ordinary microscope clearly show cell limits. Electron microscopic observations show that the nuclei are almost free of indentation. The clearly developed nucleoli are a striking feature. The doubly contoured nuclear membrane shows delicate pores like an open diaphragm. This finding indicates the morphological mechanism for the facilitation of transport between the karyoplasm and cytoplasm. Unlike the syncytium, the Langhans cell proves poor in structures under the electron microscope (Fig. 3.28). The more conspicuous, therefore, are

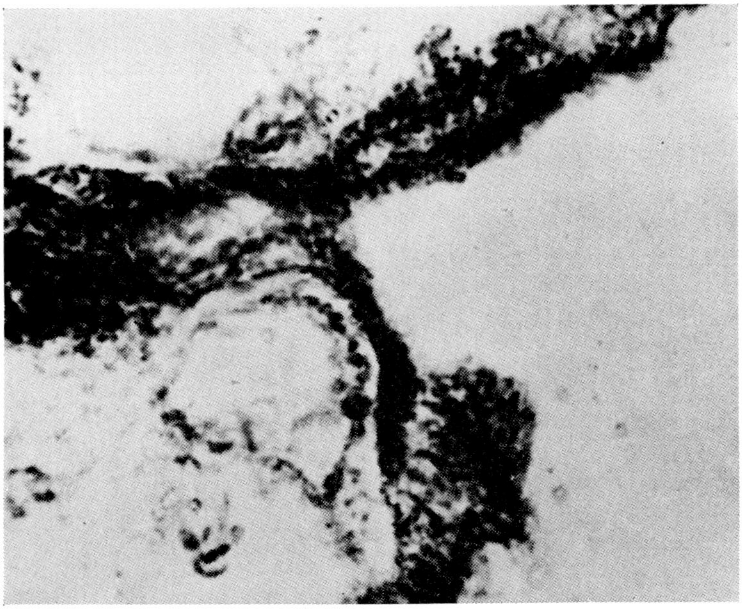

FIG. 3.27. A demonstration of DPN in the syncytio-vascular metabolic membrane. There is a negatively reacting zone between the positive zones of the capillary endothelium and the syncytium. The same applies also to TPN preparations. Strauss & Hiersche (1962).

the irregularly formed mitochondria distributed over the cytoplasm. The lamellar structures have transverse diameters of 250 mμ and longitudinal diameters of 500 mμ (Bargmann & Knoop 1959). Because of the lack of structures in the Langhans cells, it is easy to see the membrane of the Golgi apparatus (Fig. 3.28). The ergastoplasm is composed of granulated membranes and canaliculi. In spaces enclosed by ergastoplasm one finds many cloudy inclusions of low optical density. Palades granules occur not only in the membranes but also in groups in the cytoplasm (Bargmann & Knoop 1959). This finding is connected with the wealth of ribonucleoproteins in the cytoplasm, established by Dempsey &

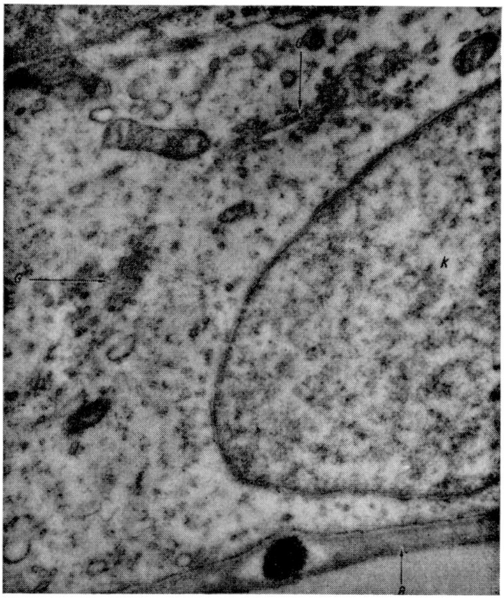

FIG. 3.28. Electron photomicrograph of a Langhans cell. B: Basal membrane with an inclusion. G: Golgi apparatus. K: Nucleus. (Enlarged 3,800 times.) After Bargmann & Knoop (1959).

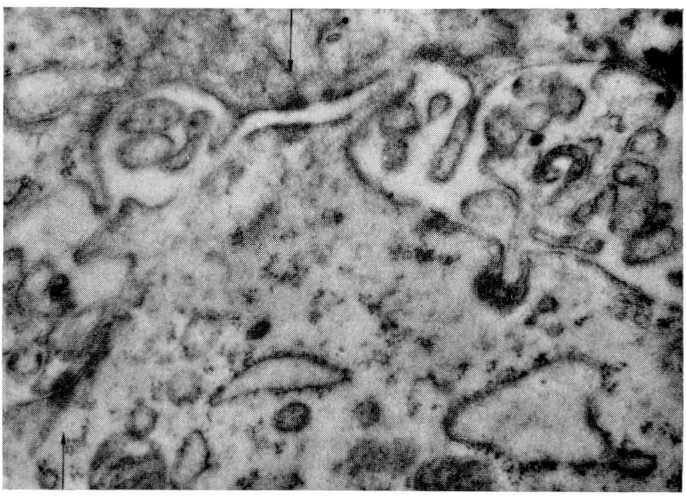

FIG. 3.29. Interdigitations between Langhans cells by means of cytoplasmatic projections. The upper arrow shows an adhesive plate. (Enlarged 56,000 times.) After Bargmann & Knoop (1959).

Wislocki (1945) and Dempsey (1948). Whether this finding has any bearing on the production of HCG is under discussion.

In the areas where two neighbouring Langhans cells are in contact, there are found protuberances which resemble microvilli, which enhance the contact between two cells by interdigitation and anchoring (Fig. 3.29). Similar protuberances project into the intercellular space which divides the cytotrophoblast from the syncytiotrophoblast. The adhesive plates

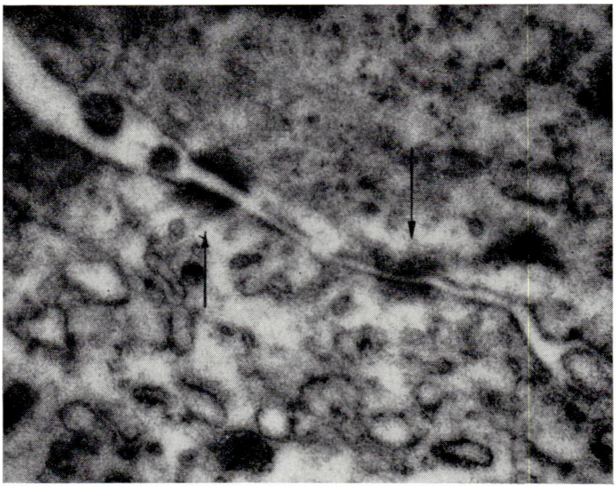

FIG. 3.30. Connections between the syncytiotrophoblast (above right) and the cytotrophoblast (below left) by means of an adhesive plate. (Enlarged 38,000 times.) After Bargmann & Knoop (1959).

constitute a further contact between two Langhans cells and also between the cytotrophoblast and syncytiotrophoblast. Here we are concerned with thickenings of the cell borders about 800 to 2,000 Å in length. True contact does not, however, take place. Two areas of thickening are separated from each other by an intercellular space of 300 Å (Fig. 3.30). They are sometimes hemispherical, present a strongly osmiophilic zone directly beneath the cell borders and project 200–300 Å into the cytoplasm. At the base of some areas of syncytium, there can also be found small, irregularly shaped protuberances which project into indentations in the top layer of the Langhans cells.

The cytotrophoblast is poor in structures and biochemical activity in comparison with the syncytium which is so rich in these. It is, however, striking to find a lot of glycogen and RNA in the cytotrophoblast of the immature villus. More recent observations show that as the villus develops, the glycogen in the Langhans layer disappears. The ribonucleic acid was supposed to produce basophilia (Bargmann 1957) and metachromasia although acid mucopolysaccharides could not be shown to occur in Langhans cells. Ortmann (1959) found no basophilia in the Langhans cells.

The reactions for glycoproteins and sudanophilic substances prove to be negative. On the other hand, the Langhans cell is rich in iron and in this resembles the foetal cells and cell columns, the shell of the trophoblast and the maternal islands and septae. The placenta as a whole has a high iron content (Göltner & Stark 1957).

The so-called functional iron is found mainly in the vicinity of the nuclear membranes. It is very likely that in this perinuclear iron we are concerned with the iron of the cytochromoxydase system. When the placental tissue is fractionated, ferritin (depot-iron) is found only in the cytoplasmic fraction and not in the nucleus. The cytoplasm contains 64 per cent of the ferritin and the microsomes have the remaining 36 per cent. The cell nucleus and mitochondria are free of ferritin (Göltner & Stark 1957 and 1960). The Langhans cells have no phosphatases, nucleotidases DPN-diaphorases and TPN-diaphorases (see Table 3.1).

Basal membrane

The trophoblast of the villus has a basal membrane about 150 mμ wide. Electron microscopy shows a space of about 250 Å between this membrane and the adjoining Langhans cells. This space is filled with an amorphous mass of low optical density. This membrane is composed of two relatively optically dense layers with a third less dense layer in between. Here especially osmiophilic spherical inclusion bodies can be seen (Bargmann & Knoop 1959, Bourne 1962).

Connective tissue

The matrix of the mature villus consists of a conglomeration of mesenchymal cells which under the microscope have a reticulated appearance together with open capillary vessels. Between them one can see delicate, often matted, fibres, some lying in no particular order and some making a lattice work. The stromal oedema extends into this. The mesenchymal cells are single cells with marked branching. The electron microscope shows that there are connections between the individual cells provided by end to end and side to side attachments of the delicate offshoots of the cells and by interdigitation of the cell extensions (see Figs. 3.2 and 3.3). A true syncytical union of cells does not exist. The nuclei of the connective tissue are oval or polymorphous. Definite, thick, large mitochondria are found in the cytoplasm. The ergastoplasm is sack-shaped (diameter: 300–400 mμ). Defined accumulations of osmiophilic granules can also be found in the cytoplasm. They most often lie in the peri-karyotic area. In size, shape and optical density these granules correspond to the palisade granules on the membrane of the ergastoplasm. In the area of the cytoplasm, one also finds vesicles with a diameter of from 40 to 120 Å. Their significance has not yet been elucidated but there are strong indications, (apart from their concentration near the cell borders), that we are here concerned with a metabolic function, (pinocytosis).

These results of electron microscopic observations may be of a great importance for the understanding of metabolism of transport of material in the villus. Contrary to the earlier concept, that support and maintenance were the only functions of the stroma, we must now regard it as a metabolically active tissue. The positive 5′nucleotidase reactions in the stroma of the villus must be seen in the same light (see Fig. 3.23). Although the metabolic activity of the connective tissue has been demonstrated, we find it relatively poor in histochemical reactions. Alkaline and acid phosphatase are lacking (Thomsen 1955a, 1955b, Strauss & Hiersche 1962). Lipids, on the other hand, are present (Thomsen & Lorenzen 1956). More especially in the larger villi, the single globules are arranged like strings of beads and more or less follow the grain of the connective tissue. They are probably components of the cell membrane or else lie very close to it. It is rare to find Sudan Black positive globules in the area of the stromal nuclei. It is striking that sudanophil substances are plentiful in the syncytiotrophoblast, not in the cellular trophoblast of the villus. It has been suggested that the fat taken up from the maternal blood can pass directly into the stroma of the villus via the syncytial cell extensions which are found between the individual Langhans cells (see Figs. 3.15 and 3.24). It is not possible to relate different diseases to particular patterns of fat distribution (Thomsen & Lorenzen 1956).

Vessels of the villus

A cross section of a mature resorption villus is almost entirely occupied by a large capillary system. It should be noted that, as the placenta matures, the capillaries of the villus are oriented to its periphery, until the syncytio-capillary membranes develop after the loss of a continuous layer of Langhans cells.

During the developmental period, the capillary network increases greatly. The stroma of the villus is supplanted and ends up as no more than a thin layer of connective tissue in the form of a narrow syncytial

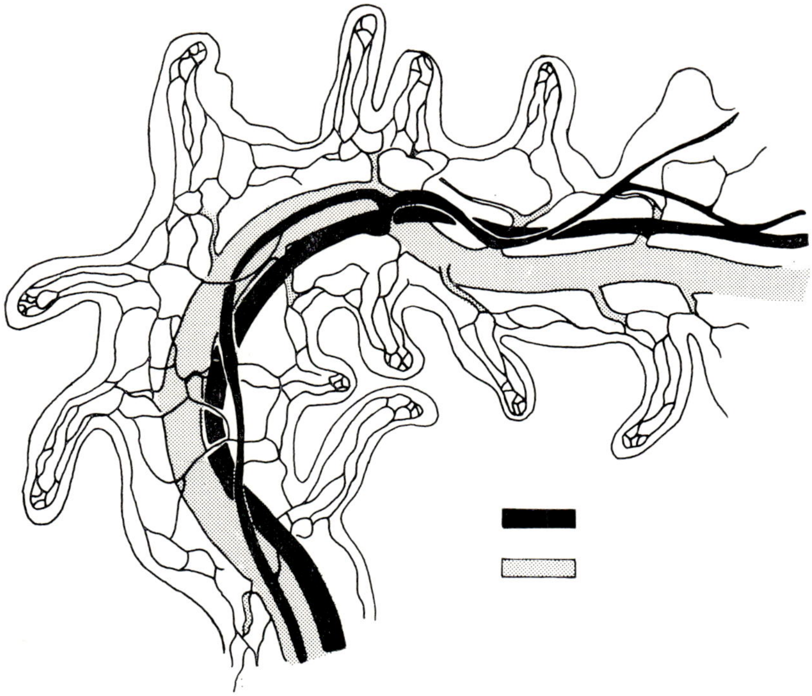

FIG. 3.31. Perivascular capillary network. According to Bøe (1954).

strip. The supplanting of the stroma by the vessels and its peripheral orientation are significant signs of maturity for the placenta. In the region of the syncytio-capillary metabolic membrane, the narrowed syncytium (in this area free of nuclei) merges with the endothelium of the capillaries. This layer is often by now only 2 μ thick and provides an optimal exchange of material between maternal and foetal blood (Figs. 3.16 and 3.17).

The capillaries of the villus consist of two separate systems (Bøe 1954): (1) the sinusoids of the villus, (2) the perivascular capillaries (Fig. 3.31). The latter are capillaries that branch out of both larger and smaller arteries; they extend in the neighbourhood of the larger vessels and then combine into venous vessels to run into a larger trunk vein. There has recently been much discussion as to whether the perivascular capillaries have any circulatory physiological significance–possibly in the sense of a pressure equalization system–or whether nutritive functions can be attributed to these capillaries proceeding relatively directly compared with the sinusoids of the villus. It is possible that in particular developmental phases, the capillaries of the villus are actively involved in albumin metabolism, since a marked positive 5′nucleotidase reaction can be found between the 15th and 20th week of pregnancy (see Fig. 3.23). The electron microscope reveals intercellular lacuni (Panigel *et al.* 1964) and it is therefore to be supposed that the pore free endothelial walls of the vessels play a part in transport performances. There has been lively discussion of sphincter-like venous pads which were supposed to serve to facilitate resorption. Recent researches were unable to find them (Ortmann 1959). The total length of the foetal vascular system is about 50 kilometres (Strauss 1964 and 1967). We owe to Ramsay (1955, 1959a, 1959b, 1960 and 1962) decisive advances in the elucidation of the arrangement of the foetal vessels in the placenta. Under electron microscopy, the capillaries of the villus show the special characteristics of a wealth of mitochondria and ergastoplasm in the cytoplasm of the endothelial cells (Arnold, Geller & Sasse 1961). These authors also describe special projections of cytoplasm into the lumen, the so-called cushions of cytoplasm. It is not known if these are of any significance in the regulation of the circulation. Neither is it known whether the vessels of the villus have vasomotor constrictory properties. Fischer & Müller (1967) were able to demonstrate a multi-capillary system of circulatory pathways in the placenta of the guinea pig, by bilateral perfusion of the live animals. A theoretical analysis on the basis of measured values of respiratory gas pressure in the foetal arterial and venous blood and the maternal arterial blood shows that the counter current principle cannot exist in the human placenta and that a multi-capillary system must be present.

Hofbauer-Chaletzky-Neumann cells

The Hofbauer cells arise from the chorionic mesenchyme and correspond to the histiocytes in form and function. From the fourth week onward the Hofbauer cells appear in the stroma of the villus as round cells 15 to 30 μ in size which show a larger eccentrically placed nucleus. Hofbauer (1903), and more recently Hörmann (1947), Thomsen & Netz (1955), Bautzmann & Schroder (1955a and b, 1956), Bourne (1962), Bleyl (1962) and others have described the picture presented by these cells under the light microscope. Amitotic increase of the cells is predominant but the mitotic form is also present (Hörmann 1947). The relatively high number of multi-nucleated cells confirms this finding.

Contrary to what was held earlier, Hofbauer cells can be found, not only in the first half of pregnancy, but in the placenta delivered at term. In order to identify them, however, it is necessary to use electron microscopy (Bargmann & Knoop 1959, Lister 1964), histochemical techniques (Thomsen & Netz 1955) or an artificial oedema of the villus (Bleyl 1962). In the ripe placenta there are no Hofbauer cells in the primary villi and those of a higher order. They are found especially in the substitute villi developed later.

There are two forms of Hofbauer cells, static and mobile. The first is round with an eccentric nucleus and has a spongy cytoplasm and vaccuoles containing granules. The second shows pseudopodia and cell extensions, has a spongy cytoplasm and is almost free of vacuoles and granules. There are forms intermediate between these two. The static form, predominates in the placenta.

Beside Hofbauer cells with round nuclei others are also known with lobular, irregular or creased nuclei. Complete segmentation is rare and seems to foreshadow the occurrence of a few Hofbauer cells with several nuclei.

The cytoplasm exhibits a considerable variety of forms. The mitochondria are of lamellar formation, *c.* 200 mμ wide and 1,800 mμ long (Bourne 1962). The ergastoplasm is composed of highly granular canaliculi with varying diameters and besides these, free RNA-granules. The large cells, in particular, clearly show cavities in the cytoplasm. They represent the so-called 'foam' cells and by specific stains can be shown to contain lipid material.

Among the vacuoles surrounded by a true membrane, some show optically empty cavities and others cloudy masses. However, small optically dense areas can also be seen in the vacuoles, obviously phagocytized material. Bourne (1962) described granules, not very dense, *c.* 30 to 80 mμ in size, and notable for their central transparency. It is not known if there is any functional connection between them and the small globules. As a reflection of their character as macrophages, the Hofbauer cells have the capacity to phagocytize substances such as meconium or haemosiderin, which may, of course, give rise to necrobiosis. This gave rise to the mistaken concept that the Hofbauer cells were degenerated.

The relatively high number of electron transferring enzymes (Strauss

& Hiersche 1962) suggests an active internal metabolism. However, Hofbauer cells, even those in the resorption villi of the mature placenta, always show positive evidence of acid phosphatase (Thomsen & Netz 1955, Bleyl 1962, Strauss & Hiersche 1962). On the other hand, no alkaline phosphatase could be found in fresh preparations of the Hofbauer cells. Non specific esterases are found (McKay *et al.* 1958). Moreover, the Hofbauer cell is rich in fat and diastase-resistant PAS-positive substances which are indicative of highly polymerized carbohydrates.

To the typical static and mobile forms must be added yet another with marked metachromasia (Pescetto 1952, Latta & Beber 1953). These are said to be caused by a substance similar to heparin.

The nuclear sex of the Hofbauer cells corresponds to that of the embryo so that no doubts remain as to the foetal origin of these cells.

THE CHORIONIC PLATE

The human placenta is classed with the so-called villus or 'pot' placentae. Figure 3.13 gives an outline of the architecture which gave rise to this description of the human placenta. The basal plate represents the base of the vessel and the chorionic plate the lid.

The chorionic plate is predominantly composed of connective tissue in which run the sub-divided major vessels of the umbilical cord (outlined in Fig. 3.31). Unlike Wharton's jelly, the connective tissue here is considerably more dense, has more cells and fibres and markedly little intercellular substance. After fixation, the intercellular substance is composed of granular basophil masses; histochemically they are acid mucopolysaccharides which are made up mainly of hyaluronic acid. However, chondroitin sulphate can also be found, especially at the end of intrauterine life. Scheuner (1964) differentiates between orderly and chaotic structures especially in the areas free of vessels in connection with which ordered connective tissue can be seen as a thin layer immediately below the amnion epithelium. A wider band of connective tissue is found lying above the fibrin boundary, (the 'fibrinoid' of Langhans) of the intervillous space. These bundles of fibres always lie parallel to the covering plate and also surround the vessels. Cross sections of vessels are thus surrounded by a sheath of connective tissue arranged in circles and composed of cells and fibres. It is often possible to identify several bundles of fibres running towards each other at acute angles so that the vessels lie in a system of fibres crossing over each other and shaped like a longitudinal spiral.

The disordered connective tissue lies between these ordered fibres. This tissue is composed of adhesive collagenous fibres, is very loose, large meshed and has few cells.

The vessels of the umbilical cord branch in the area of the chorion plate just before they subdivide into the vessels of the villus. The vessels are anchored to the chorionic plate by fibres of connective tissue that radiate into the muscular fibres and on the other hand are connected to the layer of ordered fibres in the chorionic connective tissue.

On the foetal side, the matrix of the connective tissue of the chorionic plate is covered by a single layer of cylindrical, (in places a tall cylindrical), amnion epithelium of about 20 μ in thickness. Between the connective tissue of the chorion and the amnion, there lies a zone well supplied with lymph which has relatively few cells or fibres. Near the intervillous space, the chorionic plate of the mature placenta is covered by a fibrin layer of varying thickness. However, at some points even in the mature placenta, a syncytial limitation layer can be recognized and seen to communicate with the covering of the villus. Here, moreover, are to be found areas of cellular trophoblast with typical dense granular basophil cytoplasm and with nucleoli 1 to 2 μ in size characterized by a high level of RNA.

BASAL PLATE, ISLANDS, SEPTAE AND COLUMNS

Whilst the chorionic plate is composed mainly of connective tissue, the basal plate on the other hand, consists almost entirely of cellular elements. It is further differentiated from the chorionic plate by the variegated picture of its architecture and the different origins of various elements.

The basal plate is composed on the one hand of a narrow strip of decidua which is also expelled at the time of delivery. Above this lies the actual zone of penetration with its Nitabuch's fibrin strips. This area is appropriately named since, during placentation many adhesive villi penetrate the decidua and anchor here (area of anchoring). The fibrin strip represents the barrier between infiltrating foetal tissue and infiltrated maternal tissue. On the side near the intervillous space, the basal plate is delimited by a more or less thick layer of trophoblast cells with many strata.

In the mature placenta, there can be found single nucleated cells, sometimes basophil, sometimes optically clear, sometimes with several nucleoli. Some multi-nucleated giant cells are also present. Those in the first group are derived from the foetal cell columns, those in the latter from the remainder of the syncytium.

The large basophil trophoblast cells are the main components of the trophoblastic shell (i.e. basal plate) and merit closer examination. They are large, round cells which become more fusiform on penetrating the decidua and can also develop long extensions. They can be distinguished from the cells of the decidua by their histochemical behaviour (see Table 3.1) and by the absence of the three dimensional argyrophil network which can always be found in the decidual cells.

The large trophoblastic cells of the mature placenta have a large easily stained nucleus with one or more basophil nucleoli. The membrane of the nucleus is very wavy. During the maturation of the placenta, the originally clearly defined chromatin structure of the nucleus decreases through loss of nucleotide. Later there is a decrease in nucleoli with a high RNA-content. During the development of the placenta, the cytoplasm of the trophoblast cells often shows small vesicles which merge into large vacuoles under pressure from the protoplasm. The formation of vacuoles can go so far that the nucleus becomes flattened.

The basophilia of the cells of the trophoblast is determined by their high content of ribonucleic acids which can be observed near the cellular and nuclear membranes of the cytoplasm, sometimes in a delicately granulated form, sometimes coarse and lumpy. These cells have a high content of substances of the carbohydrate and albumin series and less of the fat series, also many enzymes (see Table 3.1). The high metabolic activity of the trophoblast cells can be deduced from the fact that they have a high ribonucleic acid content. They have large nuclei containing RNA and nuclei with little chromatin. Intensive albumin metabolism is also indicated by the nuclear secretion in which acidophil globules are produced. It seems likely that the substance secreted is composed of the basic albumin bodies of the nucleolus of the histone-type which are carried over into the cytoplasm after being freed of their ribonucleic acids (Ortmann 1949). The high content of sulphydryl groups (Latta & Beber 1957) and the occurrence of nucleotidase and esterase also suggest participation in the metabolism of albumin.

More recently, Dallenbach-Hellweg & Nette (1963, 1964) established that intact basophil trophoblast cells of the mature human placenta contain protein inclusions which may be as large as the nucleus. Some of these lie in vacuoles and they range from 1 to 20 per cell. It is interesting that the protein inclusions can only really be observed in placentae delivered by Caesarean section before labour. Placentae delivered spontaneously have few or none of such cytoplasmatic inclusions. Histochemical and immunohistochemical reactions (Dallenbach & Dallenbach-Hellweg 1964) give rise to the supposition that we are here concerned with relaxin or its carrier substance which is used up in the process of delivery. The cytoplasm contains glycoprotein inclusions composed of a mucopolysaccharide and a basophil protein. They often lie in vacuoles, sometimes actually in the nucleus itself. Their occurrence is independent of labour (Dallenbach-Hellweg & Nette 1964). Thomsen & Williamsen (1959) detected these inclusions by the PAS reaction. Their localization and type of immunohistological reaction correspond to gonadotrophin. Whether this is the hormone at the production site or at the storage site has not been elucidated.

The so-called 'clear cells' are another structural element of the basal plate in addition to the giant cells. These are situated between the major masses of the basophil trophoblast cells arranged in groups.

As can be seen from Table 3.1 the cells of the trophoblast shell behave histochemically in the same way as those of the septae and islands. However, the cells of the islands and septae are not developmentally derived from the trophoblast but from the decidua (Klinger & Ludwig 1957, Sohval, Gaines & Strauss 1959, Austin 1962). The maternal origin of this tissue can be demonstrated by determining the sex chromatin of male foetuses. It is all the more remarkable that these maternal cells correspond morphologically to the foetal trophoblast cells and also functionally in so far as can be judged by histochemical reactions. Thus the present state of research suggests that there are three forms of trophoblast: (1) the Langhans layer of the villi, (2) the trophoblast of the cell columns and (3) the trophoblast of the basal ectoderm (trophoblast shell).

Although all three types of cell derive from the trophoblast they show some definite differences in topography and behaviour. The Langhans cells show the least metabolic activity and clearly represent either multipotent ancestral forms, or possibly substitute cells of the syncytiotrophoblast.

The cell column trophoblast and trophoblast shell have become functionally adapted and specialized (Ortmann 1955). The origin of the septae has not yet been fully elucidated. There is no evidence that they contain an active growth area. They can only be found from the 4th month on. They remain thin, delicate formations owing to the constant pressure of neighbouring circulatory units (Fig. 3.12). Even the septae of young placentae show fibrin deposits, (Rohr's 'fibrinoid'), which extend on to the cells of the trophoblast shell. Fibrin can, however, also be identified in the centre of the septae. In the centres of many it is also possible to discern cavities and groups of loosened cells, intraseptal cysts (Thomsen 1955a).

These islands might represent the structural basis of the septae. Their name is not exact as it is possible that besides cellular debris they may contain cavities filled with liquid. Unlike the septae, which are always in the basal area, 300–1,000 μ large islands can be traced throughout the placenta. They usually grow by fibrin deposits, but it is possible for several small islands to combine into a larger one.

FOETAL MEMBRANES

The membranes are composed of the amnion, the chorion, and the spongy layer. According to Hertig (1945) and Hertig, Rock & Adams (1956) it can be accepted that trophoblast cells differentiate into amniogenic cells 7 to 8 days after fertilization. The development of the amnion is dependent upon a vital embryonic streak but the further maturation of the foetus is not so dependent. We have already discussed the development of the chorion. Between these two layers there lies the spongy layer developed from the extra-embryonic coelom. The three layers are morphologically and functionally different from each other.

Owing to the greater speed of growth of the amniotic sac, about the end of the 2nd month the amnion becomes adherent to the spongy layer or directly to the chorion. There are, however, cases in which such an amalgamation is lacking.

The foetal membrane is not only the outer layer of the amnion cavity inside which the foetus can develop. Histochemistry and electron microscopy have confirmed the earlier conjecture that this membrane participates actively in the exchange of material between foetus and mother.

THE AMNION

As the inner lining of the three layered foetal membrane, the amnion is in constant contact with the amniotic fluid. Two sections are distinguished because of their localization: (1) the pars placentaris which rests on the top layer of the placenta and (2) the pars reflexa which, together with the spongy layer and the chorion, composes the actual wall of the amniotic sac. There is no fundamental histological difference between the placentary amnion and the pars reflexa. The pars placentaris rests on the vessel-bearing chorion plate. There is as yet no proof of the suggestion made by some authors that this position makes it possible for the pars placentaris to play a greater metabolic role than the pars reflexa.

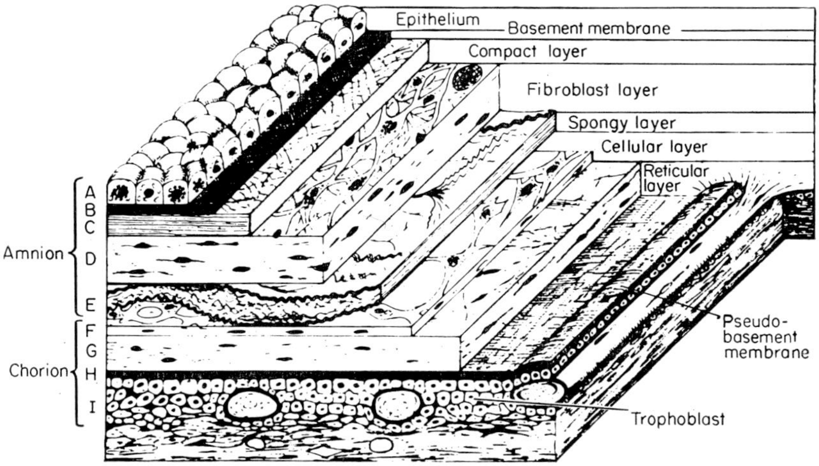

FIG. 3.32. Schematic representation of a section through the amnion and chorion. After Bourne (1962).

Contrary to the earlier findings of Keiffer (1926) and Domskikh (1957), Bourne (1962) was unable to trace blood vessels in any stage of development of the amnion. The same applies to true lymphatic pathways and clefts. The human amnion is also free of nerve and muscle fibres.

The amnion is composed of four layers (Fig. 3.32):

1 *The epithelial layer*
2 *The basal membrane*
3 *The fibrous layer*
4 *The layer of fibrocytes.*

The epithelial layer is the most important of these because of its high metabolic activity. Both the placentary and reflexa parts are composed of a single layer of cells. In the reflexa, flat epithelial forms predominate. In the pars placentaris cylindrical cells do so. The average height of the cells ranges from 1 to 25 μ. According to Bourne (1962) neither the flat cells nor the cylindrical variety are specific to a location. The cells of the epithelial layer are anchored to each other by terminal bars and intercellular bridges. Examination by light microscopy shows a brush border on the top layer which is bathed by the amniotic fluid. The electron microscope shows it to be a loose patch of microvilli (Fig. 3.33). These projections of protoplasm are club-shaped or sometimes pointed. They contained a double membrane 30 Å thick. Within the microvilli, one finds structures like canals which can be followed up to 0·5 μ into the cytoplasm so that it appears more dense at this point. The cell membranes

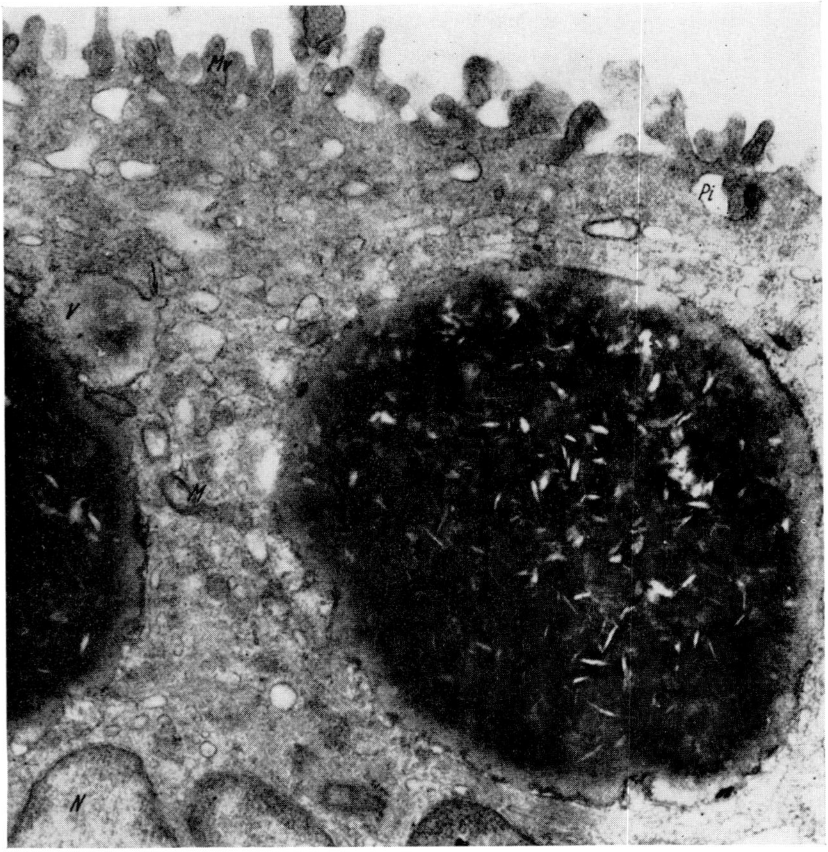

FIG. 3.33. The upper surface of a cell from the human amnion. MV: Microvilli. N: Nucleus. Pi: Pinocytic crypt. Two lipoid droplets contain crystalline inclusions. There is a vacuole (V) which has a vesicle in its upper edge (indicated by an arrow), and which comes into close contact with the membranous surround of the lipid droplet. (Enlarged 9,000 times.) After Schmidt (1963).

facing the basal membrane are not even but rather cone-shaped (Fig. 3.34). Here one can see the extensions of varying size and irregular limits anchored to the basal membrane. Apart from performing this holding function, the extensions of the cell base might make a better exchange of material possible. A system of vacuoles spreads in between the basal extensions of the epithelial layers.

In the past, research workers had described 1 to 50 vacuoles of varying sizes which in part pressed their nuclei to the cell membrane and so created the appearance of a secretory cell. Electron microscopic investigations (Bourne 1962) have shown, however, that these vacuoles are almost exclusively limited by the cell membranes of neighbouring cells. Thus we almost always have here intercellular vacuoles which make up a real intercellular lateral canal system (Fig. 3.35). These vacuoles often contain microvilli some of which are markedly branched (Fig. 3.36). Wide fusions of pairs of these vacuoles can be found and also delicate little 100 to 200 Å channels which either connect the neighbouring vesicles, or on the other hand, open into the free amnion cavity (Bourne 1962, Schmidt 1963) (Fig. 3.37).

The fact that the lateral system of vacuoles is in communication with the basal system provides the morphological conditions for the cell to be laterally and basally exposed to a flow of liquid connected with the amniotic fluid. Recent research has confirmed the importance of the exchange of material between mother and foetus taking place through the amniotic fluid. The system of canals described provides the morphological explanation for the passage of even larger particles.

The cytoplasm of the amnion epithelial cell is very granulated. The mitochondria are mostly bow-shaped. The Golgi apparatus can be clearly traced everywhere. At the maximum enlargement, small vesicles can be distinguished inside the cell as well as the lateral system of vacuoles. These are significantly smaller than those of the intercellular system. They are often so numerous that the cell takes on the appearance of a honeycomb (see Fig. 3.33). On the other hand, signs of degeneration cannot be found in the cells containing vacuoles. It is natural to infer that we have here the morphological basis for pinocytosis. The 100 Å wide small intracellular canals must also be mentioned as structures that indicate a vigorous exchange of material in the amnion epithelium. They may be connected with the small intercellular canaliculi.

Most of the polygonal amnion epithelium cells contain a single nucleus. Cells with double nuclei are not unknown, especially in the pars reflexa (Glowinski & Konecki 1962). The double nuclei are, however, sometimes simulated by the poor staining of the cell membranes. Under the light microscope, the nucleus usually appears to lie somewhat eccen-

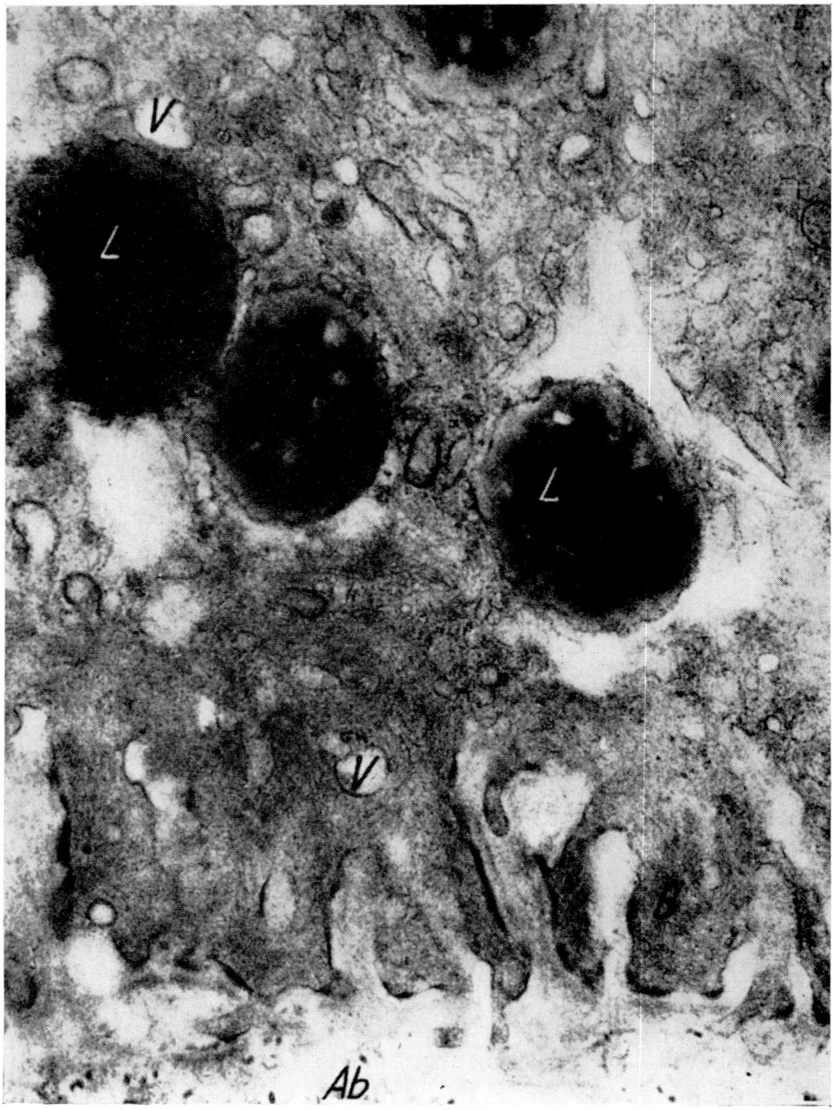

FIG. 3.34. The base of a human amnion cell with pedestals (B) lipoid droplets (L), Amniotic connective tissue (Ab) and vacuoles (V). (Enlarged 9,000 times.) After Schmidt (1963).

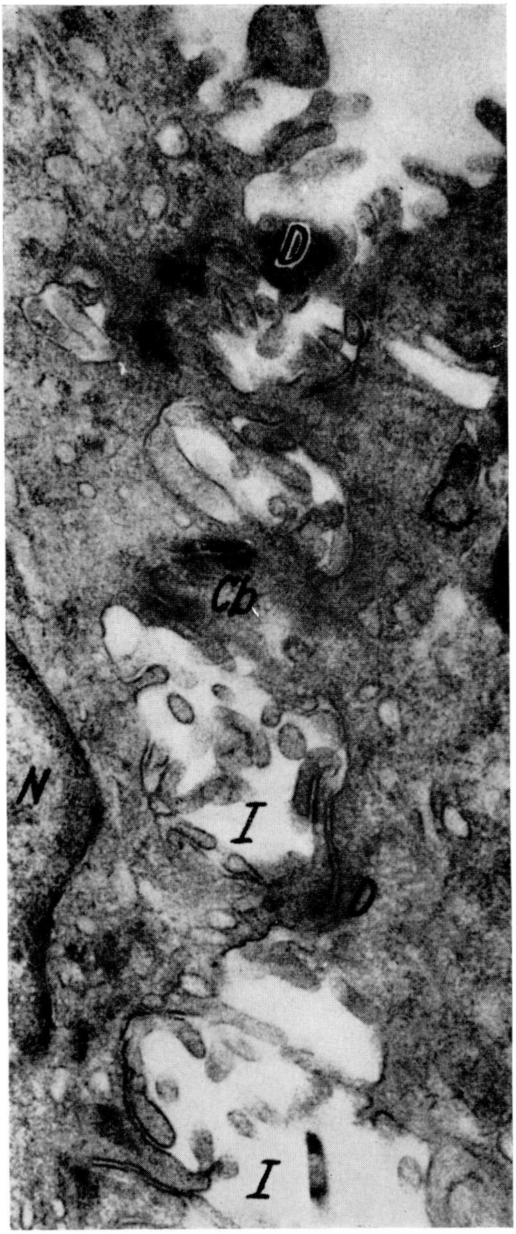

FIG. 3.35. Interdigitations and a system of lateral vacuoles between two adjacent human amnion epithelial cells. Cb: Cell bridges. D: Desmosomes. I: Intercellular space. N: Nucleus. (Enlarged 8,000 times.) After Schmidt (1963).

trically, is ball-shaped with a flat top layer and contains vacuoles. Further magnification, however, shows that the nucleus may have deep grooves and folds. It is often actually fenestrated. The nucleus is surrounded by a porous double membrane, which facilitates contact between the karyoplasm and cytoplasm. For an outline of electron microscopic findings on the human amnion cell, see Fig. 3.38.

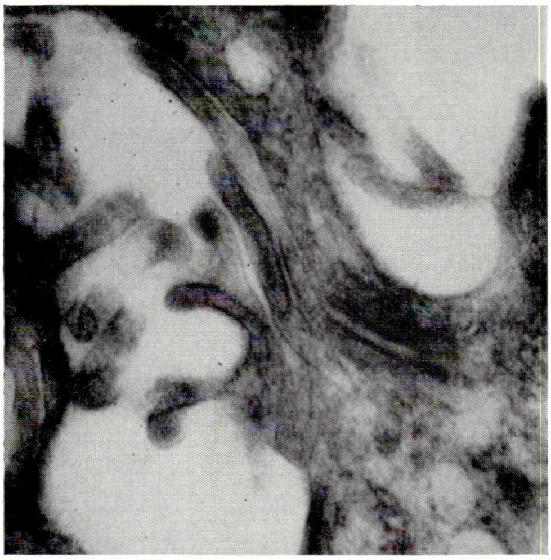

FIG. 3.36. Greatly magnified view of the amnion at the end of pregnancy. Numerous microvilli are prominent. The extensions are connected to each other by minute canals. (Enlarged 75,000 times.) After Bourne (1962).

The electron microscopic investigations of Thomas (1962) on 16 amnii from spontaneous deliveries and 16 from Caesarean sections lead him to conclude that there are two types of amnion epithelial cells differentiated by their density (Fig. 3.39). All amnii are supposed to contain both kinds of cell in differing proportions. No association was found, either with the course of the pregnancy, or with that of labour. The 'Golgi type' and the denser 'fibrillar' type are differentiated.

The fibrillar type is characterized by a fibrillar cytoplasm, the absence or infrequency of systems of endoplasmatic reticulum and a small Golgi apparatus (Fig. 3.40). This morphology and the presence of microvilli on the free surface are related to an absorptive function.

The 'Golgi type' cell contains many vacuoles, a highly developed Golgi apparatus and a very pronounced endoplasmic reticulum (Fig. 3.41). Attention should be paid to the close topographical relationship

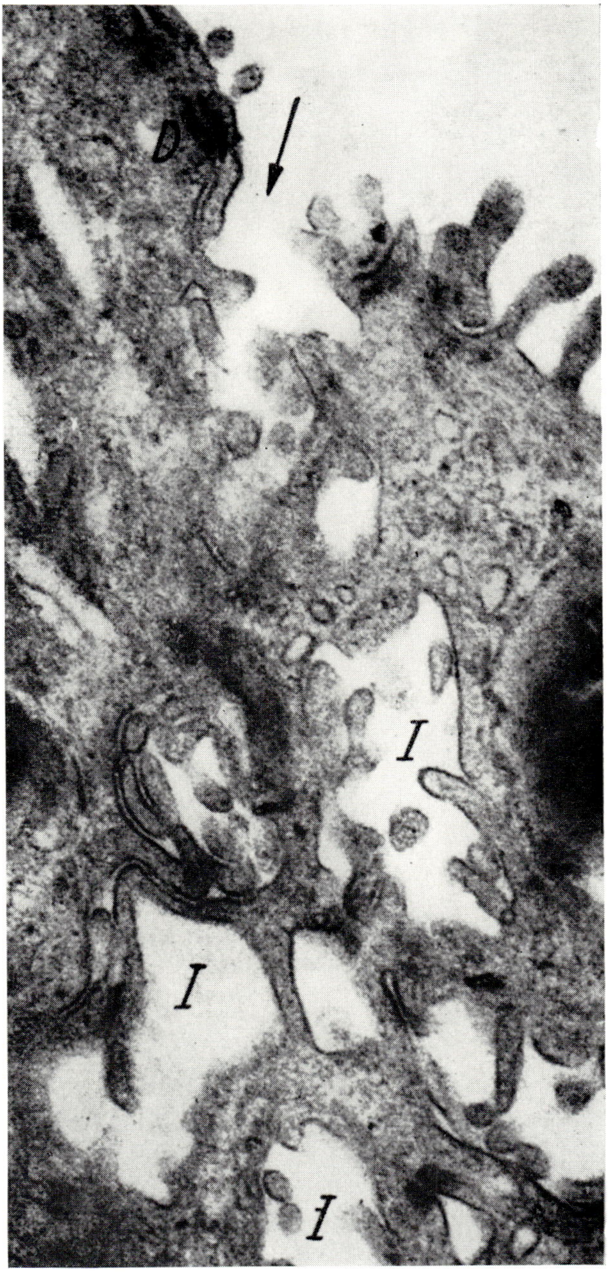

FIG. 3.37. The intercellular canal system opening into the amniotic cavity, (shown by an arrow). D: Desmosomes. I: Intercellular space. (Enlarged 12,000 times.) After Schmidt (1963).

of the vacuoles and Golgi complex to the intracellular canal system (Fig. 3.42). It is supposed that this type of cell must have an active secretory function, the secretion being discharged into the amniotic fluid through the intercellular canals (Thomas 1965).

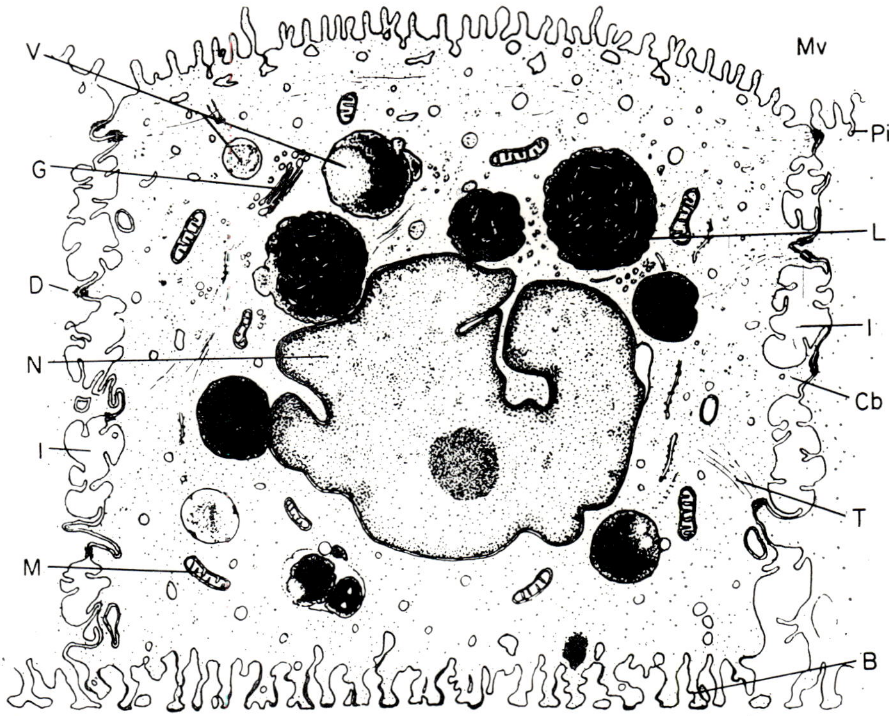

FIG. 3.38. Schematic representation of the findings by electron microscopy of the cells in the amnion of the newborn. P: Pedestals. Cb: Cytoplasmic bridges. D: Desmosomes. G: Golgi Apparatus. I: Intercellular space. N: Nucleus. Pi: Pinocytic vesicles. T: Tonofibrils. V: Vacuoles. After Schmidt (1963).

Research comparing the amnion cell of man and fowl using both light and electron microscopy (Schmidt 1963) showed that the large vacuoles which can be seen under the light microscope certainly have a share in the elaboration of the amniotic fluid and that the term amniotic fluid vacuoles is justified. These vacuoles are formed by distension of the nuclear plasma cleft and pass to the free border of the cell; there to empty their contents into the amniotic cavity. Amniotic fluid vacuoles are numerous in the embryonic stage but there are few present at the end

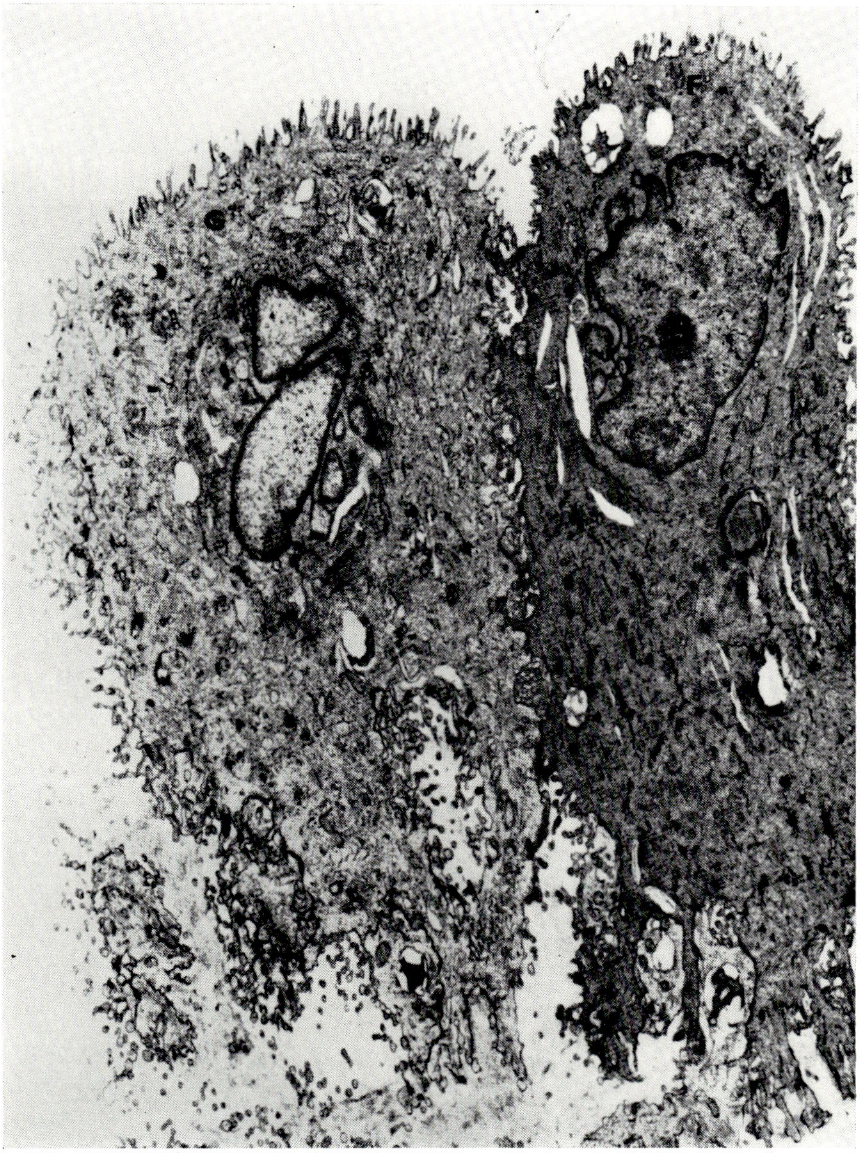

FIG. 3.39. Two different cell types in the human amniotic epithelium. G: Golgi cell type. F: Fibrillar cell type. With relatively little magnification the difference in the cytoplasmic density can clearly be seen. (Enlarged 6,560 times.) After Thomas (1962).

of pregnancy. This is interpreted as a sign of an end of production. Similarly, drop-like lipoid inclusions can be found in the amnion of man and fowl (Figs. 3.33, 3.34 and 3.38). The lipoids become mixed with the contents of the amniotic fluid vacuoles and with the amniotic fluid and reach the embryo through the intestinal canal, lungs, and the skin (Schmidt 1963). This leads to the idea that the amniotic fluid is an important nutrient fluid for the embryo and is a channel for nutrient transfer separate from the placenta (Schmidt 1963).

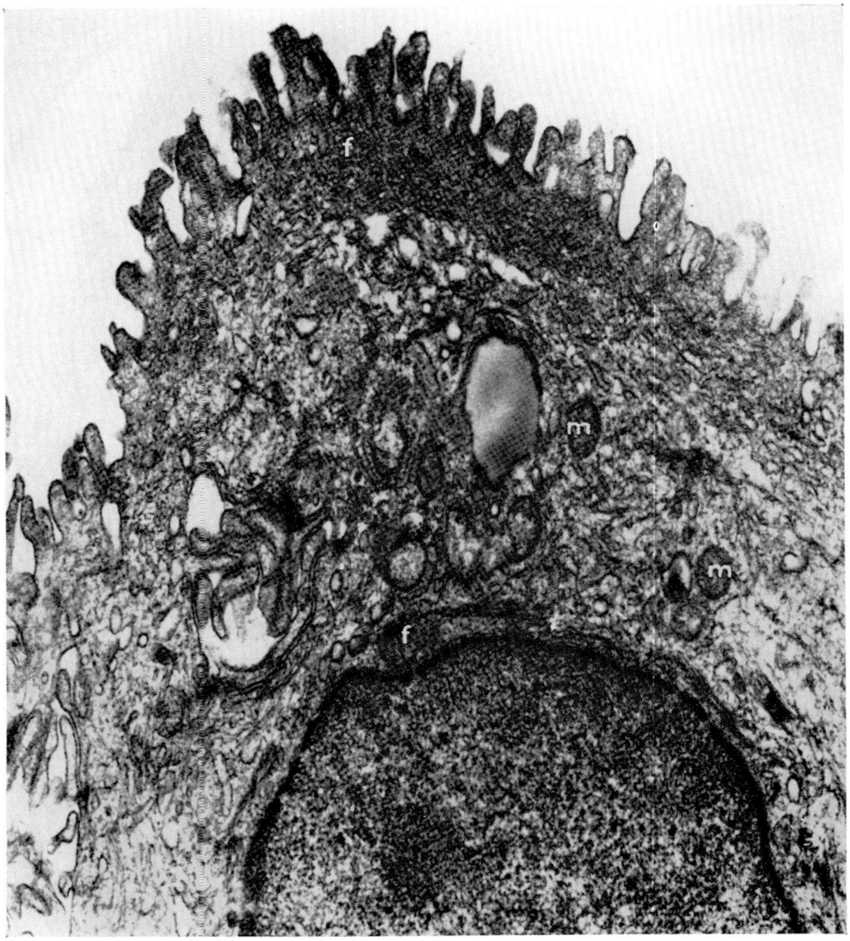

FIG. 3.40. Fibrillar type of amnion cell. The fibrillar cytoplasm is relatively dense. There are small granular mitochondria. F: Fibrillae. M: Mitochondria. (Enlarged 13,440 times.) After Thomas (1962).

On the basis of electron microscopic observations, it is suggested (Schmidt 1963) that the transport from the amniotic fluid takes place not only via the embryo but also via the amnion epithelium and the inter-

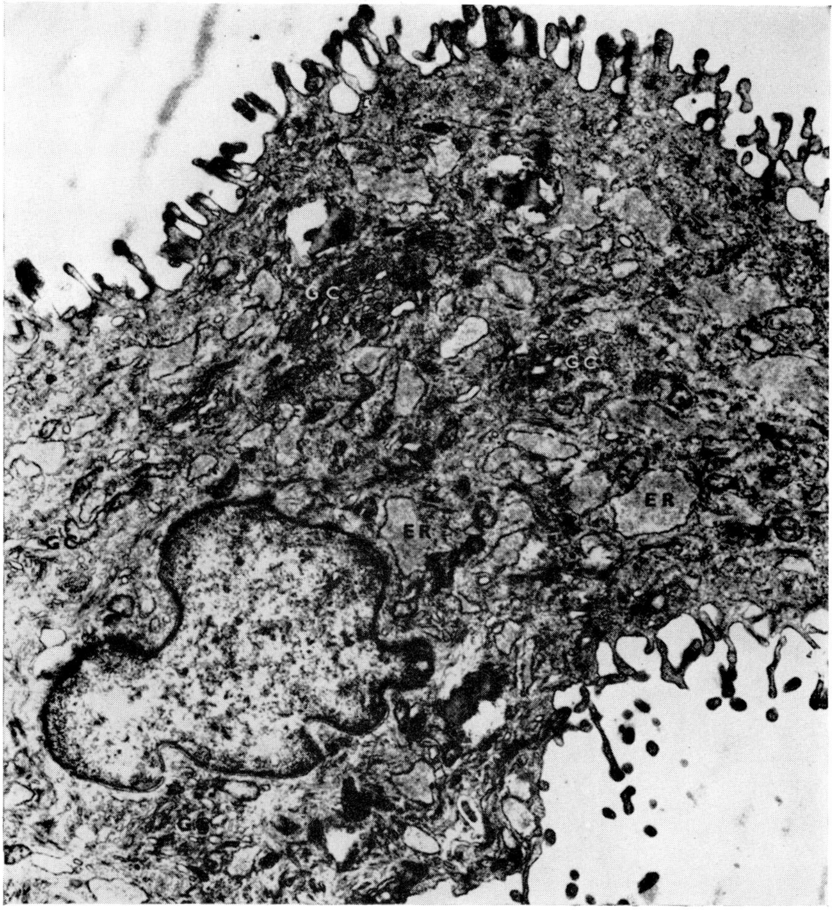

FIG. 3.41. 'Golgi' type of amnion cell. It shows a marked Golgi apparatus and dilated cysterns in the endoplasmic reticulum. GC: Golgi complex. ER: Dilated cysterns of the endoplasmic reticulum. (Enlarged 1,610 times.) After Thomas (1962).

cellular spaces. In this connection, attention must be drawn to the presence of meconium (Bourne 1962) in the intercellular spaces of the amnion epithelium.

On the basis of histochemical investigations (Galbis & Alfaro 1957), a high metabolic performance is attributed to the amnion, especially the pars placentaris (Salvi 1958). This is supported by the high content of ribonucleic acids and mitochondria besides the canalicular and vacuolar systems. Galbis & Alfaro (1957), associate this with an active secretory

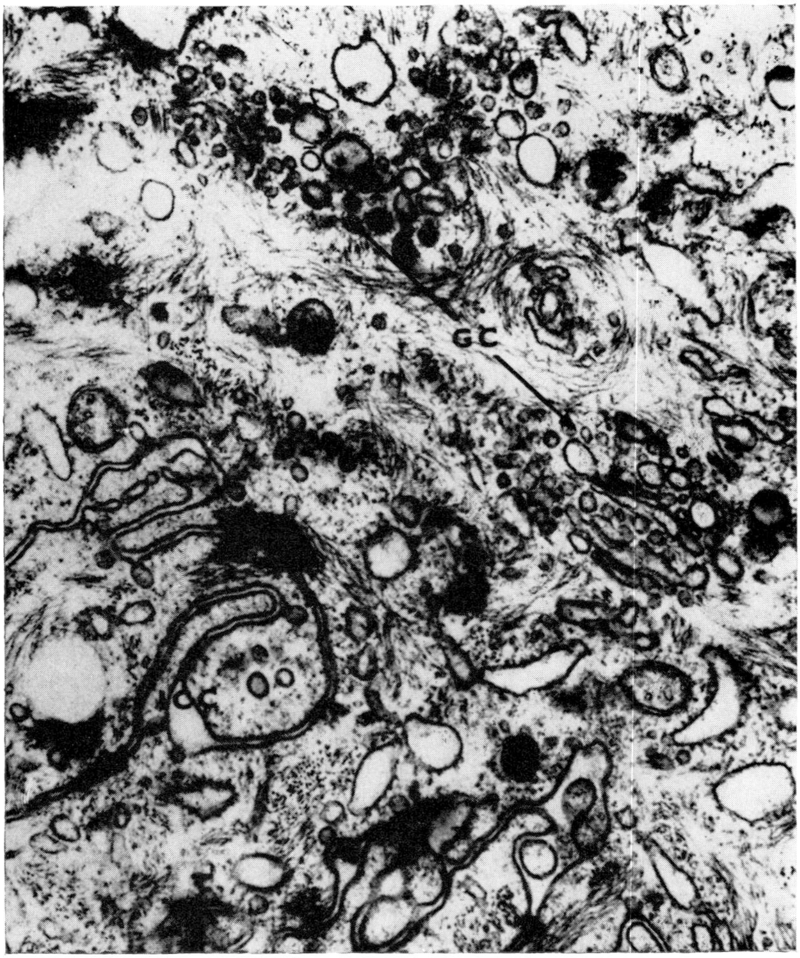

FIG. 3.42. The Golgi complex and vacuoles of the amniotic epithelium are in the close neighbourhood of the intercellular canals. (Enlarged 42,500 times.) After Thomas (1962).

performance. The latter also accept that production is predominantly of glycoproteins about the 2nd to 4th month, proteins in the 5th and 6th month and lipoids in the last three months. To demonstrate these substances, histochemically does not, however, by itself establish the secretory capacity of the amnion epithelial cells. The classification of these substances, in relation to any metabolites, has not been made clear, especially the place of glycoproteins in relation to chorionic gonadotrophin. By histochemical techniques Thiede & Chaote (1963) did, however, succeed in showing small quantities of gonadotrophin in the amnion. Diastase-resistant PAS-positive granules could be interpreted in the same way. In this connection, it is worth noting that Berle (1967) found the HCG concentration in the amniotic fluid to be twice as high as that in umbilical venous blood. The mature amnion contains glycogen. Candiani (1958) is of the opinion that glycogen is constantly excreted into the amniotic cavity as a product of cellular metabolism. In cases of hydramnios in which amniotic fluid is over-produced and the need for glycogen increased, the number of cells containing glycogen or RNA is higher than normal. In cases of postmaturity, there is a decline in substances containing glycogen RNA and SH (Candiani 1958).

The amnion is broadly anchored to the basal membrane by brush-like bundles of fibres which lie between the spaces of the cell base. Here we have a stratum of argyrophil fibres which is always clearly developed in both pars placentaris and pars reflexa (Bautzmann & Schroder 1955a, Bourne 1960).

Thick, long fasciculi of collagenous fibres are found immediately beneath the amnion epithelium and the basal membrane. They run into each other at acute angles and so compose a 'scissor' lattice. This makes it possible for the separate fasciculi of fibres to shift their positions relative to each other when changes of tension occur and this is further facilitated by the high mucus content of this stratum. This explains the elasticity of the amnion. It is supported by the anchoring of this fibrous layer (see Fig. 3.32) in the reticulum network of the fibrocyte layer. The 4th layer of the amnion is defined as the fibrocyte layer. At 0·05 to 0·5 mm it is the thickest stratum of the amnion. The cells which characterize this layer have many extensions, vary in length and diameter and show all the features of fibrocytes. The endoplasmatic reticulum of the fibrocytes is tubular but can also be lamellar and enclose a substance of variable optical density which often comprises almost the whole cell. A network of delicate fibrillae about 300 Å wide is specially noteworthy here. These fibrillae do not occur in other fibrocytes and Bourne (1962) describes in their stead small vesicles with a diameter of 500 Å. Here we probably have the intracellular formation of fibres. This assumption is further supported by the fact that the separate cell membranes are not intact and that the fibrillae lie in the lacunae and some even outside the cells. According to all appearances, they have been secreted by the cell (Fig. 3.43). The fibrocytes are surrounded by a network of fibres, which, together with the basal membrane, provide the anchoring system for the fibrous layer.

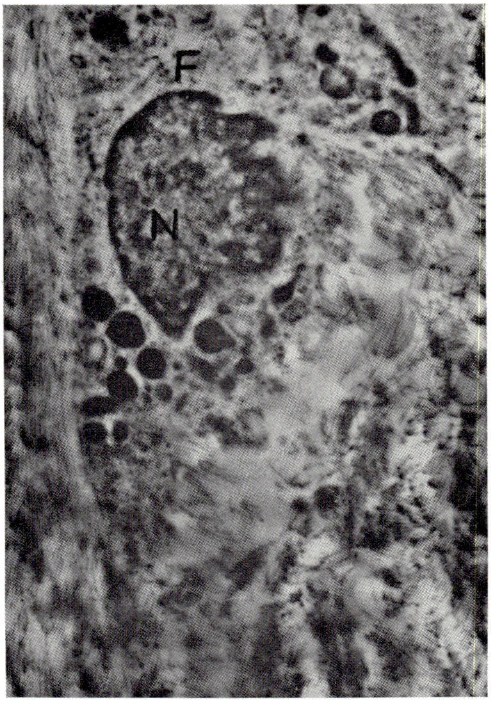

FIG. 3.43. The formation of intracellular fibrillae and their egress from the cell. F: Fibrillae. N: Nucleus. (Enlarged 12,000 times.) After Bourne (1962).

SPONGY LAYER

The spongy layer is composed of extra-embryonic coelom and must be considered the third main component of the foetal membranes, along with the amnion and the chorion. This stratum is marked off by amniotic or sometimes chorionic mesoderm and is anchored in the reticulum fibres. Here we have a layer with a high mucus content and which can store large quantities of water. Thus Petry (1954) found that 1 gm of intermediate layer binds 10 gm of water. By taking up water this stratum can increase from 5 μ to 10 mm. Isolated fibrocytes can be identified within the spongy layer. Although it was earlier thought to consist of a structureless jelly, Petry (1954) amongst others was able to show the presence of fibres and fibrillae of connective tissue which can be demonstrated by ultramicroscopic techniques. Electron microscopy revealed fibrillae 23 to 27 μ in size with transverse striation at 50 μ intervals. Using silver stained preparations one can find very long extended fibres, some of which run into each other in a star pattern and show knots at the centre. It is unlikely that these knots present crystallization centres in the development of the fibres, all the more so since Bourne (1962) was able to establish the probability of intracellular fibre formation and secretion taking place in the fibrocytes of the spongy layer. Besides these extended fibrillae, fibres forming a network of wavy forms also occur. It is possible that sometimes, under sufficient stress, the wavy forms may change into the extended form. Between the fibrillae there lie both fibrocytes and Hofbauer cells. The latter often have meconium granulae within the cell bodies. Their capacity for swelling adds to the mobility which the spongy layer lends to the amnion in contrast to the chorion which is almost rigidly bound to the decidua. It is not yet clear how far the spongy layer affects the exchange of material between mother and foetus.

THE CHORION

The chorion laeve is formed as a result of the reduction of chorionic villi on the side opposite the site of implantation. With its epithelial and connective tissue components, the chorion laeve composes the pars chorialis of the amniotic sac. The development of the chorion has already been discussed.

As in the case of the amnion, we distinguish a pars reflexa of the chorion, a pars placentaris and an area lying in front of the os uteri. There are no significant morphological differences between these three parts.

The pars reflexa of the chorion is on average 0·02 to 0·2 mm thick. It is only in the young chorion that one can distinguish four clearly defined strata (Fig. 3.32):

(1) The fibrocyte stratum
(2) The fibrous stratum
(3) The basal membrane
(4) The trophoblast stratum in contact with the decidua.

In the mature foetal membrane the first and, to some extent, the third layer have become almost indistinguishable.

In apposition to the intermediate spongy layer described above, we find the fibrocyte stratum of the chorion. It consists of a delicate meshwork of argyrophil fibres and typical fibrocytes. In the mature foetal membrane, however, the cellular part is minimal so that the network of fibres dominate the picture. Broad short strands of collagenous fibres come from the decidual trophoblast stratum and are anchored as more delicate tufts after splitting up. On the other hand, however, delicate fibres also extend outwards from the border membrane, reach as far as the trophoblast stratum and surround the chorion cells like a net. Thus, a definite fibrous layer 20 to 500 μ thick, is formed between the fibrocyte stratum and the trophoblast layer. It is especially well developed over the placenta. The connective tissue structures of the chorion have the character of columns and strands in contrast to the doubly anchored 'scissor' lattice system of the amnion, making some change of shape possible. Unlike the amnion and the spongy layer, this layer cannot be significantly displaced or stretched. This is the more so since the broad strands of fibres are arranged parallel to one another. The stratum contains typical fibrocytes and also Hofbauer cells. In the pars placentaris of the fibrous layer, the foetal vessels run into the villi. On the other hand, there are no capillaries to nourish this layer. The pars reflexa is always free of vessels. The only exceptions occur in cases of insertio velamentosa, placenta succenturiata, placenta membranacia and similar forms.

The fibrous stratum passes over into the basal membrane (see Fig. 3.32). It can be clearly traced, more especially in young foetal membrane, and is composed of a cell-free network of argyrophil fibres which blend into the wavy trophoblast stratum. The basal membrane is perforated by the collagenous bundles of fibres coming from the trophoblast stratum and going towards the amnion.

The trophoblast decidual stratum is a mechanical unit because after the trophoblast invades the mucous membrane of the uterus there later appears a well developed common supporting tissue. The development of the trophoblast to the point where villi are formed has been dealt with comprehensively elsewhere.

In the course of the development of the chorion laeve, the primary villi become atrophied. Often it is only possible to distinguish 'fern-like' remnants surrounded by decidual cells. In the mature foetal membrane, these 'ghost villi' are composed of vessel-free fibrous tissue with fibrin lamellae arranged concentrically around them. Hofbauer cells are no longer found in these villi but individual fibrocytes can still be traced. There is neither a syncytial stratum nor the remains of one in the chorion. By the demonstration of alkaline phosphatase, however, one can find in this stratum positively reacting masses of protoplasm without cell boundaries which might represent the syncytial connections (Juhos 1961).

Besides the 'ghost villi' this stratum contains a layer of varying width containing irregularly arranged trophoblast cells which go over into the decidua without a clear border and, on the other side, are anchored in the basal membrane. These cells are mainly of the clear type containing glycogen. There are also, however, cells to be found with glycoprotein inclusions. Stamm & Rioton (1958) also found diesterase-resistant and PAS-positive inclusions and droplets in these cells. Judging by the determination of the biological activity of the tissue extract the PAS positive reaction can be regarded as connected with the occurrence of gonadotrophin. Many trophoblast cells with some of their surrounding decidual cells have fallen victim to necrobiosis so that fibrin necrosis plaques have been formed. The trophoblast cells and the plaques are surrounded by a strongly argyrophil fibrous reticulum so that they lie in a thick, three dimensional meshwork which continues into the decidua. The two represent a unit designed to prevent the mechanical rupture of the amniotic membranes–the trophoblast-decidua complex. This unit is further strengthened by coarse, collagenous, pillar-like bundles of fibres which, as described earlier, originate broadly based in the decidua and after partly subdividing, are lost in the trophoblast layers. Other collagenous bundles of fibres can even be traced as far as the chorionic mesoderm on the edge of the spongy layer. The histochemical characteristics of the decidual cells are set out in Table 3.1. Only some of them occur in the form met with in the endometrium.

Some lymph spaces can be traced in the trophoblast layer. There are no real lymph channels with endothelial coverings. It is possible that these lymph spaces facilitate the foeto-maternal transport of material. They could, however, also be significant for the nourishment of the foetal membrane itself.

NOURISHMENT OF THE FOETAL MEMBRANE

The amnion, spongy layer and chorion are free of capillaries. Recent research shows that true lymph channels are also absent from the foetal membrane. Thus it may be assumed that the diffusion process takes place on the one hand from the amniotic fluid via amnion, spongy layer and chorion, and, on the other hand, from the tissue fluid out of the decidual vessels to the chorion, spongy layer and amnion. That the foetal membrane is nourished from the maternal side can, however, only be assumed

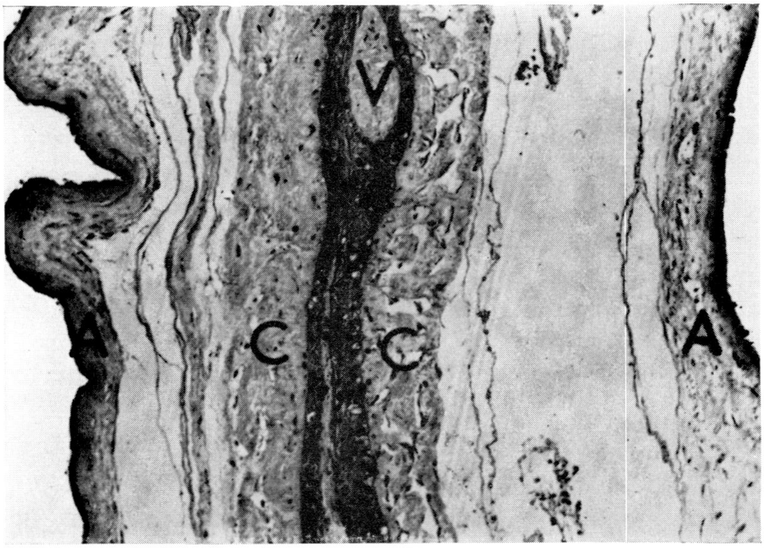

FIG. 3.44. The membranes of a dichorionic twin pregnancy. The two amnions (A) are covered by chorion. Between the two trophoblast layers is an obliterated villus (V). The right hand twin died 3 days before delivery. The amnion is necrotic, the stroma cells swollen and degenerated. On the left side the membranes are normal. (Enlarged 70 times.) After Bourne (1962).

for the chorion. A diffusion of liquor amnii seems to be required for the amnion. This view is supported by the finding that in twin foetal membranes, the separating wall is not in contact with the maternal tissue at the centre. It is therefore clearly dependent on the amniotic fluid for its nutrient supply since the diffusion path from the decidua would be too long. Moreover, the necrosis of the decidua itself does not have any major destructive effect on the foetal membrane lying above it. On the other hand, foetal death is not immediately followed by necrosis of the foetal membranes. The chorion can survive for a long time presumably through contact with the decidua. The contrary holds for the amnion which degenerates within a few days of foetal death because the nutritive function of the amniotic fluid has ceased to exist. If one of twins dies, the amnion of the dividing wall on the effected side (Bourne 1962) rapidly becomes necrotic while the parts adjacent to the decidua are only destroyed by degrees (Fig. 3.44).

THE UMBILICAL CORD

DEVELOPMENT

The umbilical cord develops out of the attaching stalk which is already clearly developed in the embryo at 21 days. The allantoic duct and the vitelline sac derive from the primitive alimentary tract and bulge into the strand of mesoderm. In man the vitelline sac does not develop beyond becoming a small umbilical vesicle. For a short period nourishment is conveyed to the embryo by the vitelline sac circulatory system thus formed. Once the chorionic allantois and vitelline sac vessels have been joined into a single system, the foeto-placental metabolism takes place through the circulatory system of the umbilical cord. In the young umbilical cord we can always see two arteries and two veins; one of the veins disappears later. In 1·1 per cent (Lyon 1960) to 1·9 per cent (Seitzmann 1964) of cases, one artery can also become atrophied. Both arteries anastamose about 1·5 cm above the point of insertion through a connecting vessel 1·5 to 2 cm long. The vein has thin walls and transports blood rich in nourishing substances from the placenta to the foetus; waste material and also foetal metabolites are carried to the placenta through the two strong muscular arteries.

MACROSCOPIC DESCRIPTION

The attaching stalk almost always develops at a position in the trophoblast stratum corresponding to the point of implantation and the implantation cell of the egg is at the same time the centre from which the sheets of the trophoblast grow out and, consequently, the attachment of the umbilical cord (49·4 per cent, Raaflaub 1959) is often centrally situated. The mature umbilical cord is from 50 to 70 cm long, and from 15 to 20 mm in diameter (Schmidt-Elmendorf 1952). The spiral form which can be ascribed to uneven growth of the two arteries is a considerable factor in the protection of vessels from occlusion. In most cases, the spiral is left-handed as seen from the foetus. The umbilical cord has the consistency of taut elastic and is blue-red in colour.

MICROSCOPIC FINDINGS

In a cross section of the mature umbilical cord, there can be seen a gelatinous mass (Wharton's jelly) covered by a stratum composed of one or more layers of flattened amnion cells with two arteries and a vein at its centre. In addition remains of the allantoic duct and parts of the vitelline sac vesicle can occasionally also be found. In the area of the umbilicus, the amnion layer merges directly into the skin of the child.

The main tissue of the cord is composed of Wharton's jelly. This is a jelly-like basophil substance transversed by a network of fibres. From the 6th to 8th week of pregnancy only oligosaccharides can be found in the Wharton's jelly. These may be precursors of hyaluronic acid. Mucopolysaccharides, however, only appear after the 8th week. These are mainly hyaluronic acids. At term, chondroitin sulphuric acid also occurs in the jelly (Schoenberg *et al.* 1960). Before the 20th week, electron microscopy reveals in this basic substance, fibrillae from 50 to 100 Å in diameter and nodules at intervals of 2,500 Å. On the other hand, in more mature umbilical cords, the diameters are mostly less than 50 Å and there are no nodules. Collagenous fibres occur in umbilical cords at all stages of maturity. Argyrophil elements can be found in the tissue of the umbilical cord alongside the typical collagenous form.

The nourishment of the Wharton's jelly takes place through the amnion epithelium by the amniotic fluid or through the arteries and umbilical vein. A dense net of capillaries can be found in the Wharton's jelly only in the first weeks of pregnancy. There follows a rapid reduction of capillary vessels so that they can only be traced in the neighbourhood of the umbilical ring. Occasionally, however, a few remain in being and functional until delivery (Vinogradov 1959). Although the small vessels lie near the umbilical arteries, there is no connection between these two systems. Spindle and star-shaped cells can be found between the fibres in the Wharton's jelly. They have the characteristics of fibrocytes. Contrary to earlier ideas, these cells do not build up a syncytium. Finally, Hofbauer cells with the characteristics of mast cells can be identified in the Wharton's jelly.

The elements of connective tissue in the Wharton's jelly are arranged round the umbilical vessels in concentric lamellae and so compose the adventitia of the arteries and veins. Goerttler (1951), Zawisch (1955),

Scheuner (1964) were able to show that this enclosing tissue is arranged in a flattened spiral. On the other hand, its innermost layer runs in the direction of the vessels and radiates into the musculature.

With its fibres of connective tissue, the Wharton's jelly builds a support system which is important for the changing function of the musculature of the vessels. Goertler (1951) drew attention to this and described the 'structural composition peculiar to the organ' of the umbilical arteries and was able to show that the arteries of the umbilical cord have layers of muscle arranged cross-wise. In the histological preparation, one finds a narrow outer longitudinal musculature, a wide middle circular musculature and again an inner longitudinal musculature. These bundles of muscle fibre are anchored in the fibrillar stroma of the Wharton's jelly described above. A horizontal section of the outer layer of muscle fibre of an umbilical artery taken in the direction of the axis of the vessel shows that the muscle fibrils divide like the foot of a goose and only subsequently come into contact with the collagenous fibres of the Wharton's jelly. Thus the tension is spread over a large surface. The inner longitudinal layer is built into a dense network of delicate elastic fibres, a feature not found in this form in other arteries of the same calibre. Two concentrically orientated polarized shifting lamellae of connective tissue stretch between the three communicating layers of muscle.

Our knowledge of the structure and arrangement of the muscle fibres and connective tissue gives us some insight into the functioning of the artery. The fact that the muscular layer is anchored to the surrounding connective tissue makes it possible for contraction to cause a narrowing of the lumen of the vessel. On the other hand, the sharply increasing angle of the muscle fibres may enable their contraction to lead to a dilatation of the vessel which readily changes to narrowing if there is a change in the angle. Indeed, if the slope is above 45° the fibres operate as longitudinal muscles but act as circular muscles if it is less than 45°. Active widening is only possible, however, if the vessel is stretched in the direction of its longitudinal course. If there is no longitudinal tension, e.g. if the blood flow has been stopped by ligation of the cord, longitudinal folds are produced by partial contraction and lead to the closing of the vessel (Gänschirt 1949, Goerttler 1951). The oedema of the jelly is also significant in this connection. Goerttler was able to show that the contraction of the artery leads to occlusion of the vessels, even after the swelling of the Wharton's jelly has subsided. This fact is of the greatest postpartum importance. Nervous factors on the other hand, play no part in the functioning of arteries of the umbilical cord since nerve fibres are only to be found in the neighbourhood of the placental and foetal insertions of the cord, or as short locally limited elements in its middle section (Aburel *et al.* 1958).

The umbilical vein is surrounded by a collagenous fibre system arranged in a spiral. This adventitial layer is, however, thinner than that of the artery (Scheuner 1964). A muscularis similar to that of the artery is found. It is composed of three layers:

(a) Longitudinal external layer
(b) Circular layer
(c) An internal longitudinal layer.

However, Stallabrass (1963) was not always able to demonstrate the presence of the outer longitudinal layer.

Very recently (Essbach 1966), numerous valves or pads have been described in the vessels of the umbilical cord. It can, however, be confidently stated that these are artefacts. They arise from partial contractions which follow on the decrease in tension or anchoring of the vessels. The x-ray investigations of Hert (1955) are strong evidence of this. The formation of valves or pads in the pulsating vessel can never be observed by x-ray during delivery. Histologically these 'valves' are always duplications of the vessel wall which can no longer be demonstrated when the unfixed umbilical cord is dilated (see Essbach & Rose 1966 for detailed discussion of this problem).

REFERENCES

ABUREL E., VASILESCU C., EUACHESCU A. & RAU C. (1958) Innervation des Mutterkuchens, der Nabelschnur und der intra-abdominalen Nabelgefäße des Feten. *Obstet. et Ginec.* **6**, 493.

AGUERO O. (1957) *Anomalias Morfologicas de la Placenta y su Significado Clinico.* Artegrafia Caracas.

AMSTUTZ E. (1960) Beobachtungen über die Reifung der Chorionzotten in der menschlichen Placenta mit besonderer Berücksichtigung der Epithelplatten. *Acta Anat. (Basel)*, **42**, 12.

ARNOLD M., GELLER, H.-F. & SASSE D. (1961) Beitrag zur elektronenoptischen Morphologie der menschlichen Placenta. *Arch. Gynak.* **196**, 238.

ASHLEY A. (1965) Study of the human placenta with the electron microscope. *Arch. of Pathol.* **80**, 377.

AUSTIN C.R. (1962) Sex chromatin in embryonic and fetal tissue. *Acta cytol.* **6**, 61.

BARGMANN W. (1957) Über den Bildungsort der Choriongonadotropine und Placenta-steroide. *Geburtsh. and Frauenheilk.* **17**, 865.

BARGMANN W. & KNOOP A. (1959) Elektronenoptische Untersuchungen an Placentarzotten des Menschen. *Z. Zellforsch.* **50**, 472.

BAUTZMANN H. & SCHRODER R. (1955a) Vergleichende Studien über Bau und Funktion des Amnions. *Z. Anat. Entwickl. Gesch.* **119**, 7.

BAUTZMANN H. & SCHRODER R. (1955b) Über Vorkommen und Bedeutung von 'Hofbauerzellen' ausserhalb der Placenta. *Arch. Gynak.* **187**, 65.

BAUTZMANN H. & SCHRODER R. (1956) Speicherversuche zum Problem der Histiocytennatur extraplacentarer 'Hofbauerzellen' im Sauzopsiden and Säugeramnion. *Z. Zellforsch*, **43**, 543.

BECKER V. (1960) Über maturitas praecox placentae. *Verh. dtsch. Ges. Path.* **44**, 256.

BECKER V. (1962) Mechanismus der Reifung fetaler Organe. *Verh. dtsch. Ges. Path.* **46**, 309.

BECKER V. & JIPP P. (1962) Über die Trophoblastschale der menschlichen Placenta. *Geburtsh and Frauenheilk.* **23**, 466.

BELTERMANN R. & STEGNER H.-E. (1968) Elektronenmikroskopische Untersuchungen an den Ovarien neugeborener Mäuse nach Behandlung mit humanem hypophysärem Gonadotropin (HCG). *Acta Endocrinologica*, **57**, 279.

BERLE P. (1967) Untersuchungen sur HCG-Konzentration im Fruchtwasser. *Geburtsh and Frauenheilk.* **27**, 1107.

BLEYL M. (1962) Histologische, histochemische und fluorescenzmikroskopische Untersuchungen an Hofbauer-Zellen. *Arch. Gynak.* **197**, 364.

BØE P. (1954) Vascular morphology of the human placenta. *Cold Spr. Harb. Symp quant. Biol.* **19**, 29.

BOURNE G.L. (1960) The microscopic anatomy of the human amnion and chorion. *Amer. J. Obstet. Gynec.* **79**, 1070.

BOURNE G.L. (1962) *The Human Amnion and Chorion.* Lloyd-Luke Ltd, London.

BOYD D.M. (1960) *The Placenta and Fetal Membranes*, p. 214. C.A.Villee, ed. William and Wilkins, Baltimore.

BOYD J.D. & HUGHES A.F.W. (1954) Observations on human chorionic villi using the electron microscope. *J. Anat. (Lond.)* **88**, 356.

BURGOS M. & RODRIGUEZ P. (1966). Specialized zones in the trophoblast of the human term placenta. *Amer. J. Obstet. Gynec.* **96**, 342.

CANDIANI G.B. (1958) La membrana amniotica normale e patologica. *Ann. Obstet. Ginec.* **80**, 3.

CAPODACQUA A., DAMIANI N. & DEBIASI E. (1961) Vascolarizzazione sanguigna e ciclo mestruale. *Minerva Ginecol.* **13**, 1081.

CRAWFORD J.M. (1956a) The fetal placental circulation. Part III. The anatomy of the cotyledons. *J. Obstet. Gynaec. Brit. Emp.* **63**, 542.

CRAWFORD J.M. (1956b) The fetal placental circulation. Part IV. The anatomy of the villus and its capillary structure. *J. Obstet. Gynaec. Brit. Emp.* **63**, 548.

CRAWFORD J.M. (1962) Vascular anatomy of the human placenta. *Amer. J. Obstet. Gynec.* **84**, 1543.

DALLENBACH F.D. & DALLENBACH-HELLWIG G. (1964) Immunhistologische Untersuchungen zur Lokalisation des Relaxins in menschlicher Placenta und Decidua. *Virchows Arch. path. Anat.* **337**, 391.

DALLENBACH-HELLWIG G. & NETTE G. (1963) Über Proteineinschlüsse in basalen Trophoblastzellen der reifen menschlicher Placenta. *Virchows Arch. path. Anat.* **336**, 528.

DALLENBACH-HELLWIG G. & NETTE G. (1964) Morphological and histochemical observations on trophoblast and decidua of the basal plate of the human placenta at term. *Amer. J. Anat.* **115**, 309.

DEMPSEY E.W. & WISLOCKI G.B. (1945) Histochemical reactions associated with basophilia and acidophilia in the placenta and pituitary gland. *Amer. J. Anat.* **76**, 277.

DEMPSEY E.W. (1948) The chemical cytology of endocrine glands. *Recent Progr. Hormone Res.* **3**, 127.

DOMSKIKH N.V. (1957) New views on the vascularity of human amnion. *Akus. Ginek*, **33**, 93.

ESSBACH H. (1966) Pathologische Morphologie der Secundinae und ihre Beziehung zu Gedeihstörungen, zur verfruhten Geburt und zum Absterben der Leibesfrucht. *Placenta und Eihäute.* H.Essbach & J.Röse, eds. Fischer, Jena.

ESSBACH H. & RÖSE J. (1966) *Placenta und Eihäute.* Fischer, Jena.

FISCHER W.M. & MÜLLER G. (1967) Das Strombahnsystem und der Austausch der Atemgase in der Meerschweinchenplacenta. *Anatom. Anz.* (in press).

FREESE U.E. (1966) The fetal-maternal circulation of the placenta. I. Histomorphologic, plastoid injection, and x-ray cinematographic studies on human placentas. *Amer. J. Obstet. Gynec.* **94**, 354.

FREESE U.E., RANNINGER K. & KAPLAN H. (1966) The fetal-maternal circulation of the placenta. II. An x-ray cinematographic study of pregnant rhesus monkeys. *Amer. J. Obstet. Gynec.* **94**, 361.

GALBIS M. & ALFARO L. (1957) Investigaciones histologicas e histoquimicas sobre el epitelio amniotico. *Rev. espan Obstetr.* **16**, 319.

GANSCHIRT H. (1949) Bau und Funktion menschlicher Nabelschnurartierien. *Morph. Jb.* **90**, 59.

GEDIGK F. (1952) Histochemische Darstellung von Kohlehydraten. *Klin. Woschr.* **30**, 1057.

GLOWINSKI M. & KONECKI J. (1962) Histological examinations of a mature human amnion epithelium. *Ginek. pol.* **33**, 739.

GOERTTLER K. (1951) Die Bedeutung der funktionellen Struktur der Gefäßwand. I. Untersuchungen an der Nabelschnurarterie des Menschen. *Morph. Jb.* **91**, 368.

GÖLTNER E.C. & STARK G. (1957) Die Lokalisation des Territius in der Placentazelle. *Arch. Gynak.* **188**, 210.

GÖLTNER E.C. & STARK G. (1960) Das Gewebesesen in der Placenta und in den fetalen Organen. *Zeitschr. Geburtsh. Gynak.* **156**, 94.

GROSSER O. (1927) *Fruhentwicklung, Eihautbildung und Placentation des Menschen und der Säugetiere.* J.F.Bergmann, München.

HAMILTON W.J. & MOSSMAN H.W. (1962) *Human embryology*. W.Heffer & Sons, Ltd, Cambridge.

HASHIMOTO M., KOSAKA M., MORI Y., KOMORI A. & AKASHI K. (1960) Electron microscopic studies on the epithelium of the chorionic villi of the human placenta (Report I). *J. Jap. Obstet. Gynaec. Soc.* 7, 44.

HASHIMOTO M., KOSAKA M., SHIMOYAMA T., HIRASAWA T., KOMORI A. & KAWASAKI T. (1960) Electron microscopic studies on the epithelium of the chorionic villi of the human placenta. *J. Jap. Obstet. Gynaec. Soc.* 7, 122.

HENDRICKS C.H. (1964) Patterns of fetal and placental growth. *Obstet. Gynec.* **24**, 357.

HERT J. (1955) O. circularnich rasach v pupecnikovych a placentaruich cevach. *Cs. Morfol.* **3**, 302.

HERTIG A.T. (1945) On the development of the amnion and exocoelomic membrane in the pre-villous human ovum. *Yale J. Biol. Med.*, **18**, 107.

HERTIG A.T. (1960) Pathological aspects. In *The Placenta and Fetal Membranes*, p. 213. C.A.Villee, ed. William and Wilkins, Baltimore.

HERTIG A.T., ROCK J. & ADAMS E.C. (1956) A description of 34 human ova within the first 17 days of development. *Amer. J. Anat.* **98**, 435.

HOFBAUER J. (1903) Uber das konstante Vorkommen bisher unbekannter zelliger Form elemente im der Chorionzotte der menschlichen Placenta. *Wien klin. Wschr.* **16**, 871.

HÖRMANN G. (1947) Haben die soegenannten Hofbauerzellen der Chorionzotten funktionelle Bedeutung? *Zbl. Gynak.* **69**, 1199.

HÖRMANN G. (1948) Die Reifung der menschlichen Chorionzotte im Lichte ökonomischer Zweckmäßigkeit. *Zbl. Gynak.* **70**, 625.

HÖRMANN G. (1950) Der Durchmesser menschlicher Chorionzotten als Ausdruck ihrer Reifung und Entwicklung. *Verh. anat. Ges.* (*Jena*), 48 Vers. ersch. 1951.

HÖRMANN G. (1951) Lebenskurve normaler und entwicklungsunfähiger Chorionzotten. *Arch. Gynak.* **181**, 36.

HÖRMANN G. (1953) Ein Beitrag zur funktionellen Morphologie der menschlichen Placenta. *Arch. Gynak.* **181**, 29.

HOWORKA E. (1956) Trophoblast of human ovum in cultures *in vitro*. *Prace Komisji Med. Doswiadez.* **13**, 1.

HOWORKA E. (1960) Lozysko i Blony Plodowe I. Poznanskie towarzystowo przyjaciol nauk wydzial lekarski. *Prace Komisji Medycyny doswiadczalnej.* **19**, 111.

HUMKE W. (1963) Untersuchungen über die alkalische Phosphatase in der menschlichen Placenta. *Gynacologia*, **155**, 400.

IKAWA A. (1959) Observations on the epithelium of human chorionic villi with the electron microscope. *Jap. Obstet. Gynec. Soc.* **6**, 219.

JUHOS D. (1961) Nachweis von alkalischer Phosphatase in Fruchtblassen. *Magy. Noorv. Lap.* **24**, 140.

KANEMATSU T. (1961) Supravital and histochemical observation on the human chorionic villi. *Tokushima J. Exp. Med.* 7, 235.

KEIFFER H. (1926) Recherches sur la physiologie de l'amnios humain. *Gynec. et Obstet.* **14**, 1.

Kleine U. (1966) Neuere Untersuchungen über den Lipidstoffwechsel reifer menschlicher Placentazotten. *Arch. gynak.* **204**, Heft. 2/3.

Kleine U. (1967a) Studies on the lipid metabolism of villi of mature human placentas. *Clin. Chim. Acta*, **17**, 95.

Kleine U. (1967b) Der In-vitro-Einbau von (1-^{14}C)acetat in Neutralfette, Phosphatide und Cholesterin reifer menschlicher Placentazotten. *Hoppe-Seyler's Z. Physiol. Chem.* **348**, 891.

Kleine U. (1967c) Gaschromatographische Untersuchungen der Fettsäuren, der Neutralfette, Phospholipide und Cholesterinesterreifer menschlicher Placentazotten in vitro. *Clin. Chim. Acta*, **17**, 479.

Klinger H.P. & Ludwig K.S. (1957) Sind die Septen und großzelligen Inseln der Placenta aus mütterlichen oder kindlichem Gewebe aufgebaut? *Z. Anat. Entw. Gesch.* **120**, 95.

Knoop J. (1960) Das Wachstum der Chorionzotte vom II. Monat. *Z. Anat. Entw. Gesch.* **122**, 42.

Latta S. & Beber C.R. (1953) Cells with metachromatic cytoplasmatic granules in the stroma of human chorionic villi. *Science*, **117**, 498.

Lemtis H. (1966) Thesis, Berlin.

Lister U.M. (1964) Ultrastructure of the early human placenta. *J. Obstet. Gynaec. Brit. Cwlth.* **71**, 27.

Ludwig K.S. (1959) Die Rolle des Fibrius bei der Bildung der menschlichen Placenta. *Acta Anat. (Basel)*, **38**, 323.

Lyon F.A. (1960) Fetal abnormalities associated with umbilical cords containing one umbilical artery and one umbilical vein. *Obstet. and Gynec.* **16**, 719.

McKay D.G. (1960) In *The Placenta and Fetal Membranes*, p. 109. C.A.Villee, ed. William and Wilkins, Baltimore.

McKay D.G., Hertig A.T., Adams E.C. & Richardson M.V. (1958) Histochemical observations on the human placenta. *Obstet. & Gynec.* **12**, 1.

Marcus G.J., Kraicher P.F. & Shelesnyak M.C. (1963) Studies on the mechanism of decidualization. II. Histamine-releasing action of pyrathiazine. *J. Reprod. Fertil.* **5**, 409.

Mossmann H.W. (1937) Comparative morphogenesis of the fetal membranes and accessory uterine structures. *Contrib. to Embryol.* **26**, 129.

Mossmann H.W. (1959) General Discussion. In *Gestation, Transactions of the Fifth Conference*. C.A.Villee, ed. J.Macy Jr. Foundation, New York.

Ortmann R. (1949) Uber Kernsekretion, Kolloid- und Vakuolenbildung in Beziehung zum Nucleinsauregehalt in Trophoblast-Riesenzellen der menschlichen Placenta. *Z. Zellforsch*, **34**, 562.

Ortmann R. (1955) Histochemische Untersuchungen am menschlicher Placenta mit besonderer Berücksichtigung der Kernkugeln (Kerneinschlüsse) und der Plasmalipoideinschlüsse. *Zschr. Anat. Entw. Gesch.* **119**, 28.

Ortmann R. (1959) Morphologie der Placenta. *Verh. anat. Ges. (Jena)*, **106/107**, 27.

Page E.W. (1957) Transfer of materials across the human placenta. *Amer. J. Obstet. Gynec.* **74**, 705.

Page E.W. (1960) Physiology of the human placenta at term. *Clin. Obstet. Gynec.* **3**, 279.

PANIGEL M., NGUYEN J. & SUH H. (1964) Ultrastructure des villa sites placentaires humaines. *Path et Biol.* **12**, 927.

PESCETTO G. (1952) Osservazioni istologiche ed istochimiche sulla cellula di Hofbauer del villo choriale umano. *Riv. Biol. N.S.* **44**, 231.

PETRY G. (1954) Studien über die morphologischen Grundlagen des Blasensprunges. *Zbl. Gynak.* **76**, 655.

RAAFLUB W. (1959) Zur Kausalität der Nabelschnurkomplikationen. *Gynaecologia (Basel)*, **148**, 145.

RAMSEY E.M. (1954) Circulation in the Maternal placenta of primates. *Amer. J. Obstet. Gynec.* **67**, 1.

RAMSEY E.M. (1955) Vascular patterns in the endometrium and the placenta. *Angiol.* **6**, 321.

RAMSEY E.M. (1959a) Circulation in the placenta. In *Gestation*, p. 77. C.A.Villee, ed. J.Macy Jr. Foundation, New York.

RAMSEY E.M. (1959b) Vascular adaptions of the uterus to pregnancy. *Ann. N.Y. Acad. Sci.* **75**, 726.

RAMSEY E.M. (1960) The Placental Circulation. In *The Placenta and Fetal Membranes*, p. 36. C.A.Villee, ed. Williams and Wilkins, Baltimore.

RAMSEY E.M. (1962) Circulation in the intervillous space of the primate placenta. *Amer. J. Obstet. Gynec.* **84**, 1649.

SADOVSKY A., SERR D.M. & KOHN G. (1957) Composition of the placental septa as shown by nuclear sexing. *Science*, **126**, 609.

SALVI P. (1958) Alcuni aspetti istochimici delle membrane ovulari umane in condizioni normali e pathologiche. *Minerva Ginec.* **10**, 799.

SAWASAKI C., MORI T., INOUE R. & SCHIMNI K. (1957) Observations on human placental membrane by the electron microscope. *Endocrin. jap.* **4**, 1.

SCHEUNER G. (1964) Über die Verankerung der Nabelschnur an der Placenta. *Morph. Jb.* **106**, 73.

SCHMIDT W. (1963) Struktur und Funktion des Amnionepithels von Mensch und Huhn. *Z. Zellforsch*, **61**, 642.

SCHMIDT-ELMENDORF H.R. (1952) Anatomie, Physiologie und Pathologie der Decidua, Eihäute und Nabelschnur einschließlich vorzeitigen Blasensprungs. In *Biologie und Pathologie des Weibes*, p. 282. Seitz-Amreich, ed. Urban and Schwarzenberg, Berlin.

SCHMIDT-MATTHIESEN H. (1963) *Das normale menschliche Endometrium.* G.Thieme Verlag, Stuttgart.

SCHMIDT-MATTHIESEN H. (1968) Endometrium und Nidation beim Menschen. *Zschr. f. Gebh. u. Gyn.*, **168**, 113.

SCHOENBERG M.D., HINMANN A. & MOORE R.D. (1960) Studies on connective tissue. V. Fiber formation in Wharton's jelly. *Lab. Invest.* **9**, 350.

SCHWARTZ W. & MERKER H.J. (1965) Die Hodenzwischenzellen der Ratte nach Hypophysektomie und nach Behandlung mit Choriongonadotropin und Amphenon B. *Z. Zellforsch.* **65**, 272.

SCOTT J.S. (1960) Placenta extrachorialis (placenta marginata and placenta circumvallata). A factor in antepartum haemorrhage. *J. Obstet. Gynaec. Brit. Emp.* **67**, 904.

SEITZMANN L. (1964) The single umbilical artery. *J. Newark Beth Israel Hosp.* **15**, 21.

SHELESNYAK M.C. (1959) Mechanism of implantation and its control. *Rep. Proc. of the 6th Inter. Conf. on Planned Parenthood*, pp. 151.

SHELESNYAK M.C. & KRAICHER P.F. (1963) The role of estrogen in nidation. *Delayed implantation*, pp. 265. A.C.Enders, ed. University of Chicago Press, Chicago.

SHETTLES M. & SCHMIDT-MATHIESSEN H. (1963) Endometrium und Nidation. In *Das normale menschliche Endometrium*, p. 294. H.Schmidt-Matthiessen, ed. Thieme Verlag, Stuttgart.

SOHVAL A.R., GAINES J.A. & STRAUSS L. (1959) Chromosomal sex detection in the human newborn and fetus from examination of the umbilical cord, placental tissue and fetal membranes. *Ann. N.Y. Acad. Sci.* **75**, 902.

STALLABRASS P. (1963) Observations on the muscular coat of the human umbilical blood vessels. *J. Obstet. Gynec. Brit. Emp.* **70**, 1042.

STAMM O. & RIOTTON G. (1958) Ein Beitrag sur funktionellen Morphologie der Eihäute. *Geburtsh. and Frauenheilk*, **18**, 310.

STARCK D. (1955) Die Placentation des Menschen. In *Embryologie*, p. 289. Gg Thieme, Stuttgart.

STARK G. & JUNG W. (1956) Phosphatasen in der Placenta und ihren einzelnen Zellfraktionen. *Arch. Gynak.* **187**, 398.

STARK G. & JUNG W. (1959) Phosphatasen in den Zellstrukturen der Placenta bei pathologischen Schwangerschaften. *Arch. Gynak.* **191**, 201.

STEGNER H.E. & BELTERMANN R. (1967) Die Ultrastruktur der Zwischenzellen des Kaninchenovar nach Uberstimulierung mit Gonadotropinen. *Z. Zellforsch.* (in press).

STRAUSS F. (1964) Bau und Funktion der menschlichen Placenta. *Fortsch Geburtsh. und Gynak.* **17**, 3.

STRAUSS F. (1967) Die normale Anatomie der menschlichen Placenta. In *Handbuch der speziellen Pathologischen Anatomie und Histologie.* F.Strauss, K.Benirschke & S.G.Driscoll, eds. Springer-Verlag, Berlin.

STRAUSS G. & HIERSCHE H.D. (1962) Untersuchungen zur Problematik der histochemischen Fermentlokalisation in der Placenta. *Arch. Gynak.* **198**, 187.

STRAUSS G. & STARK G. (1960) Zur Histo- und Cytotopik der unspezifischen alkalischen Phosphatase. *Histochem.* **2**, 87.

SUHRING J.L., GREEN J.W., ROCHLIN D.B. & BLACKMORE W.S. (1961) Transfer of maternal erythrocytes across the human placenta. *Obstet. & Gynec.* **18**, 673.

TENZER W. (1962) Graphsche Rekonstruktion des bindegewebigen Stutzaskeletts der menschlichen Placenta. Inaug. Diss (Med.) Kiel.

THIEDE H.A. & CHOATE J.W. (1963) Chorionic gonadotropin localisation in the human placenta by immunofluorescent staining. *Obstet. and Gynec.* **22**, 433.

THOMAS C.R. (1962) The ultrastructure of Human Amnion Epithelium. *J. Ultrastructure Research*, **13**, 65.

THOMSEN K. (1955a) Uber die Aktivität der alkalischen Phosphatase in der menschlichen Placenta. *Arch. Gynak.* **187**, 1.

THOMSEN K. (1955b) Histochemische Untersuchungen über die saure Phosphatase in der menschlichen Placenta. *Arch. Gynak.* **187**, 264.

THOMSEN K. (1959) *Histochemie der Placenta*. Thieme Verlag, Leipzig.

THOMSEN K. & BLANKENBURG H. (1956) Über die Entwicklung und Rückbildung der Langhansschen Zellschicht in der menschlichen Placenta. *Arch. Gynak.* **187**, 638.

THOMSEN K. & LORENTZEN CH. (1956) Untersuchungen über die Lokalisation sudanophiler Substanzen in der menschlichen Placenta. *Arch. Gynak.* **187**, 462.

THOMSEN K. & NETZ L. (1955) Über Fermentaktivität in Hofbauerzellen. *Arch. Gynak.* **185**, 794.

THOMSEN K. & WILLEMSEN R. (1959) Histochemische Untersuchungen über die Produktionsorte der Choriongonadotropine. *Acta Endocr.(Kbh).* **30**, 161.

VILLEE C.A. (1960) In *The Placenta and Fetal Membranes*, p. 29. Williams and Wilkins, Baltimore.

VINOGRADOV V.V. (1959) The capillaries of the Wharton's jelly of human umbilical cord. *Akus. i. Ginek.* **35**, 63.

WAKITANI T. (1961) Electronmicroscopic observation on the chorionic villi of the normal human placenta and chorio-epithelioma malignum. I. Electron microscopic observations on the chorionic villi of the normal human placenta. *J. Jap. Obstet. Gynaec. Soc.* **8**, 208.

WILKIN P. (1960) La vascularisation de l'endometre humain au cours de la phase progestive du cycle menstruel et au cours de la nidation ovulaire. In *Les Fonctions de Nidation Uterine et leurs Troubles*, p. 331. J.Ferin & M.Gaudefray, eds. Masson et Cie, Paris.

WINDLE W.F. (1940) *Physiology of the Fetus. Origin and Extent of Function in Prenatal Life.* W.B.Saunders, Philadelphia.

WISLOCKI G.B. & DEMPSEY E.W. (1948) The chemical histology and cytology of the human placenta and decidua with reference to mucopolysaccharides, glycogen, lipids and acid phosphatase. *Amer. J. Anat.* **83**, 1.

WISLOCKI G.B. & DEMPSEY E.W. (1955) Electron microscopy of the human placenta. *Anat. Rec.* **123**, 133.

YAMAGUCHI R., OKUDA Y., ANEYA K. & NAKAUS M. (1960) Experimental studies on the passage of fat through the human placenta. Observations by light and electron microscope. *J. Jap. obstet. gynaec. Soc.* **7**, 35.

ZAWISCH C. (1955) Die Whartonsche Sulze und die Gefässe. *Z. Zellsorsch*, **42**, 94.

ZSCHIESCHE W. & GERLACH H. (1963) Biometrische Untersuchungen über die Placenta und die Beziehungen zwischen Placenta und Frucht. *Arch. Gynak.* **199**, 199.

4

Three Topics in Placental Transport Amino acid transport: Oxygen transfer: Placental Function during Labour

MAUREEN YOUNG

AMINO ACID TRANSPORT

The basic metabolic processes concerned with the growth of the placenta and with its transport activity, have been the Cinderellas of both physiologists and biochemists. In contrast, the hormonal control of reproduction holds an established position of its own and absorbs the energies of countless laboratories. However, the function of the hormones in relation to the metabolic activity of the placenta and the foetus can only become clearer when the understanding is more equally divided between the basic processes and their controlling mechanisms.

Page (1957) pointed out that one of the most important biochemical patterns during intra-uterine differentiation and growth, was the maintenance of higher concentrations of essential materials in the foetal than in the maternal extracellular fluids. Some of the factors concerned with the establishment of a high foetal : maternal concentration ratio for riboflavine (Lust, Hagerman & Villee 1954), free amino acids (Page, Glendenning, Margolis & Harper 1957) and for Vitamin C (Raiha 1958) are well established. In the last ten years most of the interest has centered around the amino acids. Recently, it has been found that regulation of the free amino acid environment of the human infant continues into the post-term period for, in the third trimester, no differences were observed between the umbilical venous level of each of the amino acids in premature, term and post-term infants; further, the amino acid environment is not the limiting factor for growth and welfare in 'small-for-dates' infants, for the umbilical venous plasma values are similar to those in infants with a normal birth weight and of comparable age.

Umbilical venous-arterial differences for the amino acids have been shown to change during gestation in the human subject; the venous levels were always higher than the arterial in the second trimester, demonstrating the expected transfer from the mother to the foetus but, at term, some of the acids were present in higher concentrations in the umbilical arterial blood suggesting their synthesis by the foetus.

High concentrations of free amino acids are present in the trophoblast, and a further increase in concentration has been demonstrated during transport, in the direction from the maternal to the foetal circulation only. The capture of amino acids by the guinea pig placenta at term was swift and amounted to about 40 per cent of a single injection of labelled amino acid given to the mother. This suggested that the plasma disappearance rate of a suitable substance, with a large clearance into the foetus, might provide an indication of placental function which could be related to gestational age. Such a plasma clearance test, depending primarily upon placental and foetal metabolic activity, might have greater significance than the measurement of the excretory products of hormones in the maternal urine in determining whether a foetus was 'small for dates' and therefore a high perinatal mortality risk (Dawkins 1965).

MATERNAL AMINO ACID ENVIRONMENT

NORMAL PREGNANCY

The early observations of Bonsnes (1947) and of Clemetson & Churchman (1954) on the changes in total α amino nitrogen concentration in the ante-cubital vein plasma of pregnant woman are well known: they found an average non-pregnant level of 4·3 mg per cent with a reduction to 3·2 mg per cent by the end of the first trimester, which was sustained until term; the level returned to the normal non-pregnant value within two days of delivery. The relative parts played by foetal demand, the hormones (Landau & Lugibihl 1961, Zinneman, Seal & Doe 1967), and increased maternal urinary wastage of amino acids during pregnancy, particularly of glycine and glutamic acid (Christensen, Date, Schonheyder & Volquartz 1957) in causing the fall in plasma amino nitrogen during gestation have not been investigated. The onset of the fall coincides with the onset of other changes in blood chemistry, and the changes in blood volume and circulation associated with the early growth and development of the placenta (Hytten & Leitch 1964). At the end of the third trimester the low level is partly dependent upon the umbilical circulation, for a rise towards the non-pregnant level was observed during cord occlusion (Clemetson & Churchman 1954): this suggests another method for investigating foetal welfare *in utero*, and a rise in maternal plasma amino nitrogen level may prove to be an early indication for an infant at risk.

A fuller analysis of maternal antecubital vein blood at term, using ion exchange column chromatography with an automatic analyser, was first made by Glendenning, Margolis & Page (1961) and extended by Ghadimi & Pecora (1964), Lindbland & Baldestan (1967) and Young & Prenton (1969). Confirming Zinneman *et al.* (1967) the latter found that the concentrations of the basic amino acids tended to be reduced more than the other amino acids, in the venous plasma of the pregnant woman in comparison with that of the non-pregnant woman. A small reduction in the levels of the neutral amino acids, particularly glycine, also occurred, but only small changes were found for the other amino acids, and the concentration of threonine, an essential amino acid was raised. All these changes were present by 16–19 weeks' gestation and no differences were found between the bloods of conscious and anaesthetized subjects known to be in the post-absorbative state. The standard errors of the mean values were relatively large as is normally found in any group of plasma amino acid analyses. These results are illustrated for lysine in Fig. 4.1.

The concentration of amino acids in uterine vein blood has been compared with that in the brachial artery at Caesarian section for disproportion or placenta praevia. The levels are slightly higher in the uterine venous than in the systemic arterial blood and the differences are comparable with venous-arterial differences across the human forearm in the post-absorbative state (London, Foley & Webb 1965). The negative nitrogen balance across the uterus when the mother is in the post-absorbative state during surgery must be larger than across a comparable weight of skeletal muscle because of the higher uterine blood flow in comparison with the forearm, but may not necessarily apply to the placenta itself, for the proportions of venous drainage from the uterine muscle and placenta are not known. Uterine arterial α amino nitrogen is slightly higher than in the uterine vein, in the goat (Setnikar 1957).

ABNORMAL PREGNANCIES

The maternal plasma levels of individual amino acids in three groups of abnormal pregnancies were compared with normal controls, delivered vaginally at 39–40 weeks, and by Caesarian section, at 37–39 weeks' gestation; each group consisting of five to six subjects. Two of the abnormal groups were delivered vaginally, the first prematurely at 34–38 weeks' gestation and the second post-term between 42–45 weeks' gestation; the third group consisted of mothers of dysmature infants of 37–40 week's gestational age delivered by Caesarean section. No significant differences for any of the amino acids could be shown between the groups. This is illustrated by lysine in Fig. 4.1. In a preliminary study of the plasma amino acid levels in postmaturity in the Guernsey cow, Foley, Holm, London & Young (1967) also found no differences between the normal cow and those bearing calves 13–55 days post-term: however, Clemetson & Churchman (1954) found a rise in the total α amino nitrogen in the last trimester in women with toxaemia of pregnancy.

FOETAL AMINO ACID ENVIRONMENT

DURING GESTATION

Crumpler, Dent & Lindan (1950) and Clemetson & Churchman (1954) found a higher total α amino nitrogen content in the umbilical venous than in maternal antecubital vein plasma at term with an average foetal : maternal plasma ratio of the order of 1·8. With a fuller analysis of the individual amino acids, by paper chromatography (Crumpler *et al.* 1950) and by ion exchange chromatography (Glendenning *et al.* 1961, Ghadimi & Pecora 1964, Lindbland & Baldestan 1967, and Young & Prenton 1969), in umbilical vein blood collected from normal deliveries at term, each amino acid was found to be higher than in the maternal venous plasma. Each had a different foetal : maternal plasma ratio, which varied from 1·2–4·0, and of the essential amino acids only lysine had a high ratio, between 2·5–4·0. Ghadimi & Pecora (1964), and Young & Prenton (1969) found a tendency for higher umbilical venous levels early in the second trimester, when the growth rate starts to accelerate, than at term. No significant difference was found for the majority of the amino acids in the umbilical venous plasma in the two normal groups, the one delivered vaginally, and the second by Caesarian section: this is illustrated for lysine, again (Fig. 4.1). The variations in concentration were greater than in the maternal venous plasma. Some significant linear relationships between maternal and foetal levels were found, which were related to the transport group of the amino acid, but not to whether it was essential for growth. A linear relationship, over a wide range of concentration, has also been shown for phenylalanine in monkeys fed a diet high in phenylalanine (Kerr, Chamove, Harlow and Waisman 1968).

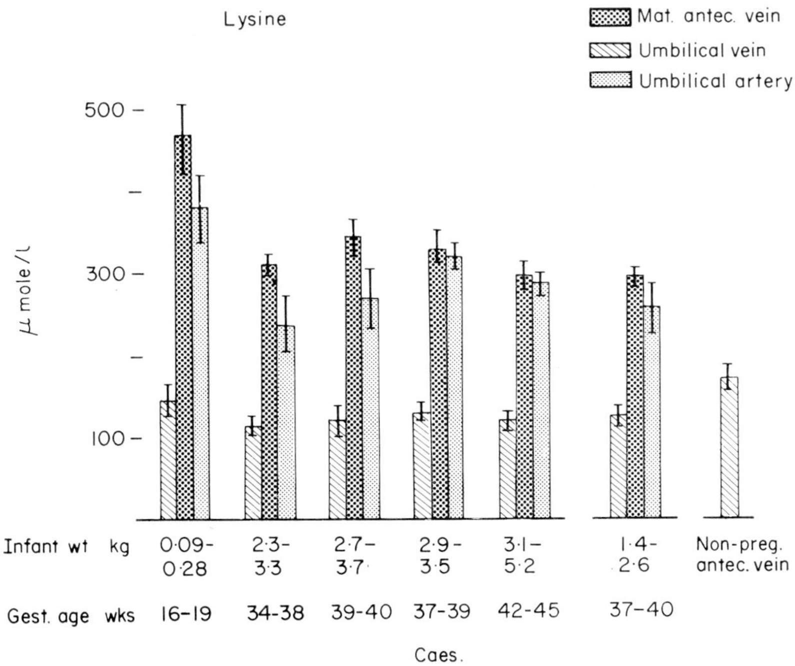

FIG. 4.1. Plasma lysine concentration, demonstrating the relationship between maternal venous and umbilical vein and artery levels during gestation, in different types of delivery and 'small for dates' infants.

ABNORMAL GESTATION

The levels of free amino acids in the umbilical vein plasma of the premature, postmature, and dysmature groups already described did not differ from those in the normal controls at term (Fig. 4.1). These observations suggest that regulation of the amino acid environment continues into the post-term period, and that it is not impaired and therefore not a limiting factor for growth, in the small-for-dates infant. These small infants had a mean birth weight of 2·0 kg in comparison with 3·1 kg for the normal infant of comparable age delivered in the hospital.

The placentas were also small, but no impairment of histological structure was found in the placentas from similar cases by Aherne & Dunnill (1966). These findings are in contrast with bovine postmaturity, in which gross impairment of placental histological structure occurs (Holm, Salvatore & Zeek-Minning 1964): low levels of some amino acids were found in the umbilical venous plasma of these calves, which were also two thirds of their expected weight when delivered by Caesarian section, 13 to 55 days post-term (Foley *et al.* 1967). Impairment of other metabolic activities of the placenta was found (Holm & Galligan 1962).

UMBILICAL VENOUS-ARTERIAL DIFFERENCES DURING GESTATION

Differences between the umbilical vein and artery plasma levels of the amino acids vary widely. At 16–19 weeks, the concentration of each amino acid is usually higher in the umbilical vein than in the artery, and the differences larger than at any other time in gestation; this is shown in Fig. 4.2 for the six amino acids, threonine, glycine, alanine, leucine, lysine and arginine. The umbilical V-A differences are small in post-term infants and those delivered by Caesarian Section. In 'small for dates' infants the differences are comparable with term infants (Prenton & Young 1969). At the end of the third trimester the V-A differences for glycine, serine and glutamic acid are frequently reversed, with higher concentrations in the artery than the vein. Rooth & Nilsson (1964) also observed higher concentrations of glutamic acid in the umbilical artery plasma than in the vein plasma at term. Horska, Janda, Stembera & Novak (1966) found α amino nitrogen to be about 8 per cent higher in umbilical artery plasma than in the umbilical vein plasma.

TRANSPORT CHARACTERISTICS

The active nature of the transport of amino acids across the placental membrane was suggested by Christensen & Streicher (1948) who first established the high foetal : maternal plasma α amino acid ratios. At term these were found to range from 5 : 1 in the guinea pig, to 2 : 1 in the rabbit and in the human; Huggett & Slater (1966) have found a ratio of 2–3 : 1 in the sheep. The total amino nitrogen concentration in the fluid of hydatidiform moles is similar to that in the umbilical vein (McKay, Roby, Hertig & Richardson 1955), suggesting placental regulation of foetal plasma amino acid levels. The part played by the maternal : foetal plasma amino acid differences in causing the trans-placental electrical potential measured in goats is not known (Meschia, Wolkoff & Barron 1958).

The transport mechanisms are qualitatively similar to those in other tissues. Competition between the mechanisms for glycine and histidine,

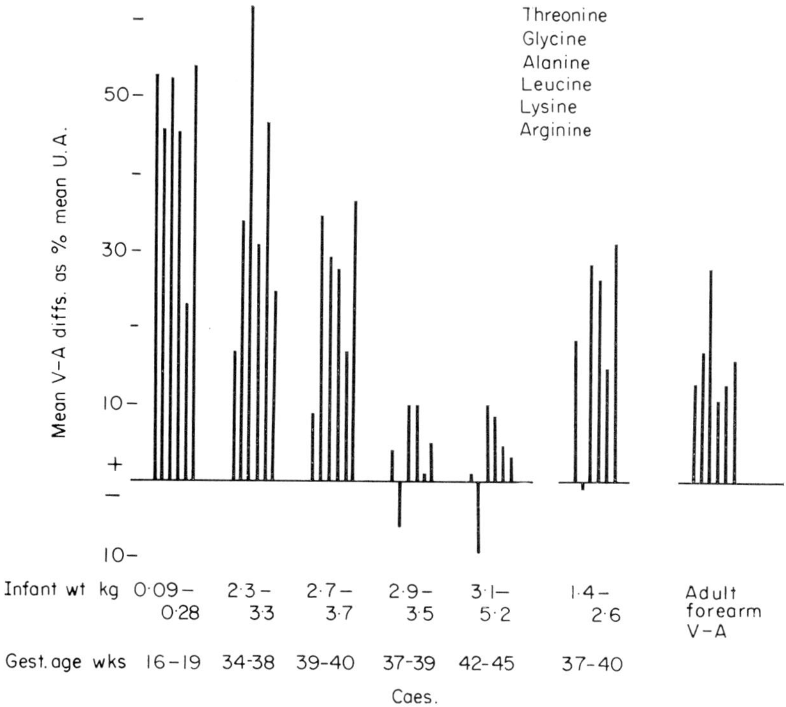

FIG 4.2. Mean umbilical V-A differences for six amino acids, expressed as a percentage of the mean umbilical artery value during gestation, in different types of delivery and 'small for dates' infants.

methionine and proline, but not glutamic acid have been demonstrated (Christensen & Streicher 1948); saturation of the transport mechanism for histidine has been shown by Dancis, Olson & Folkart (1958). Selective transport of the natural L isomer of histidine was observed in the human subject, by Page, Glendenning, Margolis & Harper 1957 and confirmed by Mischel (1963). It would be interesting to know whether cystine was transferred across the placenta in the homozygous offsprng of cystinuric patients, for it is known that the transport defect occurs in the small intestine as well as in the renal tubule (Milne, Asatoor, Edwards & Doughridge 1961).

Concentration of amino acids by the placenta during transport has been demonstrated using labelled compounds (Hayter, Hutchinson, Karvonen & Young 1964, Dancis, Money, Springer & Levitz 1968) as was shown for phosphate using P^{32} (Fuchs 1957) and iron (Bothwell, Pribilla, Mebust & Finch 1958). The free amino acid concentration in the trophoblast is 40–50 mg per cent in the guinea pig and the sheep (Reynolds & Young 1968), higher than in the foetal plasma and midway between that of the foetal skeletal muscle (Christensen & Streicher 1948) and foetal liver. Transport from the maternal to the foetal blood stream is accompanied by a further increase in concentration in the placenta, which does not occur if the labelled amino acid is injected into the foetal blood stream; this demonstrates that active accumulation occurs on the maternal side of the placenta and access to the foetal blood stream probably takes place by simple diffusion from the trophoblast down the concentration gradient. The rise in foetal plasma glycine and glutamic acid concentrations have been shown to be greater than in the maternal plasma after feeding (Christensen & Streicher 1948).

The rate of transfer of amino nitrogen, across the goat's placenta, has been calculated from uterine A-V differences and blood flow measurements (Setnikar 1957). Net accumulation in the foetus during a given period has been used to study some of the mechanisms controlling transport (Hayter *et al.* 1964, Young 1965): the method measures the combined influence of transport capacity and blood flow. A single intravenous injection of α amino isobutyric acid (A.I.B.) was given to unanaesthetized guinea pigs: this model amino acid is transported as glycine by the small intestine (Akedo & Christensen 1962) but not metabolized and, therefore, simple to recover quantitatively (Noall, Riggs, Walker & Christensen 1957). It can be seen in Table 4.1 that the amount transferred was proportional to the weight of the foetus and placenta but, if a runt was only half the average litter weight, the uptake might be only 15 per cent of that of the largest foetus. Varying capacities for amino acid uptake were also found in individual foetuses and placentae of the same weight in a litter. Clemetson & Churchman (1955) showed differences in the levels of the total α amino nitrogen in the umbilical venous plasma of twins, and differences in concentration of the individual amino acids also occurs. Foetal uptake of amino acids was reduced when the metabolic inhibitors ouabain, penicillamine and pentobarbitone were given to the mother, but neither oestrogen nor progesterone influenced uptake. Quinto, Orlandi & Bottiglioni (1964) also found that progesterone was without effect on the transport of ^{14}C labelled amino acids across the placenta in the rat, though cortisone caused a marked decrease in transport. This suggests that hormones influence transport only indirectly through their action on muscular structures in the blood

TABLE 4.1

The placental transfer of α amino isobutyric acid in relation to placental and foetal weight in the guinea pig.

Litter mates	1	2	3	1	2	3	4
Placental weight in g.	6·4	5·9	5·4	8·5	5·8	3·8	6·7
Foetal weight in g.	65	67	62	72	66	34	67
Conc. A.I.B. ^{14}C c/sec:							
Foetal plasma	139	368	284	128	150	85	153
Placenta	170	403	394	203	230	142	217
Foetal liver	172	508	234	274	234	95	213
Total transferred to foetus c/sec × 10^3	23·0	38·8	30·9	18·7	12·7	2·5	13·0
		48 hr			$2\frac{1}{2}$ hr		

vessels and uterus allowing for increased blood flow and accommodation to the foetus. Oestrogen has been shown to increase amino acid uptake by the young rat uterus *in vivo* (Roberts & Szego 1953, Noall *et al.* 1957, Williams & Needham 1964) and by the human endometrium *in vitro* (Robertson, Hagerman, Richardson & Villee 1961). The influence of growth hormone on the placental transport of amino acids has not been studied nor that of the growth hormone-like lactogen produced by the placenta (Josimovitch & Brande 1965). Inhibition of protein synthesis in the foetus by puromycin or actinomycin D, and the inhibition of the production of thyroid hormone by thiouracil were all without effect on foetal amino acid uptake, suggesting that placental transport is independent of the requirements of the foetus.

PLASMA DISAPPEARANCE RATE AS A TEST FOR PLACENTAL FUNCTION

The capture of labelled amino acid by the conceptus, following a single injection into the maternal blood stream, was swift and amounted to

30–40 per cent of the injected dose within an hour in the term guinea pig. Hayter *et al.* (1964). This suggested the possibility of using the maternal plasma disappearance rate of a suitable substance as a clinical test for placental function during gestation. Ideally, such a substance should be cleared relatively slowly from the maternal plasma in order to make

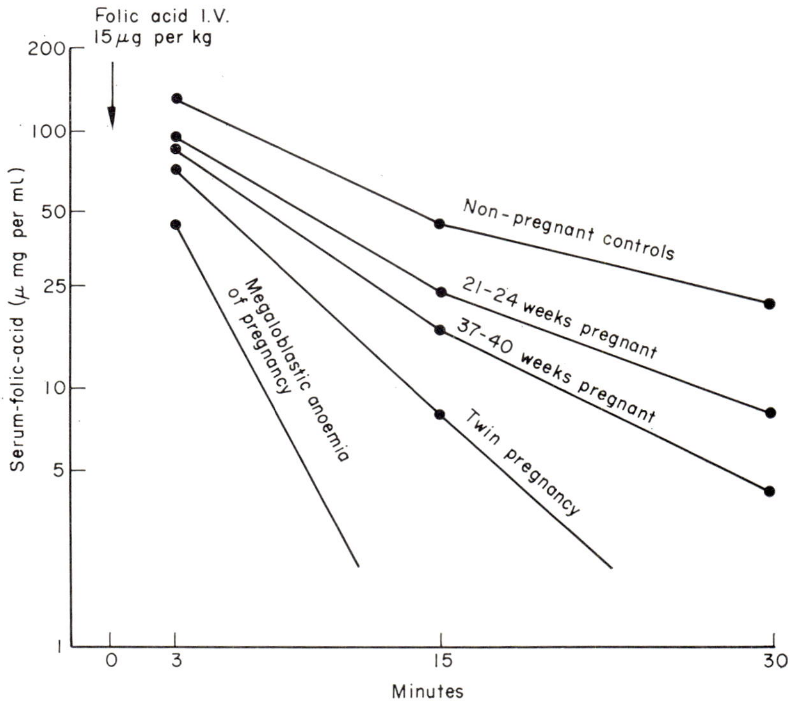

FIG. 4.3. Plasma disappearance curves for exogenous folic acid in the non-pregnant and pregnant woman, at 21–24 and 37–40 weeks' gestation; in twin pregnancies and megaloblastic anaemia of pregnancy. [Chanarin I. *et al.* (1959). Reproduced by kind permission of the authors and the editor of the *Lancet*.]

accurate measurements and, as completely as possible into the foetus, the metabolic activity of which is to be measured: minimal quantities would have to be used so that the transport mechanisms were not interfered with. Radioactively labelled compounds would be unsuitable and the maternal body pool for the test substance should not alter during gestation. The test should be simple and repeatable without discomfort to the mother.

Preliminary observations in rabbits using the model amino acid, amino isobutyric acid labelled with ^{14}C, showed that amino acids would be unsuitable because their half life in the plasma is less than a minute: the conceptus influenced the final slow portion of the plasma disappearance curve, only marginally, at the end of term. Riboflavin, folic acid, and Vit B_{12} and Vit C which are also known to have high foetal :

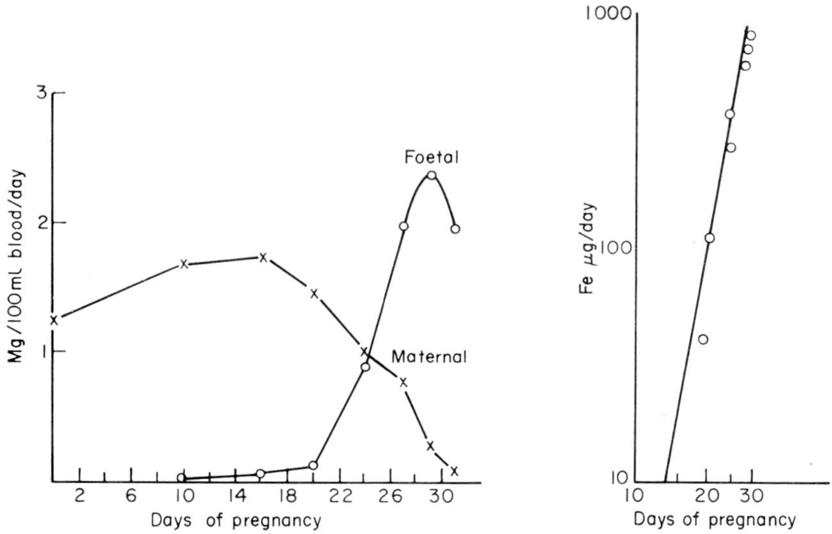

FIG. 4.4. A. Plasma iron turnover during pregnancy in the rabbit. Iron assimilated by maternal and foetal tissues. B. Placental transport of iron: iron uptake, derived from analysis of foetus and from maternal plasma iron turnover and per cent foetal iron uptake. [Bothwell T.H., Pribilla W.F., Mebust W. & Finch C.A. (1958). Reproduced by kind permission of the authors and the editor, *American Journal of Physiology*.]

maternal plasma ratios (Hagerman & Villee 1960, Widdas 1961, Dancis 1960) might be suitable but have the disadvantage that their body pools are not regulated and are subject to deficiencies, primarily dietic, which may be enhanced by the demands of the developing foetus. During a study of megaloblastic anaemia in pregnancy, Chanarin, MacGibbon, O'Sullivan & Mollin (1959) have shown that the maternal plasma clearance of a single dose of exogenous unlabelled folic acid was related to gestational age. The marked increase in plasma disappearance rate during the first 20 weeks of gestation might have been related to placental growth, but the further increase between 20 and 40 weeks was unexpectedly small as can be seen in Fig. 4.3.

Observations on the rabbit suggest that iron has the two properties most required for testing placental function, a long plasma half life and a foetal clearance related to gestational age. Bothwell *et al.* (1958) found that 5 per cent of an injected dose of ^{59}Fe was transferred across the placenta to the foetus at 19 days' gestation, in comparison with 90 per cent at term. Their findings are summarized in Fig. 4.4. Renton (personal communication) also has preliminary evidence that plasma ^{59}Fe

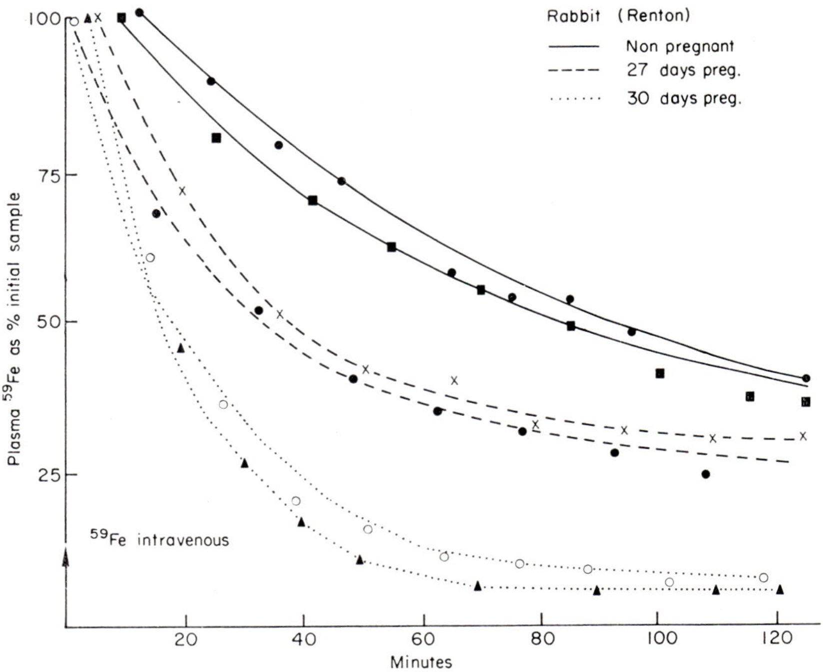

FIG. 4.5. The increase in plasma disappearance rate of ^{59}Fe during gestation in the rabbit. (From data kindly supplied by Dr. J.Renton.)

disappearance curves are related to gestational age in the rabbit. Figure 4.5 shows the slow clearance in the non-pregnant rabbit, with the increase at 27 and 30 days' gestation, when the initial slope of the disappearance curve is steeper and the final level in the plasma smaller. Whether such a relationship exists in the human is not known. The plasma clearance may also be complicated by iron deficiency. However, it is possible that investigation of plasma clearance rates during pregnancy may provide a simple and reliable test for assessing the metabolic activity of the foeto-placental unit *in utero*, and may replace that of urinary hormone excretion, which is known to represent only 10–20 per cent of their turnover rate.

OXYGEN TRANSFER

There have been many interesting advances in placental physiology during the last three years, and most have been concerned primarily with gaseous exchange and have been demonstrated in animal preparations. The observations pertain to general biological phenomena which will probably only differ quantitatively amongst the species and, moreover, the principles involved are applicable to the maternal-foetal exchange whether it be dependent upon the active nature of the placental membrane or upon simple diffusion.

Pride of place must be given to Barron and his colleagues, at Yale, who have developed a technique for chronic implantation of catheters in the umbilical vessels, in sheep foetuses *in utero*, so that sampling may be carried out in the unanaesthetized animal in its natural posture. This opens up the possibility of investigating the whole intra-uterine environment and the controlling mechanisms in the undisturbed foetus; further, a comparison between the values observed by this method and those found at Caesarian section and following normal deliveries in animals, may help in the definition of the intra-uterine environment of the human foetus where sampling is only possible during or after delivery. The constancy of the umbilical venous blood flow, for two minutes after delivery of the human infant, observed by Stembera and his colleagues in Prague, may also provide additional evidence for the relative value of umbilical vein blood samples at delivery as representing the intra-uterine environment.

Secondly, comes the establishment by Dawes and his colleagues in Oxford of the high oxygen consumption of the placenta, which is about 10 ml/kg/min and double that of the foetus itself. They also demonstrated the part which this high oxygen consumption plays in the fall in oxygen tension gradient across the placenta; from the practical point of view this observation is important in any attempt to increase the oxygen supply to the foetus during delivery. Utilization of other metabolites by the placenta must similarly affect the maternal-foetal gradients, which the activity of the membrane maintains for essential constituents.

Thirdly, Aherne & Dunnill have, from histological specimens, provided further values for the capillary and chorionic villous surface areas available for exchange in the normal human placenta, together with a comparison of the differences which may be found in diseased states. Finally, Metcalfe has demonstrated, by perfusion techniques, that a proportion of the blood flow passes through non-exchanging areas on the foetal side of the sheep's placenta.

OXYGEN UTILIZATION OF THE FOETUS COMPARED WITH THAT OF THE PLACENTA

The oxygen requirements of the early human foetus have been calculated from umbilical V-A oxygen differences and umbilical vessel blood flow measured with an electromagnetic flow meter (Assali, Rauramo & Peltonen 1960). An oxygen consumption of 4–6 ml/kg/min was observed at 9–28 weeks' gestation and is comparable with that observed at term for the whole uterus by Romney, Reid, Metcalf & Burwell (1955), who measured uterine A-V oxygen differences and uterine blood flow by the nitrous oxide technique, at Caesarian section. These values are comparable with that for the human adult, the full term foetal lamb (Acheson, Dawes & Mott 1957) and foetal goat (Huckabee, Metcalfe, Prystowsky & Barron 1962).

Assali *et al.* (1960) consider the oxygen consumption of the human placenta *in situ* to be high because the total uterine oxygen consumption increases at a faster rate than that of the foetus alone, between 18 and 28 weeks' gestation. Their findings are shown in Fig. 4.6. The oxygen consumption was calculated from uterine A-V oxygen differences and uterine blood flow measured with an electromagnetic flow meter; the evidence is slender because of the relatively few measurements it was possible to make. Campbell, Dawes, Fishman, Hyman & James (1966) have measured the oxygen consumption of the perfused sheep placenta *in situ* after arrest of the maternal circulation, and find a rate of 10 ml O_2/kg/min. This has recently been confirmed by Meschia, Cotter, Makowski & Barron (1967). Full term, isolated perfused human placentae consume oxygen at the rate of only 0·2–1·0 ml/kg/min (Nyberg & Westin 1957) and similar values are observed for placental tissue slices in many species. Friedman & Sachtleben (1960) have provided the most recent supporting evidence in these preparations of the human placenta and found that the rate of oxygen consumption decreased as gestation advanced; these results are yet another reminder of the quantitative and, possibly, qualitative inadequacy of techniques involving isolated tissues. Beaconsfield, Ginsberg & Panigel (1968) have electron microscopic evidence that the syncytiotrophoblast, from three-month placentas, disintegrates within minutes in incubation medium, the cytotrophoblast remaining intact. There are no observations on the term placenta.

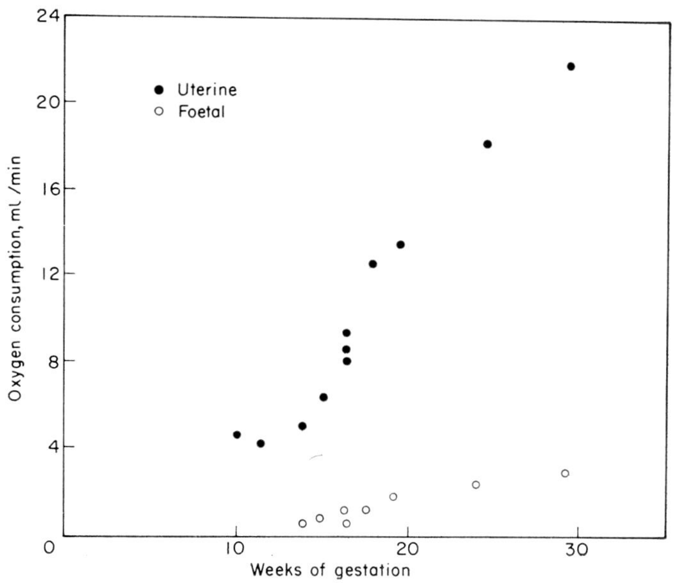

FIG. 4.6. A comparison of the total oxygen consumption of the foetus, and uterus and conceptus, from 10–30 weeks' gestation. [Assali N.S., Rauramo L. & Peltonen T. (1960) Reproduced by kind permission of the authors and the editor, *American Journal of Obstetrics and Gynaecology*.]

At term the oxygen requirements of a 3 kg foetus is probably about 15 ml/min and of the 600 g placenta about 6 ml/min, nearly one-third of the total oxygen consumption of the conceptus. The oxygen requirements of the uterus are unknown.

Zeuthen (1953) showed that whole body O_2 uptake in a variety of species varied with size according to an equation which contained a constant found experimentally to be about 0·7. Aherne (1966) also observed in the human subject that the foetal : placental weight relationship could be expressed by the formula $w = 2{\cdot}1\ W^{0{\cdot}67}$, where w = placental weight and W = foetal weight. Since the chorionic villous surface was found to vary as the placental weight throughout gestation (Aherne & Dunnill 1966) it may be concluded that the foetal O_2 consumption is also related to the $\frac{2}{3}$ power of the chorionic villous surface during intra-uterine life.

FOETAL OXYGEN ENVIRONMENT AND CHARACTER OF THE FOETAL CIRCULATION

There is now little doubt that the oxygen tension in the umbilical vein blood *in utero* is considerably lower than in the maternal arterial blood. Quilligan, Katigbak & Hofschild (1965) found a mean figure of 30.9 mm Hg O_2 in umbilical vein blood following vertex deliveries, in which the foetal heart rate was monitored continuously during labour with no changes being observed. Freda & Adamsons (1964) found 37 mm Hg O_2 in the femoral arterial blood of a $27\frac{1}{2}$ week foetus at hysterotomy for intra-uterine exchange transfusion. Until recently it was not possible to tell how representative these values were of the intra-uterine environment, because no comparison could be made with samples obtained without any disturbance of the placental circulation. Meschia, Cotter, Breathnach & Barron (1965) have developed a technique for chronic implantation of catheters into the tributaries of the umbilical vessels in the sheep and goat foetus *in utero* so that serial blood samples could be studied from unanaesthetized animals unrestrained and in their natural posture; there was a good measure of agreement between the blood gas values obtained by this method and those found at Caesarian section in these species.

What is the availability of oxygen to the foetal tissues *in utero* with an umbilical venous O_2 tension of 30 mm Hg in comparison with the maternal arterial tension of 95 mm Hg? This has been measured in animals under nembutal anaesthesia by Misrahy, Beran, Spradley & Garwood (1960); diffusion limited polarographic electrodes, 100 μ in diameter and with a circumferential recording surface 2 mm in width, were inserted into the foetus without incising the uterine wall and with minimal disturbance of the placental circulation. In the brain and kidney the oxygen availability so measured was 18–30 per cent of the diffusion current in air, corresponding to 30–45 mm Hg oxygen tension for both foetal and maternal tissue. This equality of availability of oxygen to the foetal tissues, in spite of the low arterial oxygen tension is made possible by the particular adaptations of the foetal blood and the foetal circulation.

The differences between the maternal and foetal blood for gas transport are well known and are shown in Fig. 4.7 in their application to the human subject. The foetal oxygen capacity ranges from 20–25 vols per cent oxygen while the maternal is decreased during pregnancy and at term may be 15 vols per cent (Hytten & Leitch 1964). The position of the oxygen dissociation curves *in vivo* are separated only by the influence of

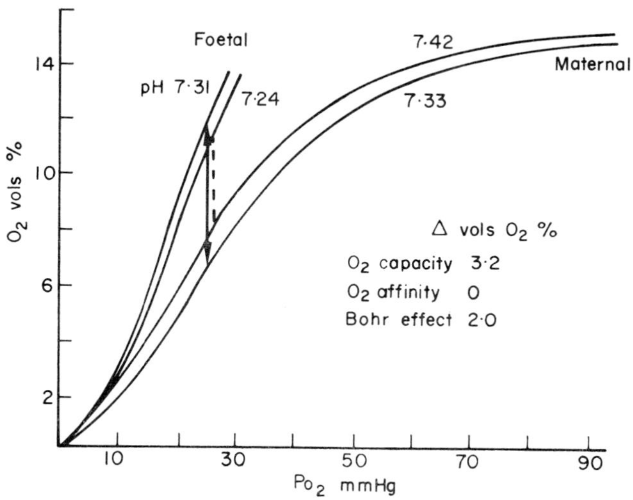

FIG. 4.7. The parts played by oxygen capacity, oxygen affinity and Bohr effect, during oxygen transport from maternal to foetal blood in the human. [Bartels H. & Metcalfe J. (1965) Reproduced by kind permission of the authors and the editor, *Proceedings of the International Union of Physical Science.*]

the different pH in the two body fluids: this was long disputed in the human, because, though the affinities of the two haemoglobins in solution are different, the environment of the red cells makes the two oxygen dissociation curves identical at the same pH. At the placental site the curves are separated further by the simultaneous exchange of carbon dioxide, the Bohr effect influencing the curves in opposite directions and ensuring a three volumes O_2 per cent content difference in favour of the foetus in the 20–30 mm Hg oxygen tension range. The steepness of the foetal oxygen dissociation curve provides a large volume supply to the foetal tissues over small oxygen tension differences. The average foetal venous-arterial oxygen differences across the maternal and foetal placenta are similar, 6·8 vols per cent, and similar to the foetal vessels at delivery (Metcalfe, Bartels & Moll 1967).

The circulatory characteristics of the human foetus *in utero* are not so well known as those for the foetal blood and have to be inferred from those of the newly born infant (Young 1966). Once the temporary disturbances due to delivery are over, the mean arterial pressure of the newborn infant measured in the lower aorta is the same as in the umbilical artery at term, 70/40 mm Hg: the cardiac output is about 540 ml/min, or 180 ml/kg body weight, which is at least double that of the adult; and the evidence for peripheral blood flow suggests that this also is high, 4–6 ml/100 g/min. These properties of the circulation, a low perfusion pressure and high conductance are adaptations suitable to maintain the foetal oxygen supply at adult levels in spite of the low arterial oxygen tension. The high cardiac output probably also rules out the possibility of any further increase to maintain the arterial pressure and peripheral flow during acute asphyxia. In the newborn infant, it is known that the arterial pressure is not maintained when the oxygen supply is halved, in spite of the tachycardia and, as bradycardia follows when the reduction in oxygen supply is continued for 6 minutes, the arterial pressure falls profoundly (James & Rowe 1957). However, a decrease in total oxygen consumption has been demonstrated in experimental animals at low arterial oxygen tensions (Cross, Dawes & Mott 1959): this is possibly due to the peripheral vasoconstriction which occurs, enabling the cerebral and coronary flows to be maintained at the expense of the less vital tissues; the bradycardia may conserve the oxygen requirements of the heart as in the diving animal (Korner 1959).

PLACENTAL TRANSFER OF OXYGEN

FOETAL PLACENTAL BLOOD FLOW

CAPILLARY AND VILLOUS SURFACE AREAS

Though primarily dependent on the maternal circulation the foetal heart and circulation is responsible finally for ensuring the transport and exchange of all the metabolites across the placental membrane. Barron (1944) and Barcroft (1946) drew attention to the ever-changing proportions of the foetal cardiac output flowing through its own organs and the placenta, which must alter both quantitatively and relatively to each other during development. Figure 4.8 demonstrates the static aspects of this relationship between the human foetus and placenta: before 12 weeks of

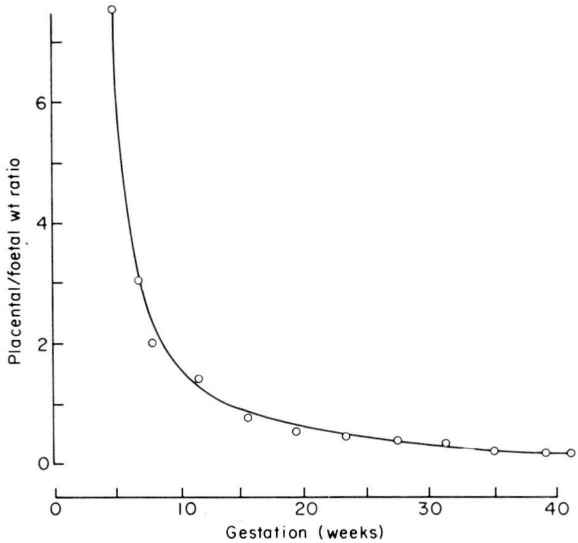

FIG. 4.8. The relationship of the placental/foetal weight ratio to gestational age. [Aherne W. (1966) Reproduced by kind permission of the author and the editor, *Biologia Neonatorum*.]

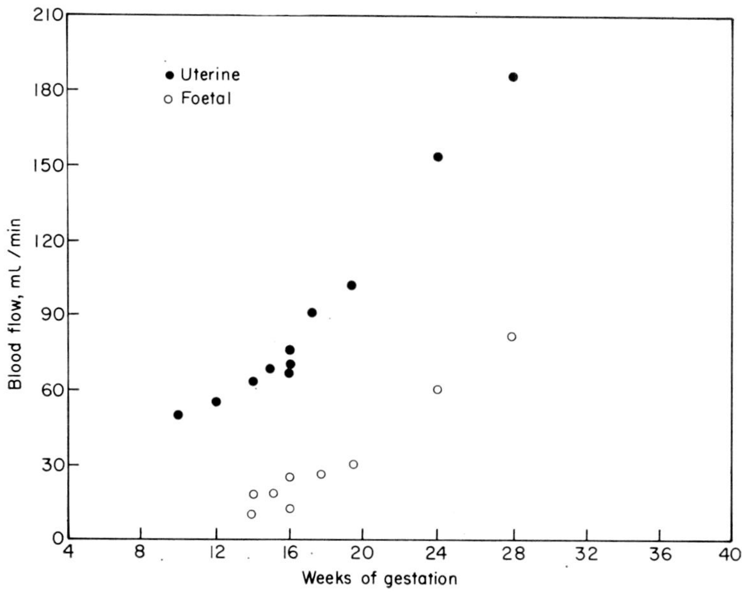

FIG. 4.9. A comparison of the uterine blood flow with that of the foetus from 10–30 weeks' gestation. [Assali N.S., Rauramo L. & Peltonen T. (1960) Reproduced by kind permission of the authors and the editor, *American Journal of Obstetrics and Gynaecology*.]

age the foetus is smaller than the placenta, and thereafter increasingly larger (Aherne 1966).

Assali *et al.* (1960) using an electromagnetic flow meter on the umbilical vein observed flows which ranged from 8·5 ml/min for an 80 g human foetus at 12 weeks' gestation, to 80 ml/min for a 650 g foetus at 28 weeks as shown in Fig. 4.9. The foetal placental blood flow was

TABLE 4.2

Summary of placental morphometry in normal and abnormal pregnancies. Figures in brackets indicate standard deviation. [Reproduced from Aherne & Dunnill (1966).]

	Normal*	Maternal hypertension†	Abnormally small infants‡
Placental volume (ml)	488 (99)	363 (77)	350 (65)
Non-parenchyma (%)	20·8 (3·6)	21·6 (1·7)	29·0 (7·4)
Volume proportions of parenchyma:			
Intervillous space	35·8 (3·2)	39·2 (5·7)	35·8 (4·9)
Chorionic villi	57·9 (5·7)	60·7 (6·1)	61·4 (6·2)
Fibrin	4·3 (2·1)	2·7 (1·0)	4·1 (2·0)
Villous surface area (m^2)	11·0 (1·3)	7·7 (1·6)	6·4 (1·4)
Capillary surface area (m^2)	12·2 (1·5)	10·3 (2·9)	6·8 (1·6)
Proportion of villus occupied by trophoblast	25·3 (1.9)	18·8 (1·0)	22·3 (3·7)

* Mean values of 10 cases at 39–40 weeks' gestation.
† Mean values of 7 cases at 39–40 weeks' gestation.
‡ Mean values of 6 cases at 39–40 weeks' gestation.

calculated to be 11 ml/100 g/min as the placental weight increases from 50–400 g during this period of gestation.

The foetal blood flow increases five-fold during the last trimester while the final increase in placental weight is small. The umbilical blood flow at term is probably in the region of 250–300 ml (Stembera, Hodr & Janda (1965), which represents a high blood flow of the order of 50 ml/100 g placenta/min, equivalent to adult cerebral and liver blood flows. This increase in flow is brought about by the rising foetal arterial pressure and, possibly, a decrease in chorionic capillary resistance. Dawes (1962) has shown that, in the sheep, the effective perfusion pressure at term is still relatively small: in the human foetus the umbilical arterial blood pressure increases from 40/20 mm Hg at 5 months to 70/45 mm Hg at term (Woodbury, Robinow & Hamilton 1938); the umbilical venous pressure is high, about 24 mm Hg and the effective perfusion is therefore 25–30 mm Hg, less than half that across the intervillous space.

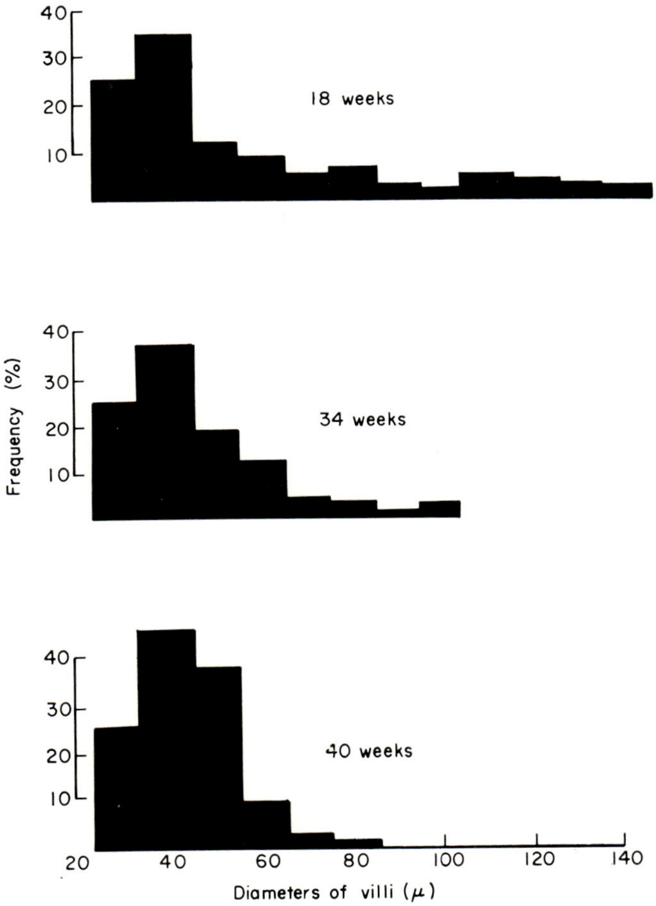

FIG. 4.10. Frequency distribution histogram of villous diameters at 18, 34 and 40 weeks' gestation. [Aherne W. & Dunnill M.S. (1966) Reproduced by kind permission of the authors and the editor, *British Medical Bulletin*.]

Quantitation of the surface area of living tissues is limited by suitable methods for sampling, fixing and measuring the histological structures. Recently, Aherne & Dunnill (1966) have been able to make suitable corrections for artifarcts introduced by fixation and embedding and,

6*

borrowing from the pulmonary physiologists and petrographers, they have used the mean linear intercept method and an equidistant point grid for calculating parenchyma volumes, and villous and capillary surface areas in the human placenta. A summary of the placental morphometry in normal and abnormal pregnancies is shown in Table 4.2. The mean value for the villous surface of $11 \pm 1{\cdot}3$ m_2 in 10 normal term placentas

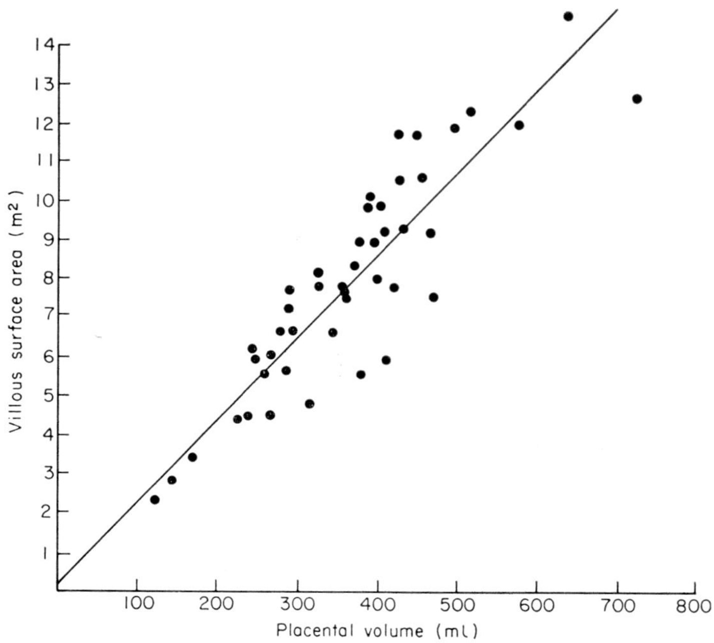

FIG. 4.11. The relation of chorionic villous surface area to placental volume. The regression line follows the equation $S = 0{\cdot}231 + 0{\cdot}0209\,V$; where S = the villous surface area in square metres, V = the total placenta volume in ml, ($r = 0{\cdot}894$; $P < 0{\cdot}001$). [Aherne W. & Dunnill M.S. (1966) Reproduced by kind permission of the authors and the editor, *British Medical Bulletin*.]

is lower than that given by Wilkin (1960), probably because care was taken to distinguish between the parenchyma and non-parenchyma volumes of the placenta; the contribution of the microvilli to the surface area is not included. The formation of new chorionic villi is responsible for the increase in weight of both the early and late placenta (Kline 1951), and the frequency distribution of villous diameters is constant from 18–40 weeks, with a modal diameter at 40–49 μ as shown in Fig. 4.10.

The villous surface area increases threefold during the last trimester but the volume proportions of villous tissue and intervillous space remain constant as the placenta enlarges. In the normal placenta there is a direct relationship ($r = 0{\cdot}894$), between villous surface area and placental volume which is demonstrated in Fig. 4.11.

In term placentas the mean foetal capillary volume was 45 ml, which represents about 10 per cent of the placental volume; this is small in comparison with the 70–100 ml found by Kayser (1955) using the dilution of ^{32}P, and about half that found by Fuchs (1957) in the guinea pig. The capillary surface area ranged from 0·4 m^2 to 1·8 m^2 during the last trimester; it depended upon the vascular filling but corresponded closely to the villous surface area.

MATERNAL PLACENTAL BLOOD FLOW

INTERVILLOUS SPACE

Enlargement of the uterine arteries can be demonstrated radiologically by the 3rd month of gestation, and their diameters may exceed the non-pregnant size, two to three fold, at term (Fernstrom 1955). The female hormones are partly responsible for this enlargement and the influence of exogenous oestrogen on uterine artery diameter has been demonstrated in secondary amenorrhoea. But what makes the uterine vessels particularly susceptible to hormonal influence at this time? Is there a common stimulus which is also partly responsible for the development of the increased blood supply to malignant growths, or to the development of collateral circulations?

At term the maternal placental flow is probably 600–700 ml/min. This flow is high, about 100 ml/100 g placenta/min: the value has been obtained both with the uterine wall intact and during Caesarian section; Browne & Veall (1953) used radioactive sodium disappearance from the decidual space and Romney *et al.* (1955) and Assali, Douglass, Baird, Nicholson & Suyemoto (1953) the nitrous oxide method with catheterization of the uterine vein. On a few occasions, between 12–28 weeks' gestation Assali *et al.* (1960) used an electro-magnetic flow meter on the uterine artery; the observed flows were comparable with the term pregnancies, in relation to the placental weight.

The effective perfusion pressure of the maternal placental circulation is high, about 80 mm Hg since the spiral artery funnels open directly into the base of the choriodecidual space, where the pressure is not more than 10 mm Hg (Hendricks, Quilligan, Tyler & Tucker 1959). The projection of the arterial blood between the villi has been demonstrated radiologically in the human subject, following retrograde injection of radio-opaque material into the femoral artery (Borell, Fernstrom & Westman 1958).

Both Aherne & Dunnill (1966) and Wilkin (1960) have calculated from histological specimens that the intervillous space occupies about 34–37 per cent of the placental parenchyma at term, which corresponds to a mean volume of 144 ml blood. This volume is high in comparison with the 70–100 ml found by ^{32}P dilution (Kayser 1955); similarly, the

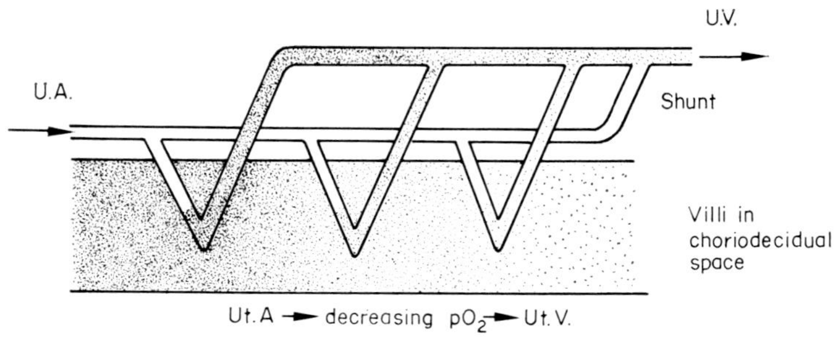

FIG. 4.12. Schematic diagram showing the effect of the inhomogeneity of the intervillous space upon the composition of blood in the chorionic villi and umbilical vein. [Bartels H. & Metcalfe J. (1965) Reproduced by kind permission of the authors and the editor, *Proceedings of the International Union of Physical Sciences*.]

guinea pig placenta only contains 20 per cent by volume of maternal blood which is equal to its foetal blood content at term (Fuchs 1957). The available evidence at present suggests a 1 : 2 ratio between the foetal and maternal blood contents of the human placenta at term.

The anatomical relation of the two placental circulations has been fully discussed in Chapter 1. From the functional point of view, Bartels (1959) has compared the foetal capillaries in the intervillous space with the pulmonary capillaries in the alveoli: but, while the pulmonary capillaries equilibrate with a practically homogenous gas phase in the alveoli, the foetal capillaries are bathed by maternal blood moving continuously, which will not alter greatly in composition as it passes each villus; moreover, this maternal blood will vary in composition depending upon the position of the villus in relation to the arterial and venous ostia, a situation which is analogous to unequal ventilation perfusion relationships in the adult lung. These relationships are schematically shown in Fig. 4.12. The composition of the umbilical vein blood will depend upon contributions from all these villi and will alter as the perfusion relations change. The inhomogeneity of the intervillous space has been demonstrated in the human subject by Fuchs, Spackman & Assali (1963) by sampling simultaneously from different sites.

DIFFUSION GRADIENT ACROSS THE PLACENTAL MEMBRANE

The most complete account of the factors concerned in the physiology of gas transport across the placenta together with the reasons for the large tension difference between the maternal and foetal arterial blood have been provided by Bartels, Moll & Metcalfe (1962) and Bartels & Metcalfe (1965). No data exists making it necessary to consider mechanisms other than simple diffusion of oxygen from the maternal to the foetal blood.

The anatomical factors concerned in gas transport across the placental membrane are the thickness of this membrane, the area of the diffusing surface and the spatial relation of the foetal and maternal vessels; their effectiveness depends upon the directions and volume flow of the two blood streams together with the properties of the dissociation curves. Attempts have been made to calculate the overall efficiencies of the mechanism for the transport of oxygen, that is the "diffusing capacity" or the ml of gas transferred per mm oxygen tension difference per minute, using Fick's diffusion equation,

$$\frac{dm}{dt}=\frac{Df}{b}(C_1-C_2)$$

where:

$\frac{dm}{dt}$ = the amount crossing per unit time, in the steady state.

D = the diffusion co-efficient, which is dependent upon the properties of the membrane and diffusing substances; this is not known for the placenta, and the value for skeletal muscle is usually used, $2{\cdot}7\times 10{\cdot}7$ cm^2/sec. Atm at 37°C.

f = the diffusing surface; the capillary and villous surface areas have been defined previously.

b = the thickness of the membrane and the layers of maternal and foetal blood through which diffusion or transport takes place. Electron microscope studies show that the thickness of the placental membrane is of the order of 25 μ at 10 weeks' gestation and the reduction to 4–5 μ at term suggests an increased diffusing efficiency as gestation proceeds. The total distance through which the gases must diffuse also includes the thin layers of both foetal and maternal blood; in the foetal capillaries this is probably small and equivalent to the distance in the lungs, about 1 μ, but on the maternal side it is difficult to estimate. Histological studies suggest that the intervillous channels are broad, 20–30 μ, which would make the diffusing distance large; but artifacts due to a reduction in intervillous volume on delivery and to histological shrinkage are difficult to estimate. Substituting reasonable values for oxygen transport/min and the partial pressure difference for O_2 between maternal and foetal blood, into the Fick equation, Adamsons (1965) has calculated a possible total diffusing distance of 50–75 μ.

$C_1 - C_2$ = concentration difference across the membrane, which is $(P_1 - P_2)$ for a gas: these concentrations are maintained by the blood flow on each side of the placenta.

Bartels *et al.* (1962) point out that the only values which are known with certainty are the partial pressures of the respiratory gases in the maternal and in the foetal blood entering each side of the placenta, in the uterine and umbilical arteries. The changes in partial pressure due to gas exchange on the foetal side of the placenta have not been measured, for umbilical vein blood contains blood shunted through areas of placenta which do not take part in gaseous exchange; similarly on the maternal side of the placenta uterine vein blood is a mixture of true placental blood flow, blood which may have been shunted in the placenta and is, in addition, mixed with the uterine muscle blood flow. Moreover, the physiological conditions may be changed by the method of sampling; Wulf (1962) and Dawes (1965) review the range of values which can be obtained for the partial pressure of oxygen in the uterine and umbilical vessels in the human and in animals. The mean partial pressure differences across the placental membrane are therefore not known with certainty: the value for oxygen must be low, about 20 mm Hg, in comparison with 60 mm across the alveolar membrane.

Considering the efficiency of the placenta in comparison with the lung, Adamsons (1965), points out that the low tension in the intervillous space, about 40 mm Hg O_2, must set a limit to the amount of oxygen transferred; however, increased demands of the order of those found during exercise in the adult do not occur in intra-uterine life. On the other hand, the maternal placental blood flow, per ml O_2 transported to the foetus, is similar to the ventilation, per ml O_2 taken up by the pulmonary blood in the lungs, about 20 ml for each. Similarly, the coefficient of oxygen utilization, in ml per 100 ml, is comparable for both placental blood and inspired gas.

INFLUENCE OF PLACENTAL OXYGEN REQUIREMENTS

Recently, further difficulties in the way of calculating the diffusing capacity of the placenta have been demonstrated. Firstly, Bartels (1959) had suggested, on theoretical grounds, that the oxygen consumption of the placenta would influence any calculation of the diffusion gradient as though it were a maternal shunt. It is interesting that so little attention has previously been paid to this fact, because the active nature of the placental membrane is not in question and there has been indirect evidence for its high oxygen requirements for some time. This property of the placental membrane implies that a proportion of the metabolites being transferred must also be utilized and, their retention by the placenta will exceed transport to the foetus during the early development of the conceptus. Placental tissue is only unique from other secretory organs in that it must also exchange the respiratory gases and waste products of the foetus. Secondly, shunting of blood through non-exchanging areas of the placenta has also been suspected of influencing the diffusion gradient. Bøe (1954) has demonstrated possible channels on the foetal side of the human placenta, by injection techniques and Metcalfe, Moll, Bartels, Hilpert & Parer (1965) have, by a perfusion technique, demonstrated that 20 per cent of the blood on the foetal side of the sheep's placenta passes through non-exchanging areas.

Campbell *et al.* (1966) have provided experimental proof of the extent to which oxygen utilization of the placenta, and placental shunts, both maternal and foetal, may reduce the oxygen tension gradient across the placenta in the sheep. This was demonstrated in two ways. Firstly, the foetal placenta was perfused *in situ*, after removal of the foetus so that there could be no oxygen utilization from this source. At equilibrium the oxygen tension in the foetal blood was about 30 mm Hg below the maternal arterial oxygen tension. Secondly, the oxygen consumption of mature lambs with an intact placental circulation was met by positive pressure ventilation, providing an identical tension in both femoral arterial and umbilical vein blood which was, again, 30–40 mm Hg below the maternal arterial level. The oxygen utilization of the placenta is in series with the foetus and Campbell *et al.* consider it to account for practically the whole gradient between the maternal arterial and umbilical vein blood in the sheep, with a smaller contribution by the blood shunted in parallel through both sides of the placental and the foetal membranes. Longo, Power & Forster (1967) have determined the carbon monoxide diffusing capacity of the placenta in experimental animals.

These findings also provide a further explanation for the poor results obtained in any attempt to increase the oxygen supply to the distressed foetus by the administration of 100 per cent oxygen to the mother; the placental oxygen consumption is computed to be about one third of the oxygen consumption of the whole conceptus and, as it lies in series between the maternal and foetal circulation, its oxygen debt is likely to be satisfied before that of the foetus.

INFLUENCE OF CHANGES IN MATERNAL ENVIRONMENT

High altitudes

At 15,000 feet, both maternal and foetal adaptations take place to maintain the diffusing capacity of the placenta for oxygen: the maternal arterial pO_2 was found to be 45 mm Hg and the maternal placental blood flow 35 per cent above that in ewes at sea level (Huckabee, Metcalfe, Prystowsky, Hellegers, Meschia & Barron 1959). The haemoglobin at term is also higher than in foetuses born to mothers at sea level (Prystowsky, Hellegers, Meschia, Metcalfe, Huckabee & Barron 1960).

Experimental reduction in the amount of placental tissue is relatively easy in the sheep because the cotyledons may be plucked off the uterine wall without impairment of the remaining organ: Alexander (1964) has shown that there is a compensatory increase in size of the remaining cotyledons, which involves both foetal and maternal tissue.

Hypertensive disease. Small infants

In placentas associated with maternal hypertension the placental volume and the chorionic villous and foetal capillary surface areas were shown to be significantly reduced at term by Aherne & Dunnill (1966) (Table 4.2), moreover the proportion of villous structure occupied by trophoblast may be only 50 per cent of the normal quantity; Hertig (1960) found premature degeneration of the syncytial trophoblast, with nuclear disappearance, involving 90–100 per cent of the villi in toxaemia of pregnancy, as compared with 10–40 per cent of the villi in normal term placentas. In similar cases to those just described occlusive vascular lesions of the maternal placental bed have been described by Dixon & Robertson (1958). A reduction in intervillous blood flow to one-third of normal was also observed by Browne & Veall (1953) and, since the infants were born alive and survived, this suggests that the placental reserve is three times the normal demand. In animal experiments bradycardia does not occur until the oxygen supply is reduced to one-third (Young 1963). In a few infarcted placentas of stillborn foetuses the villous surface area was reduced to at least a third of the normal value (Aherne & Dunnill 1966).

In the placentas of abnormally small infants, whose birth weight fell below two standard deviations of that expected for their age, the mean placental volume was small and the mean villous surface area only half that of normal term placentas. The proportion of non-parenchymal components was relatively high and the incidence of infarction small, suggesting the absence of occlusive vascular lesions (Aherne & Dunnill 1966). These authors also found a 50 per cent increase in villous surface area in two placentas of infants with haemolytic disease; hyperplasia was observed in one case associated with maternal diabetes and a normal area found in one case of idiopathic hydrops.

Hormones. Maternal arterial gas tensions

It is possible that the uterine vessels are particularly susceptible to changes in their environment during pregnancy and, thus liable to occlusive lesions, firstly, because of their hormonal environment and, secondly, because the newly formed vessels may not be innervated. It has been shown in the guinea pig (Martin & Young 1960) that both oestrogen and progesterone sensitize the maternal placental blood vessels to the vasoconstrictor substances adrenaline and noradrenaline. Though this could not be confirmed for the uterine vessels in the rabbit (Martin & Young 1963) there is good evidence for the interaction of vasoactive substances and the steroid hormones which can be demonstrated in the human subject (Haigh, Kitchin & Pickford 1963) as well as in animals (Lloyd 1959).

The influence of the maternal arterial gas tensions and acid base balance on placental gas exchange and, indirectly, blood flow has been studied recently, in relation to the maternal administration of oxygen during foetal distress, and in relation to maternal hyperventilation during labour. Some authors have found an increase in umbilical vein oxygen

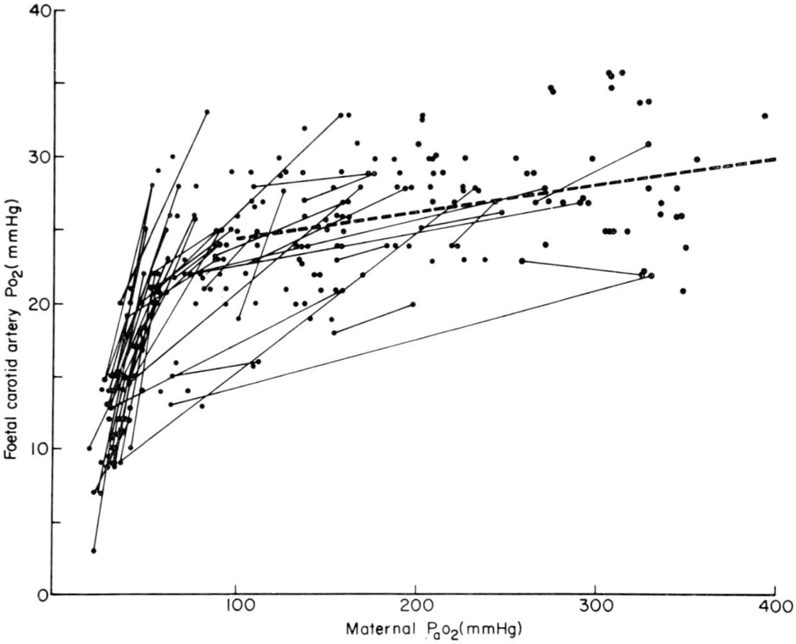

FIG. 4.13. Relation between maternal P_aO_2 and foetal carotid Po_2: maternal pH 7·20–7·60. Connected points represent multiple observations in one experiment.---- shows correlation between maternal and foetal values at maternal P_aO_2 100–400 mm Hg. [Ricard G., Motoyama E.K., Acheson F.M., Cook C.D. & Reynolds E.O.R. (1967) Reproduced by kind permission of the authors and the editor, *American Journal of Obstetrics and Gynaecology*.]

content with supplemental oxygen, given to the parturient woman or, added to the anaesthetic gas during Caesarian section: but Saling (1963a) observed a fall in Po_2 with a rise in Pco_2 in the umbilical vein blood at delivery, suggesting that a raised maternal arterial oxygen tension caused a reduction in placental blood flow; similar results have been observed in the ewe by Harned, Rowsham, Mackinney & Sugioka (1964).

These discrepancies may partly be explained by the influence of changes in acid-base balance due to labour and to maternal hyperventilation.

In a large series of anaesthetized pregnant sheep, in their last trimester, the relations of the maternal arterial and umbilical vein Po_2 were studied without the complications of alterations in the placental circulation due to labour by Rivard, Motoyama, Acheson, Cook & Reynolds (1967). Their results are shown in Fig. 4.13. A rise in maternal Po_2 of 10 mm Hg caused a rise in umbilical vein Po_2 of 4 mm Hg when the maternal Po_2 was less than 60 mm Hg, but a rise of only 0·5 mm Hg O_2 in the umbilical vein when the maternal Po_2 was above 60 mm Hg; the latter result is not surprising since the amount of oxygen in the maternal arterial blood can only be increased by 1 vol per cent, though the oxygen tension may be increased fivefold when 100 per cent is breathed. Finally, an increase in maternal arterial oxygen tension of 183 mm Hg, at a constant pH and Pco_2 raised the umbilical vein Po_2 by 14 mm Hg but reduced the umbilical arterial flow by about 9 per cent.

Moderate hyperventilation during labour was found by Moya, Morishima, Shnider & James (1965), to cause a slight alkalosis in the foetus as well as the mother in the human subject: but when the maternal alveolar Pco_2 was reduced to 17 mm Hg, the foetus became acidotic suggesting vasoconstriction and a reduction in placental blood flow. These observations have also been confirmed in guinea pigs (Morishima, Moya, Bossers & Daniels 1964) and in the lamb (Motoyama, Acheson, Rivard & Cook 1966). Low CO_2 tensions may be reached more readily during hyperventilation or assisted respiration in the pregnant woman because of her low resting Pco_2.

PLACENTAL FUNCTION DURING LABOUR

Studies of the metabolic relationships between the mother and her offspring during labour have been greatly stimulated in the last ten years by the work of James in New York, Saling in West Berlin, and Stembera in Prague: estimations made on maternal venous and umbilical vein blood, peripheral blood sampled repeatedly from the presenting part of the infant during labour, and umbilical V-A differences have been related to the foetal heart rate during labour, the passage of meconium and to the condition of the infant at birth. It is well established that during a normal labour there is minimal disturbance of acid-base balance in both mother and foetus; during prolonged labours, foetal oxygen debt occurs and the acid products of metabolism reduce the foetal plasma pH. This pH change, measured in the peripheral blood of the foetus, is some guide to the clinician for it has been found that the infant is unlikely to be depressed if the value falls, from the normal level of pH 7·30 to pH 7·20; however, the exact relationship between further metabolic acidosis and either the conventional methods of assessing foetal distress or the postnatal condition of the infant is still uncertain; the reason probably lies in the site and time of sampling and in the unknown factor of the duration of asphyxia and, therefore, exhaustion of energy sources before the indications for blood sampling.

The experimental demonstrations in the laboratory, by Dawes & Shelley at Oxford, of the influence of hypoxia on glycogen storage in the foetus has extended the primary interest, in the exchange of respiratory gases and elimination of the acid products of metabolism during labour, to the transport of glucose from the mother, for the maintenance of energy requirements in the foetus. The further demonstration, of the influence of extracellular fluid pH on the utilization of energy sources in the foetus, and the growing evidence in the human subject, for the vasoconstrictor effect of an impaired maternal acid-base balance on the uterine circulation, extends the field into the maintenance of acid-base balance in both the mother and foetus, by the administration of alkali or buffer to the mother during labour.

BLOOD SAMPLING

The inter-relationships of both oxygen and carbon dioxide with acid-base balance make the site of blood sampling most important in assessing the transport events. It is unusual to take blood from the maternal brachial artery during labour: that from the ante-cubital vein can only contribute an approximate assessment of standard bicarbonate and base excess or deficit in the blood plasma supplying the uterus. Any alteration from the normal, during the course of labour, represents the sum of all oxygen debts with little indication of the proportion due to specific uterine contributions. Uterine vein samples have rarely been obtained at Caesarian section and their value is doubtful because of the complexity of the venous drainage of the uterus and the difficulty of knowing the proportion of placental and uterine components at the site sampled.

Umbilical vein blood values provide an indication of placental efficiency which is determined by maternal supply to the trophoblast and trophoblastic activity, and may also be influenced by foetal placental blood flow. They are, however, only an approximate measure of the plasma buffer supply to the foetal tissues because of the interposition of the liver circulation. The umbilical artery contains a mixture of the venous drainage from the upper half of the body, which is shunted by the ductus arteriosus across the lungs, and arterialized blood from the aorta; its character will be influenced by umbilical vein levels of metabolites, the foetal blood flow and foetal utilization or production. Umbilical A-V or V-A differences indicate the direction of foetal-placental exchange. The part played by the metabolic activity of the placenta itself in precluding any simple relationship between the maternal and foetal blood levels has already been discussed in the previous section. Umbilical samples are usually terminal and show the cumulative effects of changes in both the maternal and foetal circulations upon both the placenta and foetus, but give little indication of the duration of these changes.

The sampling of capillary blood from the presenting scalp has the primary advantage of being repeatable from a cervical dilation of 2 cm to delivery. The site is questionable, firstly, because of possible harm to the infant's head and, secondly, because of impairment of the circulation due to engagement of the head. Two foetal deaths from head injuries have been reported (Beard, Morris & Clayton 1966). The reproducibility of changes observed by two different groups (Saling 1963b, 1964, Beard & Morris 1965), during normal labour, suggests that the scalp circulation, which is known to be good, is probably not greatly impaired. The reliability of the method during hypoxia may well be questioned for it is well known that constriction of the skin blood vessels occurs (Celander 1966). The small volume of blood obtainable is a minor disadvantage with the micro methods for plasma pH and gas tension measurement now available.

ACID-BASE BALANCE

PREGNANCY

In healthy women the mean tension of carbon dioxide in the alveolar air and arterial blood is 38 mm Hg: the arterial plasma pH is 7·40 and the total carbon dioxide content 25·3 m Eq/litre (Loeschcke 1954). In the pregnant woman the acid-base characteristics of the extracellular fluid are already altered by the 50–60th day of gestation, (Prystowsky, Hellegers & Bruns 1961). The course of the fall in the standard bicarbonate of the arterial blood during pregnancy is shown in Fig. 4.14. This change and the fall in $Paco_2$ are thought to be partly related to the increased progesterone production for similar changes in blood

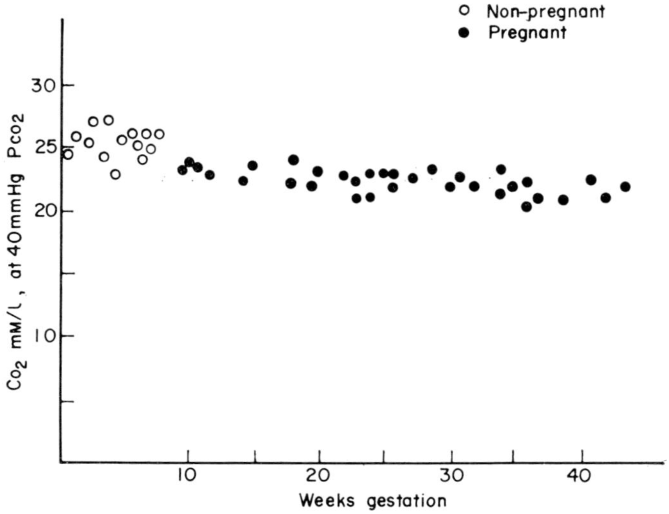

FIG. 4.14. Plasma carbon dioxide binding capacity in non-pregnant women, and during gestation. [Prystowsky H., Hellegers A. & Bruns P.D. (1961) Reproduced by kind permission of the authors and the editor, *American Journal of Obstetrics and Gynaecology*.]

chemistry can be brought about by the administration of progesterone to the non-pregnant woman (Tyler 1960). The concentrations of many other constituents of maternal plasma are also reduced long before the foetus is large enough to make a metabolic demand. The V-A bicarbonate differences, between the antecubital vein and brachial artery are reduced during pregnancy; this is probably due to the increased blood flow in skin (Hytten & Leitch 1964). By term the mean tension of carbon dioxide in the alveolar air is reduced to 32 mm Hg; the total carbon dioxide content of the arterial plasma is 22·2 m Eq/litre, and the pH 7·34. A similar fall in these values may also be demonstrated in ante-cubital vein blood (Seeds, Battaglia & Hellegers 1964).

Little is known of the acid-base characteristics of the infant throughout gestation; at hysterectomy Freda & Adamsons (1964) found the femoral arterial pH to be 7·34, the P_{CO_2} 38 mm Hg, and total carbon dioxide 22 m Eq/litre in one infant of 27½ weeks gestational age.

NORMAL LABOUR

The relationships of the maternal and foetal plasma acid-base characteristics during normal labour are shown in Fig. 4.15. Maternal blood was

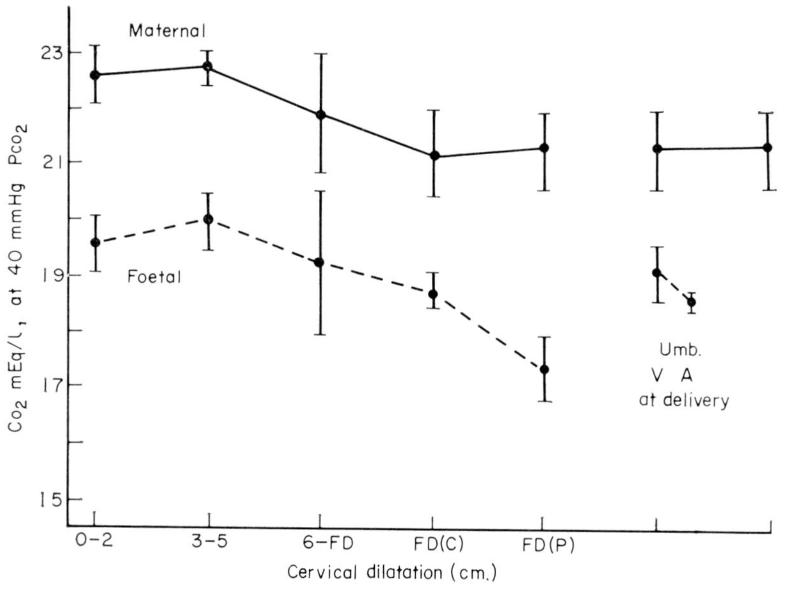

FIG. 4.15. Plasma carbon dioxide binding capacity in mother (antecubital vein) and foetus (presenting scalp) during labour. [Beard R.W. & Morris E.D. (1965) Reproduced by kind permission of the authors and the editor, *Journal of Obstetrics and Gynaecology of the British Commonwealth*.]

taken from the ante-cubital vein, and foetal blood from the presenting scalp by Saling's technique. At 2 cm dilation the total carbon dioxide in the maternal plasma is 3–4 m Eq/litre higher than the foetal, the pH is 0·1 unit higher and the foetal plasma P_{CO_2} 7 mm Hg higher than the maternal (Saling 1964, Beard & Morris 1965, Bretscher & Saling 1967). Thereafter a small metabolic acidosis develops in both; the fall in total carbon dioxide in the maternal plasma amounts to 1 m Eq/litre and occurs mostly during the second stage of labour: it accounts for the fall in pH from 7·39 to 7·35 while the P_{CO_2} falls from 44 to 40 mm Hg. In the foetus the total carbon dioxide and base excess of the plasma show a small rise until the middle of the second stage, which Saling (1963b) attributes to an increase in the uteroplacental circulation caused by the contractions: the fall which follows, continues through full dilation and while the head is on the perineum; foetal plasma pH falls from 7·29 to 7·25 during labour while the mean P_{CO_2} rises from 44 mm Hg at 2 cm in dilation, to 52 mm at full dilation. Minimal metabolic and respiratory acidosis has also been observed in umbilical venous blood at normal delivery by James, Weisbrot, Prince, Holiday & Apgar (1958) and Quilligan, Katigbak & Hofschild (1965). Saling (1963b) also measured the oxygen content of the blood samples obtained, finding an average saturation of 42 per cent and a tension of 20 mm Hg at the onset of labour; a decrease to 30 per cent saturation and 17 mm Hg oxygen tension was observed at delivery. The oxygen content of the blood obtained during a uterine contraction was slightly higher than during relaxation. The oxygen content and acid base characteristics of the peripheral blood lie between those of the umbilical artery and vein, about 25–40 per cent above the umbilical arterial levels.

The minimal oxygen debt occurring in both the mother and the foetus, demonstrates that maternal energy requirements are only moderate (Gemzell, Robbe, Stern & Ström 1957, Stern 1968) and that the overall disturbance of the placental exchange does not exceed the reserve of this organ. The plasma lactate in the umbilical vein at delivery is only slightly elevated from the normal levels of 1 m Eq/litre; it doubles during the first postnatal minutes, as it is washed out of the tissues, but returns to normal levels within half an hour (James 1959). Rooth & Nilsson (1964) observed that the foetal V-A difference in base excess was largely due to the oxygenation of the blood, and that the production of lactate only accounted for 20 per cent of the acidosis in both the maternal and foetal blood during labour.

DURING PROLONGED LABOUR AND FOETAL DISTRESS

Clinically, foetal blood sampling from the presenting scalp during delivery is usually not carried out until the classical signs of foetal distress are present; the results on 306 cases have been reported by Bretscher & Saling (1967) and on 24 by Beard & Morris (1965). A plasma pH of 7·20 is regarded by both as borderline and an indication for further sampling after five minutes. If, in this interval, a further fall of 0·05 pH is observed, very frequent observations are required and when pH 7·10 is reached a Caesarian section is performed. If the changes are slow, stationary or improving a 15- to 30-minute interval may be left before further sampling. The pH of the sample as collected indicates the degree of acidosis and the change after equilibration at a standard 40 mm Hg P_{CO_2} whether this is due to stasis or metabolic acidosis.

Although a pronounced foetal acidosis is more likely to be associated with a depressed infant (Saling 1964, Beard & Morris 1965), the relationship between metabolic acidosis, whether observed by continuous sampling during labour or in the umbilical blood at birth, and the condition of the infant is uncertain. This must be due to the multiplicity of causes for the changes in heart rate during labour (Caldeyro-Barcia, Mendes-Bauer, Poseiro, Escarcena, Pose, Bieniarz, Arnt, Gulin & Althabe 1966) and, also, to the difficulty of knowing the duration of asphyxia before the clinical signs of foetal distress become apparent and biochemical investigations are started.

Sampling continuously during labour Saling (1966) found metabolic disturbance in 18 per cent of cases in which meconium was passed, but in which no changes in foetal heart rate could be observed, in 24 per cent of cases in which the heart rate rose above 160/minute, and in 40 per cent of cases in which the foetal heart rate fell below 100/minute. Quilligan, Katigbak & Hofschild (1965) found an umbilical arterial acidosis in infants with bradycardia during contractions: when the bradycardia continued in between the contractions the umbilical arterial acidosis was greater and venous acidosis also developed, suggesting a reduction in uterine blood flow. Brady, James & Baker (1963) demonstrated that persistent tachycardia between contractions was also associated with marked metabolic acidosis in the umbilical arterial blood and depression at birth. No change in heart rate may occur with scalp samples of very low pH (Saling 1964). Saling has suggested that this may be due to vasoconstriction particularly in the skin, caused by the low oxygen and high carbon dioxide tension in the plasma as the peripheral blood flow is reduced to maintain a circulation to the heart and brain. Celander (1966) has shown that the foot and calf blood flow in the newborn child is reduced by one third when 13 per cent O_2 is breathed: the systemic arterial pressure is just maintained with such a decrease in inspired oxygen (Young & Cottom 1966).

MATERNAL : FOETAL LACTATE RELATIONSHIPS

Maternal venous lactate does not appear to rise during gestation. During labour the observed rise probably originates primarily from the oxygen debt in the uterine muscle, with a small contribution from skeletal muscle. Otey, Stenger & Eitzman (1964) found at elective Caesarian section that uterine vein blood contained 0·3 m Eq/litre more lactate than the uterine artery. Foetal plasma lactate owes its origin to overall foetal asphyxia; primarily due to impairment of the maternal oxygen supply. It has been demonstrated in the monkey (Friedman, Gray, Grynfogel, Hutchinson, Kelly & Plentl 1960) that labelled lactate diffuses freely in either direction across the placenta but no equivalent data exists in the human subject. It has also been shown *in vitro* that 9–15-week and term placentas can produce lactate, probably from glucose since the glycogen is not depleted (Ginsburg & Jeacock 1964); if this occurs *in vivo* the lactate produced may contribute to both the foetal and maternal levels. However, the value of such measurements has been questioned by Beaconsfield, Ginsburg & Panigel (1968) who have shown by electron microscopy, complete disintegration of the syncytium in slices of early placenta, after only short periods in incubation media.

The first observations on maternal-foetal lactate inter-relationships during labour were made by Bell, Cunningham & Jouett (1928); they found foetal levels at delivery higher than maternal venous, with higher umbilical arterial than venous levels and considered that the foetal lactate diffused across the placenta into the maternal blood stream. Their observations were confirmed by Hendricks (1957) but not by Eastman & McLane (1931) and Vedra (1963) who observed higher levels in maternal venous blood than in the foetal with no umbilical A-V differences. Loeser (1932) also found the levels higher in the maternal than foetal plasma, with higher umbilical venous than umbilical arterial values suggesting the placenta as the foetal source of lactate. Recently, Bell's findings have been confirmed and related more fully with the type of labour and the condition of the infant at birth. Following normal deliveries both Derom (1964) and Stembera & Hodr (1966) found the maternal venous lactate slightly lower than in the foetal plasma, with a direction relationship between the two (Fig. 4.16a). The former observed no umbilical V-A differences and the latter small differences in favour of the artery; with low mean values the umbilical venous level might be larger than the arterial but the umbilical arterial levels were always higher than the umbilical venous when labour was prolonged. During moderate and severe asphyxia, resulting in prolonged bradycardia and delayed respiration at birth, the lactate rose to 4 m Eq/litre in the umbilical artery: the umbilical venous level was also elevated and the A-V differences increased (Fig. 4.16b); the maternal level was slightly

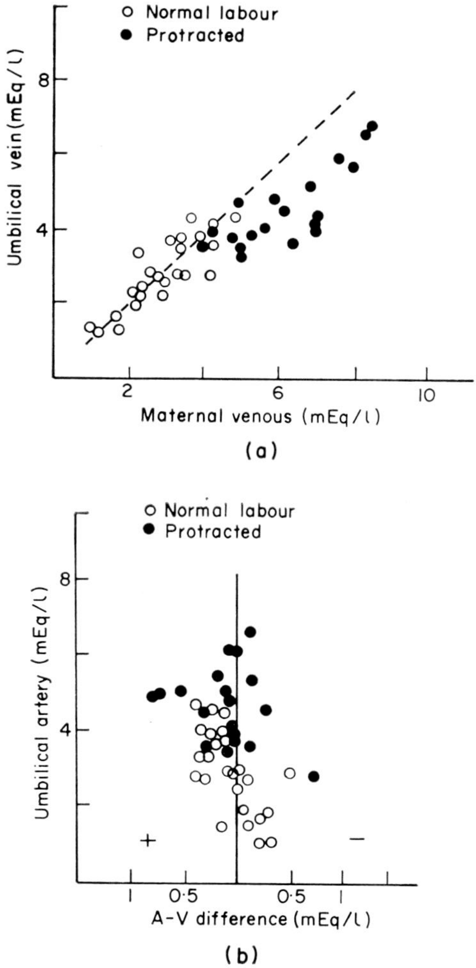

FIG. 4.16a. Relation of maternal and umbilical venous blood lactate at delivery.

FIG. 4.16b. Relation of umbilical arterio-venous lactate difference to umbilical arterial levels, at delivery. [Stembera Z.K. & Hodr J. (1966) Reproduced by kind permission of the authors and the editor, *Biologia Neonatorum*.]

elevated. These findings suggest a net diffusion of lactate from the foetus to the mother during asphyxia. This, together with the observations that even during normal labour the maternal and foetal levels are inter-related provide support for Rooth & Nilsson's suggestions that the acid-base status of the foetus might be monitored by the maternal lactate level. This has never been fully explored and it is strange that Beard & Morris (1965) should, recently, have related clinical findings to foeto-maternal acid-base differences, rather than to the absolute levels of each. However, again, the duration of asphyxia and depletion of foetal glycogen stores is an unknown factor for lactate may be metabolized at different rates in the mother and the foetus. Stembera & Hodr (1961) have some evidence that the administration of glucose to the mother during labour reduces maternal plasma pyruvate levels, but only if she is given 100 per cent oxygen to breathe simultaneously. Less maternal lactic acid is formed during prolonged labours (Stembera, Hodr & Friedlandrova 1961) if she has taken exercise during her pregnancy.

The duration of asphyxia could, possibly, be estimated by the neonatal changes in plasma lactate. In moderately asphyxiated infants the levels may be double the normal value at birth, 2 m Eq/litre, and in prolonged labours 4 m Eq/litre or more; the values rise after delivery, as lactate is washed out of the tissues, and may not return to normal for many hours (James 1959). These changes would be enhanced by respiratory depression, itself a result of intra-uterine asphyxia. A metabolic acidosis also depresses the metabolic rate and lowers the oxygen consumption, and the usual fall in body temperature observed during the first eight hours of life is enhanced and the return to the normal body temperature slower (Burnard & Cross 1958); the neonatal fall in blood glucose is, similarly, more profound and reaches normal levels more slowly (Shelley & Nelligan 1966).

GLUCOSE TRANSPORT AND UTILIZATION

Recently, Stembera & Hodr (1966) have confirmed the considerable variability in maternal venous glucose found at delivery, known from previous studies. The umbilical venous glucose is also variable, a little lower than the maternal, and directly related to it in both normal and prolonged labours (Fig. 4.17a). The umbilical V-A differences for glucose are also directly related to the umbilical venous level, suggesting greater glucose utilization. During moderate asphyxia both the maternal and umbilical venous blood glucose rise, but as Fig. 4.17b shows, the umbilical V-A differences decrease and the arterial levels may be greater than the venous. The high glucose results from the mobilization of glycogen stores, but utilization is probably inhibited at the low pH, and mother (Sabata, Stembera, Hodr & Novak 1964). Women who are

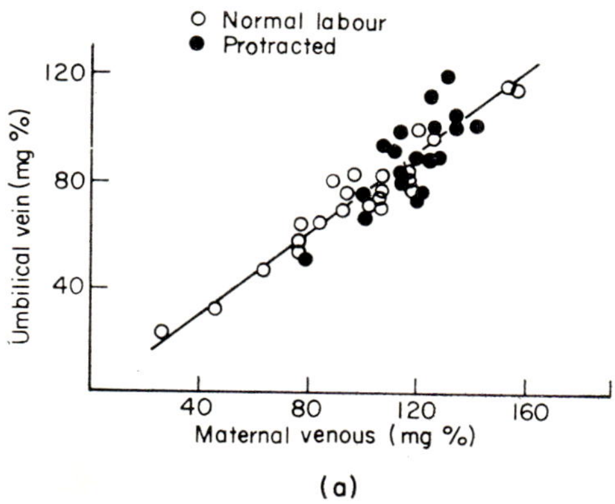

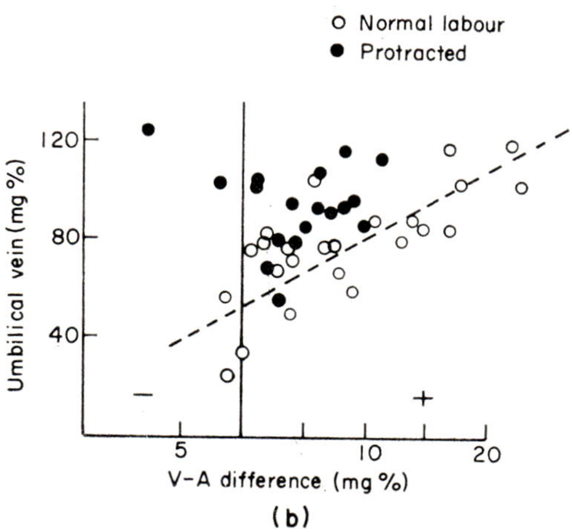

FIG. 4.17a. Relation of maternal and umbilical venous blood glucose at delivery. [Stembera Z.K. & Hodr J.]

FIG. 4.17b. Relation of umbilical veno-arterial glucose difference to umbilical venous levels at delivery. [Stembera Z.K. & Hodr J. (1966) Reproduced by kind permission of the authors and the editor, *Biologia Neonatorum*.]

eventually some glucose is even lost from the foetus to the mother. With very severe asphyxia resulting in perinatal mortality the foetal blood glucose is very low and unrelated to the maternal level.

During normal labour, the umbilical V-A difference of unsaturated non-esterified fatty acid suggests transport from the mother while that for the saturated fatty acids suggests transport from the foetus to the

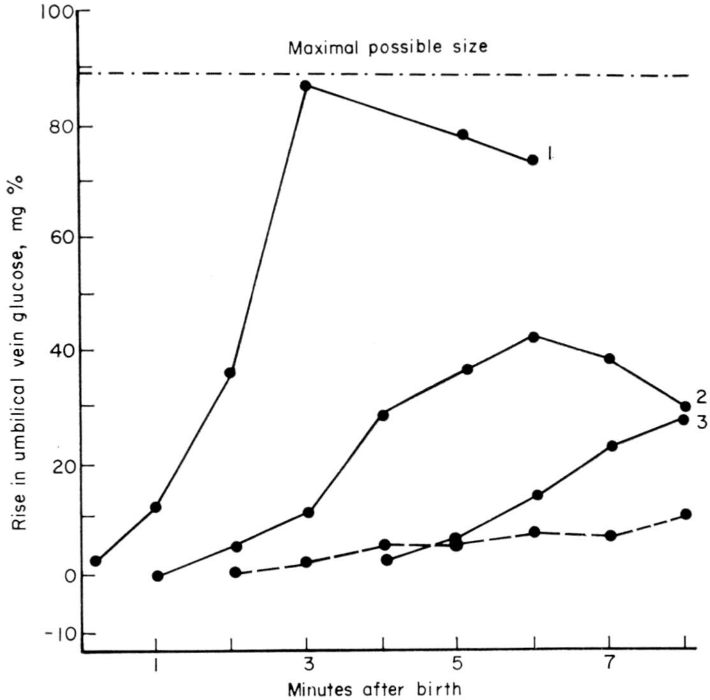

FIG. 4.18. Appearance of glucose in umbilical venous blood following intravenous administration of glucose to the mother: 1. One minute before delivery; 2. Two minutes after delivery; 3. Three minutes after delivery. --- control, no glucose to mother. [Stembera Z.K. & Hodr J. (1962) Reproduced by kind permission of the authors and the editor, *Gynakolgentagung*.]

starved before labour have a lower blood glucose and higher non-esterified fatty acid content at delivery. Non-esterified fatty acids are higher in the cord blood of large diabetic infants and associated with higher lactate levels (Sabata, Stembera & Hodr 1965). A continuous infusion of glucose during the second stage of labour, to raise the maternal plasma level to 300 mg per cent causes a doubling of the foetal plasma glucose values together with an increased umbilical V-A difference: both maternal and foetal saturated fatty acids are elevated, but the maternal plasma levels of unsaturated fatty acids fall unexpectedly as the foetal level rises.

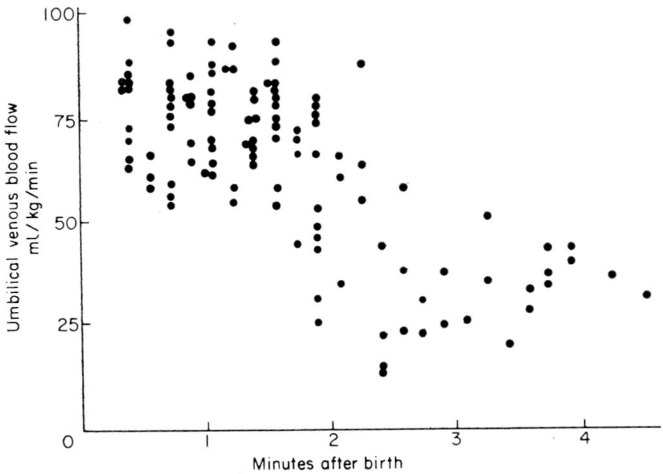

FIG. 4.19. Umbilical venous blood flow during the first four minutes after delivery of the infant: the cord was intact and the placenta *in situ*. [Stembera Z.K., Hodr J. & Janda J. (1965) Reproduced by kind permission of the authors and the editor, *American Journal of Obstetrics and Gynecology*.]

FUNCTION OF THE *IN SITU* PLACENTA AFTER DELIVERY OF THE FOETUS

Stembera & Hodr (1959) have found that glucose is transferred freely from the maternal to the foetal circulation for the first two minutes after the birth of the infant. This evidence was obtained by giving the mother glucose intravenously before and at intervals after delivery. Figure 4.18 shows that when the glucose was given 1 minute before delivery the level of glucose in the umbilical vein 2 minutes after delivery was equal to that expected, but fell subsequently. Injections after delivery gave a slower rise and a smaller final level. Measurement of the umbilical blood flow using the thermo-dilution technique, following the swift insertion of a fine needle and thermocouple sensor downstream from the needle, demonstrated that flow is constant for 2 minutes after birth; a decrease is observed when separation of the placenta takes place (Stembera *et al.* 1965) (Fig. 4.19). Although the blood flow is probably lower than *in utero* the constancy would suggest that umbilical blood samples taken at delivery are fairly representative of the placental foetal exchange at the time of sampling. The umbilical blood flows were 250–300 ml/min within 20 seconds of delivery which is about 60 per cent of the cardiac output of the newborn child (Young 1966); this is an interesting figure because it would suggest that placental blood flow, at term, is the same proportion of the cardiac output in the human infant as in the lamb (Dawes 1962 and 1968).

ACKNOWLEDGEMENTS

The author gratefully acknowledges support from the Medical Research Council for her own work on amino acid transport.

REFERENCES

Acheson G.H., Dawes G.S. & Mott J.C. (1957) Oxygen consumption and the arterial oxygen saturation in newborn lambs. *J. Physiol., Lond.* **135**, 623.

Adamsons C. (1965) Transport of organic substances and oxygen across the placenta. *Birth Defects Original Article series*, **1**, 27. The National Foundation, March of Dimes.

Aherne W. (1966) A weight relationship between the human foetus and placenta. *Biologia Neonat.* **10**, 113.

Aherne W. & Dunnill M.S. (1966) Morphometry of the human placenta. *Br. med. Bull.* **22**, 1.

Akedo H. & Christensen H.N. (1962) Transfer of amino acids across the intestine: a new model. *J. biol. Chem.* **237**, 113.

Alexander G. (1964) Studies on the placenta of the sheep. *J. Reprod. Fert.* **7**, 289.

Assali N.S., Douglass R.A., Baird W., Nicholson D.B. & Suyemoto R. (1953) Measurement of uterine blood flow and uterine metabolism; results in normal pregnancy. *Am. J. Obstet. Gynec.* **66**, 248.

Assali N.S., Rauramo L. & Peltonen T. (1960) Uterine and foetal blood flow and oxygen consumption in early human pregnancy. *Am. J. Obstet. Gynec.* **79**, 86.

Barcroft J. (1946) *Researches on Pre-Natal Life.* Blackwell, Oxford.

Barron D.H. (1944) The changes in the foetal circulation at birth. *Physiol. Rev.* **24**, 277.

Bartels H. (1959) Chemical factors affecting oxygen carriage and transfer from maternal to foetal blood. In *Oxygen Supply to the Human Foetus.* Blackwell, Oxford.

BARTELS H. & METCALFE J. (1965) Some aspects of the comparative physiology of placental gas exchange. *Proc. Int. Union Phys. Sci.* **4**, 34.

BARTELS H., MOLL W. & METCALFE J. (1962) Physiology of gas exchange in the human subject. *Am. J. Obstet. Gynec.* **84**, 1714.

BEACONSFIELD P., GINSBURG J. & PANIGEL M. (1968) *Effect of Different Incubation Conditions on Placental Ultrastructure.* To be published.

BEARD R.W. & MORRIS E.D. (1965) Foetal and maternal acid-base balance during normal labour. *J. Obstet. Gynaec. Br. Commonw.* **72**, 496.

BEARD R.W., MORRIS E.D. & CLAYTON S.G. (1966) Haemorrhage following foetal blood sampling. *J. Obstet. Gynaec. Br. Commonw.* **73**, 860.

BELL W.B., CUNNINGHAM L. & JOUETT M. (1928) The metabolism and acidity of the foetal tissues and fluids. *Br. med. J.* **1**, 126.

BØE F. (1954) Vascular morphology of the human placenta. *Cold Spring Harbor Symposia on Quantitative Biology*, **19**, 29. Cold Spring Harbor, New York.

BONSNES R.W. (1947) The plasma amino acid and amino nitrogen concentration during normal pregnancy, labor, and early puerperium. *J. biol. Chem.* **168**, 345.

BORELL U., FERNSTROM I. & WESTMAN A. (1958) Hormonal influences on the uterine arteries. An arteriographic study in the human. *Acta obstet. gynec. scand.* **32**, 271.

BOTHWELL T.H., PRIBILLA W.F., MEBUST W. & FINCH C.A. (1958) Iron metabolism in the pregnant rabbit. Iron transport across the placenta. *Am. J. Physiol.* **193**, 615.

BRADY J., JAMES L.S. & BAKER M.A. (1963) Fetal electrocardiographic studies. *Am. J. Obstet. Gynec.* **86**, 785.

BRETSCHER J. & SALING E. (1967) pH values in the human fetus during labor. *Am. J. Obstet. Gynec.* **97**, 906.

BROWNE J.C.M. & VEALL N. (1953) Maternal placental blood flow in normotensive and hypertensive women. *J. Obstet. Gynaec. Br. Commonw.* **60**, 141.

BURNARD E.D. & CROSS K.W. (1958) Rectal temperature in the newborn after birth asphyxia. *Br. med. J.* **2**, 1197.

CAMPBELL A.G.M., DAWES G.S., FISHMAN A.P., HYMAN A.I. & JAMES G.B. (1966) The oxygen consumption of the placenta and foetal membranes in the sheep. *J. Physiol.* **182**, 439.

CALDEYRO-BARCIA R., MENDEZ-BAUER C., POSEIRO J.J., ESCARCENA L.A., POSE S.V., BIENIARZ J., ARNT L., GULIN L. & ALTHABE O. (1966) Control of human fetal heart rate during labour. In *The Heart and Circulation in the Newborn and Infant.* D.E.Cassels, ed. Grune and Stratton, N.Y .

CELANDER O. (1966) Studies of the periph eral circulation. In *The Heart and Circulation in the Newborn and Infant.* D.E.Cassels, ed. Grune and Stratton, N.Y.

CHANARIN I., MACGIBBON B.M., O'SULLIVAN W.J. & M OLLIN D.L. (1959) Folic acid deficiency in pregnancy. The pathogenesis of megaloblastic anaemi c of pregnancy. *Lancet*, **2**, 634.

CHRISTENSEN H.N. & STREICHER J.A. (1948) Association between rapid growth a nd elevated cell concentrations of amino acids. I. In foetal tissues. *J. biol. Chem.* **175**, 95.

CHRISTENSEN P.J., DATE J.W., SCHONHEYDER F. & VOLQUARTZ K. (1957) Amino acids in blood plasma and urine during pregnancy. *Scand. J. clin. Lab. Invest.* **9**, 54.

CLEMETSON C.A.B. & CHURCHMAN J. (1954) The placental transfer of amino acids in normal and toxaemic pregnancy. *J. Obstet. Gynaec. Br. Commonw.* **61**, 364.

CLEMETSON C.A.B. & CHURCHMAN J. (1955) Plasma amino acid levels following protein ingestion by pregnant and non-pregnant subjects. *J. Obstet. Gynaec. Br. Commonw.* **62**, 390.

CROSS K.W., DAWES G.B. & MOTT J.C. (1959) Anoxia, oxygen consumption and cardiac output in newborn lambs and adult sheep. *J. Physiol., Lond.* **146**, 316.

CRUMPLER H.R., DENT C.E. & LINDAN O. (1950) The amino acid pattern in human foetal and maternal plasma at delivery. *Biochem. J.* **47**, 223.

DANCIS J. (1960) Placental function and fetal nutrition. In *The Placenta and Fetal Membranes*, p. 85. C.A.Villee, ed.

DANCIS J., MONEY W.L., SPRINGER D. & LEVITZ M. (1968) Transport of Amino Acids by Placenta. *Am. J. Obstet. Gynec.* **101**, 820.

DANCIS J., OLSEN G. & FOLKART G. (1958) Transfer of histidine and xylose across the placenta and into the red blood cells and amniotic fluid. *Am. J. Physiol.* **194**, 44.

DAWES G.S. (1962) The umbilical circulation. *Am. J. Obstet. Gynec.* **84**, 1634.

DAWES G.S. (1965) Oxygen supply and consumption in late fetal life, and the onset of breathing at birth. *Handbook of Physiology*, **2**, III, 1313. W.O.Fenn & H.Rahm, eds.

DAWES G.S. (1968) Foetal and Neonatal Physiology. Year Book Medical Publishers Inc., Chicago.

DAWKINS M.J.R. (1965) The 'Small for Dates' Baby. In Gestational Age, Size, and Maturity. Heinemann Medical Books Ltd.

DEROM R. (1964) Anaerobic metabolism in the human fetus. *Am. J. Obstet. Gynec.* **89**, 241.

DIXON H.G. & ROBERTSON W.B. (1958) A study of the vessels of the placental bed in normotensive and hypertensive women. *J. Obstet. Gynaec. Br. Commonw.* **65**, 803.

EASTMAN N.Y. & MCLANE C.M. (1931) Foetal blood studies. II. The lactic acid content of umbilical cord blood under various conditions. *Bull. Johns Hopkins Hosp.* **48**, 261.

FERNSTRÖM I. (1955) Arteriography of the uterine artery. Its value in the diagnosis of uterine fibromyoma, tubal pregnancy, adrenal tumour, and placental site localisation in cases of intra-uterine pregnancy. *Acta radiol. suppl.* **122**, 1.

FOLEY T.H., HOLM L.W., LONDON D.R. & YOUNG I.M. (1967) Preliminary observations on free amino acids in cow and calf plasma in prolonged gestation. *Am. J. Obstet. Gynec.* (In press).

FREDA V.J. & ADAMSONS K. (1964) Exchange transfusion *in utero*–Report of a case. *Am. J. Obstet. Gynec.* **89**, 817.

FRIEDMAN E.A. & SACHTLEBEN M.R. (1960) Placental oxygen consumption *in vitro*. I. Baseline studies. *Am. J. Obstet. Gynec.* **79**, 1058.

FRIEDMAN E.A., GRAY M.J., GRYNFOGEL M., HUTCHINSON D.L., KELLY W.T. & PLENTL A.A. (1960) The distribution and metabolism of C14 labelled acetic acid and bicarbonate in pregnant primates. *J. clin. Invest.* **39**, 227.

FUCHS F. (1957) *Studies on the Passage of Phosphate between Mother and Foetus in the Guinea Pig*. Ejnar Munksgaard, Copenhagen.

FUCHS F., SPACKMAN T. & ASSALI N.S. (1963) Complexity and Nonhomogeneity of the intervillous space. *Am. J. Obstet. Gynec.* **86**, 226.

GEMZELL C.A., ROBBE H., STERN B. & STRÖM G. (1957) Observations on circulatory changes and muscular work in normal labour. *Acta obstet. gynec. scand.* **36**, 75.

GHADIMI H. & PECORA P. (1964) Free amino acids of cord plasma as compared with maternal plasma during pregnancy. *Pediatrics*, **33**, 500.

GINSBURG J. & JEACOCK M.J. (1964) Pathways of glucose metabolism in human placental tissue. *Biochim. biophys. Acta*, **90**, 166.

GLENDENNING M.B., MARGOLIS A.J. & PAGE E.W. (1961) Amino acid concentrations in foetal and maternal plasma. *Am. J. Obstet. Gynec.* **81**, 591.

HAGERMAN D.D. & VILLEE C.A. (1960) Transport functions of the placenta. *Physiol. Rev.* **40**, No. 2, 313.

HAIGH A.L., KITCHIN A.H. & PICKFORD M. (1963) The effect of oxytocin and hand blood flow in man following the administration of progesterone and isoprenaline. *J. physiol. Lond.* **169**, 161.

HARNED H.S., ROWSHAM H., MACKINNEY L.G. & SUGIOKA K. (1964) Relations of Po_2, Pco_2, and pH to onset of breathing of the term lamb. *Pediatrics*, **33**, 672.

HAYTER C.J., HUTCHINSON E.A., KARVONEN M.J. & YOUNG M. (1964) Placental transport of amino isobutyric acid in the unanaesthetized guinea pig. *J. Physiol., Lond.* **175**, 11.

HENDRICKS C.H. (1957) Studies on lactic acid metabolism in pregnancy and labour. *Am. J. Obstet. Gynec.* **73**, 492.

HENDRICKS C.H., QUILLIGAN E.J., TYLER C.W. & TUCKER G.J. (1959) Pressure relationships between intervillous space and the amniotic fluid in human pregnancy. *Am. J. Obstet. Gynec.* **77**, 1028.

HERTIG A.T. (1960) In *The Placenta and Fetal Membranes*, p. 109. C.A.Villee, ed. Williams and Wilkins, Baltimore, Md.

HOLM L.W. & GALLIGAN S.J. (1962) Blood chemistry and tissue glycogen in post-term Guernsey foetuses with adenohypophyseal aplasia. *Biologia Neonat.* **4**, 75.

HOLM L.W., SALVATORE C. & ZEEK-MINNING P. (1964) The histology of the post-term bovine placenta. *Am. J. Obstet. Gynec.* **88**, 479.

HORSKA S., JANDA J., STEMBERA Z.K. & NOVAK M. (1966) Comparison of amino nitrogen in maternal plasma and in umbilical vessels. Exerpta Medica Symposium in Prague 'Intra-Uterine dangers to the foetus', p. 36.

HUCKABEE W., METCALFE J., PRYSTOWSKY H., HELLEGERS A., MESCHIA G. & BARRON D. (1959) Uterine blood flow and metabolism in pregnant sheep at high altitude. *Fed. Proc. Fedn. Am. Socs exp. Biol.* **18**, 281.

HUCKABEE W.E., METCALFE J., PRYSTOWSKY H. & BARRON D.H. (1962) Movements of lactate and pyruvate in pregnant uterus. *Am. J. Physiol.* **202**, 193.

HUGGETT A. & SLATER J.S. (1966) The non-protein nitrogenous constituents of the maternal blood and foetal body fluids in the sheep. *Biochem. J.* **98**, 43.

HYTTEN F.E. & LEITCH I. (1964) *The Physiology of Human Pregnancy*. Blackwell, Oxford.

JAMES L.S. (1959) Biochemical aspects of asphyxia at birth. *Report of the 31st Ross Conference on Paediatric Research*, 66. Ross Laboratories, Columbus, Ohio.

JAMES L.S. & ROWE R.D. (1957) Pattern of response of pulmonary and systemic arterial pressures in newborn and older infants to short periods of hypoxia. *J. Pediat.* **51**, 5.

JAMES L.S., WEISBROT I.M., PRINCE C.E., HOLIDAY D.H. & APGAR V.A. (1958) The acid base status of human infants in relation to birth asphyxia and the onset of respiration. *J. Pediat.* **52**, 379.

JOSIMOVICH J.B. & BRANDE B.L. (1964) Chemical properties and biological effects of human placental lactogen (H.P.L.). *Trans. N.Y. Acad. Sci.* **27**, 161.

KAYSER H.W. (1955) Investigaciones sobre la circulacion sanguinea de la placenta humana mediante fosforo radioactivo. *Acta Gynec, scand.* **6**, 299.

KERR G.R., CHAMOVE A.S., HARLOW H.F. & WAISMAN H.A. (1968) Fetal PKU: the effect of material hyperphenylalaninemia during pregnancy in the rhesus monkey (Macaca Mulatta) *Pediatrics* **42**, 27.

KLINE B.S. (1951) Microscopic observations of the development of the placenta. *Am. J. Obstet. Gynec.* **61**, 1065.

KORNER P.I. (1959) Circulatory adaptations in hypoxia. *Phys. Rev.* **39**, 687.

LANDAU R.L. & LUGIBIHL K. (1961) The catabolic and natriuretic effects of progesterone in man. *Recent Progr. Hormone Res.* **17**, 249.

LINDBLAND B.S. & BALDESTAN A. (1967) Normal venous plasma free amino acid levels of non-pregnant women and of mother and child during delivery. *Acta paediat. Stockh.* **56**, 37.

LLOYD S.M. (1959) Changes in the vascular responses of the rat during pregnancy. *J. Physiol.* (*Lond.*) **149**, 589.

LOESCHCKE H.H. (1954) Uber die wirkung von steroid hormonen auf die lungenbeluftung. *Klin. Wschr.* **32**, 441.

LOESER A. (1932) Atmung und Gärung der überlebenden Plazenta des Menschen sowie deren Beeinflussung durch Hormone nebst dem Milchsäurestoffwechsel der lebenden Plazenta im trächtigen Tiere. *Arch. Gynaek.* **148**, 118.

LONDON D.R., FOLEY T.H. & WEBB C.G. (1965) Evidence for the release of individual amino acids from the resting human forearm. *Nature, Lond.* **208**, 588.

LONGO L.D., POWER G.G. & FORSTER R.E. (1967) Respiratory function of the placenta as determined with CO in sheep and dogs. *J. Clin. Invest.* **46**, 812.

LUST J.E., HAGERMAN D.D. & VILLEE C.A. (1954) Transport of riboflavin by human placenta. *J. clin. Invest.* **33**, 38.

MARTIN J.D. & YOUNG I.M. (1960) Influence of gestational age and hormones on experimental foetal bradycardia. *J. Physiol.* **152**, 1.

MARTIN J.D. & YOUNG I.M. (1963) Experimental foetal bradycardia during postmaturity in the rabbit. *Aust. N.Z. J. Obstet. Gynaec.* **3**, 56.

MCKAY D.G., ROBY C.C., HERTIG A.T. & RICHARDSON M.V. (1955) Studies of the function of early human trophoblast. I. Observations on the chemical composition of the fluid of hydatidiform moles. *Am. J. Obstet. Gynec.* **69**, 722.

MESCHIA G., COTTER J.R., BREATHNACH C.S. & BARRON D.H. (1965) The hemoglobin, oxygen, carbon dioxide and hydrogen ion concentrations in the umbilical bloods of sheep and goats as sampled via indwelling plastic catheters. *Q. Jl. exp. Physiol.* **50**, 185.

MESCHIA G., COTTER J.R., MAKOWSKI E.L. & BARRON D.H. (1967) Simultaneous measurement of uterine and umbilical blood flows and oxygen uptakes. *Q. Jl. exp. Physiol.* **52**, 1.

MESCHIA G., WOLKOFF A.S. & BARRON D.H. (1958) Difference in electrical potential across the placenta of goats. *Proc. natn. Acad. Sci. U.S.A.* **44**, 483.

METCALFE J., BARTELS H. & MOLL W. (1967) Gas Exchange in the pregnant uterus. *Physiol. Rev.* **47**, 782.

METCALFE J., MOLL W., BARTELS H., HILPERT P. & PARER J.T. (1965) Transfer of carbon monoxide and nitrous oxide in the artificially perfused sheep placenta. *Circulation Res.* **16**, 95.

MILNE M.D., ASATOOR A.M., EDWARDS K. & LOUGHRIDGE L.W. (1961) Intestinal absorption defect in cystinuria. *Gut*, **2**, 323.

MISCHEL W. (1963) Der diaplacentare transport stereoisomerer Aminosäuren. *Arch. Gynäk.* **198**, 181.

MISRAHY G.A., BERAN A.V., SPRADLEY J.F. & GARWOOD V.P. (1960) Foetal brain oxygen. *Am. J. Physiol.* **199**, 959.

MORISHIMA H.O., MOYA F., BOSSERS A.C. & DANIEL S.S. (1964) Adverse effects of maternal hypocapnea on the newborn guinea pig. *Am. J. Obstet. Gynec.* **88**, 524.

MOTOYAMA E.K., ACHESON F., RIVARD G. & COOK C.D. (1966) Adverse effect of maternal hyperventilation on the foetus. *Lancet*, **1**, 286.

MOYA F., MORISHIMA H.O., SHNIDER S.M. & JAMES L.S. (1965) Influence of maternal hyperventilation on the newborn infant. *Am. J. Obstet. Gynec.* **91**, 76.

NOALL M.W., RIGGS T.R., WALKER L.M. & CHRISTENSEN H.N. (1957) Endocrine control of amino acid transfer. Distribution of an unmetabolizable amino acid. *Science, N.Y.* **126**, 1002.

NYBERG R. & WESTIN B. (1957) The influence of oxygen tension and some drugs on human placental vessels. *Acta physiol. scand.* **39**, 216.

OTEY E., STENGER V. & EITZMAN D. (1964) Movements of lactate and pyruvate in the pregnant uterus of the human. *Am. J. Obstet. Gynec.* **90**, 747.

PAGE E.W. (1957) Transfer of materials across the human placenta. *Am. J. Obstet. Gynec.* **74**, 705.

PAGE E.W., GLENDENNING M.B., MARGOLIS A.J. & HARPER H.A. (1957) Transfer of D and L-histidine across the human placenta. *Am. J. Obstet. Gynec.* **73**, 589.

PRENTON M. & YOUNG M. (1969) Umbilical vein-artery and uterine arterio-venous plasma amino acid differences (in the human subject). *J. Obstet. Gynaec. Br. Commonw.* in press.

PRYSTOWSKY H., HELLEGERS A., MESCHIA G., METCALFE J., HUCKABEE W. & BARRON D.H. (1960) The blood volume of foetuses carried by ewes at high altitude. *Q. Jl. exp. Physiol.* **45**, 292.

PRYSTOWSKY H., HELLEGERS A.E. & BRUNS P.D. (1961) A comparative study of the alkali reserve of normal and pregnant women. *Am. J. Obstet. Gynec.* **82**, 1295.

QUILLIGAN E.J., KATIGBAK E. & HOFSCHILD J. (1965) Correlation of fetal heart rate patterns and blood gas values. *Am. J. Obstet. Gynec.* **91**, 1123.

QUINTO P., ORLANDI C. & BOTTIGLIONI F. (1964) Effects of ovarian and adrenal steroids on placental passage of amino acids. In *Biological and Clinical Aspects of Placental Steroidgenesis*, p. 119. F.Polvani & A. Bompiani, eds. Karger Basle.

RAIHA N. (1958) On the placental transfer of Vitamin C. *Acta physiol. scand.* **45**, Suppl. 155.

REYNOLDS M. & YOUNG M. (1968) *Placental Transport of Amino Acids in the Guinea Pig.* To be published.

RIVARD G., MOTOYAMA E.K., ACHESON F.M., COOK C.D. & REYNOLDS E.O.R. (1967) The relation between maternal and foetal oxygen tensions in sheep. *Am. J. Obstet. Gynec.* **97**, 925.

ROBERTS S. & SZEGO C.M. (1953) Steroid interaction in the metabolism of reproductive target organs. *Physiol. Rev.* **33**, 593.

ROBERTSON G.L., HAGERMAN D.D., RICHARDSON G.S. & VILLEE C.A. (1961) Oestradiol stimulation of glycine incorporation by human endometrium in tissue culture. *Science*, **134**, 1986.

ROMNEY S.J., REID D.E., METCALFE J. & BURWELL C.S. (1955) Oxygen utilization by the human foetus *in utero*. *Am. J. Obstet. Gynec.* **70**, 791.

ROOTH G. & NILSSON I. (1964) Studies on foetal and maternal metabolic acidosis. *Clin. Sci.* **26**, 121.

SABATA V., STEMBERA Z.K., HODR J. & NOVAK M. (1964) Die wirkung von Glukoseinfusionen auf den Lipoid und Kohlenhydratstoffwechsel der Gebarended und der Frucht. *Z. Geburtsch. Gynak.* **162**, 253.

SABATA V., STEMBERA Z.K. & HODR J. (1965) Lipidovy a glycidovy metabolismus plodu rodicek trpicich diabetem. *Cs. Gynek.* **30**, 9, 688.

SALING E. (1963a) Die wirkung einer O_2-Atmung der mutter auf die blutgase und den saure-basen-haushalt des feten. *Geburtsch. Frauenheilk.* **23**, 528.

SALING E. (1963b) Die blutgasverhaltnisse und der Saure-Basen-Haushalt des feten bei ungestortem Geburtsablauf. *Z. Geburtsh. Gynak.* **161**, 262.

SALING E. (1964) Microblutuntersuchungen am feten, klinischer einsatz und este ergebnisse. *Z. Geburtsh. Gynak.* **162**, 56.

SALING E. (1966) A new method for safeguarding the life of the foetus before and during labour. *J. Int. Fed. Gynaec. Obstet.* **3**, 101.

SEEDS A., BATTAGLIA F.C. & HELLEGERS A.E. (1964) Effects of pregnancy on the pH, Pco_2 and bicarbonate concentrations of peripheral venous blood. *Am. J. Obstet. Gynec.* **88**, 1086.

SETNIKAR I. (1957) Trasporto di sostanze azotate dalla madre al feto. *Bolletino della Societa Italiana di Biologia Sperimentale*, **33**, 1636.

SHELLEY H.J. & NELLIGAN G.A. (1966) Neonatal Hypoglycaemia. *Br. med. Bull.* **22**, 34.

STERN R. (1968) *Oxygen Consumption during Labour.* To be published.

STEMBERA Z.K. & HODR J. (1962) Uber die Zirkulationsverhaltnisse in dem intervillosen Raum der plazenta in der nachgeburtsperiode. *Gynakolgentagung*, Thieme, Leipzig p. 81.

Stembera Z.K. & Hodr J. (1961) Effect of oxygen inhalation on the carbohydrate metabolism of parturient women during protracted labour. *Rev. Czech. Med.* **7**, 227.

Stembera Z.K. & Hodr J. (1966) The relationship between the blood levels of glucose, lactic acid and pyruvic acid in the mother and in both umbilical vessels of the healthy foetus. *Biologia Neonat.* **10**, 227.

Stembera Z.K., Hodr J. & Friedlandrova B. (1961) L'influence de la gymnastique de grossesse sur le metabolisme des glycides chez les meres. *Medicina dello*

Stembera Z.K., Hodr J. & Janda J. (1965) Umbilical blood flow in healthy newborn infants during the first minutes after birth. *Am. J. Obstet. Gynec.* **91**, 568.

Tyler J.M. (1960) The effect of Progesterone on the respiration of patients with emphysema and hypercapnia. *J. Clin. Invest.* **39**, 24.

Vedra B. (1963) Partial anaerobiosis in the human foetus. *Am. J. Obstet. Gynec.* **86**, 1088.

Widdas W.F. (1961) Transport mechanisms in the foetus. *Brit. med. Bull.* **17**, 107.

Wilkin P. (1960) *Le Placenta Humain*, p. 229. J.Snoek, ed. Masson et Cie, Paris.

Williams J.M. & Needham D.M. (1964) Amino acids and growth of the pregnant uterus. *Biochem. J.* **90**, 489.

Woodbury R.A., Robinow M. & Hamilton W.F. (1938) Blood pressure studies on infants. *Am. J. Physiol.* **122**, 472.

Wulf H. (1962) Der Gasaustausch in der reifen Plazenta des menschen. *Z. Geburtsh. Gynak.* **158**, 117, 269.

Young M. (1963) The fetal and neonatal circulation. Chapter 46 of *Handbook of Physiology*, Vol. 2, Section II, 1619. W.F.Hamilton & P.Row, eds. American Physiological Society, Washington D.C.

Young M. (1965) Amino acid exchange between the mother and foetus. *J. Reprod. Fertil.* **10**, 293.

Young M. (1966) Responses of the systemic circulation of the newborn infant. *Brit. med. Bull.* **22**, 70.

Young M. & Cottom D. (1966) Arterial and venous blood pressure responses during a reduction in blood volume and hypoxia and hypercapnia in infants during the first two days of life. *Pediat.* **37**, 733.

Young M. & Prenton M.A. (1969) Maternal and foetal plasma amino acid concentrations during gestation and in retarded foetal growth. *J. Obstet. Gynaec. Br. Commonw.* in press.

Zeuthen E. (1953) Oxygen uptake as related to body size in organisms. *Q. Rev. Biol.* **28**, 1.

Zinneman H.H., Seal U.S. & Doe R. (1967) Urinary amino acids in pregnancy following progesterone, and oestrogen-progesterone. *J. clin. Endocr.* **27**, 397.

5
Oestrogen Metabolism in Pregnancy

E. DICZFALUSY & S. MANCUSO

'To observations which ourselves we make,
We grow more partial for th'observer's sake.'
Alexander Pope: *Moral Essays*

INTRODUCTION

During pregnancy in the human there is a spectacular rise in the urinary oestrogen excretion, reflecting a greatly increased secretion (e.g. Diczfalusy & Lauritzen 1961, Klopper & Billewicz 1963, Paulsen 1965). The evidence pointing to the contents of the pregnant uterus as the most likely source of these oestrogens has been reviewed on several occasions (e.g. Diczfalusy & Troen 1961, Diczfalusy *et al.* 1961d, Schwers 1964). These reviews attribute the principal role in the biosynthesis of oestrogens to the *placenta*, whereas the developing *foetus* is generally regarded as an active site of intermediary metabolism, but not of biogenesis.

During the past five years a considerable amount of information has accumulated on a new aspect of the problem, namely the biosynthesis, catabolism, conjugation and transport of oestrogens in the *foeto-placental unit*. It became evident that the human foetus is a most active partner of the placenta in oestrogen synthesis and that the metabolic activities of the two are mutually complementary. Most of this information has been obtained *in vivo* at midpregnancy, utilizing tracer methodology and a variety of experimental approaches that hitherto had not been applied to the problems in question.

In this way it became possible to get some insight into the metabolic changes taking place in the foetal, placental and maternal compartments and to formulate a new concept of oestrogen metabolism in pregnancy. This concept, which is part of a general concept of steroid metabolism in the foeto-placental unit (e.g. Diczfalusy 1962, 1964a and b, 1965, 1969,

TABLE 5.1

Trivial names and systematic names of the steroids mentioned in this chapter.

Androstenedione	Androst-4-ene-3,17-dione
Retroandrostenedione	8β,9β,10α-Androst-4-ene-3,17-dion
15α-Hydroxy-androstenedione	15α-Hydroxyandrost-4-ene-3,17-dione
16α-Hydroxy-androstenedione	16α-Hydroxyandrost-4-ene-3,17-dione
16-Oxo-androstenediol	3β,17β-Dihydroxyandrost-5-en-16-one
Androstenetriol (Hirschmann's triol)	Androst-5-ene-3β,16α,17β-triol
Cholesterol	Cholest-5-en-3β-ol
Dehydroepiandrosterone	3β-Hydroxyandrost-5-en-17-one
Dehydroepiandrosterone sulphate	17-Oxoandrost-5-en-3β-yl sulphate
7α-Hydroxy-dehydroepiandrosterone sulphate	7α-Hydroxyandrost-5-en-17-on-3β-yl sulphate
16α-Hydroxy-dehydroepiandrosterone	3β,16α-Dihydroxyandrost-5-en-17-one
16α-Hydroxy-dehydroepiandrosterone sulphate	16α-Hydroxyandrost-5-en-17-on-3β-yl sulphate
Oestrone	3-Hydroxyoestra-1,3,5(10)-trien-17-one
Oestrone sulphate	Oestra-1,3,5(10)-trien-17-on-3-yl-sulphate
Oestrone glucosiduronate	Oestra-1,3,5(10)-trien-17-on-3-yl-β-D-glucopyranosiduronate
2-Hydroxy-oestrone	2,3-Dihydroxyoestra-1,3,5(10)-trien-17-one
2-Methoxy-oestrone	2-Methoxy-3-hydroxyoestra-1,3,5(10)-trien-17-one
6α-Hydroxy-oestrone	3,6α-Dihydroxyoestra-1,3,5(10)-trien-17-one
6β-Hydroxy-oestrone	3,6β-Dihydroxyoestra-1,3,5(10)-trien-17-one
11β-Hydroxy-oestrone	3,11β-Dihydroxyoestra-1,3,5(10)-trien-17-one
15α-Hydroxy-oestrone	3,15α-Dihydroxyoestra-1,3,5(10)-trien-17-one
15β-Hydroxy-oestrone	3,15β-Dihydroxyoestra-1,3,5(10)-trien-17-one
16α-Hydroxy-oestrone	3,16α-Dihydroxyoestra-1,3,5(10)-trien-17-one
16β-Hydroxy-oestrone	3,16β-Dihydroxyoestra-1,3,5(10)-trien-17-one
16-Oxo-oestrone	3-Hydroxyoestra-1,3,5(10)-triene-16,17-dione
16α-Hydroxy-oestrone sulphate	16α-Hydroxyoestra-1,3,5(10)-trien-17-on-3-yl sulphate

TABLE 5.1—*contd.*

18-Hydroxy-oestrone	3,18-Dihydroxyoestra-1,3,5(10)-trien-17-one
17β-Oestradiol	Oestra-1,3,5(10)-triene-3,17β-diol
17β-Oestradiol 3-sulphate	17β-Hydroxyoestra-1,3,5(10)-trien-3-yl sulphate
2-Methoxy-17β-oestradiol	2-Methoxyoestra-1,3,5(10)-triene-3,17β-diol
6α-Hydroxy-17β-oestradiol	Oestra-1,3,5(10)-triene-3,6α,17β-triol
15α-Hydroxy-17β-oestradiol	Oestra-1,3,5(10)-triene-3,15α,17β-triol
15β-Hydroxy-17β-oestradiol	Oestra-1,3,5(10)-triene-3,15β,17β-triol
16-Oxo-17β-oestradiol	3,17β-Dihydroxyoestra-1,3,5(10)-trien-16-one
11-Dehydro-17α-oestradiol	Oestra-1,3,5(10),11-tetraene-3,17α-diol
Oestriol	Oestra-1,3,5(10)-triene-3,16α,17β-triol
Oestriol 3-sulphate	16α,17β-Dihydroxyoestra-1,3,5(10)-trien-3-yl sulphate
Oestriol 3-glucosiduronate	16α,17β-Dihydroxyoestra-1,3,5(10)-trien-3-yl-β-D-glucopyranosiduronate
Oestriol 16-glucosiduronate	3,17β-Dihydroxyoestra-1,3,5(10)-trien-16α-yl-β-D-glucopyranosiduronate
Oestriol 3-sulphate, 16-glucosiduronate	17β-Hydroxyoestra-1,3,5(10)-trien-3-yl-sulphate, 16α-yl-β-D-glucopyranosiduronate
2-Methoxy-oestriol	2-Methoxyoestra-1,3,5(10)-triene-3,16α,17β-triol
6α-Hydroxy-oestriol	Oestra-1,3,5(10)-triene-3,6α,16α,17β-tetrol
15α-Hydroxy-oestriol	Oestra-1,3,5(10)-triene-3,15α,16α,17β-tetrol
16-Epi-oestriol	Oestra-1,3,5(10)-triene-3,16β,17β-triol
17-Epi-oestriol	Oestra-1,3,5(10)-triene-3,16α,17α-triol
16,17-Epioestriol	Oestra-1,3,5(10)-triene-3,16β,17α-triol
Oestratetrenol	Oestra-1,3,5(10),16-tetraen-3-ol
Pregnanediol	5β-Pregnane-3α,20α-diol
Pregnenolone	3β-Hydroxypregn-5-en-20-one
17α-Hydroxy-pregnenolone	3β,17α-Dihydroxypregn-5-en-20-one
Progesterone	Pregn-4-ene-3,20-dione
17α-Hydroxy-progesterone	17α-Hydroxypregn-4-ene-3,20-dione
Testosterone	17β-Hydroxyandrost-4-en-3-one
Retrotestosterone	17β-Hydroxy-8β,9β,10α-androst-4-en-3-one
15α-Hydroxy-testosterone	15α,17β-Dihydroxyandrost-4-en-3-one
16α-Hydroxy-testosterone	16α,17β-Dihydroxyandrost-4-en-3-one

Diczfalusy *et al.* 1965, Diczfalusy & Mancuso 1965), postulates that the placenta and foetus are two specialized compartments of an integrated functional unit, with a characteristic distribution of the essential steroidogenic enzyme systems between the two compartments.

HORMONAL CHANGES DURING PREGNANCY

Pregnancy in the human species is characterized by a gradually increasing urinary elimination of various oestrogens (e.g. Brown 1956, Diczfalusy & Lauritzen 1961, Jayle 1965). From late pregnancy urine some 20 oestrogens have been isolated thus far and at least an additional 7 have been detected in this source. The trivial names and systematic names of these oestrogens together with those of other steroids mentioned in this review are summarized in Table 5.1. The isolation and approximate quantities of various oestrogens in pregnancy urine at term are shown in Table 5.2. The oestrogens present in highest concentration are those substituted at carbon atom 16; among these oestriol accounts for some 90 per cent of the total. With the exception of oestrone, all other 16-desoxy-oestrogens isolated so far seem to be present in concentrations of less than 1·0 mg/24 hr. Compared with the oestrogen excretion by non-pregnant women, it appears that in late pregnancy the increase in the elimination of oestriol is some 1,000-fold and that of oestrone almost 100-fold. It is of considerable interest that some of these compounds (specially the products of 15α-hydroxylation) are predominantly of foetal origin (Gurpide *et al.* 1966).

The increased urinary excretion of oestrogen in pregnancy urine is accompanied by elevated oestrogen levels in maternal blood (Roy & MacKay 1962, Smith & Arai 1963, Maner *et al.* 1963, Smith 1965), in the amniotic fluid (Diczfalusy & Magnusson 1958) and cord blood (Roy 1962, Maner *et al.* 1963) and by highly elevated oestriol excretion in the urine (Diczfalusy *et al.* 1957a and b) and meconium (Diczfalusy *et al.* 1959) of the newborn.

The oestrogen pattern of these last two sources is dominated by oestriol, and other oestrogens are present only in very low amounts (e.g. Diczfalusy & Lauritzen 1961, Thorsen *et al.* 1964). The same can be said with regard to the pattern of oestrogens in various foetal tissues (Diczfalusy & Magnusson 1958). On the other hand, the oestrogen pattern of placental tissue is more or less in agreement with that of maternal blood (Diczfalusy & Lindqvist 1956, Schmidt-Elmendorff 1961). The available figures representing the conditions at term are

TABLE 5.2

Oestrogens isolated from or detected in human pregnancy urine, and their approximate quantities at term.

	References	Approximate quantities (mg/24 hr)
Oestrogens isolated		
Oestriol	Marrian 1929	25·0–35·0
Oestrone	Doisy *et al.* 1929	1·20–1·40
16α-Hydroxy-oestrone	Marrian *et al.* 1957	0·60[c]–1·60[b]
16-Epi-oestriol	Marrian & Bauld 1955	0·35[a]–0·80[b]
16β-Hydroxy-oestrone	Layne & Marrian 1958	0·10[c]–0·72[b]
16-Oxo-17β-oestradiol	Layne & Marrian 1958	0·20[c]–1·10[b]
17β-Oestradiol	Huffmann *et al.* 1940	0·42–0·60
2-Methoxy-oestrone	Loke & Marrian 1958	0·17[d]–0·60[b]
6-Hydroxy-oestriol	Breuer *et al.* 1966	0·05[g]–0·50[g]
17-Epi-oestriol	Breuer 1960a	0·01[e]–0·12[b]
16,17-Epi-oestriol	Breuer & Pangels 1959	0·04[f]–0·15[b]
2-Methoxy-oestriol	Breuer 1964	0·30[b]
11-Dehydro-17α-oestradiol	Luukkainen & Adlercreutz 1965	—
18-Hydroxy-oestrone	Loke *et al.* 1957	—
15α-Hydroxy-oestrone	Knuppen *et al.* 1965	—
6α-Hydroxy-oestrone	Knuppen *et al.* 1966a	—
15β-Hydroxy-oestrone	Knuppen *et al.* 1966b	—
15β-Hydroxy-17β-oestradiol	Knuppen *et al.* 1966b	—
15α-Hydroxy-17β-oestradiol	Lisboa *et al.* 1967	—
15α-Hydroxy-oestriol	Zucconi *et al* 1967b	—
Oestrogens detected		
Oestratetrenol	Breuer 1964	1·60[b]
6α-Hydroxy-17β-oestradiol	Breuer 1964	0·80[b]
2-Methoxy-17β-oestradiol	Frandsen 1959	0·20[b]
2-Hydroxy-oestrone	Notchev & Stimmel 1962	0·12[h]
16-Oxo-oestrone	Serchi 1953	—
6β-Hydroxy-oestrone	Breuer 1964	—
11β-Hydroxy-oestrone	Breuer 1964	—

[a] Watson & Marrian 1956. [b] Breuer 1964. [c] Layne & Marrian 1958. [d] Hobkirk & Nilsen 1962. [e] Breuer 1960a. [f] Breuer & Pangels 1959. [g] Breuer *et al.* 1966. [h] Notchev & Stimmel 1962.

summarized in Table 5.3 and those referring to midpregnancy in Table 5.4. An assessment of the data of Tables 5.3 and 5.4 indicates a high concentration of oestriol contrasted to the paucity or lack of oestrone and 17β-oestradiol in all foetal tissues and body fluids. On the

TABLE 5.3

Concentration of oestrone, 17β-oestradiol and oestriol in tissues and body fluids at term. Values are expressed as μg/100 ml and μg/100 gr, respectively.

Oestrogen	Maternal urine*	Maternal blood	Umbilical cord		Placenta	Amniotic fluid	Blood (newborn)	Urine (newborn)	Meconium
			Artery	Vein					
Oestrone	100·0	6·3[a]	1·0[a]	1·3[a]	35·8[c]	0·6[d]	—	0·7[f]	0·0
17β-Oestradiol	35·0	1·3[a]	0·3[a]	0·4[a]	113·5[c]	0·5[d]	—	0·1[f]	0·0
Oestriol	1500·0	9·1[a]	81·0[b]	79·0[b]	202·0[c]	88·0[d]	25·0[e] 40·0[h]	700·0[f]	9700·0[g]

* Assuming an average urine output of 1500 ml per 24 hr.

[a] Geometric means from Roy & Brown 1960 and Maner *et al.* 1963. [b] Geometric means from Roy & Brown 1960, Maner *et al.* 1963 and Klausner & Ryan 1964. [c] Geometric means from Diczfalusy & Lindkvist, 1956 and Schmidt-Elmendorff 1961. [d] From: Diczfalusy & Magnusson 1958. [e] From: Diczfalusy & Lauritzen 1961 (2 hours after birth). [f] From: Diczfalusy *et al* 1957a. [g] From: Diczfalusy *et al.* 1959. [h] From: Troen *et al.* 1961.

other hand, in the placental tissue and maternal blood there seems to be almost as much oestrone and 17β-oestradiol as oestriol. The high concentration of oestriol in the urine of newborns and in the meconium seems to reflect a gradual accumulation of this compound in the foetal organism and the absence of oestrone and 17β-oestradiol suggests their rapid catabolism.

TABLE 5.4

Concentration of oestrone, 17β-oestradiol and oestriol in mother and foetus during the second trimester of pregnancy. Values are expressed as μg/100 ml.

Oestrogens	Maternal urine[a]	Maternal blood[b]	Foetal blood[c]	Amniotic fluid[c]	Placenta μg/100 gr[a]
Oestrone	12·6	2·70	0·47	0·38	6·4
17β-Oestradiol	4·7	1·40	0·11	0·17	3·2
Oestriol	236·6	3·50	20·5	3·70	12·0

For maternal urine average 24-hr output is calculated as 1500 ml.
[a] Cassmer 1959. [b] Cédard 1964. [c] Diczfalusy & Magnusson 1958.

SITES OF OESTROGEN FORMATION

What is the origin of the high amounts of oestrogens present during pregnancy? Until fairly recently it was believed that the placenta was the major, if not exclusive, source of these oestrogens (e.g. Diczfalusy & Troen 1961).

This was based *i.a.* on the evidence that the removal of other oestrogen-producing glands of the mother (such as the ovaries and adrenals) did not abolish the high urinary oestrogen levels (e.g. Diczfalusy & Borell 1961, Harkness *et al.* 1966), whereas after delivery or removal of the placenta, the urinary oestrogen excretion rapidly returned to non-pregnancy levels. Also in many cases of hydatidiform mole or chorio-epithelioma (e.g. Frandsen & Stakemann 1964b, MacNaughton 1965), a relatively elevated urinary oestrogen excretion was reported.

Other data, such as the claims that human term placental tissue is capable of producing oestrogen when cultivated in tissue culture (DeClerc 1958), when implanted into the eyes of castrated rabbits (Stewart 1951), or perfused with radioactive acetate (Levitz *et al.* 1955) provided only ambiguous evidence of the mechanism of oestrogen synthesis in pregnancy (e.g. Frandsen & Stakemann 1963), the more

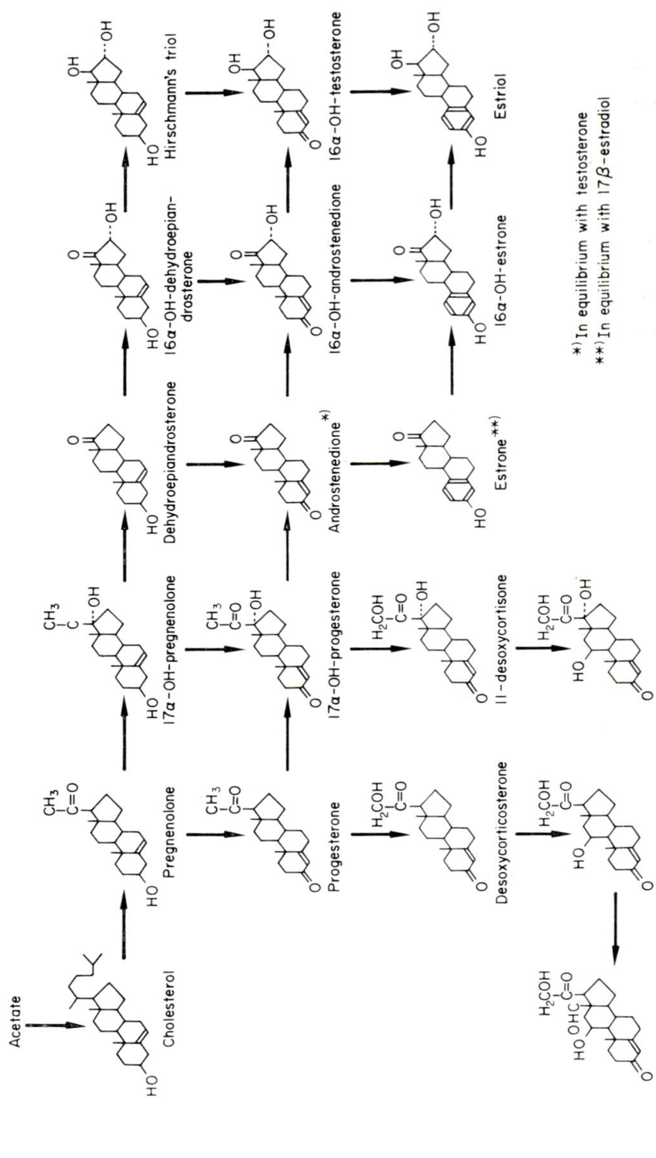

FIG. 5.1. Some of the most important steps of steroidogenesis in the human organism. (According to Diczfalusy 1964a.)

so as the conversion of acetate by perfused placentas was not confirmed later (Levitz *et al.* 1962).

The inadequacy of previous interpretations should probably be sought in their nature, which was anatomico-biological, rather than biochemical. Interpretations were based on the general assumption that a certain endocrine gland either produces a biologically active steroid hormone, or not, and the possibility was not envisaged that the different enzyme reactions involved in the synthesis of any biologically active steroid may be complementary and localized in anatomically different structures. Furthermore, the possibility was not considered that the human foetus might be endowed with a marked ability to carry out certain enzyme reactions which are essential for the synthesis of several steroid hormones.

In contrast, the concept of the foeto-placental unit (e.g. Diczfalusy *et al.* 1965, Diczfalusy 1967, 1969) considers that the steroidogenesis of pregnancy takes place in two 'compartments' of the same system, the foetal and placental compartments.

This theory states that at midpregnancy both the foetus and placenta represent deficient but mutually complementary steroidogenic systems, which complement each other in such a fashion that the foeto-placental unit is capable of carrying out the synthesis of practically all biologically active steroid hormones.

GENERAL PATHWAY OF OESTROGEN BIOSYNTHESIS

Discussion of the peculiarities of the foeto-placental oestrogen producing system may be greatly facilitated by a short recapitulation of the general pathways leading to the synthesis of steroid oestrogens. A necessarily incomplete scheme with some of the key reactions involved in the biosynthesis of the most important steroid hormones is presented in Fig. 5.1.

This scheme may be considered as representing one of several cross-sections of a three-dimensional system, in which each of the steroids indicated may give rise to several products of conjugation, hydroxylation and/or reduction, situated below and above the plane of the paper, but not indicated in the scheme.

This group of 'forgotten' steroids also includes biologically important products of dehydrogenation, such as testosterone and 17β-oestradiol. These compounds and also androst-5-ene-3β,17β-diol are in dynamic equilibrium with their 17-oxo counterparts. Thus in order to be converted into oestrogen, acetate has to be transformed into cholesterol, and the latter into pregnenolone. As shown in Fig. 5.1, both pregnenolone and progesterone might give rise to oestrogens, the former via 17α-hydroxy-pregnenolone and dehydroepiandrosterone, the latter via 17α-hydroxy-progesterone and androstenedione. However, the balance

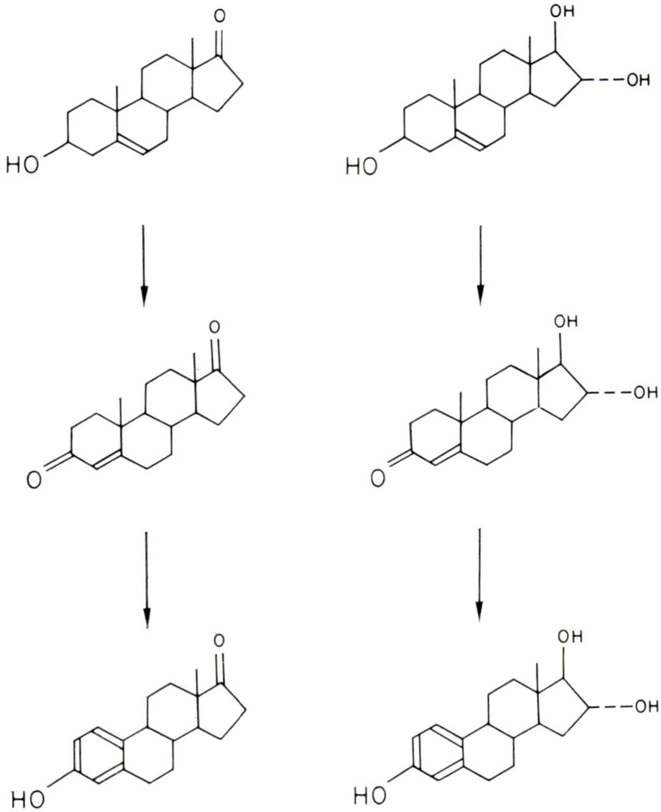

FIG. 5.2. The most characteristic steps of oestrogen biogenesis in the human placenta.

of evidence available at present indicates that androstenedione is an obligatory intermediate in the conversion of dehydroepiandrosterone to oestrogens, or in more general terms that the α,β-unsaturated 3-ketosteroids with 19 carbon atoms are obligatory intermediates in the conversion of β,γ-unsaturated steroids into the corresponding ring A aromatic steroids. This is illustrated by two characteristic examples shown in Fig. 5.2. The examples shown in Fig. 5.2 are schematic and do not indicate the intermediary products formed in connection with the removal of the angular methyl group at carbon atom 10. These reactions have been discussed *i.a.* by Ryan (1963b) and by Wilcox & Engel (1965a and b).

PLACENTAL BIOGENESIS *IN VITRO*

A 'true' oestrogen producing organ is capable of utilizing all the important precursors for oestrogen biosynthesis. Thus it was demonstrated that human ovarian tissue *in vitro* can synthesize 17β-oestradiol and/or oestrone in good yield from acetate (Ryan & Smith 1961a), cholesterol (Ryan & Smith 1961b), pregnenolone (Ryan 1963a), progesterone (Ryan & Smith 1961c, Ryan 1963a), androstenedione (Smith & Ryan 1961, Axelrod & Goldzieher 1965) and testosterone (Wotiz *et al.* 1956, Baggett *et al.* 1959, Axelrod & Goldzieher 1965).

It was also shown that human ovarian tissue can convert androstenedione and testosterone into oestriol (Axelrod & Goldzieher 1965). These results indicate that the human ovary is endowed *i.a.* with the 16α-hydroxylating and aromatizing enzyme systems. In addition, it is also capable of carrying out 17α-hydroxylation of pregnenolone and progesterone and it can remove the side chain of both 17α-hydroxypregnenolone and 17α-hydroxy-progesterone.

When it comes to the assessment of the steroid biogenetic potential of the placenta, there is no doubt that it has a most potent aromatizing enzyme system and is capable of converting a wide variety of neutral C-19 steroids into the corresponding oestrogens, as indicated in Table 5.5. Perusal of the data of Table 5.5 reveals that hydroxylation at the positions 1β-, 2β-, 7α-, 7β- and 11α- does not interfere with aromatization, whereas compounds hydroxylated at 1α-, 2α-, 11β- positions, as well as 7-oxo- and 11-oxo- compounds are not aromatized. Furthermore Δ^6-compounds cannot be aromatized, whereas the Δ^1-, Δ^4-, Δ^5-, Δ^7 and Δ^{16}-compounds are converted into steroid oestrogens. Finally, the 8β, 9β, 10α-, or 8α, 9α, 10α-configurations exclude aromatization, whereas the 8β, 9β, 10β- and 8β, 9α, 10β-configurations do not interfere with the removal of the angular methyl group at C-10.

The balance of evidence indicates that if enzymic reactions required for side-chain cleavage are present at all in placental tissue, the extent of these reactions must be minimal. Thus no conversion of pregnenolone,

TABLE 5.5

Aromatization of various steroids by human placental preparations.

Aromatized		Not aromatized	
19-Nor-17β-hydroxyandrost-4-en-3-one	Gual *et al.* 1962	3-Oxoandrost-4-ene-17β-yl sulphate	Baulieu *et al.* 1965
10β-Carboxyoestr-4-ene-3,17-dione	Morato *et al.* 1961	5α-Androst-1-ene-3,17-dione	Gual *et al.* 1962, Ryan 1963b
Oestr-4-ene-3,17-dione	Gual *et al.* 1962		
		17β-Hydroxyandrostan-3-one	Ryan 1963b
17β-Hydroxyoestr-4-en-3-one[a]	Ryan 1959a	17β-Hydroxy-8β,9β,10α-androst-4-en-3-one[g]	Walop & de Lange 1966
Androst-4-ene-3,17-dione[b]	Ryan 1959a		
Androsta-1,4-diene-3,17-dione	Ryan 1959a	8α,9α,10α-Androst-4-ene-3,17-dione	Walop & de Lange 1966
Androsta-4,7-diene-3,17-dione	Stárka *et al.* 1966a	2α-Hydroxyandrost-4-ene-3,17-dione	Ryan 1963b
Androsta-4,16-diene-3,17-dione	Knuppen & Breuer 1963	6α-Fluoro-17β-hydroxyandrost-4-en-3-one	Gual *et al.* 1962
3β-Hydroxyandrost-5-en-17-one[b]	Ryan 1959a	6β-Fluoro-17β-hydroxyandrost-4-en-3-one	Gual *et al.* 1962
3β-Hydroxyandrosta-5,7-diene-17-one	Starka *et al.* 1966a	3β,17β-Dihydroxyandrost-5-en-7-one	Cédard *et al.* 1964
17β-Hydroxyandrost-4-en-3-one[b, c]	Ryan 1959a	11β-Hydroxyandrost-4-ene-3,17-dione	Breuer 1962
17α-Hydroxyandrost-4-en-3-one	Ryan 1963b	Androst-4-ene-3,11,17-trione	Ryan 1959a
17β-Acetoxyandrost-4-en-3-one	Walop & de Lange 1966	11β,17β-Dihydroxyandrost-4-en-3-one	Ryan 1963b
17α-Methyl-17β-hydroxyandrost-4-en-3-one	Ryan 1963b	5α-Androstane-3,17-dione	Gual *et al.* 1962
		1α-Hydroxyandrost-4-ene-3,17-dione	Gual *et al.* 1962
17β-Hydroxyandrosta-1,4-dien-3-one	Ryan 1963b	1α,3β-Dihydroxyandrost-5-en-17-one	Gual *et al.* 1962
17β-Hydroxyandrosta-4,6-dien-3-one	Walop & de Lange 1966	Androsta-4,6-diene-3,17-dione	Gual *et al.* 1962
8β,9β,10β-Androst-4-ene-3,17-dione	Walop & de Lange 1966	Androsta-1,4,6-triene-3,17-dione	Gual *et al.* 1962

1β,17β-Dihydroxyandrost-4-en-3-one	Ryan 1963b	Pregn-4-ene-3,20-dione	Ryan 1959a
2β-Hydroxyandrost-4-ene-3,17-dione	Ryan 1963b, Gual *et al.* 1962	3β-Hydroxypregn-5-en-20-one	Ryan 1959a
		17α-Hydroxypregn-4-ene-3,20-dione	Ryan 1959a
6α-Hydroxyandrost-4-ene-3,17-dione	Breuer 1960b		
6β-Hydroxyandrost-4-ene-3,17-dione	Breuer 1960b		
3β,7α-Dihydroxyandrost-5-en-17-one	Cédard *et al.* 1964 Starka *et al.* 1966b		
3β,7β-Dihydroxyandrost-5-en-17-one	Cédard *et al.* 1964		
Androst-5-ene-3β,7β,17β-triol	Cédard *et al.* 1964		
9α,17β-Dihydroxyandrost-4-en-3-one	Gual *et al.* 1962		
9α-Fluoroandrosta-1,4-diene-3,17-dione	Gual *et al.* 1962		
11α-Hydroxyandrost-4-ene-3,17-dione	Gual *et al.* 1962		
11α,17β-Dihydroxyandrost-4-en-3-one	Ryan 1963b		
16α-Hydroxyandrost-4-ene-3,17-dione[d]	Ryan 1959b		
3β,16α-Dihydroxyandrost-5-en-17-one[d]	Magendantz & Ryan 1964		
16α,17β-Dihydroxyandrost-4-en-3-one[d]	Ryan 1959b		
3β,17β-Dihydroxyandrost-5-en-16-one[e]	—		
Androst-5-ene-3β,16α,17β-triol[f]	Ryan 1958		
18-Hydroxyandrost-4-ene-3,17-dione	Tan & Loke 1966		
19-Hydroxyandrost-4-ene-3,17-dione	Meyer 1955		
3β,19-Dihydroxyandrost-5-en-17-one	Wilcox & Engel 1965a		
3,17-Dioxo-androst-4-en-19-al	Morato *et al.* 1961		

Aromatization of these compounds by placentas perfused *in situ* has been demonstrated by the following authors: [a] Dell'Acqua *et al.* 1965. [b] Bolté *et al.* 1964a. [c] Bolté *et al.* 1964d. [d] Dell'Acqua *et al.* 1967b. [e] Reynolds *et al.* 1968. [f] Dell'Acqua *et al.* 1967a. [g] Dell'Acqua *et al.* 1966.

17α-hydroxy-pregnenolone, progesterone or 17α-hydroxy-progesterone into oestrogen was found following incubation with placental preparations (Ryan 1959a). Also hydatidiform moles converted in high yield dehydroepiandrosterone but not pregnenolone into oestrone and 17β-oestradiol (Van Leusden & Villee 1966). That normal placentas are not capable of converting C-21 into C-18 steroids was also shown *in vitro* by Sobrevilla *et al.* (1964) and following perfusions of midterm placentas *in situ* by Pion *et al.* (1965), Jaffe *et al.* (1965) and Palmer *et al.* (1966a and b). Furthermore, no oestrogens were found following perfusion of placental cotyledons with acetate (Levitz *et al.* 1962). On the other hand, reports have been published claiming that placental tissue is capable of removing the steroid side-chain (Little *et al.* 1963, Warren & Cheatum 1964, DeMiquel & Troen 1966, Jungmann *et al.* 1966). In several of these communications the identification of the end product was tentative. At any rate, there is a consensus of opinion that–from the quantitative point of view–the ability of the placenta to remove the steroid side-chain is insignificant. The same can be said about the 16α-hydroxylating capacity of human placental tissue, which was claimed by several investigators (e.g. Cédard *et al.* 1961, Troen 1961, Little *et al.* 1963, Slaunwhite *et al.* 1965, Jungmann *et al.* 1966), but could not be demonstrated by others, using placental slices (e.g. Ryan & Engel 1953), microsomes (e.g. Ryan 1959a, Morato *et al.* 1965), homogenates (Jackanicz & Diczfalusy 1968), term cotyledons perfused *in vitro* (Levitz *et al.* 1956), intact term placentas perfused *in vitro* (Cédard & Knuppen 1965, Alonso & Troen 1966), or midterm placentas perfused *in situ* (Bolté *et al.* 1964a, Pion *et al.* 1965, Dell'Acqua *et al.* 1966, Palmer *et al.* 1966a and b, Dell'Acqua *et al.* 1967b, Reynolds *et al.* 1968).

Obviously, it is always difficult to exclude definitely the possibility that a certain reaction product is formed in very small or trace quantities. However, it is easy to see that the quantitative significance of such a reaction is practically nil, especially if the reaction is demonstrated only *in vitro*, but the finding is not corroborated *in vivo*. Therefore, from the quantitative point of view, the 16α-hydroxylating ability of the placenta is insignificant. On the other hand, it has been demonstrated that placental preparations are capable of aromatizing in good yield 16α-substituted neutral C-19 steroids such as Hirschmann's triol (Ryan 1958), 16α-hydroxy-androstenedione, 16α-hydroxy-testosterone (Ryan 1959b), and 16α-hydroxy-dehydroepiandrosterone (Magendantz & Ryan 1964).

Thus the balance of the *in vitro* evidence (strongly supported by certain *in vivo* studies) indicates that the human placenta has a most active aromatizing enzyme system and converts in high yield both 16-desoxy- and 16-oxygenated C-19 neutral steroids into the corresponding oestrogens.

On the other hand, the side-chain splitting and 17α-hydroxylating capacity of the placenta appears to be so limited that the high concentration of oestriol and other oestrogens in pregnancy urine cannot be explained without assuming that these reactions occur mainly, if not entirely, in the foetal and maternal, but not in the placental compartment.

LIMITATIONS OF THE *IN VITRO* APPROACH

The Stockholm approach can be characterized by the philosophy that whenever possible, *in vivo* experiments should be conducted in order to obtain information under experimental conditions approaching the physiological. Some of the advantages of the *in vivo* approach are obvious, some of them are less obvious and can only be assessed in the light of the limitations of the *in vitro* approach. Thus the relative amounts of certain end-products formed *in vitro* by homogenates or purified enzymes may depend on the co-factors added and the pH employed (Henning & Zander 1962, Dorfman *et al.* 1964). Thus homogenates of foetal liver form only 17-oxo metabolites (both neutral and aromatic) from androstenedione, whereas perfusion of previable foetuses with the same compound (Mancuso *et al.* 1968) or its injection into the intact foeto-placental circulation (Benagiano *et al.* 1967) yields 17β-hydroxy- and 17-oxo-forms in approximately equal quantities and in complete equilibrium.

The presence or absence of another steroid in an *in vitro* system significantly influences the metabolism of some steroids (e.g. Dorfman *et al.* 1964, Villee & Villee 1964, Villee 1965), a major complication in the *in vitro*, but not in the *in vivo* assessment of the quantitative importance of a reaction. Furthermore, in an *in vivo* situation, enzymes can be compartimentalized in the various cell structures and different substrates may reach these 'compartments' in different quantities. Thus it was shown by Lamb *et al.* (1967) that more dehydroepiandrosterone sulphate than dehydroepiandrosterone is converted into androstenedione by mid-term placentas perfused *in situ*. Homogenization of the tissue may make the demonstration of such differences difficult, if not impossible. However, one may demonstrate important conversions by the use of *in vitro* systems, which cannot be demonstrated *in vivo* because of the general distribution, metabolism and transport of the circulating precursor in question. Thus no oestrogens were isolated from the urine of gonadotrophin-stimulated women following a long-term intravenous infusion of a combination of labelled dehydroepiandrosterone sulphate and dehydroepiandrosterone (Mancuso *et al.* 1965c), whereas steroid sulphatase (Sandberg & Jenkins 1966) activity of human ovarian tissue as well as the aromatization of dehydroepiandrosterone (Flickinger *et al.* 1967) and of 7α-hydroxy-dehydroepiandrosterone sulphate (Starka *et al.* 1966a) by human corpus luteum tissue is readily demonstrated *in vitro*.

On the other hand, *in vitro* experiments also have great merits. They were shown to be of great value for the biosynthesis of labelled steroid material to be used *in vivo* (e.g. Levitz *et al.* 1965, Goebelsmann *et al.* 1965c, Reynolds 1966). Furthermore, there seems to be a close qualitative (but not quantitative) agreement between the various products of hydroxylation found in the tissues of previable foetuses following perfusion, or *in vitro* incubation (Knuppen *et al.* 1966c, Mancuso *et al.* 1967). All products formed *in vitro* were also detected following perfusion.*

The same can be said concerning the absence of sterol sulphatase activity from the tissues of human foetuses, which was demonstrated both *in vitro* (Pulkkinen 1961, French & Warren 1965) and *in vivo* (Bolté *et al.* 1966).

Another great advantage of *in vitro* studies is that they enable the investigator to follow the kinetics of a reaction and to demonstrate the formation of important intermediary products, which are sometimes metabolized so rapidly that it may be very difficult to isolate them in an *in vivo* system. Thus it was shown that 19-hydroxylation is an obligatory intermediary reaction in the aromatization of androstenedione, using placental microsomal preparations (Wilcox & Engel 1965b), whereas no 19-hydroxylated neutral metabolites were detected following the *in situ* perfusion of placentas with dehydroepiandrosterone sulphate and dehydroepiandrosterone (Lamb *et al.* 1967).

Thus *in vitro* and *in vivo* studies of steroidogenesis are mutually

* On the other hand, several metabolites found following the incubation of foetal tissues with progesterone were not detected in perfusion studies (e.g. Bird *et al.* 1966).

complementary, and not exclusive, each of these techniques providing different but essential information.

EXPERIMENTAL APPROACH

Although *in vivo* experiments provide information which cannot always be obtained *in vitro*, even such experiments have serious limitations. It is important therefore to adopt a variety of techniques and approaches to obtain valid information. In Stockholm, we try to reach such conclusions as follows. The experiments are carried out–whenever possible–*in vivo* on volunteers who are admitted to the hospital for the interruption of gestation for social-medical indications. Permission for interruption of pregnancy is granted, upon request of the patients, by the Royal Medical Board of Sweden under the statute of 1938, amended in 1946 and 1963. The period of gestation is between the 17th and 20th week.

The general approach involves the administration of tracer doses of radioactive steroids into the various compartments of the foeto-placental unit, or perfusion of normal (e.g. Diczfalusy *et al.* 1961b, Mikhail *et al.* 1963a) or adrenalectomized (Wilson *et al.* 1966) previable foetuses. The foetuses are perfused in a single cycle with the steroid administered in diluted and oxygenated human group O, Rh negative blood. In comparative studies (*in vivo* versus *in vitro*) the foetuses are perfused as above with a labelled steroid. A part of the foetal tissues is analysed, whereas another part is incubated with the same steroid, which is labelled differently. Foetal tissue is used either as slices (Knuppen *et al.* 1966c) or homogenates (Mancuso *et al.* 1967). In order to single out organs in which important accumulation and metabolism of the steroid in question takes place, whole body autoradiography is carried out following perfusion of such foetuses with high doses of radioactive steroids (Bengtsson *et al.* 1964).

To study the processes taking place in the placental compartment, *in situ* perfusion of the placentas is performed at laparotomy following removal of the foetus (e.g. Bolté *et al.* 1964a). However, it may be questioned whether the perfusion of the previable foetuses at 20° is really equivalent to experimental conditions *in vivo*, not only because of the low temperature, but also because the composition of adult blood is different from that of the cord blood. It is realized, furthermore, that *in situ* perfusion of the placentas at laparotomy is carried out under haemodynamic conditions, which may be significantly different from those existing in an intact pregnant uterus. Therefore, the conclusions reached in foetal and placental perfusion experiments must be corroborated and completed by studies in which the intact foeto-placental unit is maintained *in situ* and the steroids to be studied are introduced into the intact foeto-placental circulation, either at laparotomy (e.g. Mikhail *et al.* 1963b), or *per vaginam* (Bolté *et al.* 1964c), or following the injection of the tracer into a uterine artery (Bolté *et al.* 1964b), or into the amniotic fluid (Diczfalusy *et al.* 1963) prior to the removal of the products of conception. Finally, in order to assess the importance of the maternal metabolism, the tracer is administered into the antecubital vein of the mother as a single injection (Wilson *et al.* 1964), or as an infusion (Goebelsmann *et al.* 1965a). Some of these experimental designs are illustrated schematically in Fig. 5.3.

The metabolites formed are then isolated from the various tissues and body fluids in a radiochemically homogeneous form.

PLACENTAL BIOGENESIS IN VIVO

In 1959 Cassmer ligated the umbilical cord in patients undergoing legal abortions and left the placenta and dead foetus *in situ* for three days. Interruption of the foeto-placental circulation resulted in a very marked and immediate drop in the urinary excretion of the three 'classical' oestrogens, oestrone, 17β-oestradiol and oestriol, whereas pregnanediol excretion showed only a slight decrease, suggesting that for placental oestrogen synthesis foetal precursors are more important than the maternal precursors. This is in agreement with the findings that the urinary oestrogen excretion in women pregnant with anencephalic monsters is low (Frandsen & Stakemann 1961, 1964a), similarly to that found in pathological pregnancies characterized by the absence of the foetus, such as hydatidiform mole and chorioepithelioma (Frandsen & Stakemann 1964b, MacNaughton 1965). Since in anencephalic monsters

FIG. 5.3. Schematic representation of some of the experimental approaches used in Stockholm. A: Perfusion of a previable foetus. B: *In situ* perfusion of a midterm placenta. C: Injection of tracers into a uterine artery. D: Simultaneous injection of tracers into the foetal and maternal circulations.

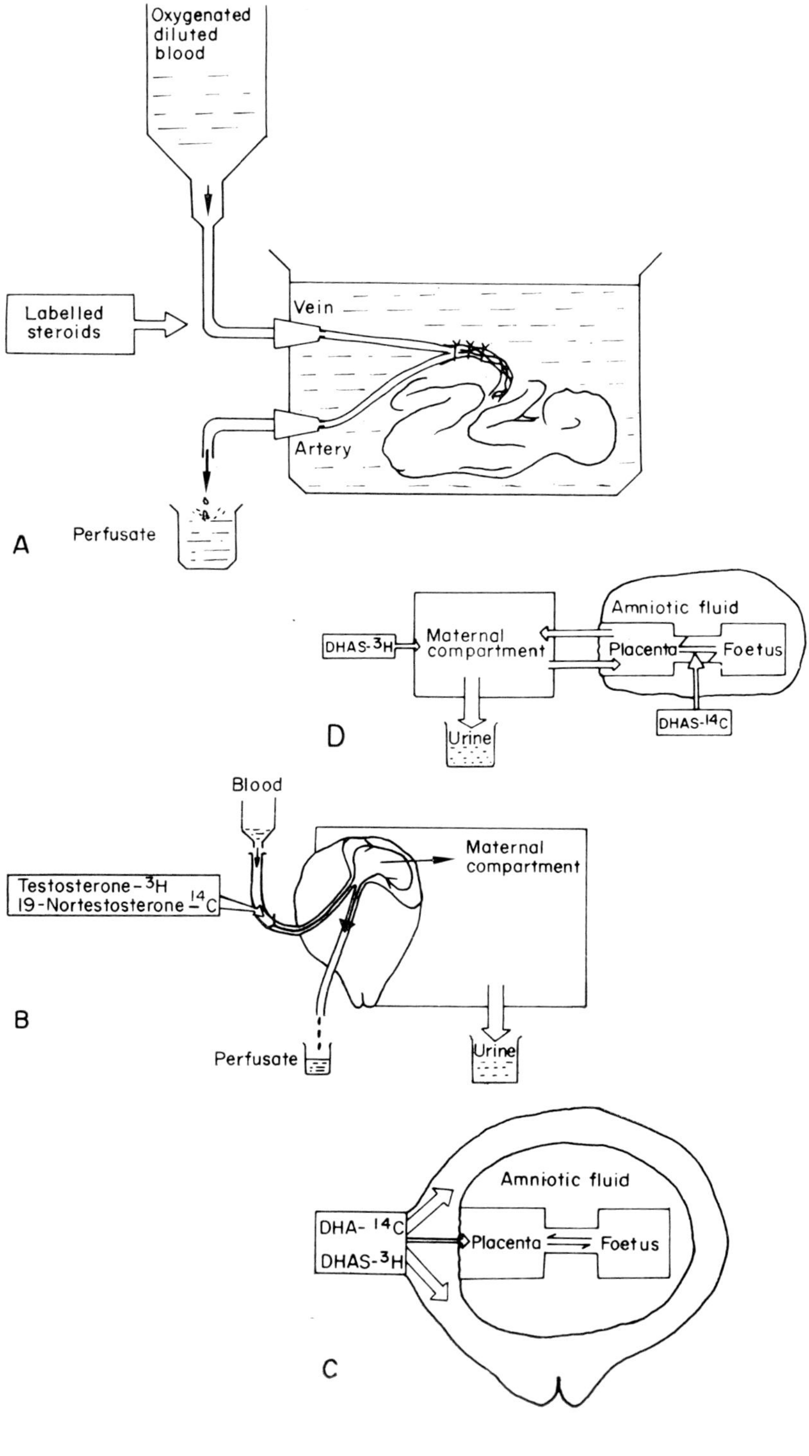

Oxygenated diluted blood
Labelled steroids
Vein
Artery
Perfusate
A
DHAS-^{3}H
Maternal compartment
Amniotic fluid
Placenta
Foetus
DHAS-^{14}C
Urine
D
Blood
Testosterone-^{3}H
19-Nortestosterone-^{14}C
Maternal compartment
B
Perfusate
Urine
Amniotic fluid
DHA-^{14}C
DHAS-^{3}H
Placenta
Foetus
C

the adrenals are usually rudimentary (Lanman 1953, Benirschke 1956), Frandsen & Stakemann suggested that in normal pregnancy the foetal adrenals are producing substantial quantities of a precursor which is converted by the placenta into oestrogens.*

That placental aromatization of various C-19 steroids is indeed involved in the elaboration of the major quantities of oestrogen in pregnant women was demonstrated following perfusion of term placentas *in vitro* (Cédard 1964, Cédard *et al.* 1966) and following the administration of radioactive compounds to pregnant women (Baulieu & Dray 1963, Siiteri & MacDonald 1963, Warren & Timberlake 1964, Bolté *et al.* 1964c).

That aromatization of foetal precursors plays a particularly important role was then shown following *in situ* perfusion of placentas at midpregnancy, using labelled androstenedione, testosterone, dehydroepiandrosterone and dehydroepiandrosterone sulphate (Bolté *et al.* 1964a and d). Perfusion with any of these precursors resulted in the formation of both oestrone and 17β-oestradiol, but no oestriol was detected (e.g. Bolté *et al.* 1964a, Dell'Acqua *et al.* 1966, Dell'Acqua *et al.* 1967b). Irrespective of the precursor, some three times more oestrone than 17β-oestradiol was isolated from the perfusates, but some three times more 17β-oestradiol than oestrone was found in the placental tissue. The same relationship was also found following the perfusion of 17β-oestradiol (Bolté *et al.* 1964a). The ratio found in the placentas and perfusates, respectively, agrees with the actual concentration of these two oestrogens in the placenta (e.g. Diczfalusy & Lindkvist 1956, Schmidt-Elmendorff 1961) and in the umbilical vein at term (Roy 1962, Maner *et al.* 1963).

The pathway of oestrone and 17β-oestradiol synthesis in the midterm placenta perfused *in situ* with various neutral C-19 steroids was in part also elucidated (Bolté *et al.* 1964d, Lamb *et al.* 1967). The results of these studies are summarized in Fig. 5.4. Dehydroepiandrosterone sulphate, which is known to be present in cord blood in high quantities (Migeon *et al.* 1955, Colás *et al.* 1964, Simmer *et al.* 1964, Eberlein 1965) is converted by the placenta into dehydroepiandrosterone and the latter into androstenedione. The major part of androstenedione is converted into oestrone and then into 17β-oestradiol, whereas a smaller part of it

* It is of some interest in this respect that human term placental tissue implanted into spayed mice was shown to convert dehydroepiandrosterone and its sulphate into oestrogens (Mancuso *et al.* 1966).

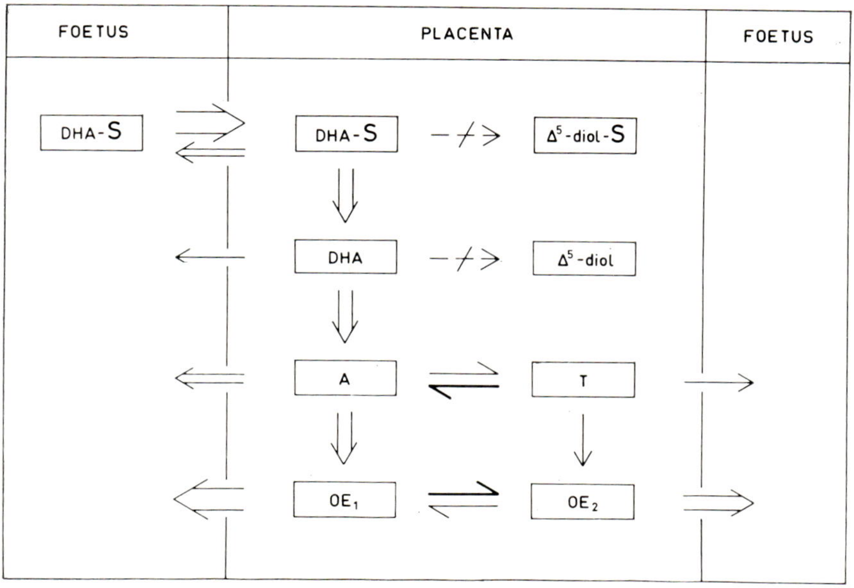

FIG. 5.4. Pathways of the metabolism of dehydroepiandrosterone sulphate (DHA-S) in the human placenta at midpregnancy; DHA is dehydroepiandrosterone, A is androstenedione, OE_1 is oestrone, Δ^5-diol-S is 17β-hydroxyandrost-5-en-3β-yl sulphate, Δ^5-diol is androst-5-ene-3β,17β-diol, T is testosterone and OE_2 is 17β-oestradiol. (According to Lamb *et al.* 1967.)

is secreted by the placenta to the foetus. Neither dehydroepiandrosterone sulphate nor dehydroepiandrosterone is converted by the placenta into the corresponding 17β-hydroxy form, and also the conversion of androstenedione into testosterone is very limited. On the other hand, significantly more oestrone is converted into 17β-oestradiol than *vice versa*.*

More oestrone than 17β-oestradiol, and a great deal more androstenedione than testosterone is secreted by the placenta to the foetal compartment.

However, oestriol was found in the urine following placental per-

* The specificity of placental 17β-hydroxysteroid dehydrogenases is further indicated by the fact that following *in situ* placental perfusion with retrotestosterone significantly more retrotestosterone than retroandrostenedione was isolated from the perfusates, whereas the reverse relationship was noted in the placenta (Dell'Acqua *et al.* 1966). That retrosteroids cannot be aromatized by placental tissue *in vitro* (Walop & De Lange 1966) or *in vivo* (Dell'Acqua *et al.* 1966) was indicated in Table 5.4.

fusion with various neutral 16-desoxy compounds (Bolté *et al.* 1964a), suggesting that this oestriol was formed in the maternal organism rather than in the placenta. Indeed, when midterm placentas were perfused *in situ* with ^{14}C-labelled 17β-oestradiol and ^{3}H-labelled 17β-oestradiol was injected into an antecubital vein immediately following the removal of the placenta, the oestriol to oestrone + 17β-oestradiol ratio was the same with respect to both labels (Bolté *et al.* 1964a). These findings are in agreement with those demonstrating that the extent of conversion of 17β-oestradiol and oestrone into oestriol is the same in pregnant and non-pregnant subjects (Pearlman *et al.* 1954, Fishman *et al.* 1962, Gurpide *et al.* 1962) and exclude the placenta as a quantitatively important site of 16α-hydroxylation.

OESTRIOL SYNTHESIS IN THE FOETO-PLACENTAL UNIT

Where and how is the oestriol synthesized in the organism of pregnant women? This is a question of paramount importance, since from the quantitative point of view, oestriol is by far more important during pregnancy than any other oestrogen. This is also a problem of considerable complexity, which must be answered in biochemical rather than anatomical terms, since this synthesis involves several steps (16α-hydroxylation, aromatization, reduction) which take place in different sequences and in different organs.

Whereas oestriol was never found in midterm placentas perfused *in situ* with 16-desoxy neutral precursors, when differently labelled dehydroepiandrosterone and dehydroepiandrosterone sulphate were injected together into a uterine artery prior to the surgical interruption of gestation, oestriol was found in the placenta and a 16α-hydroxy-oestrone-like compound was detected in the foetal tissues (Bolté *et al.* 1964b). This suggested that in the foeto-placental unit the participation of the foetal compartment is essential for the formation of oestriol. Indeed, when dehydroepiandrosterone sulphate with ^{14}C-label was injected into the foetal umbilical vein and with ^{3}H-label into the antecubital vein of the mother 6 days prior to the interruption of the gestation, much more oestriol (in relation to oestrone and 17β-oestradiol) was formed from the foetal precursor. This demonstrates that the foetal contribution to oestriol excretion is more important than the maternal one (Bolté *et al.* 1964c). The same conclusion was reached when differently labelled dehydroepiandrosterone sulphate and oestrone sulphate were injected into the foeto-placental and maternal circulations, respectively (Kirschner *et al.* 1966). Furthermore, the predominance of the foetal compartment in oestriol production is suggested by oestrogen production rate studies (Siiteri & MacDonald 1966) and by the low urinary oestriol excretion in cases of hydatidiform moles, chorio-epitheliomas (Frandsen & Stakemann 1964b, MacNaughton 1965) as

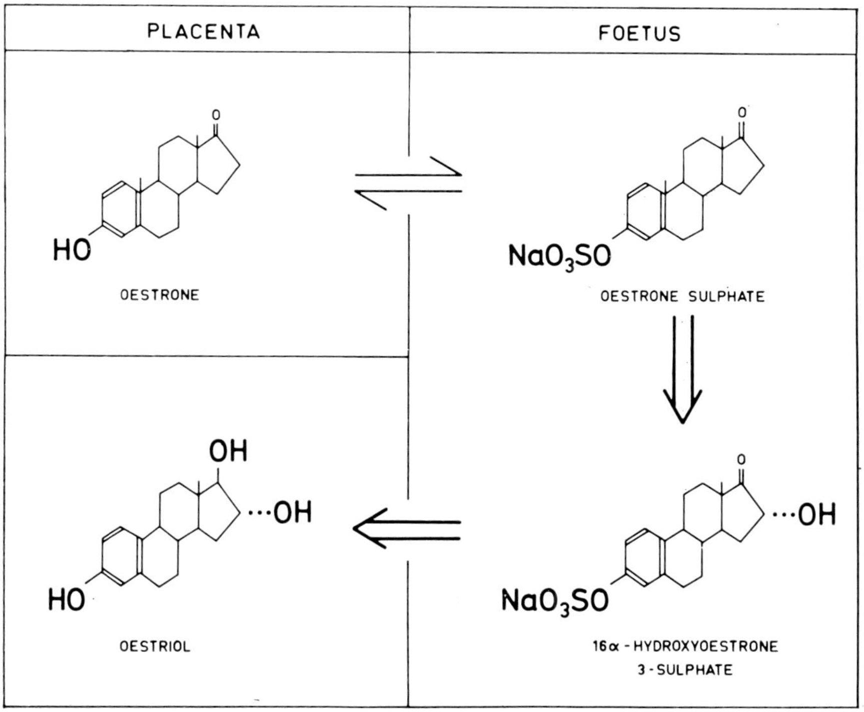

FIG. 5.5. Principal pathway of oestriol formation from oestrone in the foetal-placental unit. According to Diczfalusy (1967).

well as in women pregnant with anencephalic foetuses (Frandsen & Stakemann 1961, 1964a, Michie 1966).

Therefore the foetal organism must be a most important site of 16α-hydroxylation. Indeed, it was demonstrated by Engel *et al.* (1962) that incubation of foetal liver tissue with 17β-oestradiol yielded oestriol. Unfortunately, the *in vivo* results of the Stockholm group created some confusion at first, since in their initial studies of previable foetuses perfused with 17β-oestradiol the formation of oestriol could not be ascertained (Haynes *et al.* 1964). Whether this was due to the relatively bad condition and poor oxygenation of the foetuses perfused, or to the low amount of labelled material administered, is not clear. Continued studies in this laboratory, however, established beyond any reasonable doubt the presence of high quantities of conjugated oestriol in the liver of previable foetuses perfused with oestrone and oestrone sulphate (Emerman *et al.* 1965, Schwers *et al.* 1965b). The bulk of this material was most probably oestriol-3-sulphate (e.g. Mikhail *et al.* 1963a). No oestriol was found in the perfusate. However, considerable quantities of a ketonic intermediate (most probably the 3-sulphate of 16α-hydroxy-oestrone) were isolated.* This compound was converted into oestriol following reduction (Schwers *et al.* 1965b). Therefore the conversion of oestrone into oestriol by the foeto-placental unit can be visualized as indicated in Fig. 5.5. Furthermore, when a combination of differently labelled 17β-oestradiol and oestrone was introduced into the intact foeto-placental circulation at midpregnancy, as much as 10 per cent of the radioactive material recovered from the foetal liver was isolated in the form of oestriol (Schwers *et al.* 1965a). In this study oestriol was also isolated from the foetal carcass and the placenta. However, the isotopic ratio of the oestriol isolated from these two sources indicated that it was formed by the foetal liver. The amount of radioactive material present in the foetal adrenals was so limited that it was not possible to investigate the presence of oestriol. This fact itself seems to speak against a major role of the foetal adrenal in 16α-hydroxylation of oestrone.

Since cord blood contains much more dehydroepiandrosterone sulphate + dehydroepiandrosterone than oestrone sulphate + oestrone (e.g. Tables 5.3, 5.4 and 5.6), the possibility has to be considered that the neutral pathway (i.e. 16α-hydroxylation of dehydroepiandrosterone followed by aromatization) is quantitatively more important than the phenolic pathway (i.e. aromatization of dehydroepiandrosterone followed by 16α-hydroxylation of oestrone). Therefore previable foetuses were perfused with a combination of dehydroepiandrosterone and dehydroepiandrosterone sulphate (Bolté *et al.* 1966). Large quantities of 16α-hydroxylated intermediates (Hirschmann's triol from the liver and 16α-hydroxy-dehydroepiandrosterone from the perfusate) were isolated.

* That the foetus secretes predominantly ketonic oestrogens into the foeto-placental circulation was demonstrated also in a recent study (Mancuso *et al.* 1968). The same seems to apply to the secretion of β,γ-unsaturated C-19 steroids (Bolté *et al.* 1966).

If Hirschmann's triol or 16α-hydroxy-dehydroepiandrosterone was present in the adrenals at all, its concentration had to be less than 0·01 per cent of the radioactive material recovered. Therefore the principal–if not exclusive–site of 16α-hydroxylation for both oestrone

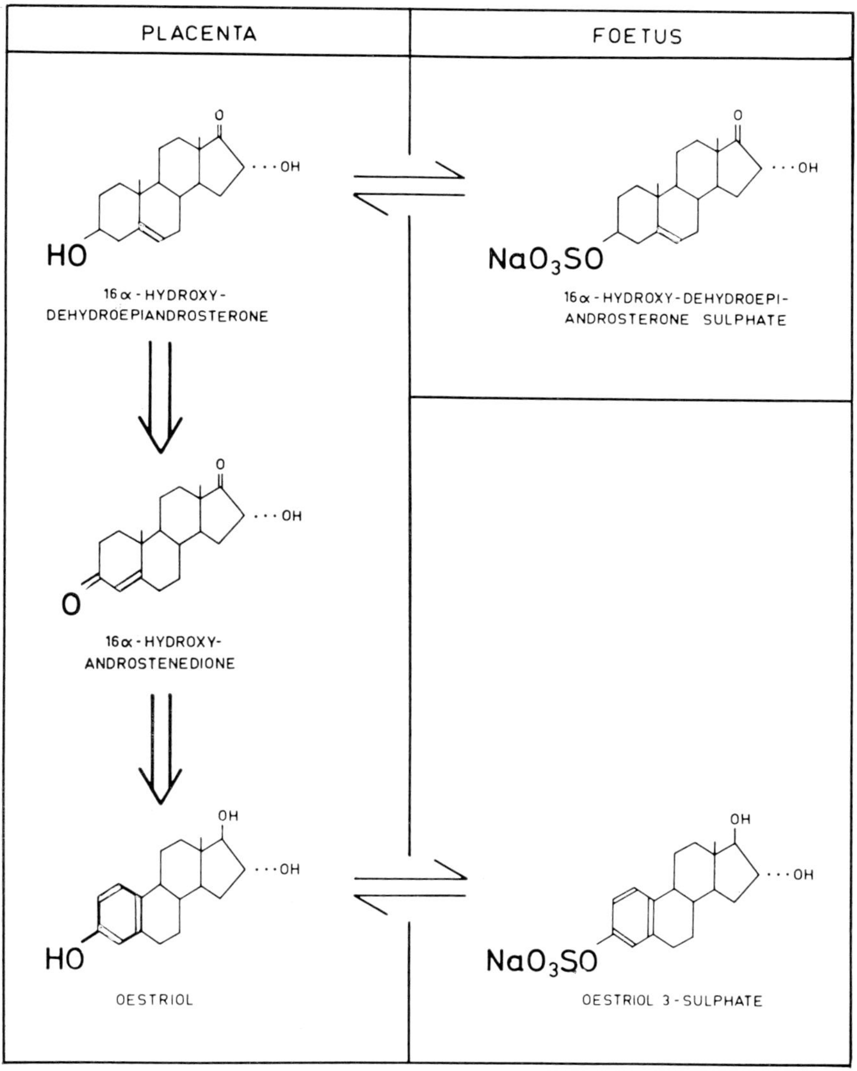

FIG. 5.6. Principal pathway of oestriol formation from 16α-hydroxy-dehydroepiandrosterone sulphate in the foeto-placental unit. According to Diczfalusy (1967).

TABLE 5.6

Approximate concentration of some 3β-hydroxy-Δ^5-steroids (oestrogen precursors) in maternal and cord blood and in the placental tissue at full term pregnancy. All values are expressed as μg/100 ml plasma, except in case of [b], where they represent μg/100 ml serum.

Precursor	Maternal blood		Cord blood				Placenta	
	Unconjugated	Conjugated	Unconjugated		Conjugated		Unconjugated	Conjugated
			Artery	Vein	Artery	Vein		
Dehydroepiandrosterone	—	12[a]	—	—	35[a]		—	—
	—		—	—	60[c]		—	—
	—	32[d]	—	—	81[d]	68[d]	—	—
	—	100[e]	—	—	162[e]	130[e]	—	—
16-Oxo-androstenediol	—	—	—	—	13[g]	10[g]	—	—
16α-Hydroxy-dehydro-epiandrosterone	6[b]	8[b]	16[b]	30[b]	254[b]	166[b]	26[b]	4[b]
	—	7[d]	—	—	134[g]	104[g]	—	—
	—	—	24[f]	17[f]	110[f]	87[f]	—	—

[a] Migeon *et al.* 1955. [b] Magendantz & Ryan 1964. [c] Eberlein 1965. [d] Colas *et al.* 1964. [e] Simmer *et al.* 1964 (corrected for losses). [f] Easterling *et al.* 1966 (uncorrected for losses). [g] Colas & LeRoy Heinrichs 1965.

and dehydroepiandrosterone (and their 3-sulphates) is the foetal liver.*

Since, furthermore, both oestriol and 16α-hydroxy-androstenedione were isolated from placentas perfused *in situ* with 16α-hydroxy-dehydroepiandrosterone (Dell'Acqua *et al.* 1967b), the second (and quantitatively much more important) pathway of oestriol synthesis in the foeto-placental unit can be depicted as indicated in Fig. 5.6.

That the neutral pathway of oestriol synthesis in the foeto-placental unit is quantitatively more important than the phenolic pathway was also demonstrated by Kirschner *et al.* (1966), who injected a combination of oestrone sulphate and dehydroepiandrosterone sulphate into the intact foeto-placental circulation and isolated oestrone, 17β-oestradiol and oestriol from the urine of the mother. However, when the same precursors were injected into the antecubital vein of the mother, urinary oestriol was mainly formed via the phenolic pathway. The importance of the neutral pathway is also supported by the high concentration of 16α-hydroxy-dehydroepiandrosterone in cord blood (Magendantz & Ryan 1964, Colás *et al.* 1964, Easterling *et al.* 1966) (see Table 5.6). That 16α-hydroxylated C-19 neutral steroids are aromatized by placental preparations *in vitro* has been shown previously (e.g. Table 5.4). To explore the oestriol precursor role of such compounds *in vivo*, midterm placentas were perfused with labelled 16α-hydroxy-dehydroepiandrosterone, 16α-hydroxy-androstenedione and 16α-hydroxy-testosterone (Dell'Acqua *et al.* 1967b). All these compounds were converted into oestriol by the placentas, although the yield from 16α-hydroxy-testosterone was poor when compared to the other precursors. Also Hirschmann's triol was found to be aromatized by the placenta following its injection into the intact foeto-placental unit. However, the extent of aromatization was relatively poor also in this case, indicating that ring D ketols are much better oestriol precursors than ring D glycols (Dell'Acqua *et al.* 1967a). A high amount of 16α-hydroxy-testosterone accumulated in the placenta following the administration of Hirschmann's triol suggested that the high concentration of this compound in term placentas (Neher & Stark 1961) may reflect an accumulation due to impeded aromatization rather than to an important function as an oestriol precursor.

* On the other hand, C-21 steroids, such as progesterone, certainly can be 16α-hydroxylated by the foetal adrenals (e.g. Bird *et al.* 1966), whereas α,β-unsaturated 3-ketosteroids with 19 carbon atoms, such as androstenedione and testosterone, are not 16α-hydroxylated in the organism of the previable human foetus to any significant extent (Mancuso *et al.* 1968).

Since no interconversion between the neutral ring D ketols and glycols could be demonstrated in these experiments, it is likely that the oestriol synthesis in the placenta from 16α-substituted C-19 steroids takes place as indicated in the scheme shown in Fig. 5.7.

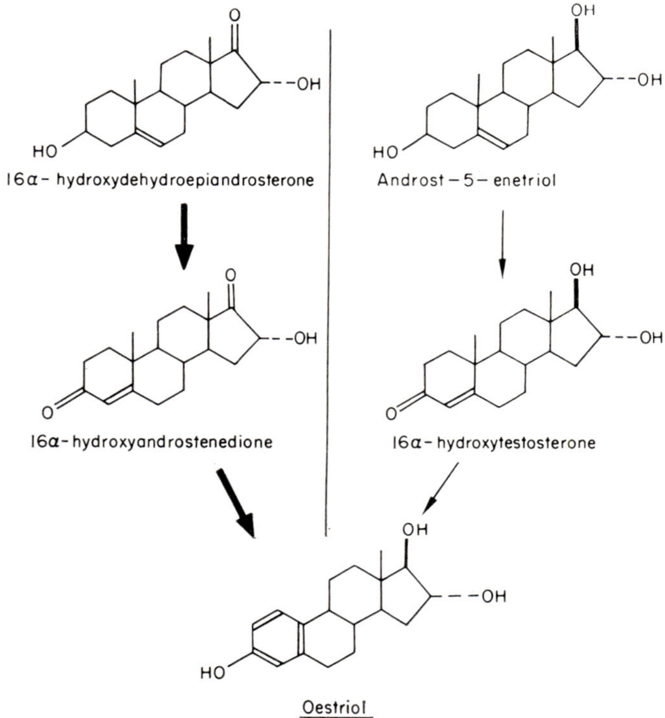

FIG. 5.7. Present concept of oestriol formation from 16α-hydroxylated neutral precursors by human placentas perfused *in situ* at midpregnancy. (According to Dell'Acqua *et al.* 1967b.)

SYNTHESIS OF 16-OXO-OESTRADIOL AND 16-EPIOESTRIOL

Perusal of the data of Table 5.1 reveals that 16-oxo-17β-oestradiol and 16-epioestriol are quantitatively fairly important constituents of pregnancy urine. These compounds are also present in placental tissue (Diczfalusy & v. Münstermann 1959, Diczfalusy & Halla 1958).

It was also shown that perfused previable foetuses are capable of converting 17β-oestradiol, oestrone, oestrone sulphate (Schwers *et al.* 1965a and b, Knuppen *et al.* 1966c) as well as androstenedione and testosterone (Mancuso *et al.* 1968) into 16-oxo-17β-oestradiol and/or 16-epioestriol. The major, if not the exclusive site of the formation of these compounds was the foetal liver. Thus one pathway for the formation of 16-oxo-17β-oestradiol and 16-epioestriol involves the conversion of placental oestrone into these two compounds in the foetal liver. The evidence available strongly suggests that this reaction takes place in the form of aryl sulphates. This pathway would then be the counterpart of the 'phenolic' pathway of oestriol formation (Kirschner *et al.* 1966).

A neutral pathway also seems to be operative: 3β,17β-dihydroxy androst-5-en-16-one is a normal constituent of the urine of newborn infants (Reynolds 1964) and cord plasma at term (Colás & LeRoy Heinrichs 1965); indeed, perfusion of midterm placentas with labelled 3β,17β-dihydroxy-androst-5-en-16-one resulted in the formation of major quantities of 16-oxo-17β-oestradiol, 16-epioestriol and oestriol (Reynolds *et al.* 1968).

FOETAL BIOGENESIS OF OESTROGENS *IN VIVO*

As indicated in Fig. 5.4, midterm placentas perfused with dehydroepiandrosterone and dehydroepiandrosterone sulphate convert these compounds into androstenedione and also into small amounts of testosterone. These androgens are then secreted by the placenta into the umbilical circulation (Lamb *et al.* 1967). Thus considerable quantities of androstenedione and some testosterone may reach the foetal organism at midpregnancy. To study the fate of these androgens, previable foetuses were perfused with labelled androstenedione and testosterone, whereas other foetuses were perfused with a combination of dehydroepiandrosterone and androstenedione.

These studies revealed that a part of the androstenedione and testosterone was aromatized by foetuses of both sexes. From the liver of the perfused foetuses not only oestrone and 17β-oestradiol (Mancuso *et al.* 1965a), but also oestriol, 15α-hydroxy-17β-oestradiol and 16-epioestriol were isolated (Mancuso *et al.* 1965b, 1968). Furthermore, since no 15α- or 16α-hydroxy-androstenedione or testosterone was found in any of the tissues of these foetuses, it may be suggested that 15α- and 16α-hydroxylation occurred following aromatization of androstenedione and testosterone as indicated in Fig. 5.8. Therefore, if 16α-hydroxy-androstenedione is present in the foetal organism, it must have been formed mainly in the placenta from 16α-hydroxy-dehydroepiandrosterone (Dell'Acqua *et al.* 1967b). However, no dehydroepiandrosterone whatsoever was converted by perfused foetuses into oestrogens (Mancuso *et al.* 1965a, 1968). Lack of oestrogen formation was also demonstrated in another study involving perfusion of foetuses with dehydroepiandrosterone and dehydroepiandrosterone sulphate (Bolté *et al.* 1966).

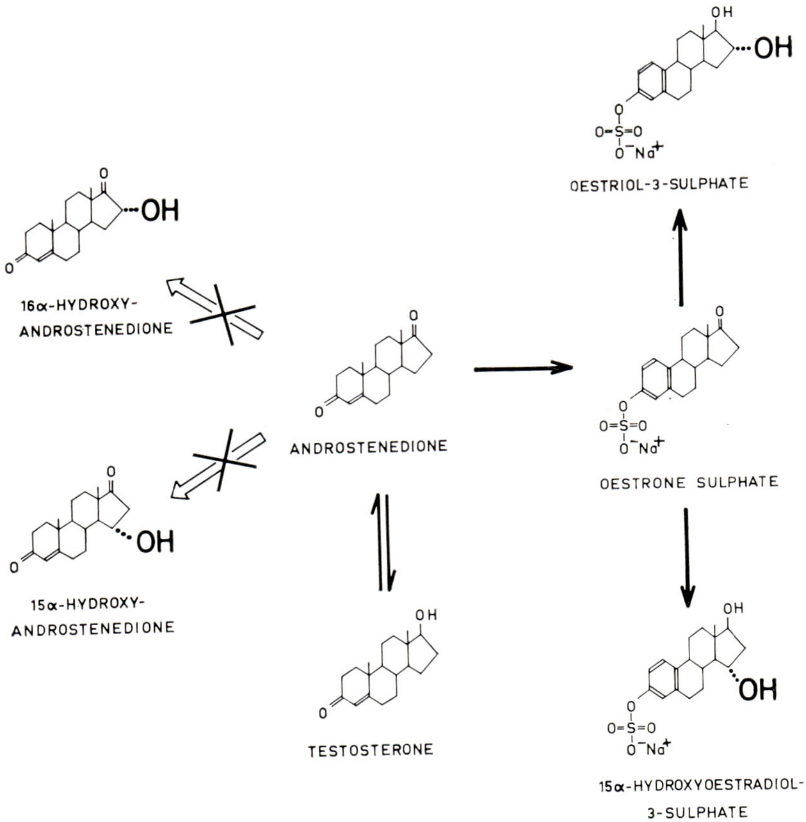

FIG. 5.8. Mechanism of 15α- and 16α-hydroxylation in the liver of previable foetuses perfused with androstenedione and testosterone. (According to Mancuso *et al.* 1968).

It appears therefore that the midterm foetus is capable of producing oestrogens from α,β-unsaturated C-19 3-ketosteroids but not from dehydroepiandrosterone and dehydroepiandrosterone sulphate. Since oestrogens were isolated in good yield from the liver but were not detected in other tissues of the perfused foetuses and since incubation of homogenates of the liver but not those of foetal adrenals resulted in the formation of oestrogens (Mancuso *et al.* 1968), it appears that the liver is the principal, if not exclusive, site of this reaction in the foetal organism.* Thus, the suggestion of earlier investigators (Lelong *et al.* 1951) that the foetal adrenals synthesize oestrogens, could not be verified.

Furthermore, since plenty of androstenedione but little or no dehydroepiandrosterone was converted into oestrogens by the liver of a perfused anencephalic monster at term (Mancuso *et al.*, to be published), it appears likely that this foetal capacity persists at least until the time of parturition† and that the corresponding 3β-hydroxy steroid-dehydrogenase and $\Delta^4 \leftarrow \Delta^5$-isomerase activities are virtually absent from the foetal organism from the fourth month of gestation to term.‡ Aromatization of testosterone by homogenates of foetal liver was also demonstrated by Slaunwhite *et al.* (1965), and Jungmann *et al.* (1966) claimed that such homogenates convert progesterone and 17α-hydroxy-pregnenolone into oestrogens.

PRESENT CONCEPT OF OESTROGEN SYNTHESIS IN MIDPREGNANCY

In Fig. 5.9 an attempt is made to present our general concept of the principal pathways of oestrogen synthesis in the foeto-placental unit. The figure indicates two hypothetical foetal compartments, one containing the quantitatively important reactions (right column) and another one with the metabolism of the 17β-hydroxylated compounds, which is quantitatively much less important (left column). Evidence is available indicating an interconversion of the various Δ^5- (Bolté *et al.* 1966), Δ^4- (Benagiano *et al.* 1968) and aromatic (Schwers *et al.* 1965a, Emerman *et al.* 1965) 17-oxo- and 17β-hydroxy steroids in the foetal compartment (especially in the foetal liver). These interconversions, or the secretion of steroids to the maternal compartment are not illustrated in Fig. 5.9.

* The possible aromatizing ability of the foetal testicles remains to be evaluated.

† The aromatizing ability of the human liver may persist throughout adult life as well (e.g. West *et al.* 1956).

‡ Recent evidence strongly suggests the existence of *several* substrate specific 3β-hydroxysteroid dehydrogenase systems; some of them do function in the organism of midgestation foetuses (e.g. Pasqualini *et al.* 1968).

The scheme indicates that aromatization takes place both in the placental and foetal compartment, but that aromatization in the foetus is restricted to α,β-unsaturated 3-ketosteroids. On the other hand, the 3β-hydroxy-Δ^5- precursors are converted into the corresponding oestrogens in the placenta via the formation of the corresponding α,β-unsaturated 3-ketones, as intermediates. Furthermore, 16α-hydroxylation* of the C-19 and C-18 compounds takes place only in the foetal compartment, more exactly in the foetal liver. However, among the C-19 compounds, only those with a 3β-hydroxy-Δ^5- configuration can be 15α- or 16α-hydroxylated. The symbols in squares indicate those compounds which are secreted by the placenta to the mother and to the foetus, whereas those encircled represent the principal precursors.† The balance of evidence available at present indicates that the placenta secretes far more oestrogens to the maternal than to the foetal compartment (Kirschner *et al.* 1966, Lamb *et al.* 1967).

Generally speaking, the relative quantitative importance of the various precursors of aromatization is a function of their concentration in the blood reaching the placenta and the foetus. Therefore, in Table 5.6 we have compiled some of the information available on the concentration of the major precursors in cord blood at term.

The concentration of 16α-hydroxy-oestrone is not yet known, although this compound seems to be the major 16α-hydroxylated aromatic intermediate secreted by the foetus to the placenta (Schwers *et al.* 1965b). Furthermore, the impeded aromatization of the ring B glycols (e.g. Dell'Acqua *et al.* 1967a and b) seems to minimize the quantitative importance of this pathway. Thus it can be concluded that the major foetal precursors of the oestrogens elaborated in the foeto-placental unit are dehydroepiandrosterone sulphate 16α-hydroxy-dehydroepiandrosterone sulphate and 16-oxo-androstenediol (Dell' Acqua *et al.* 1967b, Reynolds *et al.* 1968).

* This statement can be enlarged as to include hydroxylations in all positions with the exception of carbon atoms 6 and perhaps 2 (e.g. Diczfalusy 1967).

† The synthesis of dehydroepiandrosterone sulphate by the foetus has been studied. The available evidence indicates that it is formed by the foetus from placental pregnenolone (e.g. Pion *et al.* 1967).

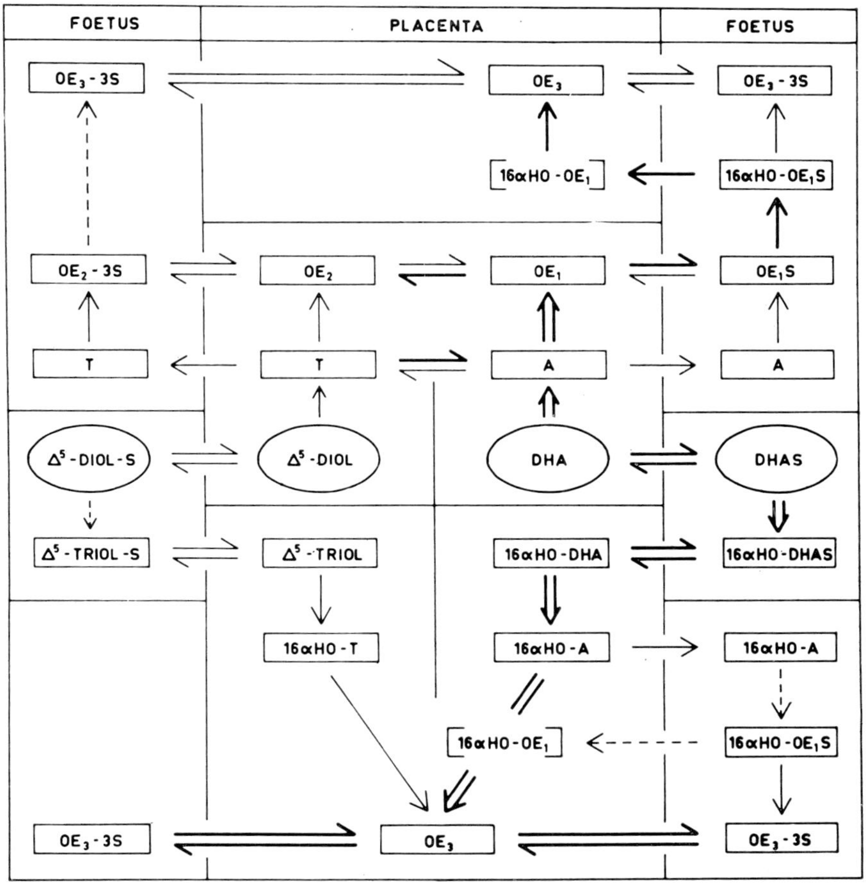

FIG. 5.9. General concept of the principal pathways of oestrogen synthesis in the foeto-placental unit. OE_3-3S: oestriol-3-sulphate; OE_2-3S: 17β-oestradiol 3-sulphate; T: testosterone; Δ^5-DIOL-S: androst-5-ene-3β,17β-diol 3-sulphate; Δ^5-TRIOL-S: androst-5-ene-3β,16α,17β-triol 3-sulphate; OE_2: 17β-oestradiol; Δ^5-DIOL: androst-5-ene-3β,16α,17β-diol; Δ^5-TRIOL: androst-5-ene-3β,16α,17β-triol; 16αHO-T: 16α-hydroxy-testosterone; OE_3: oestriol; 16αHO-OE_1: 16α-hydroxy-oestrone; OE_1: oestrone; A: androstenedione; DHA: dehydroepiandrosterone; 16αHO-DHA: 16α-hydroxy-dehydroepiandrosterone; 16αHO-A: 16α-hydroxy-androstenedione; 16αHO-OE_1S: 16α-hydroxy-oestrone-3-sulphate; OE_1S: oestrone sulphate; DHAS: dehydroepiandrosterone sulphate; 16αHO-DHAS: 16α-hydroxy-dehydroepiandrosterone sulphate.

FOETAL AND PLACENTAL METABOLISM OF CONJUGATES

In 1953 it was noted that whereas in the placenta oestrogens were mainly present in the unconjugated form, there was a high concentration of conjugated oestrogens in the foetal liver. It was suggested therefore that human foetuses at midpregnancy are capable of conjugating oestrogens (Diczfalusy 1953). Continued studies revealed that the oestrogen pattern of all foetal tissues was indeed dominated by the conjugated forms (Diczfalusy & Magnusson 1958) and that this was also the case in the amniotic fluid, cord blood (Diczfalusy & Magnusson 1958, Troen *et al.* 1961) and meconium (Diczfalusy *et al.* 1959). It was also demonstrated that a considerable proportion of the conjugated oestriol in these sources was oestriol-3-sulphate (Diczfalusy *et al.* 1961c, Troen *et al.* 1961, Menini & Diczfalusy 1961b), a conjugate which was first isolated from the meconium (Menini & Diczfalusy 1961b). Oestriol glucosiduronate was also isolated from the meconium (Menini & Diczfalusy 1961a), amniotic fluid and cord blood (Troen *et al.* 1961). However, the exact position of glucosiduronation (C-16 or C-17) could not be established at that time (cf. Goebelsmann *et al.* 1965b).

That conjugation of oestrogen takes place in virtually every foetal tissue was then demonstrated by incubation experiments (Diczfalusy *et al.* 1961b, Wengle 1964) as well as following the injection of oestrogens into the amniotic fluid prior to the surgical interruption of gestation (e.g. Diczfalusy 1958), or following perfusion of previable foetuses with oestradiol and oestriol (Diczfalusy *et al.* 1961a). The bulk of the conjugated oestrogen formed under these conditions was isolated and identified as the aryl sulphates of oestrone, 17β-oestradiol and oestriol (Diczfalusy *et al.* 1961c).

When the various types of experiments were repeated by the use of labelled compounds, it became possible to assess these reactions more precisely. Thus following perfusion of previable foetuses with labelled oestriol, more than 90 per cent of the radioactive material recovered from the foetal tissues was in a conjugated form, mainly as oestriol-3-sulphate (Mikhail *et al.* 1963a) and following the perfusion of labelled 17β-oestradiol mainly as oestrone sulphate and 17β-oestradiol-3-sulphate (Haynes *et al.* 1964). However, from the foetuses perfused with oestriol also oestriol-16-glucosiduronate and a double conjugate, oestriol-3-sulphate,16-glucosiduronate, were isolated (Mikhail *et al.* 1963a). This confirms the earlier isolation of oestriol glucosiduronate following the incubation of 17β-oestradiol with foetal liver (Engel *et al.* 1962) and indicates that the human foetus at midpregnancy possesses a well developed oestrogen glucosiduronating enzyme system.

On the other hand, when foetuses were perfused with oestrone sulphate, no evidence of hydrolysis was found (Emerman *et al.* 1965, Schwers *et al.* 1965b) indicating the lack of any appreciable *in vivo* aryl sulphatase activity.

Thus it appears that the human foetus at midterm possesses a most powerful and extensive aryl sulphurylating system, but no appreciable aryl sulphatase activity. Therefore the oestrogen metabolism of the foetus takes place predominantly in the form of oestrogen sulphates. It was demonstrated for instance that 17β-oestradiol-3-sulphate is converted by the liver of previable foetuses into oestriol-3-sulphate without any prior hydrolysis (Emerman *et al.* 1965, Schwers *et al.* 1965b).

The midterm foetus is also endowed with an oestrogen glucosiduronating and some β-glucuronidase enzyme systems; the latter is, however, very limited. Thus, whereas some oestriol-16-glucosiduronate was shown to be converted by the foetus into oestriol-3-sulphate (Goebelsmann *et al.* 1966b), the direct conversion of oestrone glucosiduronate into oestriol-3-glucosiduronate could also be demonstrated (Zucconi *et al.* 1967a). It has also been demonstrated that the formation of oestriol-3-sulphate,16-glucosiduronate in the foetus takes place exclusively via the sulphurylation of oestriol-16-glucosiduronate (Goebelsmann *et al.* 1966b). It seems reasonable to conclude, therefore, that the principal pathway of oestrogen metabolism in the midterm foetus proceeds along the sulphoconjugated forms and a minor one along the glucosiduronates.

How is the foetal conjugation mechanism at term? The only information available so far was obtained following the intravenous injection of labelled oestriol into an anencephalic monster. Ten to twelve minutes after injection more than 98 per cent of the circulating radioactive material was conjugated. Seventy-five per cent of this was oestriol-3-sulphate and 20 per cent oestriol-3-sulphate,16-glucosiduronate, whereas in the urine some 50 per cent of the excreted material was isolated as oestriol-16-glucosiduronate, some 16 per cent as oestriol-3-sulphate and more than 25 per cent as oestriol-3-sulphate,16-glucosiduronate (Diczfalusy *et al.* 1964).

The corresponding enzyme pattern of the *placenta* is markedly different from that of the midterm foetus. This follows from several types of experiments. Thus, following the injection of labelled oestrone, 17β-oestradiol and oestriol into the intact foeto-placental unit, or amniotic fluid, the oestrogen pattern of the foetal tissues was always dominated by conjugated forms (mainly sulphates), whereas unconjugated oestrogens prevailed in the placenta and membranes (Mikhail *et al.* 1963b, Haynes *et al.* 1964, Diczfalusy *et al.* 1963, Schwers *et al.* 1965a). The same was also true following the intra-amniotic administration of oestrone sulphate (Diczfalusy *et al.* 1963) or oestriol-3-sulphate (Goebelsmann *et al.* 1966b). Furthermore, *in situ* perfusion of midterm placentas with oestriol-3-sulphate also resulted in a high concentration of unconjugated oestriol in the placenta (Levitz *et al.* 1967). These findings are in agreement with the earlier *in vitro* demonstration of aryl sulphatase activity in placental tissue (Pulkkinen 1961, Warren & Timberlake 1962) and in the membranes (Katz *et al.* 1965). The aryl sulphurylating activity of midterm placentas perfused *in situ* appears to be little, if any (Levitz *et al.* 1967). Although some activity has been reported following the *in vitro* perfusion of placentas with oestriol (Troen *et al.* 1966), the balance of evidence indicates that if there is *in situ* such an activity at all, its extent must be very limited, perhaps because of the predominance of the aryl sulphatase activity.

On the other hand, no *in vivo* β-glucuronidase or glucuronyl transferase activity is present in the midterm placenta or in the membranes (Goebelsmann *et al.* 1966a, 1968a, Levitz *et al.* 1967, Zucconi *et al.* 1967a).

Thus, at midpregnancy, the glucuronyl transferase (E.C.2.4.I.17) and β-glucuronidase (E.C.3.2.1.31.) activities seem to be restricted to the foetal compartment. Furthermore, there is a differential distribution of aryl sulphotransferase (E.C.2.8.2.1.) and aryl sulphatase (E.C.3.1.6.1.) activities between the foetus and placenta. In the foetal tissues the abundance of sulphotransferase activity is contrasted with the absence of sulphatases, whereas in the placenta there is a most active aryl sulphatase system associated with very little aryl sulphotransferase activity. The physiological significance of this arrangement appears to be at least three-fold, (a) protection of the foetus from the effect of the biologically active placental oestrogens, (b) regulation of the amount available for foetal, placental and maternal metabolism and (c) facilitation of the tissue uptake of certain oestrogens (e.g. the specific uptake of oestrone sulphate by the liver (Schwers *et al.* 1965b, Kirschner *et al.* 1966). Whether, in addition to these functions, oestrogen sulphates are also involved in the regulation of foetal growth processes, e.g. by stimulation of protein and nucleic acid synthesis, remains to be elucidated.

INTERMEDIARY OESTROGEN METABOLISM IN THE FOETUS

The preponderance of oestriol associated with very little oestrone and 17β-oestradiol (e.g. Table 5.4) in the various tissues of midterm foetuses (Diczfalusy & Magnusson 1958), in the urine of the newborn (Diczfalusy *et al.* 1957a) and meconium (Diczfalusy *et al.* 1959) suggested earlier the existence of an extensive foetal metabolism of oestrone and 17β-oestradiol of placental origin. This was also supported by the rapid disappearance from the various foetal tissues of intra-amniotically administered 17β-oestradiol (Diczfalusy *et al.* 1961d) or by the extremely limited urinary excretion of oestrone and 17β-oestradiol following the administration of 17β-oestradiol to newborn infants (Diczfalusy *et al.* 1957b), or to infants (Barr *et al.* 1961). It is reasonable to assume that the rapid elimination of the biologically highly active oestrogens takes place via a variety of hydroxylation reactions, leading to the formation of 'highly polar' oestrogen metabolites (e.g. Diczfalusy *et al.* 1961d, Hagen *et al.* 1965).

The demonstration of oestriol formation from 17β-oestradiol by human foetal liver tissue *in vitro* (Engel *et al.* 1962) and *in vivo* (Schwers *et al.* 1965a) has been mentioned previously. This oestriol formation represents one (albeit a quantitatively very important one) of the numerous hydroxylation reactions taking place in the foetal organism, mainly in the foetal liver. The oestriol and 16α-hydroxy-oestrone formed by human foetuses perfused with 17β-oestradiol (Schwers *et al.* 1965a), oestrone (Schwers *et al.* 1965b) and oestrone sulphate (Schwers *et al.* 1965b, Kirschner 1966) was recovered exclusively in a conjugated form. It is likely that the bulk of this material is oestriol-3-sulphate.

Hydroxylation in position 16 is not restricted to the 16α-orientation, since 16-epi-oestriol, 16β-hydroxy-oestrone and 16-oxo-17β-oestradiol have also been isolated (Schwers *et al.* 1965a, Knuppen *et al.* 1966).

Other hydroxylated metabolites isolated from previable foetuses perfused with oestrone and 17β-oestradiol were: 2-methoxy-oestrone, 2-methoxy-oestriol, 6α-hydroxy-oestrone, 6α-hydroxy-oestriol, 17-epi-oestriol (Knuppen *et al.* 1966).

Another foetal hydroxylation reaction, which from the quantitative point of view may be almost as important as the 16α-hydroxylation, is 15α-hydroxylation (Schwers *et al.* 1965c). Midterm foetuses perfused with oestrone, oestrone sulphate, 17β-oestradiol (and even androstenedione and testosterone (Mancuso *et al.* 1967)) form large quantities of 15α-hydroxy-17β-oestradiol and 15α-hydroxy-oestrone (Schwers *et al.* 1965a, b, c, Knuppen *et al.* 1966). 15α-Hydroxy-17β-oestradiol was also isolated from the liver of an anencephalic monster injected with 17β-oestradiol (Roth *et al.* unpublished data).

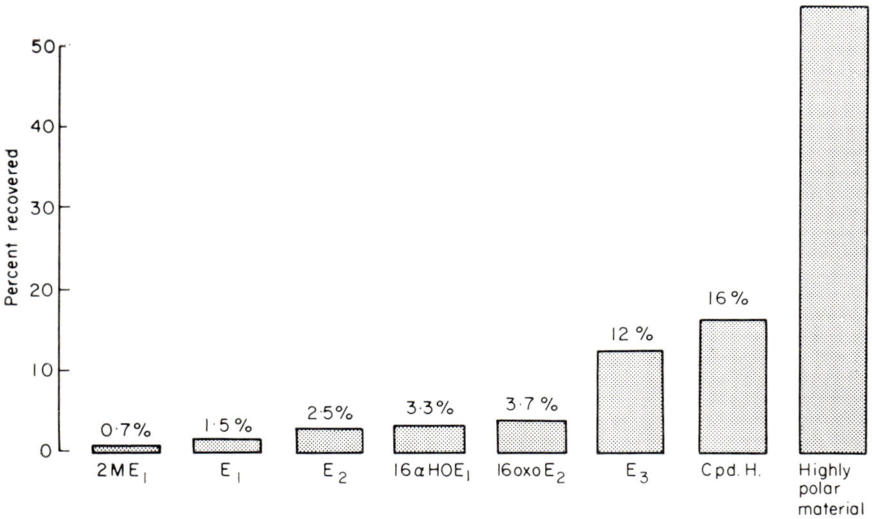

FIG. 5.10. Distribution of the urinary metabolites of labelled 17β-oestradiol in three malformed children. $2ME_1$: 2-methoxy-oestrone; E_1: oestrone; E_2: 17β-oestradiol; 16αHOE_1: 16α-hydroxy-oestrone; 16oxoE_2: 16oxo-17β-oestradiol; E_3: oestriol; Cpd H: Compound 'H' = 15α-hydroxy-oestriol. Calculated from the data published by Hagen *et al.* 1965.

Recently, another highly polar oestrogen metabolite was identified in the urine of malformed infants injected with 17β-oestradiol. This compound, which is an oestrogenic tetrol, was excreted in the urine in larger quantities than oestriol (Hagen *et al.* 1965) (indicated as Cpd.H in Fig. 5.10). It was also a major and gradually increasing metabolite in the blood of an anencephalic monster injected with 17β-oestradiol, as shown in Fig. 5.11 (Roth *et al.* unpublished data). This compound was recently isolated from the urine of newborn infants and also from pregnancy urine, and was identified as 15α-hydroxy-oestriol (Zucconi *et al.* 1967b). The importance of the formation of 15α-hydroxylated metabolites by the foetal organism appears to be considerable; their oestrogenic activity appears to be extremely low (e.g. Laskin *et al.* 1964).

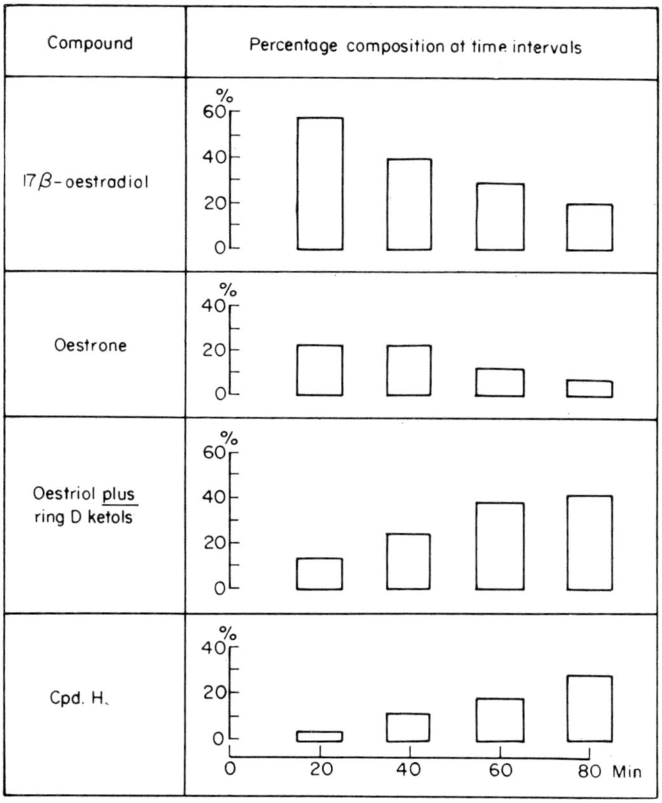

FIG. 5.11. Distribution of 17β-oestradiol, oestrone, oestriol + ring D ketols and Cpd H (15α-hydroxy-oestriol) in the conjugated fraction of the blood of an anencephalic monster at different intervals following the intravenous administration of labelled 17β-oestradiol. (According to Roth *et al.*, unpublished data.)

Furthermore, 15α-hydroxylation seems to be a predominant foetal reaction (Gurpide *et al.* 1966). It is possible, therefore, that the excretion of 15α-hydroxylated oestrogens in pregnancy urine offers another indicator for the assessment of foetal viability, perhaps even more useful than the presently employed estimation of oestriol.

TRANSPORT BETWEEN FOETUS AND MOTHER

Only a few studies have been reported in which the transfer of oestrogen from the mother to the foetus was investigated, and the evidence available at present indicates that the transfer in this direction is very limited (Diczfalusy *et al.* 1961a, Wilson *et al.* 1964), even following the administration of massive doses of oestrogens to the mother (Diczfalusy *et al.* 1961a).

However, the transport from the foetal to maternal compartment has been more extensively studied, using several approaches.

When midterm placentas were perfused *in situ* with the three possible combinations of oestriol-3-sulphate, oestriol-16-glucosiduronate and oestriol, it became apparent that unconjugated oestriol was transferred to the mother across the placenta at a rate of at least 10 times greater than the conjugates. Oestriol-3-sulphate was hydrolysed by the placenta but oestriol-16-glucosiduronate was not. Consequently, the transfer of oestriol-3-sulphate was more rapid than that of oestriol-16-glucosiduronate (Levitz *et al.* 1967).

The results of other studies involving the administration of oestriol-3-sulphate and oestriol-16-glucosiduronate into the amniotic fluid indicate that the foetal membranes behave similarly in this respect (Diczfalusy *et al.* 1963, Goebelsmann *et al.* 1966a).

That the transplacental passage of oestrogen glucosiduronates takes place without hydrolysis in an unchanged form was then demonstrated following the administration of double-labelled oestrone-glucosiduronate into the foeto-placental circulation and the re-isolation of this compound with the same isotopic ratio from the urine of the mother (Zucconi *et al.* 1967a) as well as following placental perfusion with oestriol-3-glucosiduronate (Goebelsmann *et al.* 1968a). The information which is available at present on the metabolism and transfer of oestriol in the foeto-placental unit can be summarized schematically as shown in Fig. 5.12 (e.g. Goebelsmann *et al.* 1966a). The bulk of oestriol synthesized by the placenta mainly from 16α-hydroxylated neutral and phenolic precursors of foetal origin is secreted predominantly to the mother (Kirschner *et al.* 1966, Levitz *et al.* 1967) and to a smaller extent to the foetus. The major portion of oestriol reaching the foetus is converted irreversibly to oestriol-3-sulphate (Mikhail *et al.* 1963a and b), which seems to be the principal end-product of foetal oestrogen metabolism. Part of the oestriol-3-sulphate formed by the foetus is released to the placenta, where it is subjected in part to hydrolysis (Mikhail *et al.* 1963b, Levitz *et al.* 1967). This constitutes the foeto-placental oestriol-3-sulphate cycle, consisting of foetal sulphurylation and placental desulphurylation. Some oestriol-3-sulphate is excreted by the foetus into the amniotic fluid (Troen *et al.* 1961, Diczfalusy *et al.*

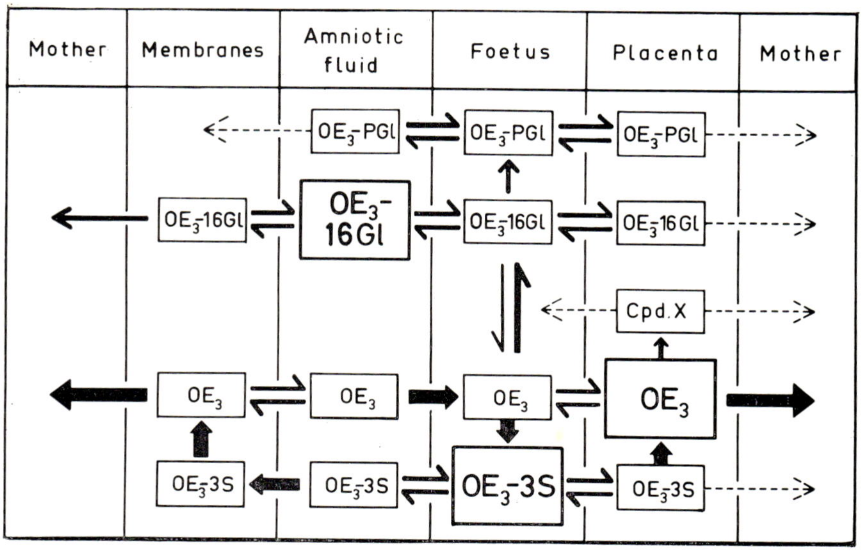

FIG. 5.12. Present concept of the metabolism and transport of oestriol in the human foeto-placental unit at midterm. Large boxes: quantitatively most significant forms of oestriol in the compartment. Heavy arrows: quantitatively major pathways. Light arrows: quantitatively minor pathways. Dotted arrows: probable, but not yet proven pathways. OE_3-PGl: a polar conjugate of oestriol (mostly oestriol-3-sulphate,16-glucosiduronate); OE_3-16Gl: oestriol-16-glucosiduronate; OE_3: oestriol; OE_3-3S: oestriol-3-sulphate. Cpd X is an unknown polar metabolite. According to Goebelsmann *et al.* (1966a).

1964). It reaches the membranes, where it becomes in part hydrolysed (Diczfalusy *et al.* 1963, Katz *et al.* 1965), and the liberated oestriol is transferred both to the maternal and foetal organism (Diczfalusy *et al.* 1963). Whether smaller amounts of oestriol-3-sulphate are also transferred across the placenta and membranes in an unchanged form, remains to be discovered.

Some oestriol is converted by the foetus into oestriol-16-glucosiduronate (Mikhail *et al.* 1963a). A part of this reaches the placenta and also the amniotic fluid (Troen *et al.* 1961, Diczfalusy *et al.* 1963). It is not hydrolysed by the placenta (Levitz *et al.* 1967) or by the membranes (Goebelsmann *et al.* 1966a) but is transferred to the maternal organism in an unchanged form. A substantial part of the oestriol-16-glucosiduronate is converted by the foetus into 'polar conjugates' (Goebelsmann *et al.* 1966a). The principal constituent of this fraction was isolated recently in the form of oestriol-3-sulphate,16-glucosiduronate (Goebelsmann *et al.* 1966b). The foetal metabolism of this compound remains to be studied; it has been shown, however, that this double conjugate is a quantitatively important constituent of pregnancy plasma, but not of pregnancy urine (Goebelsmann *et al.* 1968b).

A small part of the oestriol is converted by the placenta into an unidentified compound (Cpd X in Fig. 5.12). Whether this is a 6-hydroxylated polar metabolite is not known. Human placentas have been shown, however, to hydroxylate steroid oestrogens at C-6 (Cédard & Knuppen 1965, Alonso & Troen 1966).

Both oestriol-3-sulphate and oestriol-16-glucosiduronate (and also unconjugated oestriol) are taken up from the amniotic fluid by the foetus via the oral route, and a part of oestriol enters via the foetal skin as well (Diczfalusy *et al.* 1963). A small part of the oestriol-16-glucosiduronate formed by the foetus is hydrolysed by the foetal liver and/or gastrointestinal tract, and the bulk of the oestriol liberated is sulphurylated (Goebelsmann *et al.* 1966a and b).

METABOLISM IN THE MATERNAL COMPARTMENT

Most of the studies conducted so far have been limited to the investigation of the three classical oestrogens, oestrone, 17β-oestradiol and oestriol. With the exception of one report (Davis *et al.* 1963), most authors agree that the intermediary oestrogen metabolism in pregnant women does not differ essentially from that of non-pregnant subjects (Beer & Gallagher 1955, Fishman *et al.* 1962, Gurpide *et al.* 1962).

The metabolism of oestriol and of its various conjugates by pregnant women has been studied more recently in Stockholm following intravenous injections or infusions of tracers (Wilson *et al.* 1964, Goebelsmann *et al.* 1965a and b, Goebelsmann *et al.* 1966a, Goebelsmann *et al.* 1968a and b). These studies indicated that there is a gradually changing pattern of excretion of conjugated oestriol following the administration of oestriol (Wilson *et al.* 1964, Goebelsmann *et al.* 1965a and b), that oestriol-3-glucosiduronate is excreted most rapidly (Goebelsmann *et al.* 1966c) and oestriol-3-sulphate, 16-glucosiduronate most slowly (Goebelsmann *et al.* 1968b).

Circulating oestriol was converted into oestriol-3-sulphate, but very little oestriol-3-sulphate was excreted in the urine. The bulk of urinary metabolites was excreted as oestriol-16-glucosiduronate and 'polar' glucosiduronate (Wilson *et al.* 1964), identified later by Goebelsmann *et al.* (1965a) as oestriol-3-glucosiduronate. Small quantities of oestriol-

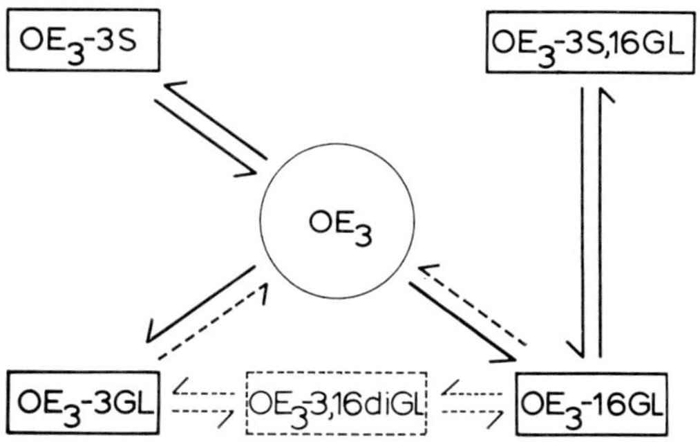

FIG. 5.13. Present concept of oestriol metabolism in midpregnancy. OE_3: oestriol, OE_3-3S: oestriol-3-sulphate, OE_3-3S,16Gl: oestriol-3-sulphate,16-glucosiduronate, OE_3-16Gl: oestriol-16-glucosiduronate, OE_3-3Gl: oestriol-3-glucosiduronate and OE_3-3,16diGl: oestriol-3,16-diglucosiduronate. Solid arrows indicate established pathways, broken arrows unproven pathways. Although the interconversion of OE_3-16Gl and OE_3-3Gl is established, it is not yet known whether it takes place *via* OE_3 or a so far hypothetical OE_3-3,16diGl. (According to Goebelsmann *et al.* 1968b.)

3-sulphate,16-glucosiduronate were also found (Wilson *et al.* 1964). Following the infusion of oestriol-3-sulphate, only small amounts were excreted unchanged in the urine. The bulk of urinary radioactive material was eliminated as oestriol-16-glucosiduronate and oestriol-3-glucosiduronate (Goebelsmann *et al.* 1965b). Following the infusion of oestriol-16-glucosiduronate or oestriol-3-glucosiduronate (Goebelsmann *et al.* 1966c) no oestriol-3-sulphate was detected in the urine, probably because both compounds are excreted very rapidly. Following the infusion of each of these two conjugates the only urinary metabolite isolated was the other glucosiduronate. However, whereas almost 20 per cent of oestriol-16-glucosiduronate was converted into oestriol-3-glucosiduronate (Goebelsmann *et al.* 1965a, b, 1966c), only some

2 per cent of the oestriol-3-glucosiduronate was excreted in the urine as oestriol-16-glucosiduronate. Following the infusion of oestriol-3-sulphate, 16-glucosiduronate some 50 per cent of the urinary excretion products consisted of oestriol-3-glucosiduronate, some 30 per cent was oestriol-16-glucosiduronate and 20 per cent was excreted in an unchanged form (Goebelsmann *et al.* 1968b).

On the basis of these results, the metabolism of oestriol in pregnant women (at midpregnancy) can be summarized as shown in Fig. 5.13.

It appears from the data of Fig. 5.13 that this metabolism is characterized by the central position of unconjugated oestriol. Indeed, with the exception of the formation of oestriol-3-sulphate, 16-glucosiduronate, which takes place exclusively via oestriol-16-glucosiduronate (Levitz *et al.* 1965, Goebelsmann *et al.* 1966b), all other compounds must undergo hydrolysis followed by reconjugation. There is reason to believe that the various hydrolytic steps and conjugations take place in different organs. The extent of this hydrolysis and reconjugation depends *i.a.* on renal filtration and thus on the amount of conjugate retained in the circulation; therefore the further metabolism of oestriol-3-sulphate is the most extensive and that of oestriol-3-glucosiduronate is minimal.

CONCLUDING REMARKS

Pregnancy in the human species is characterized by a gradually increasing secretion and elimination of a large number of steroid oestrogens; thus at term the excretion of one of them, that of oestriol, exceeds 1,000 times the levels found in non-pregnant women. The bulk of these oestrogens is produced by the foeto-placental unit. In the present state of affairs, the biosynthesis, catabolism and transport of these oestrogens must necessarily be interpreted in terms of steroid enzymology.

It is emphasized that the human placenta is an incomplete oestrogen producing organ, which depends for its oestrogen synthesis mainly upon neutral steroid precursors reaching it from the foetal and maternal circulations. The available evidence indicates that the foetal precursors are quantitatively more important than the maternal ones.

The principal oestrogen precursors are the 3-sulphates of various 3β-hydroxy-androst-5-ene derivatives and the essential enzyme systems required for oestrogen (and especially oestriol) synthesis are distributed between the placenta and foetus in a characteristic manner. Thus aryl sulphatase (E.C.3.1.6.1.) and the corresponding 3β-hydroxysteroid dehydrogenase (E.C.1.1.1.-51.) and $\Delta^4 \leftarrow \Delta^5$-isomerase activities (acting on C-19 steroids) are only present in the placenta, whereas the corresponding 16α-hydroxylating enzyme system (acting on C-18 and C-19 steroids) is only present in the foetal liver. Finally, the aromatizing enzyme system is present both in the placenta, and in the foetus. Thus the foetus and placenta form a functional unit, carrying out together the synthesis of the major part of oestrogens excreted in pregnancy urine.

There is a most extensive aryl sulphokinase (E.C.2.8.2.1.) activity in the foetal organism. This activity does not seem to be present in significant quantities in the placenta. Since no *in vivo* aryl sulphatase activity is present in the foetus, the foetal oestrogen-sulphurylating mechanism coupled with the extensive hydroxylation of oestrogen sulphates at various carbon atoms seems to be capable of providing the foetus with an endocrinologically 'oestrogen-free' milieu at a time when the maternal organism is under the influence of highly elevated amounts of biologically active oestrogens. It is possible that the oestrogen sulphates formed also have specific functions in the rapidly developing foetal organism. There is also a considerable glucuronyl transferase (E.C.2.4.1.17.) and some β-glucuronidase (E.C.3.2.1.31.) activity in the foetal liver and/or intestinal tract. These enzymic activities do not seem to be present in the placenta.

The placenta releases a great deal more oestrogen to the maternal than to the foetal compartment. In addition, oestrogen sulphates reaching the placenta with the foetal circulation are hydrolysed by the placenta and transferred rapidly to the maternal compartment. Nevertheless, considerable quantities of conjugated oestrogens are accumulated in various foetal tissues and by the end of gestation, the concentration of conjugated oestriol in the urine of the newborn and in the meconium is exceptionally high.

The oestrogen transfer from the maternal to the foetal compartment is limited; most of the transfer takes place in the opposite direction. Unconjugated oestrogens are transferred more rapidly than sulphates and sulphates more rapidly than glucosiduronates. The transplacental passage of oestrogen glucosiduronates does not involve hydrolysis of the conjugated form.

Placental secretion of oestriol to the mother is followed by a metabolism involving extensive conversion of unconjugated oestriol, oestriol-3-sulphate,16-glucosiduronate and oestriol-3-sulphate into oestriol-16-

and then into oestriol-3-glucosiduronate. The balance of evidence suggests that most of the dynamic changes in the pattern of conjugation take place in the form of repeated hydrolysis and reconjugation, rather than the conversion of one conjugate into another. An exception is the conversion of oestriol-16-glucosiduronate into oestriol-3-sulphate,16-glucosiduronate.

Research efforts of the past two decades resulted in a considerable clarification of the biogenesis, catabolism, transport and elimination of the oestrogens during pregnancy. However, the raison d'être of the high amounts of oestrogens secreted by the foeto-placental unit is still obscure and seems to offer a most fascinating field for continued research.

REFERENCES

ALONSO C. & TROEN P. (1966) Perfusion studies of the human placenta. V. Metabolism of estrone-^{3}H,sulfate-^{35}S and 17β-estradiol-^{14}C at midpregnancy. *Biochemistry*, **5**, 337.

AXELROD L.R. & GOLDZIEHER J.W. (1965) The polycystic ovary. V. Alternate pathways of steroid aromatization in normal, pregnancy and polycystic ovaries. *J. Clin. Endocr. Metab.* **25**, 1275.

BAGGETT B., ENGEL L.L., BALDERAS L., LANMAN G., SAVARD K. & DORFMAN R.I. (1959) Conversion of ^{14}C-testosterone to ^{14}C-estrogenic steroids by endocrine tissues. *Endocrinology*, **64**, 600.

BARR M., DICZFALUSY E. & TILLINGER K.-G. (1961) Studies on oestrogen metabolism in infants and children. *Acta endocr.* (*Kbh*), **37**, 241.

BAULIEU E.E. & DRAY F. (1963) Conversion of ^{3}H-dehydroisoandrosterone (3β-hydroxy-Δ^{5}-androsten-17-one) sulfate to ^{3}H-estrogens in normal pregnant women. *J. Clin. Endocr. Metab.* **23**, 1298.

BAULIEU E.E., CORPÉCHOT C., DRAY F., EMILIOZZI R., LEBEAU M.C., MAUVAIS-JARVIS P. & ROBEL P. (1965) An adrenal-secreted 'androgen': dehydroisoandrosterone sulfate. Its metabolism and a tentative generalization on the metabolism of other steroid conjugates in man. *Recent Progr. Hormone Res.* **21**, 411.

BEER C.T. & GALLAGHER T.F. (1955) Excretion of estrogen metabolites by humans. II. The fate of large doses of estradiol-17β after intramuscular and oral administration. *J. Biol. Chem.* **214**, 351.

BENAGIANO G., KINCL F.A., ZIELSKE F., WIQVIST N. & DICZFALUSY E. (1967) Studies on the metabolism of C-19 steroids in the human foeto-placental unit. 2. Metabolism of androstenedione and testosterone in the intact foeto-placental unit. *Acta endocr.* (*Kbh*) **56**, 203.

BENAGIANO G., MANCUSO S., MANCUSO F.P., WIQVIST N. & DICZFALUSY E. (1968) Studies on the metabolism of C-19 steroids in the human foeto-placental unit. 3. Dehydrogenation and reduction products formed by previable foetuses perfused with androstenedione and testosterone. *Acta endocr.* (*Kbh*) **57**, 187.

BENGTSSON G., ULLBERG S., WIQVIST N. & DICZFALUSY E. (1964) Autoradiographic studies on previable human foetuses perfused with radioactive steroids. 1. Distribution of radioactive material following perfusion of progesterone-4-^{14}C. *Acta endocr.* (*Kbh*), **46**, 544.

BENIRSCHKE K. (1956) Adrenals in anencephaly and hydrocephaly. *Obstet. Gynec.* **8**, 412.

BIRD C.E., WIQVIST N., DICZFALUSY E. & SOLOMON S. (1966) Metabolism of progesterone by the perfused previable human fetus. *J. Clin. Endocr. Metab.* **26**, 1144.

BOLTÉ E., MANCUSO S., ERIKSSON G., WIQVIST N. & DICZFALUSY E. (1964a) Studies on the aromatisation of neutral steroids in pregnant women. 1. Aromatisation of C-19 steroids by placentas perfused *in situ*. *Acta endocr.* (*Kbh*), **45**, 535.

BOLTÉ E., MANCUSO S., ERIKSSON G., WIQVIST N. & DICZFALUSY E. (1964b) Studies on the aromatisation of neutral steroids in pregnant women. 2. Aromatisation of dehydroepiandrosterone and its sulphate administered simultaneously into a uterine artery. *Acta endocr.* (*Kbh*), **45**, 560.

BOLTÉ E., MANCUSO S., ERIKSSON G., WIQVIST N. & DICZFALUSY E. (1964c) Studies on the aromatisation of neutral steroids in pregnant women. 3. Over-all aromatisation of dehydroepiandrosterone sulphate circulating in the foetal and maternal compartments. *Acta endocr.* (*Kbh*), **45**, 576.

BOLTÉ E., MANCUSO S., DRAY F., BAULIEU E.E. & DICZFALUSY E. (1964d) Conversion of testosterone-17α-^{3}H into 17β-estradiol-17α-^{3}H by human placentas perfused *in situ*. *Steroids*, **4**, 613.

BOLTÉ E., WIQVIST N. & DICZFALUSY E. (1966) Metabolism of dehydroepiandrosterone and dehydroepiandrosterone sulphate by the human foetus at mid-pregnancy. *Acta endocr.* (*Kbh*), **52**, 583.

BREUER H. (1960a) Isolation of 17-Epioestriol from the urine of pregnant women. *Nature*, **185**, 613.

BREUER H. (1960b) Biogenese und Stoffwechsel 6-substituierter Oestrogene beim Menschen. *Symp. Deut. Ges. Endokrin.* **7**, 273.

BREUER H. (1962) Metabolism of the natural estrogens. *Vitamins and Hormones*, **20**, 285.

BREUER H. (1964) Occurrence and determination of the newer oestrogens in human urine. *Research on Steroids*, **1**, 133. C. Cassano (Ed.) Il pensiero scientifico, Rome.

BREUER H. & PANGELS C. (1959) Isolation of oestriol-3,16β,17α, from the urine of pregnant women. *Biochim. Biophys. Acta*, **36**, 572.

BREUER J., BREUER F., BREUER H. & KNUPPEN R. (1966) Isolierung von 6-Hydroxy-östriol aus dem Urin schwangerer Frauen. *Hoppe-Seyler's Z. Physiol. Chemie*, **346**, 279.

BROWN J.B. (1956) Urinary excretion of oestrogens during pregnancy, lactation and the re-establishment of menstruation. *Lancet*, **270**, 704.

CASSMER O. (1959) Hormone production of the isolated human placenta. *Acta endocr.* (*Kbh*), Suppl. 45.

CÉDARD L., YANNOTTI S. & VARANGOT J. (1961) La perfusion de placenta *in vitro* appliquée à l'étude de la biosynthèse des oestrogènes. *C.R. Soc. Biol.* (*Paris*), **155**, 458.

CÉDARD L. (1964) *Contribution à l'étude de la biosynthèse et du métabolisme des oestrogènes naturels.* Masson & Cie, ed., Paris.

CÉDARD L., FILLMANN B., KNUPPEN R., LISBOA B.P. & BREUER H. (1964) Stoffwechsel und Aromatisierung von 7-substituierten C-19 Steroiden in der Placenta. *Hoppe-Seyler's Z. Physiol. Chemie*, **338**, 89.

CÉDARD L. & KNUPPEN R. (1965) 6α-Hydroxylation in human placenta perfusion. *Steroids*, **6**, 307.

CÉDARD L., VARANGOT J. & YANNOTTI S. (1966) Biosynthèse et metabolisme des oestrogènes dans le placenta humain perfusé ou incubé *in vitro*. II. Variation des réactions enzymatiques en fonction de l'âge de la grossesse. *Eur. Journ. Steroids*, **1**, 287.

COLÁS, A., LE ROY HEINRICHS W. & TATUM H.J. (1964) Pettenkofer chromogens in the maternal and fetal circulations: Detection of 3β,16α-dihydroxyandrost-5-en-17-one in umbilical cord blood. *Steroids*, **3**, 417.

COLÁS A. & LEROY HEINRICHS W. (1965) Pettenkofer chromogens in the maternal and fetal circulations: Anencephalic pregnancies, cesarean sections, and tentative identification of 3β,17β-dihydroxyandrost-5-en-16-one in umbilical cord blood. *Steroids*, **5**, 753.

DAVIS M.E., WIENER M., JACOBSON H.I. & JENSEN E.V. (1963) Estradiol metabolism in pregnant and nonpregnant women. *Am. J. Obst. Gynec.* **87**, 979.

DE CLERC P. (1958) In *Le Placenta Humain*, p. 515. J.Snoeck, ed. Masson et Cie., Paris.

DELL'ACQUA S., MANCUSO S., ERIKSSON G. & DICZFALUSY E. (1965) Oestrogen formation from 19-nortestosterone and testosterone following *in situ* perfusion of human placentas at midterm. *Acta endocr.* (*Kbh*), Suppl. **100**, 81.

DELL'ACQUA S., MANCUSO S., ERIKSSON G. & DICZFALUSY E. (1966) Metabolism of retrotestosterone and testosterone by midterm human placentas perfused *in situ*. *Biochim. Biophys. Acta*, **130**, 241.

DELL'ACQUA S., MANCUSO S., WIQVIST N., RUSE J.L., SOLOMON S. & DICZFALUSY E. (1967a) Studies on the aromatisation of neutral steroids in pregnant women. 5. Metabolism of androst-5-ene-3β,16α,17β-triol in the intact foeto-placental unit at midpregnancy. *Acta endocr.* (*Kbh*) **55**, 389.

DELL'ACQUA S., MANCUSO S., ERIKSSON G., RUSE J.L., SOLOMON S. & DICZFALUSY E. (1967b) Studies on the aromatisation of neutral steroids in pregnant women. 6. Aromatisation of 16α-hydroxylated C-19 steroids by midterm placentas perfused *in situ*. *Acta endocr.* (*Kbh.*) **55**, 401.

DE MIQUEL M. & TROEN P. (1966) Metabolism of 17α-hydroxy-progesterone by mid-pregnancy human placentas. *Excerpta medica Internat. Congress series*, **111**, 292.

DICZFALUSY E. (1953) Chorionic gonadotrophin and oestrogens in the human placenta. *Acta endocr.* (*Kbh*), **12**, Suppl. 12.

DICZFALUSY E. (1958) Métabolisme des oestrogènes chez le foetus et le nouveau-né. *Bull. Soc. Roy. Belge Gyn. Obst.* **28**, 459.

DICZFALUSY E. (1962) Endocrinology of the foetus. *Acta Obst. Gynec. Scand.* **41**, Suppl; 1, 45.

DICZFALUSY E. (1964a) Endocrine functions of the human feto-placental unit. *Fed. Proc.* **23**, 791.

DICZFALUSY E. (1964b) *In vivo* biogenesis and metabolism of oestrogens in the foeto-placental unit. *Excerpta medica Internat. Congress series*, **83**, 732.

DICZFALUSY E. (1965) Biogenesis y metabolismo de los estrogenos en la mitad del embarazo. *Acta Ginecol. (Madrid)*, **16**, 429.

DICZFALUSY E. (1967) Oestrogen and progesterone metabolism in the human foeto-placental unit. *Mém. Acad. roy. Méd. Belg.* II. Sér. **6**, 111.

DICZFALUSY E. (1969) Steroid metabolism in the foeto-placental unit. *Excerpta medica Internat. Congress* series **183**, 278.

DICZFALUSY E. & LINDKVIST P. (1956) Isolation and estimation of 'free' oestrogens in human placentae. *Acta endocr. (Kbh)*, **22**, 203.

DICZFALUSY E., TILLINGER K.-G. & WESTMAN A. (1957a) Studies on oestrogen metabolism in newborn boys. I. Excretion of oestrone, oestradiol-17β and oestriol during the first few days of life. *Acta endocr. (Kbh)*, **26**, 303.

DICZFALUSY E., TILLINGER K.-G. & WESTMAN A. (1957b) Studies on oestrogen metabolism in newborn boys. II. A study of metabolism of exogeneous oestradiol-17β. *Acta endocr. (Kbh)*, **26**, 313.

DICZFALUSY E. & MAGNUSSON A.M. (1958) Tissue concentration of oestrone, oestradiol-17β and oestriol in the human foetus. *Acta endocr. (Kbh)*, **28**, 169.

DICZFALUSY E. & HALLA M. (1958) The detection of an epimeric oestriol in placental extracts. *Acta endocr. (Kbh)*, **27**, 303.

DICZFALUSY E., MENINI E., TILLINGER K.-G. & WESTMAN A. (1959) Studies on oestrogen metabolism in newborn boys. III. Faecal excretion of oestrogen during the first few days of life. *Acta endocr. (Kbh)*, **30**, 539.

DICZFALUSY E. & v. MÜNSTERMANN A.M. (1959) Isolation and identification of 16-oxo-oestradiol-17β in human placentae. *Acta endocr. (Kbh)*, **32**, 195.

DICZFALUSY E. & BORELL U. (1961) Influence of oophorectomy on steroid excretion in early pregnancy. *J. Clin. Endocr. Metab.* **21**, 1119.

DICZFALUSY E. & LAURITZEN C. (1961) *Oestrogene beim Menschen.* Springer Verlag, Berlin.

DICZFALUSY E. & TROEN P. (1961) Endocrine functions of the human placenta. *Vitamins and Hormones*, **19**, 229.

DICZFALUSY E., CASSMER O., ALONSO C. & DE MIQUEL M. (1961a) Oestrogen metabolism in the human foetus. I. Tissue levels following the administration of 17β-oestradiol and oestriol. *Acta endocr. (Kbh)*, **37**, 353.

DICZFALUSY E., CASSMER O., ALONSO C., DE MIQUEL M. & WESTIN B. (1961b) Oestrogen metabolism in the human foetus. II. Oestrogen conjugation by foetal organs *in vitro* and *in vivo*. *Acta endocr. (Kbh)*, **37**, 516.

DICZFALUSY E., CASSMER O., ALONSO C. & DE MIQUEL M. (1961c) Oestrogen metabolism in the human foetus. III. Nature of the conjugated oestrogen formed by the foetus. *Acta endocr. (Kbh)*, **38**, 31.

DICZFALUSY E., CASSMER O., ALONSO C. & DE MIQUEL M. (1961d) Estrogen metabolism in the human fetus and newborn. *Recent Progr. Hormone Res.* **17**, 147.

DICZFALUSY E., TILLINGER K.-G., WIQVIST N., LEVITZ M., CONDON G.P. & DANCIS J. (1963) Disposition of intra-amniotically administered estriol-16-^{14}C and estrone-16-^{14}C sulfate by women. *J. Clin. Endocr. Metab.* **23**, 503.

DICZFALUSY E., BARR M. & LIND J. (1964) Oestriol metabolism in an anencephalic monster. *Acta endocr.* (*Kbh*), **46**, 511.

DICZFALUSY E. & MANCUSO S. (1965) Biogenesi e metabolismo steroideo nell'unità feto-placentare. *Rivista di Anatomia Patologica e Oncologia*, **28**, 33.

DICZFALUSY E., PION R. & SCHWERS J. (1965) Steroid biogenesis and metabolism in the human foeto-placental unit at midpregnancy. *Arch. Micr. Anat.* **54**, 67.

DORFMAN R.I., FORCHIELLI E., ICHII S. & KOWAL J. (1964) Ovarian steroid biosynthesis. *Excerpta medica Internat. Congress series*, **83**, 1087.

DOISY E.A., VELER C.D. & THAYER S.A. (1929) Folliculin from urine of pregnant women. *Am. J. Physiol.* **90**, 329.

EASTERLING W.E. Jnr., SIMMER H.H., DIGNAM W.J., FRANKLAND M.W. & NAFTOLIN F. (1966) Neutral C-19 steroids and steroid sulfates in human pregnancy. II. Dehydroepiandrosterone sulfate, 16α-hydroxy-dehydroepiandrosterone and 16α-hydroxy-dehydroepiandrosterone sulfate in maternal and fetal blood of pregnancies with anencephalic and normal fetuses. *Steroids*, **8**, 157.

EBERLEIN W.R. (1965) Steroids and sterols in umbilical cord blood. *J. Clin. Endocr. Metab.* **25**, 1101.

EMERMAN S., DANCIS J., LEVITZ M., WIQVIST N. & DICZFALUSY E. (1965) Metabolism of estrone-6,7-^{3}H sulfate-^{35}S in the perfused human fetus. *J. Clin. Endocr. Metab.* **25**, 639.

ENGEL L.L., BAGGETT B. & HALLA M. (1962) *In vitro* metabolism of estradiol-17β by human fetal liver: formation of estriol, 16-epi-estriol, estrone and an estriol glucosiduronic acid. *Endocrinology*, **70**, 907.

FISHMAN J., BROWN J.B., HELLMAN L., ZUMOFF B. & GALLAGHER T.F. (1962) Estrogen metabolism in normal and pregnant women. *J. Biol. Chem.* **237**, 1489.

FLICKINGER G.L., WU C.-H. & TOUCHSTONE J.C. (1967) The conversion of dehydroepiandrosterone-7α-^{3}H to oestrogens by corpora lutea of early human pregnancy. *Acta endocr.* (*Kbh*), **54**, 30.

FRANDSEN V.A. (1959) The demonstration of 2-methoxy-oestrone and of 2-methoxy-oestradiol in human pregnancy urine. *Acta endocr.* (*Kbh*), **31**, 603.

FRANDSEN V.A. & STAKEMANN G. (1961) The site of production of oestrogenic hormones in human pregnancy. Hormone excretion in pregnancy with anencephalic foetus. *Acta endocr.* (*Kbh*), **38**, 383.

FRANDSEN V.A. & STAKEMANN G. (1963) The site of production of oestrogenic hormones in human pregnancy. II. Experimental investigations on the role of the foetal adrenal. *Acta endocr.* (*Kbh*), **43**, 184.

FRANDSEN V.A. & STAKEMANN G. (1964a) The site of production of oestrogenic hormones in human pregnancy. III. Further observations on the hormone excretion in pregnancy with anencephalic foetus. *Acta endocr.* (*Kbh*), **47**, 265.

FRANDSEN V.A. & STAKEMANN G. (1964b) The excretion of hormones in cases of hydatidiform mole and chorionepithelioma. *Acta endocr.* (*Kbh*), Suppl. **90**, 81.

FRENCH A.P. & WARREN J.C. (1965) Steroid-3β-sulfatase in fetal and placental tissues. *Steroids*, **6**, 865.

GOEBELSMANN U., SJÖBERG K., WIQVIST N. & DICZFALUSY E. (1965a) Oestriol-3-glucosiduronate, a major urinary metabolite of oestriol and oestriol-16(17?)-glucosiduronate. *Acta endocr.* (*Kbh*), **50**, 261.

GOEBELSMANN U., ERIKSSON G., WIQVIST N. & DICZFALUSY E. (1965b) Metabolism of oestriol-3-sulphate and oestriol-16(17?)-glucosiduronate in pregnant women. *Acta endocr.* (*Kbh*), **50**, 273.

GOEBELSMANN U., DICZFALUSY E., KATZ J. & LEVITZ M. (1965c) Biosynthesis of radioactive estriol-3-glucosiduronate by guinea pig liver homogenate. *Steroids*, **6**, 859.

GOEBELSMANN U., WIQVIST N., DICZFALUSY E., LEVITZ M., CONDON G.P. & DANCIS J. (1966a) Fate of intra-amniotically administered oestriol-15-^{3}H-3-sulphate and oestriol-16-^{14}C-16-glucosiduronate in pregnant women at mid-term. *Acta endocr.* (*Kbh*), **52**, 550.

GOEBELSMANN U., ERIKSSON G., DICZFALUSY E., LEVITZ M. & CONDON G.P. (1966b) Fate of oestriol-3-sulphate and oestriol-16-glucosiduronate in the intact foeto-placental unit at midpregnancy. *Acta endocr.* (*Kbh*), **53**, 391.

GOEBELSMANN U., COOKE I., WIQVIST N. & DICZFALUSY E. (1966c) Comparison of the metabolism of oestriol-3-glucosiduronate and oestriol-16-glucosiduronate in pregnant women. *Acta endocr.* (*Kbh*), **52**, 30.

GOEBELSMANN U., WIQVIST N. & DICZFALUSY E. (1968a) Placental transfer of oestriol glucosiduronates. *Acta endocr.* (*Kbh*), **59**, 426.

GOEBELSMANN U., WIGVIST N. & DICZFALUSY E. (1968b) Metabolism of oestriol-3-sulphate-16-glucosiduronate in pregnant women. *Acta endocr.* (*Kbh*), **59**, 595.

GUAL C., MORATO T., HAYANO M., GUT M. & DORFMAN R.I. (1962) Biosynthesis of estrogens. *Endocrinology*, **71**, 920.

GURPIDE E., ANGERS M., VANDE WIELE R.L. & LIEBERMAN S. (1962) Determination of secretory rates of estrogens in pregnant and nonpregnant women from the specific activities of urinary metabolites. *J. Clin. Endocr. Metab.* **22**, 935.

GURPIDE E., SCHWERS J., WELCH M.T., VANDE WIELE R.L. & LIEBERMAN S. (1966) Fetal and maternal metabolism of estradiol during pregnancy. *J. Clin. Endocr. Metab.* **26**, 1355.

HAGEN A.A., BARR M. & DICZFALUSY E. (1965) Metabolism of 17β-oestradiol-4-^{14}C in early infancy. *Acta endocr.* (*Kbh*), **49**, 207.

HARKNESS R.A., MENINI E., CHARLES D., KENNY F.M. & ROMBAUT R. (1966) Studies of urinary steroid excretion by an adrenalectomized woman during and after pregnancy. *Acta endocr.* (*Kbh*), **52**, 409.

HAYNES R.C. Jnr., MIKHAIL G., ERIKSSON G., WIQVIST N. & DICZFALUSY E. (1964) Oestradiol metabolism in the previable human foetus and in the foeto-placental unit. *Acta endocr.* (*Kbh*), **45**, 297.

HENNING H.D. & ZANDER J. (1962) Verwendung von Hübeners 20β-Hydroxysteroid Dehydrogenase bei mikrochemischer Identifizierung und Trennung von Steroiden. *Hoppe-Seyler's Z. Physiol. Chem.* **330**, 31.

HOBKIRK R. & NILSEN M. (1962) Observation on the occurrence of six estrogen fractions in human pregnancy urine. I. Normal pregnancy. *J. Clin. Endocr. Metab.* **22**, 134.

HUFFMANN M.N., MACCORQUODALE D.W., THAYER S.A., DOISY E.A., SMITH G.V. & SMITH O.W. (1940) The isolation of α-dehydrotheelin from human pregnancy urine. *J. Biol. Chem.* **134**, 591.

JACKANICZ, T.M. & DICZFALUSY E. (1968) Absence of 16α-hydroxylating activity in the human midterm placenta. *Steroids*, **11**, 877.

JAFFE R., PION R., ERIKSSON G., WIQVIST N. & DICZFALUSY E. (1965) Studies on the aromatization of neutral steroids in pregnant women. 4. Lack of oestrogen formation from progesterone. *Acta endocr.* (*Kbh*), **48**, 413.

JAYLE M.F. (1965) *Hormonologie de la Grossesse Humaine*, A. Soulairac & M. Marois, eds. Monographie de la Révue Européenne d'Endocrinologie.

JUNGMANN R.A., KOT E. & SCHWEPPE J.S. (1966) *In vitro* synthesis of estrogens by midterm human placenta and fetal liver. *Steroids*, **8**, 977.

KATZ S.R., DANCIS J. & LEVITZ M. (1965) Relative transfer of estriol and its conjugates across the fetal membranes *in vitro*. *Endocrinology*, **76**, 722.

KIRSCHNER M.A., WIQVIST N. & DICZFALUSY E. (1966) Studies on oestriol synthesis from dehydroepiandrosterone sulphate in human pregnancy. *Acta endocr.* (*Kbh*), **53**, 584.

KLAUSNER D.A. & RYAN K.J. (1964) Estriol secretion by the human term placenta. *J. Clin. Endocr. Metab.* **24**, 101.

KLOPPER A. & BILLEWICZ W. (1963) Urinary excretion of oestriol and pregnandiol during normal pregnancy. *J. Obst. Gynaec. Brit. Comm.* **70**, 1024.

KNUPPEN R. & BREUER H. (1963) Biogenese von Östratetraenol beim Menschen. *Acta endocr.* (*Kbh*), **42**, 129.

KNUPPEN R., HAUPT O. & BREUER H. (1965) Isolation and identification of 15α-hydroxyoestrone from the urine of pregnant women. *Biochem. J.* **96**, 33c.

KNUPPEN R., HAUPT O. & BREUER H. (1966a) The isolation of 6α-hydroxyoestrone from the urine of pregnant women. *Biochem. J.* **101**, 397.

KNUPPEN R., HAUPT O. & BREUER H. (1966b) Isolation and identification of 15β-hydroxyoestrone and 15β-hydroxyoestradiol-17β from the urine of pregnant women. *Steroids*, **8**, 403.

KNUPPEN R., BREUER H. & DICZFALUSY E. (1966c) Comparative studies on the metabolism of oestrogens by the human foetus during perfusion and *in vitro*. *Excerpta medica Internat. Congress series*, **111**, 171.

LAMB E., MANCUSO S., DELL'ACQUA S., WIQVIST N. & DICZFALUSY E. (1967) Studies on the metabolism of C-19 steroids in the human foeto-placental unit. 1. Neutral metabolites formed from dehydroepiandrosterone and dehydroepiandrosterone sulphate by the placenta at midpregnancy. *Acta endocr.* (*Kbh*) **55**, 263.

LANMAN J.T. (1953) The foetal zone of the adrenal gland. *Medicine, Baltimore*, **32**, 389.

LASKIN A.I., GRABOVIC B., JUNTA B., DELISLE MEYERS C. & FRIED J. (1964) Microbial hydroxylation of estrone and estradiol in the 6β-, 7α- and 15α-positions. *J. Org. Chem.* **29**, 1333.

LAYNE D.S. & MARRIAN G.F. (1958) The isolation of 16β-hydroxyoestrone and 16-oxo-oestradiol-17β from the urine of pregnant women. *Biochem. J.* **70**, 244.

LELONG M., VANDEL S., BORNICHE P. & JAYLE M.F. (1951) Dosage des oestrogènes dans le placenta et les organs d'enfants morts á la naissance. *Ann. Endocr. (Paris)*, **12**, 922.

LEUSDEN VAN H.A. & VILLEE C.A. (1966) Formation of estrogens by hydatidiform moles *in vitro*. *J. Clin. Endocr. Metab.* **26**, 842.

LEVITZ M., CONDON G.P. & DANCIS J. (1955) Conversion of acetate-1-^{14}C to estradiol in perfused human placenta. *Fed. Proc.* **14**, 245.

LEVITZ M., CONDON G.P. & DANCIS J. (1956) The interconversion of estrone and estradiol in the perfused human placenta. *Endocrinology*, **58**, 376.

LEVITZ M., EMERMAN S. & DANCIS J. (1962) Sterol synthesis in perfused human placenta. *Excerpta medica Internat. Congress series*, **51**, 266.

LEVITZ M., KATZ J. & TWOMBLY G.H. (1965) The biosynthesis of labeled estriol-3-sulfate, 16-glucosiduronate. *Steroids*, **6**, 553.

LEVITZ M., CONDON G.P., DANCIS J., GOEBELSMANN U., ERIKSSON G. & DICZFALUSY E. (1967) Transfer of estriol and estriol conjugates across the human placenta perfused *in situ* at midpregnancy. *J. Clin. Endocr. Metab.* **27**, 1723.

LISBOA B.P., GOEBELSMANN U. & DICZFALUSY E. (1967) Isolation of 15α-hydroxyoestradiol from human pregnancy urine. *Acta endocr. (Kbh)*, **54**, 467.

LITTLE B., SHAW A. & PURDY R. (1963) The conversion of progesterone to 16α-hydroxy-pregn-4-ene-3,20-dione and androst-4-ene-3,17-dione by human placenta *in vitro*. *Acta endocr. (Kbh)*, **43**, 510.

LOKE K.H., WATSON E.J.D. & MARRIAN G.F. (1957) The isolation of a sixth Kober chromogen from urine of pregnant women and its provisional identification as 18-hydroxyoestrone. *Biochim. Biophys. Acta*, **26**, 230.

LOKE K.H. & MARRIAN G.F. (1958) Isolation of 2-Methoxyoestrone from the urine of pregnant women. *Biochim. Biophys. Acta*, **27**, 213.

LUUKKAINEN T. & ADLERCREUTZ H. (1965) Isolation and identification of 11-dehydro-oestradiol-17α, a new type of urinary steroid, in the urine of pregnant women. *Biochim. Biophys. Acta*, **107**, 579.

MACNAUGHTON M.C. (1965) Urinary excretion of oestrogen and pregnanediol in hydatidiform mole. *J. Obst. Gynaec. Brit. Comm.* **72**, 249.

MAGENDANTZ H.G. & RYAN K.J. (1964) Isolation of an estriol precursor, 16α-hydroxydehydroepiandrosterone, from human umbilical sera. *J. Clin. Endocr. Metab.* **24**, 1155.

MANCUSO S., DELL'ACQUA S., ERIKSSON G., WIQVIST N. & DICZFALUSY E. (1965a) Aromatisation of androstenedione and testosterone by the human fetus. *Steroids*, **5**, 183.

MANCUSO S., BENAGIANO G., DELL'ACQUA S. & DICZFALUSY E. (1965b) Metabolismo degli androgeni nel feto umano. *Rivista di Anatomia Patologica e Oncologia*, **28**, 54.

MANCUSO S., MANCUSO F.P., TILLINGER K.-G. & DICZFALUSY E. (1965c) Lack of aromatisation of circulating dehydroepiandrosterone and dehydroepiandrosterone sulphate in amenorrhoeic women stimulated with human gonadotrophins. *Acta endocr. (Kbh)*, **49**, 248.

MANCUSO S., NILSSON L. & DICZFALUSY E. (1966) Oestrogen formation from dehydroepiandrosterone sulphate in spayed mice implanted with human placental tissue. *Research on Steroids*, **2**, 47. C. Cassano (Ed.) Il pensiero scientifico, Rome.

MANCUSO S., BENAGIANO G., DELL'ACQUA S., SHAPIRO M., WIQVIST N. & DICZFALUSY E. (1968) Studies on the metabolism of C-19 steroids in the human foeto-placental unit. 4. Aromatisation and hydroxylation products formed by previable foetuses perfused with androstenedione and testosterone. *Acta endocr.* (*Kbh*), **57**, 208.

MANER F.D., SAFFAN B.D., WIGGINS R.A., THOMSON J.D. & PREEDY J.R.K. (1963) Interrelationship of estrogen concentrations in the maternal circulation, fetal circulation and maternal urine in late pregnancy. *J. Clin. Endocr. Metab.* **23**, 445.

MARRIAN G.F. (1929) The chemistry of oestrin: I. Preparation from urine and the separation from an unidentified solid alcohol. *Biochem. J.* **23**, 1090.

MARRIAN G.F. & BAULD W.S. (1955) The isolation of 16-epioestriol from the urine of pregnant women. *Biochem. J.* **59**, 136.

MARRIAN G.F., LOKE K.H., WATSON E.J.D. & PANATTONI M. (1957) 16α-Hydroxy-oestrone in the urine of pregnant women. *Biochem. J.* **66**, 60.

MENINI E. & DICZFALUSY E. (1961a) Isolation and identification of estriol glucosiduronate in human meconium. *Endocrinology*, **67**, 500.

MENINI E. & DICZFALUSY E. (1961b) Isolation and identification of sodium estriol-3-sulphate in human meconium. *Endocrinology*, **68**, 492.

MEYER A.S. (1955) Conversion of 19-Hydroxy-Δ^4-androstene-3,17-dione to oestrone by endocrine tissues. *Biochim. Biophys. Acta*, **17**, 441.

MICHIE E.A. (1966) Oestrogen levels in urine and amniotic fluid in pregnancy with live anencephalic foetus and the effect of intra-amniotic injection of sodium dehydroepiandrosterone sulphate on these levels. *Acta endocr.* (*Kbh*), **51**, 535.

MIGEON C., KELLER A.R. & HOLMSTROM E.G. (1955) Dehydroepiandrosterone, androsterone and 17-hydroxy-corticosteroid levels in maternal and cord plasma in cases of vaginal delivery. *Bull. Johns Hopk. Hosp.* **97**, 415.

MIKHAIL G., WIQVIST N. & DICZFALUSY E. (1963a) Oestriol metabolism in the previable human foetus. *Acta endocr.* (*Kbh*), **42**, 519.

MIKHAIL G., WIQVIST N. & DICZFALUSY E. (1963b) Oestriol metabolism in the human foeto-placental unit. *Acta endocr.* (*Kbh*), **43**, 213.

MORATO T., HAYANO M., DORFMAN R.I. & AXELROD L.R. (1961) The intermediate steps in the biosynthesis of estrogens from androgens. *Biochem. Biophys. Res. Comm.* **6**, 334.

MORATO T., LEMUS A.E. & GUAL C. (1965) Efficiency of dehydroepiandrosterone sulphate as an estrogen precursor. *Steroids*, **5**, Suppl. 1, 59.

NEHER R. & STARK G. (1961) Nachweis von Corticosteroiden in menschlicher Placenta und Isolierung von 16α-Hydroxytestosteron. *Experientia*, **17**, 510.

NOTCHEV V.D. & STIMMEL B.F. (1962) 2-Hydroxyestrone in human pregnancy urine. *Excerpta medica Internat. Congress series*, **51**, 175.

PALMER R., ERIKSSON G., WIQVIST N. & DICZFALUSY E. (1966a) Studies on the metabolism of C-21 steroids in the human foeto-placental unit. 2. Metabolism of pregnenolone sulphate by midterm placentas perfused *in situ*. *Acta endocr.* (*Kbh*), **52**, 598.

PALMER R., BLAIR J.A., ERIKSSON G. & DICZFALUSY E. (1966b) Studies on the metabolism of C-21 steroids in the human foeto-placental unit. 3. Metabolism of progesterone and 20α- and 20β-dihydroprogesterone by midterm placentas perfused *in situ*. *Acta endocr.* (*Kbh*), **53**, 407.

PASQUALINI J.R., LOWY J., WIQVIST N. & DICZFALUSY E. (1968) Biosynthesis of cortisol from 3β,17α,21-trihydroxypregn-5-en-20-one by the intact human foetus at midpregnancy. *Biochim. Biophys. Acta*, **152**, 648.

PAULSEN C.A. (1965) *Estrogen Assays in Clinical Medicine. Basis and Methodology.* The University of Washington Press.

PEARLMAN W.H., PEARLMAN M.R.J. & RAKOFF A.E. (1954) Estrogen metabolism in human pregnancy; a study with the aid of deuterium. *J. Biol. Chem.* **209**, 803.

PION R.J., JAFFE R.B., ERIKSSON G., WIQVIST N. & DICZFALUSY E. (1965) Studies on the metabolism of C-21 steroids in the human foeto-placental unit. 1. Formation of α,β-unsaturated 3-ketones in midterm placentas perfused *in situ* with pregnenolone and 17α-hydroxy-pregnenolone. *Acta endocr.* (*Kbh*), **48**, 234.

PION R.J., JAFFE R.B., WIQVIST N. & DICZFALUSY E. (1967) Formation of dehydroepiandrosterone sulphate by previable human foetuses. *Biochim. Biophys. Acta*, **137**, 584.

PULKKINEN M.O. (1961) Arylsulphatase and the hydrolysis of some steroid sulphates in developing organism and placenta. *Acta Physiol. Scand.* **52**, Suppl. 180.

REYNOLDS J.W. (1964) The isolation of 16-ketoandrostenediol (3β,17β-dihydroxy-androst-5-en-16-one) from the urine of a newborn infant. *Steroids*, **3**, 77.

REYNOLDS J.W. (1966) 16α-Hydroxylation of pregnenolone by human liver. *Steroids*, **7**, 261.

REYNOLDS J.W., MANCUSO S., WIQVIST N. & DICZFALUSY E. (1968) Studies on the aromatisation of neutral steroids in pregnant women. 7. Aromatisation of 3β,17β-dihydroxy-androst-5-en-16-one by placentas perfused *in situ* at mid-pregnancy. *Acta endocr.* (*Kbh*), **58**, 377.

ROY E.J. (1962) The concentration of oestrogens in maternal and foetal blood obtained at cesarean section, and the effect of hospitalization on maternal blood oestrogens levels. *J. Obst. Gynaec. Brit. Comm.* **69**, 196.

ROY E.J. & BROWN J.B. (1960) A method for the estimation of oestriol, oestrone and oestradiol-17β in the blood of the pregnant woman and of the foetus. *J. Endocr.* **21**, 9.

ROY E.J. & MACKAY R. (1962) Concentration of oestrogens in blood during pregnancy. *J. Obst. Gynaec. Brit. Comm.* **69**, 13.

RYAN K.J. (1958) Conversion of Δ^5-androstene-3β,16α,17β-triol to estriol by human placenta. *Endocrinology*, **63**, 392.

RYAN K.J. (1959a) Biological aromatization of steroids. *J. Biol. Chem.* **234**, 268.

RYAN K.J. (1959b) Metabolism of C-16 oxygenated steroids by human placenta: the formation of estriol. *J. Biol. Chem.* **234**, 2006

RYAN K.J. (1963a) The conversion of pregnenolone-7-^{3}H and progesterone-4-^{14}C to oestradiol by a corpus luteum of pregnancy. *Acta endocr.* (*Kbh*), **44**, 81.

RYAN K.J. (1963b) Biogenesis of estrogens. *Proceedings of the Fifth International Congress of Biochemistry: Biosynthesis of Lipids*, Vol. VIII, p. 381, G.Popják, ed. Pergamon Press and Polish Scientific Publishers.

RYAN K.J. & ENGEL L.L. (1953) The interconversion of estrone and estradiol by human tissue slices. *Endocrinology*, **52**, 287.

RYAN K.J. & SMITH O.W. (1961a) Biogenesis of estrogens by human ovary. 1. Conversion of acetate-1-^{14}C to estrone and estradiol. *J. Biol. Chem.* **236**, 705.

RYAN K.J. & SMITH O.W. (1961b) Biogenesis of estrogens by human ovary. 3. Conversion of cholesterol-4-^{14}C in estrone. *J. Biol. Chem.* **236**, 2204.

RYAN K.J. & SMITH O.W. (1961c) Biogenesis of estrogens by human ovary. 2. Conversion of progesterone to estrone and estradiol. *J. Biol. Chem.* **236**, 710.

SANDBERG E.C. & JENKINS R.C. (1966) Aryl and steroid sulfatase in the human ovary. *Biochim. Biophys. Acta*, **113**, 190.

SCHMIDT-ELMENDORF H.W. (1961) Der Gehalt von Östron, 17β-Östradiol und Östriol in der menschlichen Placenta. *Acta endocr.* (*Kbh*), **38**, 527.

SCHWERS J. (1964) *Les Oestrogènes au Cours de la Seconde Moitié de la Grossesse.* Editions Arscin S.A., Bruxelles.

SCHWERS J., ERIKSSON G. & DICZFALUSY E. (1965a) Metabolism of oestrone and oestradiol in the human foeto-placental unit at midpregnancy. *Acta endocr.* (*Kbh*), **49**, 65.

SCHWERS J., GOVAERTS-VIDETSKY M., WIQVIST N. & DICZFALUSY E. (1965b) Metabolism of oestrone sulphate by the previable human foetus. *Acta endocr.* (*Kbh*), **50**, 597.

SCHWERS J., ERIKSSON G., WIQVIST N. & DICZFALUSY E. (1965c) 15α-Hydroxylation: a new pathway of estrogen metabolism in the human fetus and newborn. *Biochim. Biophys. Acta*, **100**, 313.

SERCHI G. (1953) La separazione di un metabolita urinario estratrienico in forma cristalline. b, Estrazione dal cromatogramma su carta. *Chimica* (*Milano*), **8**, 10.

SIITERI P.K. & MACDONALD P.C. (1963) The utilization of circulating dehydroisoandrosterone sulfate for estrogen synthesis during human pregnancy. *Steroids*, **2**, 713.

SIITERI P.K. & MACDONALD P.C. (1966) Placental estrogen biosynthesis during human pregnancy. *J. Clin. Endocr. Metab.* **26**, 751.

SIMMER H.H., EASTERLING W.E. Jnr., PION R.J. & DIGNAM W.J. (1964) Neutral C19-steroids and steroid sulfates in human pregnancy. 1. Identification of dehydroepiandrosterone sulfate in fetal blood and quantification of this hormone in cord arterial, cord venous and maternal peripheral blood in normal pregnancies at term. *Steroids*, **4**, 125.

SLAUNWHITE W.R., KARSAY M.A., HOLLMER A., SANDBERG A.A. & NISWANDER K. (1965) Fetal liver as an endocrine tissue. *Steroids*, **6**, Suppl. **2**, 211.

SMITH O.W. & HAGERMAN D.D. (1965) Quantitative estimation of estrogen conjugates in late pregnancy plasma. *J. Clin. Endocr. Metab.* **25**, 732.

SMITH O.W. & ARAI K. (1963) Blood estrogens in late pregnancy: an evaluation of methods with improved recovery. *J. Clin. Endocr. Metab.* **23**, 1141.

SMITH O.W. & RYAN K.J. (1961) Biogenesis of estrogens by the human ovary: the conversion of androstenedione-4-^{14}C to estrone and estradiol in high yield. *Endocrinology*, **69**, 869.

SOBREVILLA L.A., HAGERMAN D.D. & VILLEE C.A. (1964) The metabolism of pregnenolone and 17-hydroxyprogesterone by homogenates of human term placentas. *Biochim. Biophys. Acta*, **93**, 665.

STÁRKA L., BREUER H. & CÉDARD L. (1966a) Biosynthesis of equilin and related ring B unsaturated oestrogens in perfused human placenta. *J. Endocr.* **34**, 447.

STÁRKA L., JANATA J., BREUER H. & HAMPL R. (1966b) Biosynthesis of equilin and equilenin from 7α-hydroxydehydroepiandrosterone and its sulphate by human placenta maintained in organ culture. *Europ. J. Steroids*, **1**, 37.

STEWART H.L. Jnr. (1951) Hormone secretion by human placenta grown in the eyes of rabbits. *Am. J. Obst. Gynec.* **61**, 990.

TAN I.-K. & LOKE K.H. (1966) Aromatization of 18-hydroxyandrostenedione to 18-hydroxyestrone by human placenta. *Steroids*, **8**, 385.

THORSEN T., STØA K.F. & AARSKOG D. (1964) Identification of ring D α-ketolic oestrogens in the urine of newborn infants. *Acta endocr.* (*Kbh*), **45**, 415.

TROEN P. (1961) Perfusion studies of the human placenta. II. Metabolism of C^{14}-17β-estradiol with and without added human chorionic gonadotropin. *J. Clin. Endocr. Metab.* **21**, 895.

TROEN P., NILSSON B., WIQVIST N. & DICZFALUSY E. (1961) Pattern of oestriol conjugates in human cord blood, amniotic fluid, and urine of newborns. *Acta endocr.* (*Kbh*), **38**, 361.

TROEN P., DE MIQUEL M. & ALONSO C. (1966) Perfusion studies of the human placenta. IV. Conjugation of oestriol-16-^{14}C. *Biochemistry*, **5**, 332.

VILLEE D.B. (1965) Influence of progesterone on steroid metabolism in fetal adrenals. *Excerpta medica Internat. Congress series*, **99**, 182.

VILLEE D.B. & VILLEE C.A. (1964) Synthesis of corticosteroids in the fetal-placental unit. *Excerpta medica Internat. Congress series*, **83**, 709.

WALOP J.N. & DE LANGE N. (1966) Dependence of the biochemical aromatization of C-19 steroids on the configuration at carbon atoms 8, 9 and 10. *Biochim. Biophys. Acta*, **130**, 249.

WARREN J.C. & TIMBERLAKE C.E. (1962) Steroid sulfatase in the human placenta. *J. Clin. Endocr. Metab.* **22**, 1148.

WARREN J.C. & TIMBERLAKE C.E. (1964) Biosynthesis of estrogens in pregnancy; precursor role of plasma dehydroisoandrosterone. *Obst. Gynec.* **23**, 689.

WARREN J.C. & CHEATUM S. (1964) Demonstration of a steroid 17-20 desmolase in the human placenta. *Canad. J. Biochem.* **42**, 143.

WATSON E.J.D. & MARRIAN G.F. (1956) Observations on the occurrence of 16-*epi*oestriol in urine. *Biochem. J.* **63**, 64.

WENGLE B. (1964) Ester sulfates. XXI. Sulfate conjugation in fetal human tissue extracts. *Acta Soc. Med. Upsalien.* **69**, 105.

WEST C.D., DAMAST B.L., SARRO S.D. & PEARSON O.H. (1956) Conversion of testosterone to estrogens in castrated, adrenalectomized human females. *J. Biol. Chem.* **218**, 409.

WILCOX R.B. & ENGEL L.L. (1965a) The aromatization of 10-methyl and 10-hydroxymethyl steroids by human placental microsomes. *Steroids*, **6**, Suppl. **2**, 249.

WILCOX R.B. & ENGEL L.L. (1965b) Kinetic studies on the role of 19-hydroxyandrost-4-ene-3,17-dione in estrogen biosynthesis. *Steroids*, **5**, Suppl. **1**, 49.

WILSON R., ERIKSSON G. & DICZFALUSY E. (1964) Oestriol metabolism in pregnant women. *Acta endocr.* (*Kbh*), **46**, 525.

WILSON R., BIRD C.E., WIQVIST N., SOLOMON S. & DICZFALUSY E. (1966) Metabolism of progesterone by the perfused adrenalectomized human fetus. *J. Clin. Endocr. Metab.* **26**, 1155.

WOTIZ H.H., DAVIS J.W., LEMON H.M. & GUT M. (1956) Studies on steroid metabolism. *v*. The conversion of testosterone-4-^{14}C to estrogens by human ovarian tissue. *J. Biol. Chem.* **222**, 487.

ZUCCONI G., GOEBELSMANN U., WIQVIST N. & DICZFALUSY E. (1967a) Metabolism of oestrone-glucosiduronate at midpregnancy. *Acta endocr.* (*Kbh*), **56**, 71.

ZUCCONI G., LISBOA B.P., SIMONITSCH E., ROTH L., HAGEN A.A. & DICZFALUSY E. (1967b) Isolation of 15α-hydroxy-oestriol from human pregnancy urine and from the urine of newborn infants. *Acta endocr.* (*Kbh*), **56**, 413.

Neutral Steroids in Human Pregnancy: Isolation, Formation and Metabolism*

EDWARD V. YOUNGLAI & SAMUEL SOLOMON

INTRODUCTION

Shortly after the isolation of pregnanediol (see Table 6.1) from human pregnancy urine by Marrian (1929) and by Dingemanse *et al.* (1930), it was realized that it is the principal metabolite of progesterone (Browne *et al.* 1937) and that its excretion increased with progessing pregnancy (Venning 1938). It was soon realized that large amounts of progesterone were elaborated during pregnancy and that it was the placenta which was the site of its origin. Similar evidence led to the conclusion that the large amounts of estrogens elaborated during pregnancy were also formed in the placenta. The earlier evidence has been reviewed by Diczfalusy & Troen (1961) and will not be dealt with here.

Lanman (1953) in his review of the fetal zone of the adrenal gland focused attention on this important structure and it was not long before a number of investigators initiated *in vitro* studies to determine the biosynthetic pathways of steroid formation in this tissue. Similar *in vitro* incubation studies and perfusion experiments were also performed with the human placenta (Solomon *et al.* 1954, Solomon 1960) and these demonstrated that cholesterol was the precursor of progesterone and pregnenolone. These initial studies were followed by a more physiological type of approach in which the previable human fetus was perfused with ^{14}C or ^{3}H labeled precursors or the precursors were injected into the

* Supported by a research grant from the U.S.P.H.S. (AM-04329) and by a grant from the Medical Research Council of Canada (MT-1658).

TABLE 6.1

Trivial names and systematic names of steroids used in this chapter

C-18	
Estriol	Estra-1,3,5(10)-triene-3,16α,17β-triol
C-19	
Dehydroisoandrosterone	3β-Hydroxyandrost-5-en-17-one
Androstenediol	Androst-5-ene-3β,17β-diol
Androsterone	3α-Hydroxy-5α-androstan-17-one
Isoandrosterone	3β-Hydroxy-5α-androstan-17-one
Etiocholanolone	3α-Hydroxy-5β-androstan-17-one
11-Ketoetiocholanolone	3α-Hydroxy-5β-androstane-11,17-dione
11β-Hydroxyandrosterone	3α,11β-Dihydroxy-5α-androstan-17-one
16α-Hydroxyetiocholanolone	3α,16α-Dihydroxy-5β-androstan-17-one
16α-Hydroxyandrosterone	3α,16α-Dihydroxy-5α-androstan-17-one
16α-Hydroxydehydroisoandrosterone	3β,16α-Dihydroxyandrost-5-en-17-one
Androstenedione	Androst-4-ene-3,17-dione
Testosterone	17β-Hydroxyandrost-4-en-3-one
Retroandrostenedione	8β,9β,10α-Androst-4-ene-3,17-dione
Retrotestosterone	17β-Hydroxy-8β,9β,10α-androst-4-en-3-one
11β-Hydroxyandrostenedione	11β-Hydroxyandrost-4-ene-3,17-dione
11-Ketoandrostenedione	Androst-4-ene-3,11,17-trione
16α-Hydroxyandrostenedione	16α-Hydroxyandrost-4-ene-3,17-dione
16α-Hydroxytestosterone	16α,17β-Dihydroxyandrost-4-en-3-one
19-Hydroxyandrostenedione	19-Hydroxyandrost-4-ene-3,17-dione
Dehydroisoandrosterone sulfate	17-Ketoandrost-5-ene-3β-yl sulfate
Testosterone sulfate	3-Ketoandrost-4-ene-17β-yl sulfate
16α-Hydroxydehydroisoandrosterone sulfate	16α-Hydroxy-17-ketoandrost-5-ene-3β-yl sulfate
C-21	
Pregnenolone	3β-Hydroxypregn-5-en-20-one
16α-Hydroxypregnenolone	3β,16α-Dihydroxypregn-5-en-20-one
17α-Hydroxypregnenolone	3β,17α-Dihydroxypregn-5-en-20-one
20α-Dihydropregnenolone	3β,20α-Dihydroxypregn-5-en-20-one
Progesterone	Pregn-4-ene-3,20-dione
6β-Hydroxyprogesterone	6β-Hydroxypregn-4-ene-3,20-dione
6-Ketoprogesterone	Pregn-4-ene-3,6,20-trione
15α-Hydroxyprogesterone	15α-Hydroxypregn-4-ene-3,20-dione
16α-Hydroxyprogesterone	16α-Hydroxypregn-4-ene-3,20-dione
17α-Hydroxyprogesterone	17α-Hydroxypregn-4-ene-3,20-dione
20α-Dihydroprogesterone	20α-Hydroxypregn-4-ene-3,20-dione
20β-Dihydroprogesterone	20β-Hydroxypregn-4-ene-3,20-dione
17α,20α-Dihydroxyprogesterone	17α,20α-Dihydroxypregn-4-ene-3,20-dione

TABLE 6.1 (*continued*)

11-Dehydrocorticosterone	21-Hydroxypregn-4-ene-3,11,20-trione
Corticosterone	11β,21-Dihydroxypregn-4-ene-3,20-dione
Deoxycorticosterone	21-Hydroxypregn-4-ene-3,20-dione
Cortisol	11β,17α,21-Trihydroxypregn-4-ene-3,20-dione
Cortisone	17α,21-Dihydroxypregn-4-ene-3,11,20-trione
6β-Hydroxycortisol	6β,11β,17α,21-Tetrahydroxypregn-4-ene-3,20-dione
Aldosterone	11β,21-Dihydroxy-3,20-diketopregn-4-en-18-al
Pregnanolone	3α-Hydroxy-5β-pregnan-20-one
5α-Pregnanolone	3α-Hydroxy-5α-pregnan-20-one
Isopregnanolone	3α-Hydroxy-5β,17α-pregnan-20-one
5α-Pregnanediol	5α-Pregnane-3α,20α-diol
5α-Pregnanedione	5α-Pregnane-3,20-dione
5β-Pregnanedione	5β-Pregnane-3,20-dione
Pregnanetriol	5β-Pregnane-3α,17α,20α-triol
Tetrahydrocortisone	3α,17α,21-Trihydroxy-5β-pregnane-11,20-dione
5β-Dihydrocortisone	17α,21-Dihydroxy-5β-pregnane-3,11,20-trione
Cortolone	3α,17α,20α,21-Tetrahydroxy-5β-pregnan-11-one
Pregnenolone sulfate	20-Ketopregn-5-ene-3β-yl sulfate
17α-Hydroxypregnenolone sulfate	17α-Hydroxy-20-keto-pregn-5-ene-3β-yl sulfate
Pregnanolone sulfate	20-Keto-5β-pregnane-3α-yl sulfate
Pregnanediol sulfate	20α-Hydroxy-5β-pregnane-3α-yl sulfate
Corticosterone sulfate	11β-Hydroxy-3,20-diketopregn-4-ene-21-yl sulfate
Deoxycorticosterone sulfate	3,20-Diketopregn-4-ene-21-yl sulfate
11-Dehydrocorticosterone sulfate	3,11,20-Triketopregn-4-ene-21-yl sulfate
Cortisol sulfate	11β,17α-Dihydroxy-3,20-diketopregn-4-ene-21-yl sulfate
Pregnanolone glucosiduronate	20-Keto-5β-pregnane-3α-yl-β-D-glucopyronosiduronic acid
Pregnanediol glucosiduronate	20α-Hydroxy-5β-pregnane-3α-yl-β-D-glucopyronosiduronic acid
Others	
Squalene	2,6,10,15,19,23-Hexamethyltetracosa-2,6,10,14,18,22-hexaene
Mevalonate (mevalonic acid)	3,5-Dihydroxy-3-methylpentanoic acid

TABLE 6.1 (*continued*)

Lanosterol	4,4[1],14α-Trimethylcholesta-8(9),24-dien-3β-ol
Cholesterol	Cholesta-5-en-3β-ol
20α-Hydroxycholesterol	Cholesta-5-ene-3β,20α-diol
17α,20α-Dihydroxycholesterol	Cholesta-5-ene-3β,17α,20α-triol

umbilical vein with the fetus *in utero*. In addition, placental metabolism of the neutral steroids was also studied by the perfusion of the placenta *in situ* at midterm or at term. Simultaneously *in vitro* incubation studies of fetal tissue and of the placenta were also being pursued and they have provided a different type of data which sometimes was in agreement with, and at other times differed from, the data obtained from the intact fetus. Both experimental approaches have yielded valuable information which, for the most part, can be reconciled and have played their role in providing us with a more complete picture of the complex metabolism of the neutral steroids in the human fetus.

Most of the data which will be discussed were obtained from the study of human fetal tissues obtained at midterm. Studies performed on tissues obtained from the newborn will not be considered in this review because we feel that they probably represent a separate experimental situation.

ISOLATION OF NEUTRAL STEROIDS FROM THE PLACENTA

In Table 6.2 are shown the neutral steroids isolated or detected from human placental tissue. Although androgenic activity, using bioassay procedures, has been demonstrated in extracts of placental tissue (Goecke *et al.* 1933, Cunningham & Kuhn 1941, Riess 1952), Dorfman (1948) was unable to detect any androgens in placental tissue. The only C-19 steroid isolated from this tissue is 16α-hydroxytestosterone (Neher & Stark 1961). As much as 35 μg of 16α-hydroxytestosterone was isolated from 30 Kg of tissue and it was suggested that this steroid may be an intermediate in the synthesis of estriol.

Progestational activity, as detected by bioassays, has been demonstrated in placental tissue by a number of workers (Adler *et al.* 1934, McGinty *et al.* 1936, van Lankeren 1936, Smith & Kennard 1937, Haffner 1938, Fujii *et al.* 1956). Using physiochemical methods, progesterone has

TABLE 6.2

Neutral steroids isolated from human placenta

Steroid isolated	Reference
16α-Hydroxytestosterone	Neher & Stark (1961)
Progesterone	Pearlman & Cerceo (1952a), Pearlman & Cerceo (1953), Salhanick *et al.* (1952, 1956), Noall *et al.* (1953)
5β-Pregnane-3α,20α-diol	Pearlman & Cerceo (1952b)
5α-Pregnane-3β,20α-diol	Pearlman & Cerceo (1952b)
3β-Hydroxy-5α-pregnan-20-one	Pearlman & Cerceo (1952b)
20α-Dihydroprogesterone	Zander *et al.* (1958), Zander (1959)
20β-Dihydroprogesterone	Zander *et al.* (1958), Zander (1959)
16α-Hydroxyprogesterone (placental blood)	Zander *et al.* (1962a)
Cortisol	Neher & Stark (1961)
Cortisone	Berliner *et al.* (1956), Neher & Stark (1961)
17α,20α,21-Trihydroxypregn-4-ene-3,11-dione	Neher & Stark (1961)
17α,20β,21-Trihydroxypregn-4-ene-3,11-dione	Neher & Stark (1961)

been isolated from placenta (Pearlman & Cerceo 1952a and 1953, Salhanick *et al.* 1952, Noall *et al.* 1953). By means of isotope dilution techniques, Pearlman (1957a and b) calculated the production of progesterone in late pregnancy to be about 250 mg per day, which was confirmed by Short & Eton (1959). This value is approximately the same as that, (190–280 mg in 24 hours), previously derived by Zander & von Munstermann (1956) from the concentration of progesterone entering the maternal organism from the placenta via the uterine vein. Zander (1959) estimated the concentration and total amount of progesterone in placentas during pregnancy. His findings, shown in Fig. 6.1, indicate that there is a steady and progressive rise in the total placental content of progesterone. The placenta has been shown to be the main source of progesterone in the absence of the fetal organism (Cassmer 1959), maternal ovaries (Diczfalusy & Borell 1961), and adrenals (Moses *et al.* 1959).

The C-21 steroids isolated from the human placenta are shown in Table 6.1. Neher & Stark (1961) isolated cortisol, cortisone and the 20α and 20β reduced products from placental tissue. Previously, Berliner *et al.* (1956) had isolated a number of corticosteroids from placental tissue and Salhanick *et al.* (1956) concluded that these steroids were concentrated in the tissue from the maternal blood. In addition to the steroids shown in Table 6.1, a number of compounds have been reported by Zander *et al.* (1962b and c) in placental blood. Among these are progesterone, 20α and 20β-dihydroprogesterone, 17α-hydroxyprogesterone, 16α-hydroxyprogesterone, 17α,20α-dihydroxypregn-4-en-3-one, 11β-hydroxyandrostenedione and 11-ketoandrostenedione. *To date no conjugated steroids have been isolated from human placental tissue.*

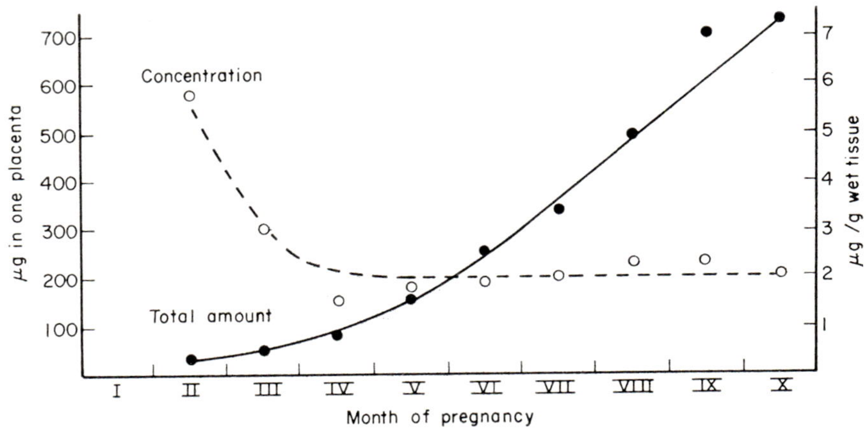

FIG. 6.1. Comparison of average values of concentrations (broken line), and of total amounts (solid line) of progesterone in eighty placentas in the 2nd to the 10th month of pregnancy. Reproduced from Zander (1959), by permission from Academic Press, New York.

METABOLISM OF NEUTRAL STEROIDS BY THE PLACENTA

Nissim & Robson (1952) were the first to study steroid metabolism in the human placenta when they showed that pregnenolone could be converted to a material with progestational activity. This material has since been identified as progesterone and the enzymic conversion of pregnenolone to progesterone in the placenta is well documented (Pearlman *et al.* 1954, Sobreville *et al.* 1964, Pion *et al.* 1965, Jaffe & Ledger 1966, Ryan *et al.* 1966, Jaffe 1967). These reactions establish the presence of an active 3β-hydroxysteroid dehydrogenase enzyme system in the placenta and it seems to be located in the syntrophoblast (Baillie *et al.* 1965a).

TABLE 6.3

Biosynthesis of neutral steroids in human placental tissue

Precursor	Tissue preparation	Products formed	Reference
Acetate	Mince	Squalene, cholesterol	Van Leusden & Villee (1965)
		Cholesterol	Zelewski & Villee (1966)
Mevalonate	Mince	Squalene, lanosterol, cholesterol	Zelewski & Villee (1966)
Cholesterol	Perfusion	Pregnenolone, progesterone	Solomon *et al.* (1954), Solomon (1960)
	Acetone powder	Pregnenolone, progesterone	Morrison *et al.* (1965)
	Homogenate and mitochondria	Progesterone	Ryan *et al.* (1966)
	In situ perfusion	Pregnenolone	Jaffe *et al.* (1965), Jaffe & Peterson (1966)
20α-Hydroxy-cholesterol	Homogenate	Pregnenolone	Shimizu *et al.* (1961)
Androstenedione	Homogenate	19-Hydroxyandrostenedione	Longchampt *et al.* (1960), Wilcox & Engel (1965)
		16α-Hydroxyandrostenedione	Jungmann & Schweppe (1967)
Testosterone	Perfusion	Androstenedione	Bolté *et al.* (1964), Dell'Acqua *et al.* (1966)
	Homogenate	16α-Hydroxyandrostenedione	Jungmann & Schweppe (1967)
Retrotestosterone	Perfusion	Retroandrostenedione	Dell'Acqua *et al.* (1966)
Dehydroisoandro-sterone	Slice	Androstenedione	Bloch & Newman (1966)
	Microsomes	Androstenedione	Morato *et al.* (1965)
	In situ perfusion	Androstenedione, testosterone	Lamb *et al.* (1967)
Androst-5-ene-3β,17β-diol	Homogenate	Testosterone	Baulieu *et al.* (1963)

TABLE 6.3 (*continued*)

Precursor	Tissue preparation	Products formed	Reference
11β-Hydroxyandrostenedione	Homogenate	11-Ketoandrostenedione	Osinki (1960)
16α-Hydroxydehydroisoandrosterone	*In situ* perfusion	16α-Hydroxyandrostenedione	Dell'Acqua *et al.* (1967b)
Androst-5-ene-3β,16α,17β-triol	*In situ* perfusion	16α-Hydroxytestosterone	Dell'Acqua *et al.* (1967a)
Pregnenolone	Mince, homogenate	Progesterone	Nissim & Robson (1952), Pearlman *et al.* (1954)
	Homogenate	Progesterone, 20α-dihydroprogesterone	Sobreville *et al.* (1964)
	Perfusion	Progesterone	Pion *et al.* (1965)
		Progesterone, 6β-hydroxyprogesterone	Jaffe & Ledger (1966)
	Homogenate and mitochondria	Progesterone	Ryan *et al.* (1966)
	Injection into the umbilical vein	Progesterone, 20α-dihydroprogesterone	Solomon *et al.* (1967)
Progesterone	Mince	6β-Hydroxyprogesterone	Berliner & Salhanick (1956)
	Perfusion	6-Ketoprogesterone	Hagopian *et al.* (1956)
	Homogenate	20α-Dihydroprogesterone	Little *et al.* (1959)
		17α-Hydroxyprogesterone	Little & Shaw (1960, 1961)
		16α-Hydroxyprogesterone, androstenedione	Little *et al.* (1963)
		Androstenedione, testosterone, 17α-hydroxyprogesterone, 16α-hydroxyprogesterone	Jungmann & Schweppe (1967)

	Homogenate and perfusion	Androstenedione	Warren & Cheatum (1964)
	In situ perfusion	20α-Dihydroprogesterone, 6β-hydroxyprogesterone	Palmer *et al.* (1966a), Kitchin *et al.* (1967)
	Injection into the umbilical vein	Pregnanolone, 3β-hydroxy-5α-pregnan-20-one, 20α-dihydroprogesterone, pregnanediol	Solomon *et al.* (1967)
17α-Hydroxy-pregnenolone	Perfusion	17α-Hydroxyprogesterone	Pion *et al.* (1965)
	Homogenate	Androst-5-ene-3β,16α,17β-triol, dehydroisoandrosterone, testosterone, androstenedione, 17α-hydroxyprogesterone	Jungmann & Schweppe (1967)
17α-Hydroxy-progesterone	Homogenate	17α,20α-Dihydroxypregn-4-en-3-one	Sobreville *et al.* (1964)
	Perfusion	17α,20α-Dihydroxypregn-4-en-3-one	De Miquel & Troen (1966)
20α-Dihydro-progesterone	*In situ* perfusion	Progesterone, 6β-hydroxyprogesterone	Palmer *et al.* (1966b)
16α-Hydroxy-progesterone	Injection into the umbilical vein	3α,16α-Dihydroxy-5β-pregnan-20-one	Solomon *et al.* (1967)
Cortisol	Homogenate	Cortisone	Osinki (1960)
	Slice	Cortisone, tetrahydrocortisone, 5β-dihydrocortisone	Meigs & Engel (1961)
Cortisone	Slice	Cortolone	Meigs & Engel (1961)
Corticosterone	Homogenate	11-Dehydrocorticosterone	Osinki (1960)

The biosynthetic conversions which have been demonstrated in the human placenta are shown in Table 6.3. As can be seen from the data in this Table, a variety of tissue preparations have been employed to demonstrate these conversions. Using a mince, van Leusden & Villee (1965) have reported a small conversion of acetate to squalene and cholesterol (0·002–0·005 per cent cholesterol conversion). Woolever *et al.* (1961) found no conversion of ^{14}C-acetate to sterols or steroids in this tissue but recently Zelewski & Villee (1966) showed that mevalonate could be converted to squalene, lanosterol and cholesterol in small yields. Cholesterol can serve as an efficient precursor of pregnenolone (Solomon *et al.* 1954, Solomon 1960, Morrison *et al.* 1965, Jaffe *et al.* 1965) and progesterone (Solomon *et al.* 1954, Solomon 1960, Morrison *et al.* 1965).

Single step conversions involving C-19 steroids have been demonstrated using a variety of starting products. Thus, the activity of the 3β-hydroxysteroid dehydrogenase has been demonstrated for dehydroisoandrosterone (Morato *et al.* 1965, Bloch & Newman 1966, Lamb *et al.* 1967), androst-5-ene-3β,17β-diol (Baulieu *et al.* 1963), 16α-hydroxydehydroisoandrosterone (Dell'Acqua *et al.* 1967b) and androst-5-ene-3β,16α,17β-triol (Dell'Acqua *et al.* 1967a) while the presence of a 19-hydroxylating enzyme (Longchampt *et al.* 1960, Wilcox & Engel 1965), 17β-hydroxysteroid dehydrogenase (Bolté *et al.* 1964, Dell'Acqua *et al.* 1966) and 11β-hydroxysteroid dehydrogenase (Osinki 1960) has been demonstrated.

A number of enzymes for the hydroxylation of progesterone have been demonstrated in placental tissue, 6β-hydroxylation (Berliner & Salhanick 1956, Palmer *et al.* 1966a and b, Kitchin *et al.* 1967), 17α-hydroxylation (Little & Shaw 1960 and 1961) and 16α-hydroxylation (Little *et al.* 1963). Reduction of the 20-ketone (Little *et al.* 1959, Sobreville *et al.* 1964, De Miquel & Troen 1966, Palmer *et al.* 1966a, Kitchin *et al.* 1967) has been well documented. Side-chain cleavage of C-21 steroids needs further confirmation since this reaction has not been demonstrated with 17α-hydroxypregnenolone in placental perfusion (Pion *et al.* 1965) or for 17α-hydroxyprogesterone in an incubation experiment (Sobreville *et al.* 1964). In contrast to these findings, Jungmann & Schweppe (1967) recently reported that a homogenate of human placenta can convert 17α-hydroxypregnenolone to dehydroisoandrosterone, testosterone, androstenedione, 17α-hydroxyprogesterone and androst-5-ene-3β,16α,17β-triol. In the same study these authors obtained similar results when they incubated progesterone with a homogenate of fetal liver.

Following the injection of pregnenolone into the umbilical vein, progesterone and 20α-dihydroprogesterone were isolated only from the placenta and not from the fetal tissue (Solomon *et al.* 1967). The same results were obtained when pregnenolone sulfate was injected into the umbilical vein. When labeled progesterone was injected into the umbili-

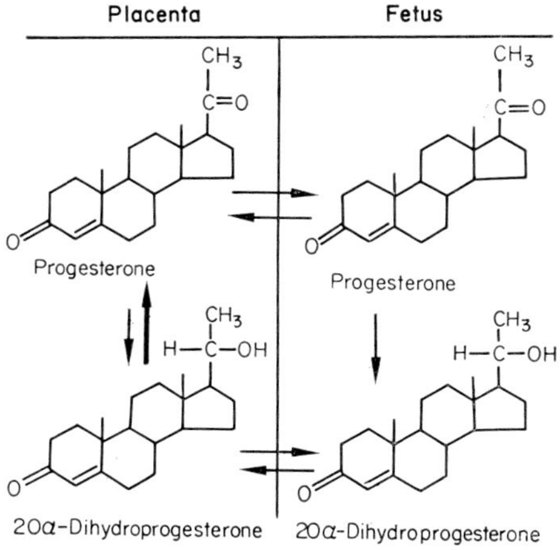

FIG. 6.2. Interconversion of progesterone and 20α-dihydroprogesterone in the human placenta and fetus.

cal vein, pregnanolone, 3β-hydroxy-5α-pregnan-20-one, 20α-dihydroprogesterone and pregnanediol were isolated from the placenta (Solomon *et al.* 1967). It was concluded from this study that the isolated metabolites were not formed in the placenta but were transported to this tissue from the fetus. In similar studies with labeled 16α-hydroxyprogesterone it was possible to isolate 3α,16α-dihydroxy-5β-pregnan-20-one which also seems to have been formed in the fetus.

When Palmer *et al.* (1966b) perfused the midterm human fetus with labeled progesterone and 20α-dihydroprogesterone, they found a sizable conversion of 20α-dihydroprogesterone to progesterone but not the reverse reaction. In Fig. 6.2 is shown the cyclic process of oxidation and reduction at C-20 in the fetus and placenta. It is possible that the feto-placental unit uses this series of reactions to conserve progesterone, as suggested by Palmer *et al.* (1966b).

With regard to the metabolism of steroid sulfates it has been demonstrated that dehydroisoandrosterone sulfate is converted to dehydroisoandrosterone, androstenedione and testosterone (Lamb *et al.* 1967) and pregnenolone sulfate is hydrolyzed to pregnenolone (Palmer *et al.* 1966a, Solomon *et al.* 1967) and oxidized to progesterone (Palmer *et al.* 1966a, Pion *et al.* 1966, Solomon *et al.* 1967).

Although the human placenta has been considered to be an incomplete organ as far as its steroid production is concerned, a scheme for the biosynthesis of neutral steroids can be compiled from the available evidence and this is depicted in Fig. 6.3.

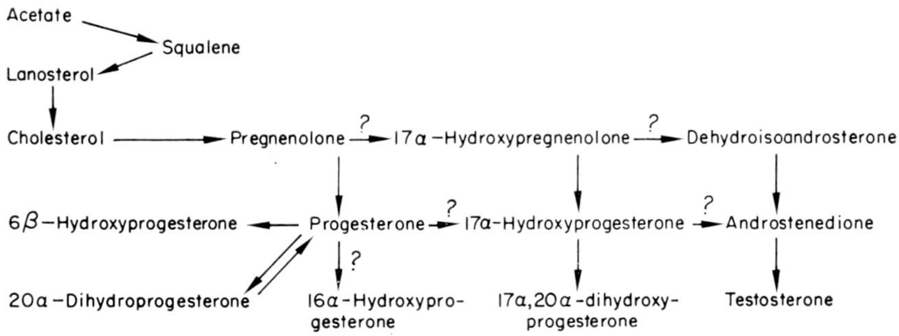

FIG. 6.3. Scheme of steroid conversions demonstrated for the human placenta.

It must be borne in mind that some of the reactions shown in Fig. 6.3 have not been confirmed and should have a question mark beside them. From the available evidence (van Leusden & Villee 1965, Zelewski & Villee 1966) it would seem that cholesterol can be formed from acetate *in vitro* by the human placenta. The formation of cholesterol is at the moment too small to account for the large amounts of progesterone and pregnenolone elaborated by the term placenta. In this connection it is of interest to note that Konrad Bloch (1945) demonstrated a large conversion of maternal cholesterol to urinary pregnanediol in a subject in the third trimester of pregnancy. Davis *et al.* (1956) also reported that labeled cholesterol was converted to urinary pregnanediol by a pregnant subject. It is thus possible that maternal cholesterol is the main precursor of placental progesterone and pregnenolone. It seems that the human placenta can hydroxylate progesterone at C_6. Whether it can hydroxylate steroids at C_{16} or C_{17} remains to be unequivocally demonstrated. It would also be important to determine if the human placenta under physiological conditions can convert 17α-hydroxyprogesterone and 17α-hydroxypregnenolone to C-19 steroids.

Considerable quantities of progesterone are transported from the placenta to both the fetal and maternal organisms. Here this hormone is extensively metabolized as will be discussed in subsequent sections.

ISOLATION OF NEUTRAL STEROIDS FROM BLOOD

(a) *Umbilical cord blood*

Arteriovenous differences in the amounts of steroid in umbilical blood are indicative of the type of steroids elaborated in the fetus or in the placenta. By means of the Zimmerman reaction Puck *et al.* (1953) found the concentration of 17-ketosteroids in cord blood to be 9·6 mg per litre and Gardner & Walton (1954) observed that the level of 17-ketosteroids was higher in cord plasma than in maternal plasma, indicating fetal production of this class of steroid. Migeon *et al.* (1955) demonstrated that in cases of vaginal delivery there was no difference in levels of dehydroisoandrosterone and androsterone between cord and maternal plasma. At term there is a higher concentration of 16α-hydroxydehydroisoandrosterone in the umbilical artery than in the vein (Colas *et al.* 1964, Colas & LeRoy Hendrichs 1965) indicating fetal production of this intermediate.

TABLE 6.4

Neutral steroids isolated from human cord blood

Steroid isolated	Reference
16α-Hydroxydehydroisoandrosterone	Magendantz & Ryan (1964), Colas *et al.* (1964), Colas & LeRoy Heinrichs (1965), Easterling *et al.* (1966)
3β,17β-Dihydroxyandrost-5-en-16-one	Colas & LeRoy Heinrichs (1965)
Dehydroisoandrosterone sulfate	Simmer *et al.* (1964), Easterling *et al.* (1966)
16α-Hydroxydehydroisoandrosterone sulfate	Easterling *et al.* (1966)
Progesterone	Zander (1959), Zander (1961), Zander *et al.* (1962b), Runnebaum & Zander (1962)
20α-Dihydroprogesterone	Zander (1959), Zander (1961), Zander *et al.* (1962b), Runnebaum & Zander (1962)
20β-Dihydroprogesterone	Zander (1961), Zander *et al.* (1962b), Runnebaum & Zander (1962)
Pregnenolone sulfate	Conrad *et al.* (1967)

In Table 6.4 are shown the neutral steroids isolated from cord blood. Several C-19 steroids have been isolated recently. Progesterone, 20α and 20β-dihydroprogesterone have been detected and measured by physio-chemical methods (Zander 1959, Zander 1961, Zander *et al.* 1962b, Runnebaum & Zander 1962) but definitive identification of these steroids has not been accomplished. In addition, Eberlein (1965) has published on the isolation of steroids from placental blood. Pregnenolone, dehydroisoandrosterone, 17α-hydroxypregnenolone and pregn-5-ene-3β,17α,20ξ,21-tetrol have been identified and a partial identification was obtained for 19 other steroids and five sterols.

With regard to conjugated steroids the concentrations of dehydro-isoandrosterone sulfate in cord arterial plasma were found to be 162·0 ± 62·5 μg per 100 ml and in cord venous plasma, 130·5 ± 59·5 μg per 100 ml, suggesting an uptake by the placenta and probable production in the fetus (Simmer *et al.* 1964). A similar arteriovenous difference has been observed for 16α-hydroxydehydroisoandrosterone sulfate–110 μg per 100 ml cord arterial plasma, 87 μg per 100 ml cord venous plasma (Easterling *et al.* 1966). Pregnenolone sulfate has also been found in cord blood (Conrad *et al.* 1967). Thus it seems probable that the fetus produces sizable amounts of dehydroisoandrosterone sulfate and 16α-hydroxydehydroisoandrosterone sulfate and that the pregnenolone reaching the fetus from the placenta is converted to pregnenolone sulfate.

(b) *Maternal blood*

Progesterone concentration in plasma is elevated during pregnancy (Zander & Simmer 1954) and rises with progessing gestation (Oertel *et al.* 1959, Futterweit *et al.* 1962, Lurie *et al.* 1966). Seal & Doe (1966) and Sandberg *et al.* (1966) found that transcortin, (CBG, corticosteroid-binding globulin), has a high affinity for progesterone. Estrogens can stimulate the synthesis of transcortin (Sandberg & Slaunwhite 1959) and the levels of this binding protein are elevated during pregnancy (Slaunwhite & Sandberg 1959, Doe *et al.* 1964).

Very recently Pearlman & Crèpy (1967) found that testosterone was bound to a plasma protein which was not transcortin (Pearlman *et al.* 1967). Testosterone binding increases with progressing pregnancy up to the 20th week of gestation and then levels off to term and was at a low level after delivery (Pearlman *et al.* 1967). It would be of some interest to know whether this binding protein is also present in the fetal circulation.

It has long been known that there is a progressive rise in the maternal level of plasma 17-hydroxycorticosteroids during pregnancy (reviewed by Sandberg *et al.* 1957). This rise in plasma 17-hydroxycorticosteroids is not due to an elevated secretion of adrenal steroid but rather to the increased level of transcortin (Slaunwhite & Sandberg 1959, Doe *et al.* 1964) whose production is induced by estrogens during pregnancy.

ISOLATION OF NEUTRAL STEROIDS FROM FETAL TISSUE

There have been very few reports on the isolation of neutral steroids from endocrine tissues of the human fetus. Using paper chromatographic procedures Bloch *et al.* (1955, 1956) and Benirschke *et al.* (1956) provided presumptive evidence for the presence of androstenedione, 11β-hydroxy-androstenedione, dehydroisoandrosterone and cortisol in extracts of human fetal adrenal. Benirschke & Bloch (1960) could not find C-19 steroids in extracts of human fetal testes. It would be of great interest to determine the endogenous levels of the biologically active steroid hormones in fetal tissue at different periods of gestation.

NEUTRAL STEROIDS IN MECONIUM AND AMNIOTIC FLUID

Human meconium, the intestinal contents of the fetus, has been a source for the isolation of a number of steroids–dehydroisoandrosterone (Francis *et al.* 1960), 3β-hydroxypregn-5,16-dien-20-one (Francis *et al.* 1962) 5β-pregnane-3α,20α-diol (Francis & Kinsella 1966) and 5α-pregnane-3α,20α-diol (Francis & Kinsella 1967). Progesterone has been detected in the pregnant myometrium (Kumar *et al.* 1962) and in the amniotic fluid (Zander & Munstermann 1956). Klopper & MacNaughton (1959) found pregnanediol in amniotic fluid.

METABOLISM OF NEUTRAL STEROIDS BY HUMAN FETAL TISSUES

(a) *Adrenals*

A functional role for the human fetal adrenals during pregnancy has long been favoured because of the relatively large size of these glands and the characteristic fetal zone present in this tissue. Numerous studies conducted during the past fifteen years have defined the biosynthetic capacity

TABLE 6.5

Formation of neutral steroids in human fetal adrenals

Precursor	Tissue preparation	Products formed	Reference
Acetate	Slice	Dehydroisoandrosterone, androstenedione, 11β-hydroxyandrostenedione, pregnenolone	Bloch & Benirschke (1959)
		Cholesterol, cortisol, androstenedione	Bloch & Benirschke (1960, 1962)
20α-Hydroxycholesterol	Slice	17α,20α-Dihydroxycholesterol dehydroisoandrosterone, cortisol	Shimizu *et al.* (1965)
Dehydroisoandrosterone	Homogenate	Androstenedione	Bloch *et al.* (1962b)
Testosterone	Perfusion of fetus	Testosterone sulfate	Mancuso *et al.* (1967)
Pregnenolone	Injection into the umbilical vein	Dehydroisoandrosterone, pregnenolone sulfate, 17α-hydroxypregnenolone sulfate, dehydroisoandrosterone sulfate	Solomon *et al.* (1967)
	Homogenate, slice	Dehydroisoandrosterone, 16α-hydroxypregnenolone	Villee *et al.* (1962)
	Mince	Androstenedione, 11β-hydroxyandrostenedione	Villee & Driscoll (1965)

17α-Hydroxy-pregnenolone	Perfusion of fetus	17α-Hydroxypregnenolone sulfate, dehydroisoandrosterone sulfate	Pion *et al.* (1967)
Progesterone	Homogenate	Androstenedione, 17α-hydroxy-progesterone	Solomon *et al.* (1958)
		Cortisol	Villee *et al.* (1959)
	Slice, homogenate	16α-Hydroxyprogesterone, 17α-hydroxy-progesterone, deoxycorticosterone	Villee *et al.* (1961)
	Mince	11β-Hydroxyandrostenedione, cortisol, 16α-hydroxyprogesterone	Villee & Driscoll (1965)
	Organ culture	Cortisol	Bloch *et al.* (1965)
	Perfusion of fetus or injection into the umbilical vein	20α-Dihydroprogesterone, 6β-hydroxy-progesterone, 16α-hydroxyprogesterone, 17α-hydroxyprogesterone, cortisol	Bird *et al.* (1966), Solomon *et al.* (1967)
		Corticosterone sulfate, deoxycortico-sterone sulfate, 11-dehydrocorticosterone sulfate, cortisol sulfate	Bird *et al.* (1965), Solomon *et al.* (1967)
Endogenous	Organ culture	Cortisol	Stark *et al.* (1965)

of the fetal adrenal and these are listed in Table 6.5. Using histochemical techniques a number of investigators have studied enzymes involved in the metabolism of neutral C-19 steroids. Thus Dawson *et al.* (1961) were able to demonstrate 3β-hydroxysteroid dehydrogenase activity in adrenal glands from fetuses after the 11th week of gestation. With dehydroisoandrosterone as substrate similar data was obtained by others (Bloch *et al.* 1962b, Niemi & Baillie 1965, Goldman *et al.* 1966). However, it is doubtful that 3β-hydroxysteroid dehydrogenase enzymes demonstrated by these techniques are active *in vivo* because of the large number of 3β-hydroxy-5-ene-steroids which are isolated in an unaltered form from the adrenal. It has been postulated that this deficiency may account for the hyperplasia of the fetal adrenal gland (Klevit 1966).

Bengtsson *et al.* (1964) perfused the previable human fetus with labeled progesterone and found by autoradiography that the highest uptake of radioactivity was in the adrenal glands. This gives further weight to the investigations carried out by several workers on the metabolic fate of progesterone in the fetal adrenals. By means of *in vitro* techniques, it was shown that fetal adrenals can convert progesterone to various corticosteroids (Lanman & Silverman 1957, Villee *et al.* 1959, Hillman *et al.* 1962, Villee & Driscoll 1965). Shimizu *et al.* (1965) showed that 20α-hydroxycholesterol is converted by fetal adrenal slices to 17α,20α-dihydroxycholesterol, dehydroisoandrosterone and a number of 4-ene-ketosteroids. Previously, Villee *et al.* (1959) could find no Porter-Silber chromogens after incubating acetate or cholesterol with fetal adrenal homogenates. In later studies it was found that 16α-hydroxyprogesterone, 17α-hydroxyprogesterone and deoxycorticosterone were formed from progesterone but no neutral steroids could be derived from acetate, mevalonate or cholesterol (Villee *et al.* 1961). This is in contrast to the variety of conversions from acetate reported by Bloch & Benirschke (1959, 1960, 1962). However, it should be pointed out that only very small conversions were observed and in some instances radiochemical purity could not be obtained because of the small amount of radioactivity incorporated into the products of incubation. Solomon *et al.* (1967) also found very small conversions of acetate and cholesterol to neutral steroids in the adrenals of the perfused previable human fetus.

When (7α-^{3}H)pregnenolone was injected into the umbilical vein at the time of therapeutic abortion, labeled dehydroisoandrosterone, pregnenolone sulfate, 17α-hydroxypregnenolone sulfate and dehydroisoandrosterone sulfate were isolated in radiochemically pure form

(Solomon 1966, Solomon *et al.* 1967). There was no evidence for the formation of 4-ene-3-ketosteroids from pregnenolone in these studies. Villee *et al.* (1962) and Villee & Driscoll (1965) obtained conflicting results when pregnenolone was incubated with fetal adrenal slices, minces and homogenates. With the homogenate and slice, these authors obtained 3β-hydroxy-5-ene steroids but with the adrenal mince they obtained 4-ene-3-ketosteroids.

It is generally accepted that steroid hydroxylation reactions take place as early as the 15th week of gestation. One such reaction which is quantitatively important is 16α-hydroxylation (Villee *et al.* 1961, 1962, Villee & Villee 1964, Solomon *et al.* 1964, Villee & Driscoll 1965, Villee *et al.* 1965, Bird *et al.* 1966). This activity appears early in gestation and may be an important mechanism for providing precursors for the biosynthesis of estriol by the placenta (Diczfalusy 1964). Evidence has also been provided for the presence of hydroxylases for C_{17} (Solomon *et al.* 1958, Villee *et al.* 1961, Solomon *et al.* 1964, Shimizu *et al.* 1965, Bloch *et al.* 1965, Villee *et al.* 1965, Bird *et al.* 1966, Solomon *et al.* 1967), C_{11} (Villee & Driscoll 1965, Bird *et al.* 1965, Bird *et al.* 1966) and C_{21} (Villee & Driscoll 1965, Bird *et al.* 1965, Bird *et al.* 1966, Solomon *et al.* 1967).

It is important to note that labeled androstenedione was not isolated from fetal tissues in the study where the previable human fetus was perfused with labeled progesterone (Bird *et al.* 1966) or when the labeled hormone was injected into the umbilical vein with the fetus *in utero* (Solomon *et al.* 1967). It was also found that when labeled 17α-hydroxyprogesterone was injected into the umbilical vein neither androstenedione or testosterone were isolated from the adrenals or the testes (Solomon *et al.* 1967). These findings are in marked contrast to the *in vitro* results cited above.

A large number of conjugated metabolites have been isolated from human fetal adrenals following perfusion of the previable midterm fetus with labeled progesterone or when the labeled hormone was injected into the umbilical vein (Bird *et al.* 1965, Solomon *et al.* 1967). Other conjugates have been isolated after *in vitro* incubations (Villee *et al.* 1965). The same authors reported that dehydroisoandrosterone sulfate is converted by fetal adrenals to dehydroisoandrosterone, androstenedione, 11β-hydroxyandrostenedione and 16α-hydroxydehydroisoandrosterone. When pregnenolone sulfate was injected into the umbilical vein of the midterm fetus no further metabolism could be detected in the adrenals (Solomon *et al.* 1967).

Thus it is well established that the human fetal adrenal is capable of forming a variety of steroids from preformed precursors. The interpretation and correlation of the published data have been handicapped by the occasionally divergent results obtained using *in vivo* and *in vitro* techniques. Perfusion studies and injection of the steroid into the umbilical vein may be more representative of the biosynthetic pathways in the intact cell, while slices, minces and homogenates reflect the biochemical conversions of the cells whose architecture has been disrupted. This explains the formation of 4-ene-3-ketosteroids from pregnenolone and of androstenedione and 11β-hydroxyandrostenedione from progesterone when *in vitro* techniques are used and the failure to observe these conversions with whole cell systems. It is established both *in vivo* and *in vitro* that the adrenal possesses C-17-20 desmolase for 3β-hydroxy-5-ene steroids and the presence of desmolases for 4-ene-3-ketosteroids in adrenal homogenates may be a reflection of the loss of enzyme specificity of the 3β-hydroxy-5-ene steroid enzymes in disrupted cells. The synthesis of deoxycorticosterone, corticosterone and cortisol by the fetal adrenal raises some important questions concerning the role of these steroid hormones in the development and homeostasis of the human fetus.

(b) *Testes*

A number of studies have been conducted to determine the metabolic capacity of the fetal gonads during intrauterine existence. Thus a number of recent publications have appeared indicating that the human testes *in vitro* are capable of forming C-19 and C-21 steroids from suitable precursors as is shown in Table 6.6. When fetal testes were maintained in organ culture with labeled acetate, minute amounts of neutral steroids could be synthesized after eight days of incubation (Rice *et al.* 1966). The major products formed were pregnenolone, progesterone, 17α-hydroxyprogesterone and testosterone. A homogenate of interstitial cells which are well differentiated and abundant during fetal development, converted dehydroisoandrosterone to androstenedione (Bloch *et al.* 1962b). Baillie *et al.* (1965b) also demonstrated 3β-hydroxysteroid dehydrogenase activity in fetal interstitial cells.

With a mince of fetal testicular tissue, pregnenolone can be converted to dehydroisoandrosterone, androstenedione, testosterone (Acevedo *et al.* 1961, Acevedo *et al.* 1963), 17α-hydroxypregnenolone, 17α-hydroxyprogesterone and androst-5-ene-3β,16α,17β-triol (Acevedo *et al.* 1963). Ikonen & Niemi (1966) also reported that slices of fetal testes can form

TABLE 6.6

Formation of neutral steroids by human fetal testes

Precursor	Tissue preparation	Products formed	Reference
Acetate	Organ culture	Pregnenolone, progesterone, 17α-hydroxyprogesterone, testosterone	Rice *et al.* (1966)
Dehydroisoandrosterone	Homogenate (interstitial cells)	Androstenedione	Bloch *et al.* (1962b)
Pregnenolone	Mince	Dehydroisoandrosterone, testosterone, androstenedione	Acevedo *et al.* (1961)
	Mince	Testosterone, androstenedione, dehydroisoandrosterone, androst-5-ene-3β,16α,17β-triol, 17α-hydroxypregnenolone, 17α-hydroxyprogesterone	Acevedo *et al.* (1963)
17α-Hydroxypregnenolone	Slice	17α-Hydroxyprogesterone, dehydroisoandrosterone, androstenedione, androstenediol, testosterone	Ikonen & Niemi (1966)
Progesterone	Homogenate	Testosterone, 16α-hydroxyprogesterone, 17α-hydroxyprogesterone	Bloch (1964)
	Mince	Androstenedione, 16α-hydroxyandrostenedione, 17α-hydroxyprogesterone, 20α-dihydroprogesterone, 17α,20α-dihydroxypregn-4-en-3-one	Acevedo *et al.* (1963)
	Injection into the umbilical vein	Pregnanolone, 20α-dihydroxyprogesterone, 17α-hydroxyprogesterone	Solomon *et al.* (1967)
	Slice	17α-Hydroxyprogesterone, androstenedione, testosterone	Bloch *et al.* (1962a), Ikonen & Niemi (1966)

17α-hydroxyprogesterone, dehydroisoandrosterone, androstenedione, androstenediol and testosterone from 17α-hydroxypregnenolone. Using progesterone as a substrate, minces, slices and homogenates of fetal testes can effect a number of conversions including 17α-hydroxylation (Bloch *et al.* 1962a, 1964, Acevedo *et al.* 1963, Ikonen & Niemi 1966), 16α-hydroxylation (Acevedo *et al.* 1963, Bloch 1964), and side-chain cleavage as is shown by the products formed which are listed in Table 6.6. Bloch (1964) found that testosterone synthesis by testes obtained during the third trimester of pregnancy was at least seven-fold that of the younger testes and felt that this correlated well with the morphological changes observed in the interstitial cells during these periods of gestation.

When ^{14}C-progesterone was injected into the umbilical vein (Solomon *et al.* 1967) evidence was obtained for the formation of pregnanolone, 20α-dihydroprogesterone and 17α-hydroxyprogesterone in the fetal testes. An attempt was made to demonstrate side-chain cleavage of 17α-hydroxyprogesterone but no C-19 steroids could be detected in any of the studies performed (Solomon *et al.* 1967). The authors therefore concluded that at midpregnancy, testosterone and androstenedione are derived from dehydroisoandrosterone sulfate formed by the maternal adrenals or the fetal adrenals, the placenta being responsible for hydrolysing the sulfate and oxidizing the β,γ-unsaturated alcohol to the α,β-unsaturated ketone. One other explanation advanced was that the peak of activity of the desmolase in the fetal testes may be present at 12 weeks gestation as observed for 3β-hydroxysteroids dehydrogenase (Goldman *et al.* 1966), which may explain the lack of androstenedione or testosterone formation observed. One further complication is the secretion by the maternal adrenal of androstenedione which amounts to approximately 3 mg per day (Horton & Tait 1966, Tait & Horton 1966). This steroid may not be totally aromatized by the placenta and may cross to the fetus thus providing a constant source of androgens. How these observations can be reconciled with the proposed role of androgens in the embryonic development of sex characteristics in the fetus is difficult to explain at the present time.

(c) *Ovaries*

While the human fetal adrenals and testes appear to be very active sites in the formation and metabolism of steroids, the fetal ovaries are rather quiescent. Bloch (1964) found that a homogenate of fetal ovaries converted progesterone to 20α-dihydroprogesterone and this metabolite was also formed when the ovaries were maintained in organ culture with progesterone in the medium (Bloch *et al.* 1965). No other products were identified in either of these studies.

(d) *The liver*

Several groups of investigators have shown that the fetal liver is very active in the metabolism of neutral steroids and the transformations which have been effected are shown in Table 6.7. The 16α-hydroxylation of dehydroisoandrosterone is a very active process in the fetal liver as is evident from the work of Slaunwhite and associates (1965) and Bolté *et al.* (1966). In the latter study labeled dehydroisoandrosterone and dehydroisoandrosterone sulfate were perfused into the previable human fetus and androst-5-ene-3β,17β-diol sulfate, as well as androst-5-ene-3β,16α,17β-triol sulfate were isolated and identified in the liver. The formation of 16α-hydroxylated C-19 steroids in the fetal liver is important in view of the demonstration that this organ is capable of aromatizing testosterone (Slaunwhite *et al.* 1965, Mancuso *et al.* 1965).

When labeled pregnenolone was injected into the umbilical vein and the cord was clamped 20 seconds later, the liver had already metabolized the substrate to a number of products–pregnenolone sulfate, 20α-dihydropregnenolone and 16α-hydroxypregnenolone (Solomon 1966, Solomon *et al.* 1967). A similar study with pregnenolone sulfate gave only unconjugated pregnenolone (Solomon *et al.* 1967). Villee & Loring (1963) incubated ^{14}C-progesterone with a homogenate of fetal liver and demonstrated the formation of 20α-dihydroprogesterone and possibly pregnanediol. When the previable human fetus was perfused with labeled progesterone, a number of conjugated and unconjugated metabolites were isolated from the liver. The unconjugated metabolites isolated were 20α-dihydroprogesterone, pregnanolone and pregnanediol (Solomon *et al.* 1964, Bird *et al.* 1966). The conjugates isolated were pregnanolone sulfate, pregnanediol sulfate and pregnanediol glucosiduronate (Bird *et al.* 1965). In an attempt to simulate the physiological conditions *in vivo*, a number of studies were performed in which the labeled precursors were injected into the fetus via the umbilical vein (Solomon *et al.* 1967). In such studies progesterone was converted by the liver to pregnanolone, 3β-hydroxy-5α-pregnan-20-one, 20α-dihydroprogesterone, pregnanediol and the sulfate and glucosiduronate of pregnanediol, and 16α-hydroxyprogesterone was converted to 3α,16α-dihydroxy-5β-pregnan-20-one, its sulfate and glucosiduronate, and 5β-pregnane-

TABLE 6.7

Formation of neutral steroids by human fetal liver

Precursor	Tissue preparation	Products formed	Reference
Dehydroisoandrosterone	Homogenate	16α-Hydroxydehydroisoandrosterone	Slaunwhite *et al.* (1965)
Androstenedione and testosterone	Homogenate	16α-Hydroxyandrostenedione	Jungmann & Schweppe (1967)
Dehydroisoandrosterone and dehydroisoandrosterone sulfate	Perfusion of pre-viable fetus	Androst-5-ene-3β,16α,17β-triol sulfate, androst-5-ene-3β,17β-diol sulfate	Bolté *et al.* (1966)
Pregnenolone	Injection into the umbilical vein	Pregnenolone sulfate, 20α-dihydropregnenolone, 16α-hydroxypregnenolone	Solomon (1966), Solomon *et al.* (1967)
Progesterone	Homogenate	20α-Dihydroprogesterone, pregnanediol	Villee & Loring (1963)
		Androstenedione, testosterone, 17α-hydroxyprogesterone, 16α-hydroxyprogesterone	Jungmann & Schweppe (1967)
	Perfusion of pre-viable fetus or injection into the umbilical vein	20α-Dihydroprogesterone, pregnanolone, pregnanediol, 3β-hydroxy-5α-pregnan-20-one	Bird *et al.* (1966), Solomon *et al.* (1967)

		Pregnanolone sulfate, pregnanediol sulfate, pregnanediol glucosiduronate	Bird *et al.* (1965), Solomon *et al.* (1967)
	Injection into umbilical vein	20α-Dihydroprogesterone, 20β-dihydroprogesterone	Zander (1961)
16α-Hydroxyprogesterone	Injection into the umbilical vein	$3\alpha,16\alpha$-Dihydroxy-5β-pregnan-20-one, $3\alpha,16\alpha$-dihydroxy-5β-pregnan-20-one sulfate, $3\alpha,16\alpha$-dihydroxy-5β-pregnan-20-one glucosiduronate, 5β-pregnane-$3\alpha,16\alpha,20\alpha$-triol	Solomon *et al.* (1967)
17α-Hydroxypregnenolone	Homogenate	Androst-5-ene-$3\beta,16\alpha,17\beta$-triol, dehydroisoandrosterone, androstenedione, testosterone, 17α-hydroxyprogesterone	Jungmann & Schweppe (1967)

3α,16α,20α-triol. It was not possible to determine the exact location of the sulfate and glucosiduronate groups on the steroid nucleus. Thus it is established that the fetal liver is capable of conjugating neutral steroids and reducing the A/B rings of 4-ene-3-ketosteroids. Moreover, the 16α-hydroxylase enzymes are active in this tissue.

Some very interesting data have recently been published by Jungmann & Schweppe (1967). These authors incubated homogenates of fetal liver with progesterone and reported its conversion to androstenedione, testosterone, 17α-hydroxyprogesterone and 16α-hydroxyprogesterone but not to pregnanediol. When 17α-hydroxypregnenolone was incubated in the same study it was converted to androst-5-ene-3β,16α,17β-triol, dehydroisoandrosterone, androstenedione, testosterone and 17α-hydroxyprogesterone. The *in vitro* conversions noted in fetal liver by these investigators have not been reported by others using more physiological conditions.

(e) *Other fetal tissues*

Peripheral tissues show a remarkable ability to either metabolize progesterone or to concentrate its metabolites (Bird *et al.* 1966, Solomon 1966, Solomon *et al.* 1967) whereas pregnenolone and pregnenolone sulfate are not, to any extent, treated in similar fashion (Solomon *et al.* 1967). Table 6.8 shows the neutral steroids isolated from the fetal lung, kidney and intestine following perfusion of the midterm previable

TABLE 6.8

Formation of neutral steroids from progesterone by human fetal lung, kidney and intestine

Tissue	Products from progesterone	Reference
Lung	20α-Dihydroprogesterone 3β-Hydroxy-5α-pregnan-20-one 6β-Hydroxyprogesterone 17α-Hydroxyprogesterone	Bird *et al.* (1966), Solomon (1966), Solomon *et al.* (1967)
Kidney	20α-Dihydroprogesterone 3β-Hydroxy-5α-pregnan-20-one 6β-Hydroxyprogesterone 16α-Hydroxyprogesterone	Bird *et al.* (1966), Solomon (1966), Solomon *et al.* (1967)
Intestine	20α-Dihydroprogesterone Pregnanolone	Bird *et al.* (1966), Solomon (1966), Solomon *et al.* (1967)

human fetus with labeled progesterone. The presence of 20α-dihydroprogesterone was observed in all three tissues while 3β-hydroxy-5α-pregnan-20-one was isolated from lung and kidney and pregnanolone was isolated from the intestine. The isolation of the hydroxylated metabolites, 6β-hydroxyprogesterone from lung and kidney, 17α-hydroxyprogesterone from lung and 16α-hydroxyprogesterone from kidney, is of some interest.

TABLE 6.9

Neutral metabolites of progesterone in the fetal heart, thymus and thyroid after injection of the steroid into the umbilical vein

Tissue	Metabolites	Reference
Heart	Pregnanolone 3β-Hydroxy-5α-pregnan-20-one 20α-Dihydroprogesterone Pregnanediol	Solomon *et al.* (1967)
Thymus	Pregnanolone 20α-Dihydroprogesterone	Solomon *et al.* (1967)
Thyroid	Pregnanolone	Solomon *et al.* (1967)

When labeled progesterone was injected into the umbilical vein, reduced metabolites were also found in other peripheral tissues (Solomon *et al.* 1967). These are shown in Table 6.9. Pregnanolone was isolated from all three tissues. From the heart and thymus it was possible to isolate 20α-dihydroprogesterone, while pregnanediol and 3β-hydroxy-5α-pregnan-20-one were isolated from the heart. The significance of these findings remains to be established. It is still uncertain whether the isolation of these metabolites in such tissues reflect metabolism therein or mere accumulations from the circulatory system.

A summary of some of the metabolic conversions leading to the formation of neutral steroids in the fetoplacental unit is shown in Fig. 6.4, which outlines the main conversions observed during midpregnancy. The data shown in Fig. 6.4 were obtained by perfusion of the previable fetus or by injection of the precursor into the umbilical vein (Solomon *et al.* 1967). It would seem that, at midterm, maternal cholesterol is a major source of the pregnenolone and progesterone elaborated by the placenta. The fetus does not seem to utilize acetate or cholesterol for the formation of neutral steroids, but it very readily metabolizes pregnenolone and progesterone reaching it from the placenta. Pregnenolone is transformed by the fetal adrenal into pregnenolone sulfate, 17α-hydroxypregnenolone sulfate and dehydroisoandrosterone sulfate. Further metabolism of pregnenolone sulfate seems to be prevented by the presence of the sulfate group. Progesterone, synthesized by the placenta is metabolized by all the fetal tissues examined but the main sites

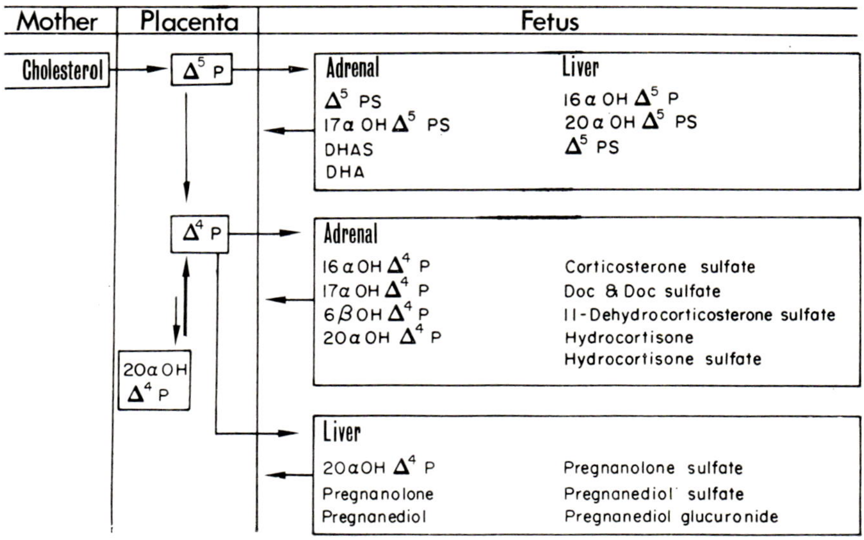

FIG. 6.4. A scheme for the metabolism of pregnenolone and progesterone in the human placenta and fetus at mid-pregnancy. Δ^5 P = pregnenolone; Δ^5 PS = pregnenolone sulfate; 17α OH Δ^5 PS = 17α-hydroxypregnenolone sulfate; DHAS = dehydroisoandrosterone sulfate; DHA = dehydroisoandrosterone; 16α OH Δ^5 P = 16α-hydroxypregnenolone; 20α OH Δ^5 PS = 20α-dihydropregnenolone sulfate; 16α OH Δ^4 P = 16α-hydroxyprogesterone; 17α OH Δ^4 P = 17α-hydroxyprogesterone; 6β OH Δ^4 P = 6β-hydroxyprogesterone; 20α OH Δ^4 P = 20α-dihydroprogesterone; DOC = deoxycorticosterone.

of metabolic transformations are the liver and adrenal. In the adrenal it is hydroxylated at C_{11}, C_{16}, C_{17} and C_{21} and converted to the sulfates of deoxycorticosterone, corticosterone and cortisol. The cyclic conversion of progesterone to 20α-dihydroprogesterone is demonstrable in the placenta. A large number of conjugated and unconjugated metabolites of progesterone are formed from progesterone by the fetal liver.

Thus the available evidence points to the high activity of the human fetus at midterm in producing a variety of steroids, some of which are biologically active in adult life. What role these steroids play in the maintenance and development of the human fetus is not presently known.

ISOLATION OF NEUTRAL STEROIDS FROM HUMAN PREGNANCY URINE

C-19 *steroids*

In the early studies of the urinary excretion of C-19 steroids during pregnancy, only crude methods were available for their analysis and as a result a confusing picture was obtained. When the urinary metabolites were isolated and identified, their excretion could be correlated with the elaboration of their precursors in the fetoplacental unit. The urinary excretion of androgens has been reported as unchanged during pregnancy using a biological assay (Dingemanse *et al.* 1937). Pincus & Pearlman (1943) and Venning (1946) found no change in the urinary levels of 17-ketosteroids when the antimony trichloride method of Pincus (1943) was used. Diczfalusy & Borell (1961) reported that the titre of 17-ketosteroids remained unaltered after removal of the maternal ovaries during pregnancy. Other workers have observed a decrease of 17-ketosteroid excretion during pregnancy (Hain 1939, Dobriner *et al.* 1948, Patti *et al.* 1963b). Studies with the use of the Zimmerman reaction, however, have yielded results which indicate a slight increase in total 17-ketosteroids (Venning 1946, Hegnauer 1952, Zondek & Finkelstein 1952, Huis in't Veld 1954, Birke *et al.* 1958) in the third trimester. In an attempt to correlate the excretion of 17-ketosteroids in pregnancy with the sex of the fetus, Burrows and associates (1943) could find no significant difference. Eagle (1952) and Birchall and associates (1961) detected dehydroisoandrosterone in the urine of premature infants but not from full-term infants, indicating that the fetus produces the precursors of the urinary 17-ketosteroids.

Dobriner and associates (1948) fractionated the 17-ketosteroids during pregnancy and found that androsterone excretion decreased to zero by the 8th month of gestation while etiocholanolone were very much reduced. Normal amounts of 11-ketoetiocholanolone was present in the urine but 11-hydroxyandrosterone was absent. From the conflicting results cited above it is doubtful whether the total amount of 17-ketosteroid excreted is changed but from the investigations of Dobriner *et al.* (1948) it would seem that the excretion of individual 17-ketosteroids is markedly altered during pregnancy.

The C-19 steroids which have been isolated from pregnancy urine in pure form are shown in Table 6.10. Androsterone was first isolated from human pregnancy urine by Marker & Lawson (1938). When dehydroisoandrosterone sulfate was injected into a subject in the third trimester of pregnancy, androsterone was isolated from both the sulfate and glucosiduronate fractions (YoungLai & Solomon 1968), while dehydroisoandrosterone was isolated only from the sulfate fraction. In 1948, Lieberman and associates isolated a variety of steroids from human pregnancy urine among which was isoandrosterone. Siiteri & MacDonald (1966) reported the isolation of 16α-hydroxydehydroisoandrosterone and androst-5-ene-3β,16α,17β-triol from the urine of pregnant subjects after the intravenous administration of ^{3}H-16α-hydroxydehydroisoandrosterone. In a similar study (YoungLai & Solomon 1967) weighable amounts of androst-5-ene-3β,16α,17β-triol were isolated from the urine of the third trimester of pregnancy. In the same study these investigators were able to identify 16α-hydroxydehydroisoandrosterone, 16α-hydroxyandrostenedione, 16α-hydroxyetiocholanolone, 16α-hydroxyandrosterone and 3α,16α-dihydroxyandrost-5-en-17-one.

C-21 steroids

During the course of pregnancy there is an increase in urinary excretion of corticosteroids as attested to by the results of many investigators (Venning 1946, Tobian 1949, Parviainen *et al.* 1950, Lloyd *et al.* 1952, Jayle *et al.* 1953, Wheeler *et al.* 1953, Devis 1954, Appleby & Norymberski 1957, Daessler 1964). This excretion reaches a peak at term and then drops after parturition. Similar changes occur in the excretion of pregnanediol (Venning 1938, Borth & de Watteville 1952, Coyle *et al.* 1956, Patti *et al.* 1963b), but at a much higher level. Pregnanetriol, a metabolite of 17α-hydroxyprogesterone and 17α-hydroxypregnenolone, is recovered from urine in increasing amounts as gestation progresses (Appleby & Norymberski 1957, Hermann & Silverman 1957, Ronan *et al.* 1960). An increase in the excretion of aldosterone also occurs during pregnancy (Venning *et al.* 1957, Laidlaw *et al.* 1958), which rapidly returns to normal following delivery (Venning *et al.* 1957). This rise in aldosterone excretion is said to be due to the increased secretion of aldosterone because of the antagonism at the renal tubular level by progester-

TABLE 6.10

Isolation of neutral steroids from human pregnancy urine

Steroid isolated	Reference
C-19	
Androsterone	Marker & Lawson (1938), YoungLai & Solomon (1968)
Isoandrosterone	Lieberman *et al.* (1948)
Dehydroisoandrosterone	YoungLai & Solomon (1968)
16α-Hydroxydehydroisoandrosterone	Siiteri & MacDonald (1966), YoungLai & Solomon (1967)
Androst-5-ene-3β,16α,17β-triol	Siiteri & MacDonald (1966), YoungLai & Solomon (1967)
16α-Hydroxyandrostenedione	YoungLai & Solomon (1967)
16α-Hydroxyetiocholanolone	
16α-Hydroxyandrosterone	
3α,16α-Dihydroxyandrost-5-en-17-one	
C-21	
Progesterone	Ismail & Harkness (1965)
5β-Pregnanedione; 5α-pregnanedione	Dobriner *et al.* (1948)
3α,6-Dihydroxy-5α-pregnan-20-one; 5α-pregn-2-en-20-one	Lieberman *et al.* (1948)
3α-Hydroxypregnane	Marker & Lawson (1938)
Pregnanolone	Marker & Kamm (1937), Lieberman *et al.* (1948), Shen *et al.* (1963)
5α-Pregnanolone	Marker *et al.* (1937); Lieberman *et al.* (1948)
3β-Hydroxy-5α-pregnan-20-one	Pearlman *et al.* (1942); Lieberman *et al.* (1948)
Isopregnanolone	Lieberman *et al.* (1948), Ruse & Solomon (1966b)
Pregnanediol	Klopper *et al.* (1955), Marrian (1929), Dingemanse *et al.* (1930)
5α-Pregnanediol	Hartmann & Locher (1935), Marker & Rohrmann (1939), Kyle & Marrian (1951)
5α-Pregnane-3β,20α-diol	Marker & Rohrmann (1939)
15α-Hydroxyprogesterone	Giannopoulos & Solomon (1967)
16α-Hydroxyprogesterone	Ruse & Solomon (1966b)
3α,16α-Dihydroxy-5α-pregnan-20-one	Ruse & Solomon (1966a)
3α,16α-Dihydroxy-5β-pregnan-20-one	Ruse & Solomon (1966a)
5α-Pregnane-3α,16α,20α-triol	Hirschmann *et al.* (1961), Ruse & Solomon (1966a)

TABLE 6.10 (*continued*)

Steroid isolated	Reference
5β-Pregnane-3α,16α,20α-triol	Hirschmann *et al.* (1961), Ruse & Solomon (1966a)
Pregnanetriol	Ronan *et al.* (1960)
6β-Hydroxycortisol	Frantz *et al.* (1960)
6β,17α,20β-21-Tetrahydroxypregn-4-ene-3,11-dione; 6β,11β,17α,20α,21-pentahydroxypregn-4-en-3-one; 6α,11β,17α,20β,21-pentahydroxypregn-4-en-3-one	Dixon & Pennington (1966)
Conjugates	
Pregnane-3β,20α-diol sulfate; 3β-hydroxy-5β-pregnan-20-one sulfate	Crépy *et al.* (1962)
Pregnanediol-3α-glucosiduronate	Odell & Marrian (1936), Venning & Browne (1936), Crépy *et al.* (1962)
Pregnanolone glucosiduronate	Crépy *et al.* (1962)

one (Martin & Mills 1956, Rinsler & Rigby 1957, Jones *et al.* 1959). As much as 16–34 μg of aldosterone is excreted per day during pregnancy (Venning & Dyrenfurth 1956).

In Table 6.10 are listed the other C-21 steroids which have since been isolated from pregnancy urine. A number of 4-ene-3-ketosteroids were isolated and identified by infrared analysis. Progesterone was isolated from a large pool of human pregnancy urine (Ismail & Harkness 1965), 15α-hydroxyprogesterone from a 14-day urine collection of a subject in the third trimester of pregnancy (Giannopoulos & Solomon 1967) and 16α-hydroxyprogesterone from 5 days' urine (Ruse & Solomon 1966b). The 16α-hydroxylated product was found in larger quantities than the 15α-hydroxylated steroid and from the results obtained by Giannopoulos & Solomon (to be published) it would appear that 15α-hydroxylation occurs in the fetus. Several other 15α-hydroxylated estrogens have been isolated but a neutral steroid with a 15α-hydroxyl group has not previously been found in urine. Frantz *et al.* (1960) reported the isolation of 6β-hydroxycortisol from the unconjugated fraction of pregnancy urine. de Courcy *et al.* (1953) found cortisol, cortisone and 3α,17α,21-trihydroxypregnan-11,20-dione which were identified by chromatographic methods, color reactions and absorption spectra, while Dixon & Pennington (1966) detected the presence of several 4-ene-3-ketosteroids having four and five hydroxyl groups.

Pregnanediol was isolated from pregnancy urine in crystalline form by Marrian (1929) and by Dingemanse *et al.* (1930) but its structure was not elucidated until later by Butenandt (1930). Pregnanolone was subsequently found by Marker & Kamm (1937). These two metabolites together with pregnanetriol seem to be excreted mainly as the glucosiduronate (Shen *et al.* 1963). There seems to be no diurnal variation in the excretion of pregnanediol during pregnancy (Bachman *et al.* 1941). The 5α-epimers of these steroids have also been isolated from human pregnancy urine–5α-pregnanolone (Marker *et al.* 1937, Lieberman *et al.* 1948), 5α-pregnanediol (Hartmann & Locher 1935, Marker & Rohrmann 1939, Kyle & Marrian 1951), 3β-hydroxy-5α-pregnan-20-one (Pearlman *et al.* 1942, Lieberman *et al.* 1948), 5α-pregnane-3β,20α-diol (Marker & Rohrmann 1939) and both pregnanediones (Dobriner *et al.* 1948, Lieberman *et al.* 1948). Ruse & Solomon (1966a) have found the 16α-hydroxylated derivatives of 5α and 5β pregnanolone, while the 16α-hydroxylated triols have been isolated by two groups of investigators (Hirschmann *et al.* 1961, Ruse & Solomon 1966b).

A small number of conjugated steroids have been isolated from human pregnancy urine. Pregnanediol glucosiduronate was isolated independently by Odell & Marrian (1936) and Venning & Browne (1936) and its configuration as the 3α-glucosiduronate was determined by Heard *et al.* (1944). Crèpy *et al.* (1962) reported the isolation of pregnanediol sulfate and the sulfate of 3β-hydroxy-5β-pregnan-20-one, whereas the 3α-epimers of these steroids were isolated as the glucosiduronates.

METABOLISM OF NEUTRAL STEROIDS DURING PREGNANCY

This section will deal with data obtained from studies where the steroids were administered to the mother and their conversion to urinary metabolites was determined. The availability of labeled precursors has provided the means by which such investigations could be carried out. In such studies the results obtained are difficult to interpret because of the possible metabolism of the precursor in the fetoplacental unit. When ^{14}C-dehydroisoandrosterone sulfate was injected with ^{3}H-16α-hydroxydehydroisoandrosterone to a subject in the third trimester of pregnancy, weighable amounts of 16α-hydroxydehydroisoandrosterone and androst-5-ene-3β,16α,17β-triol containing both labels were isolated from the sulfate fraction of the urine (YoungLai & Solomon 1968). In the same study, ^{14}C-androsterone was isolated from the sulfate and glucosiduronate fractions and it had approximately the same specific activity as that of 16α-hydroxydehydroisoandrosterone and androst-5-ene-3β,16α,-17β-triol with respect to ^{14}C. Siiteri & MacDonald (1966), using the same precursors, found an extensive 16α-hydroxylation of dehydroisoandrosterone sulfate. It is probable from the data of these two groups that 16α-hydroxylation takes place mainly in the fetal compartment. However, Fotherby *et al.* (1957) have shown that dehydroisoandrosterone can be 16α-hydroxylated by the maternal liver when they administered dehydroisoandrosterone to an ovariectomized, adrenalectomized woman and isolated 16α-hydroxydehydroisoandrosterone from the urine. The extent of the conversion was not measured.

The single major urinary metabolite of 16α-hydroxydehydroisoandrosterone was found to be 3α,16α-dihydroxyandrost-5-en-17-one (YoungLai & Solomon 1967). In addition, a number of other metabolites were isolated – 16α-hydroxyandrostenedione, 16α-hydroxyetiocholanolone and 16α-hydroxyandrosterone. It was postulated that the 3α-hydroxy-5-ene steroid originated through the inhibition of the Δ^4-isomerase enzyme by the 16α-hydroxyl group as suggested by Fukushima *et al.* (1961). In order to determine the origin of this unusual metabolite, ^{14}C-16α-hydroxyandrostenedione was injected with ^{3}H-16α-hydroxydehydroisoandrosterone in a subject in the third trimester, but no conversion of the 4-ene-3-ketosteroid to any β-γ-unsaturated alcohol was observed. Instead, a sizable conversion to A/B saturated metabolites was obtained, the 5β steroids being excreted in greater amounts than 5α steroids (YoungLai & Solomon 1968). In these studies the largest amount of 3α,16α-dihydroxyandrost-5-en-17-one was obtained from 16α-hydroxydehydroisoandrosterone and only a slight amount from dehydroisoandrosterone sulfate or 16α-hydroxydehydroisoandrosterone sulfate.

Progesterone, when administered to the pregnant mother, is converted in large part to urinary pregnanediol. It was postulated at one time that there was an increased conversion of progesterone to pregnanediol (Venning & Browne 1940, Sommerville & Marrian 1950, Guterman 1953) during pregnancy but this has not been substantiated by Klopper & Michie (1956) and by Pearlman (1957b). During pregnancy, progesterone is also converted to pregnanolone (Davis & Plotz 1958, Contractor & Pearlman 1960) and pregnanedione (Contractor & Pearlman 1960).

When labeled 16α-hydroxyprogesterone was injected intravenously into a subject in the third trimester of pregnancy, labeled isopregnanolone, 3α,16α-dihydroxy-5α and 5β-pregnan-20-one and 5α and 5β-pregnane-3α,16α,20α-triol were isolated from the urine (Ruse & Solomon 1966a). It was shown that 16α-hydroxyprogesterone could have arisen by the peripheral conversion from 16α-hydroxypregnenolone but not from progesterone (Ruse & Solomon 1966b). When ^{3}H-pregnenolone sulfate and ^{14}C-pregnenolone were injected intravenously to a subject in the third trimester of pregnancy, pregnanolone, pregnanediol and 5α-pregnane-3α,16α,20α-triol, containing both labels, were isolated from the urine (Stanczyk & Solomon, to be published), indicating that peripheral hydroxylation of the precursors must have occurred. The same authors found that progesterone can be converted to pregnanolone, pregnanediol, 3α,16α-dihydroxy-5α-pregnan-20-one and 5α-pregnane-3α,16α,20α-triol but not to urinary 16α-hydroxyprogesterone. Fotherby *et al.* (1965) have reported that progesterone can be converted to 6-oxygenated metabolites by the pregnant female. Giannopoulos & Solomon (to be published) identified 3α,15α-dihydroxy-5α-pregnan-20-one and 3α,15α-dihydroxy-5β-pregnan-20-one as urinary metabolites of 15α-hydroxyprogesterone, a steroid recently isolated from a large pool of late pregnancy urine (Giannopoulos & Solomon 1967). It is difficult from such studies to determine where the steroids administered to the mother are metabolized because of physical compartmentalization.

CONCLUSIONS

The human placenta elaborates large amounts of progesterone and pregnenolone. These neutral steroids seem to be formed from maternal cholesterol rather than from cholesterol synthesized in the placenta. Progesterone and pregnenolone are the major precursors for the large array of steroids synthesized by the fetal adrenals and liver. The available evidence indicates that acetate and cholesterol are not efficient precursors for neutral steroids in human fetal tissues.

There is *in vitro* evidence which indicates that the placenta can hydroxylate progesterone at C_{16} and C_{17} and can cleave the side-chain of 17α-hydroxyprogesterone to form androstenedione and testosterone. These conversions have not been observed after *in situ* perfusion of the placenta with progesterone or when the precursor was injected into the umbilical vein with the fetus and placenta *in utero*. It is therefore concluded that these enzymes are present in placental tissue but are not operative under more physiological conditions. It is also possible that in homogenates these conversions are noted because the specificity of the enzymes are lowered when the integrity of the cell is destroyed.

When progesterone reaches the fetus it is extensively metabolized by the fetal adrenals and the liver and by other peripheral tissues. The adrenal converts progesterone to 20α-dihydroprogesterone and hydroxylates it at C_6, C_{11}, C_{16}, C_{17} and C_{21}. In addition, a number of these hydroxylated products have been isolated from the adrenal as sulfate conjugates. Pregnanediol is the most abundant metabolite of progesterone isolated from the fetal liver but in addition its sulfate and glucosiduronate are also formed. A number of other reduced metabolites of progesterone have also been isolated from the liver. There is *in vitro* evidence for the hydroxylation of progesterone at C_{16} and C_{17} in fetal liver but these conversions have not been observed in more physiological studies.

An important difference between the results obtained from *in vitro* studies and from the studies using the intact previable fetus is side-chain cleavage of 17α-hydroxyprogesterone to form androstenedione and testosterone. This has been observed many times *in vitro* but has not been observed in numerous experiments with the intact midterm fetus. From the adrenals and testes of these latter studies, 17α-hydroxyprogesterone has been isolated but no trace of testosterone or androstenedione has been found. It is of some interest that the side-chain cleavage reaction has also been recently demonstrated in fetal liver using *in vitro* techniques but the conversion of progesterone to pregnanediol was not observed.

There is also a considerable difference between the results obtained *in vitro* and those obtained with the intact previable fetus at a comparable gestation age when the metabolism of progesterone is studied in testicular tissue. With the use of *in vitro* systems progesterone is hydroxylated at C_{16} and C_{17} and side-chain cleavage occurs, leading to the formation of androstenedione and testosterone but in the previable intact fetus progesterone is converted to 17α-hydroxyprogesterone in the testes and no side-chain cleavage to form C-19 steroids is observed.

When pregnenolone reaches the fetus it is not as extensively metabolized as was observed with progesterone. In the intact fetus pregnenolone is converted by the adrenals to dehydroisoandrosterone, pregnenolone sulfate, 17α-hydroxypregnenolone sulfate and dehydroisoandrosterone sulfate. Dehydroisoandrosterone and its sulfate are converted to 16α-hydroxydehydroisoandrosterone sulfate which serves as a major precursor of estriol in the placenta. It is also of interest to note that pregnenolone is hydroxylated at C_{16} by the fetal liver. Pregnenolone is not converted to an α,β-unsaturated ketone until it reaches the placenta and no functional evidence for the 3β-hydroxysteroid dehydrogenase enzyme can be observed in any fetal tissue. Using *in vitro* systems a number of investigators have found evidence for the 3β-hydroxysteroid dehydrogenase for pregnenolone in fetal adrenals, liver and testes. In addition, data from *in vitro* studies have indicated an extensive metabolism of pregnenolone. The products formed are much the same as those found with incubation of progesterone. In the intact previable fetus pregnenolone sulfate is not further metabolized but in the placenta it is hydrolyzed and converted to progesterone and 20α-dihydroprogesterone. Thus the absence of a 3β-hydroxysteroid dehydrogenase and the presence of a sulfokinase limits the metabolism of pregnenolone in human fetal tissues.

Studies in the last ten years have uncovered a great deal concerning the metabolism of neutral steroids in the fetus and the placenta. It is apparent that some enzyme systems are not present in fetal tissues but are very active in the placenta. It is also true that the fetal adrenals, liver and placenta complement each other in a number of metabolic conversions which each performs. This complementary function of each tissue may be an important mechanism in controlling metabolic functions in the human fetus. One important question which remains unanswered is the role of the neutral steroids in the growth and development of the human fetus.

ACKNOWLEDGEMENTS

The authors wish to thank Miss Pauline Illsley for the typing of the manuscript.

REFERENCES

ACEVEDO H.F., AXELROD L.R., ISHIKAWA E. & TAKAKI F. (1961) Steroidogenesis in the human fetal testis: the conversion of pregnenolone-7α-H^3 to dehydroepiandrosterone, testosterone and 4-androstene-3,17-dione. *J. clin. Endocr. Metab.* **21**, 1611.

ACEVEDO H.F., AXELROD L.R., ISHIKAWA E. & TAKAKI F. (1963) Studies in fetal metabolism. II. Metabolism of progesterone-4-C^{14} and pregnenolone-7α-H^3 in human fetal testes. *J. Clin. Endocr. Metab.* **23**, 885.

ADLER A., DE FREMERY P. & TAUSK M. (1934) Progestin in placental extract. *Nature*, **133**, 293.

APPLEBY J.I. & NORYMBERSKI J.K. (1957) The urinary excretion of 17-hydroxycorticosteroids in human pregnancy. *Biochem. J.* **15**, 310.

BACHMAN C., LEEKLEY D. & HIRSCHMANN H. (1941) Day and night excretion of pregnanediol glucuronidate and neutral 17-ketosteroids in pregnancy. *J. clin. Endocr. Metab.* **1**, 142.

BAILLIE A.H., CAMERON E.H.D., GRIFFITHS K. & HART D.McK. (1965a) 3β-Hydroxysteroid dehydrogenase in the adrenal gland and placenta. *J. Endocrinol.* **31**, 227.

BAILLIE A.H., NIEMI M. & IKONEN M. (1965b) 3β-Hydroxysteroid dehydrogenase activity in the human fetal testes. *Acta Endocrinol.* **48**, 429.

BAULIEU E.-E., WALLACE E. & LIEBERMAN S. (1963) The conversion *in vitro* of Δ^5-androstene-3β,17β-diol-17α-^{3}H to testosterone-17α-^{3}H by human adrenal and placental tissue. *J. Biol. Chem.* **238**, 1316.

BENGTSSON G., ULLBERG S., WIQVIST N. & DICZFALUSY E. (1964) Autoradiographic studies on previable human foetuses perfused with radioactive steroids. I. Distribution of radioactive material following perfusion of progesterone-4-^{14}C. *Acta Endocrinol.* (*Kbh*), **46**, 544.

BENIRSCHKE K., BLOCH E. & HERTIG A.T. (1956) Concerning the function of the fetal zone of the human adrenal gland. *Endocrinology*, **58**, 598.

BENIRSCHKE K. & BLOCH E. (1960) Failure to demonstrate C-19 steroids in bovine testes. *Acta Endocrinol.* (*Kbh*), **34**, 65.

BERLINER D.L. & SALHANICK H.A. (1956) The presence of 6β-hydroxylase in human placenta. *J. Clin. Endocr. Metab.* **16**, 903.

BERLINER D.L., JONES J.E. & SALHANICK H.A. (1956) The isolation of adrenal-like steroids from the human placenta. *J. Biol. Chem.* **223**, 1043.

BIRCHALL K., CATHRO D.M., FORSYTH C.C. & MITCHELL F.L. (1961) Separation and estimation of adrenal steroids in the urine of newborn infants. *Lancet*, i, 26.

BIRD C.E., SOLOMON S., WIQVIST N. & DICZFALUSY E. (1965) Formation of C-21 steroid sulphates and glucosiduronates by previable human foetuses perfused with (4-^{14}C)progesterone. *Biochim. Biophys. Acta*, **104**, 623.

BIRD C.E., WIQVIST N., DICZFALUSY E. & SOLOMON S. (1966) Metabolism of progesterone by the perfused previable human fetus. *J. clin. Endocr. Metab.* **26**, 1144.

BIRKE G., GEMZELL C.A., PLANTIN L.-O. & ROBBE H. (1958) Plasma levels of 17-hydroxycorticosteroids and urinary excretion patterns of ketosteroids in normal pregnancy. *Acta Endocrinol.* (*Kbh*), **27**, 389.

BLOCH K. (1945) The biological conversion of cholesterol to pregnanediol. *J. Biol. Chem.* **157**, 661.

BLOCH E., BENIRSCHKE K. & DORFMAN R.I. (1955) The presence of Δ^4-androstene-3,17-dione in prenatal and postnatal human adrenal glands. *J. clin. Endocr. Metab.* **15**, 379.

BLOCH E., BENIRSCHKE K. & ROSEMBERG E. (1956) C_{19} steroids, 17α-hydroxycorticosterone and a sodium retaining factor in human fetal adrenal glands. *Endocrinology*, **58**, 626.

BLOCH E. & BENIRSCHKE K. (1959) Synthesis *in vitro* of steroids by human foetal adrenal gland slices. *J. Biol. Chem.* **234**, 1085.

BLOCH E. & BENIRSCHKE K. (1960) Acetate incorporation into 3β-hydroxy-Δ^5- and Δ^4-3-ketosteroids by human foetal adrenal slices. *Acta Endocrinol.* (*Kbh*), Suppl. **51**, 691.

BLOCH E. & BENIRSCHKE K. (1962) Steroidogenic capacity of foetal adrenals *in vitro*. In *The Human Adrenal Cortex*, p. 589. A.R.Currie, T.Symington & J.K.Grant, eds. E. & S.Livingstone Ltd, London.

BLOCH E., TISSENBAUM B. & BENIRSCHKE K. (1962a) The conversion of (4-^{14}C)progesterone to 17α-hydroxyprogesterone, testosterone, and Δ^4-androstene-3,17-dione by human fetal testes *in vitro*. *Biochim. Biophys. Acta*, **60**, 182.

BLOCH E., TISSENBAUM B., RUBIN B.L. & DEANE H.W. (1962b) Δ^5-3β-Hydroxysteroid dehydrogenase activity in human fetal adrenals. *Endocrinology*, **71**, 629.

BLOCH E. (1964) Metabolism of 4-^{14}C-progesterone by human fetal testis and ovaries. *Endocrinology*, **74**, 833.

BLOCH E., ROMNEY S.L., KLEIN M., LIPPIELLO L., COOPER P. & GOLDRING I.P. (1965) Steroid synthesis by human fetal adrenals and ovaries maintained in organ culture. *Proc. Soc. Expt. Biol. Med.* **119**, 449.

BLOCH E. & NEWMAN E. (1966) Comparative placental steroid synthesis. I. Conversion of (7-^{3}H)-dehydroepiandrosterone to (^{3}H)-androst-4-ene-3,17-dione. *Endocrinology*, **79**, 524.

BOLTÉ E., MANCUSO S., DRAY F., BAULIEU E.-E. & DICZFALUSY E. (1964) Conversion of testosterone-17α-^{3}H into 17β-estradiol-17α-^{3}H by human placentas perfused *in situ*. *Steroids*, **4**, 613.

BOLTÉ E., WIQVIST N. & DICZFALUSY E. (1966) Metabolism of dehydroepiandrosterone and dehydroepiandrosterone sulphate by the human foetus at mid-pregnancy. *Acta Endocrinol.* (*Kbh*), **52**, 583.

BORTH R. & DE WATTEVILLE H. (1952) Hormone assays in obstetrics and gynecology. *Vitamins and Hormones*, **10**, 141.

BROWNE J.S.L., HENRY J.S. & VENNING E.H. (1937) The corpus luteum hormone in pregnancy. *J. Clin. Invest.* **16**, 678.

BURROWS H., MACLEOD D.H. & WARREN F.L. (1943) The excretion of ketosteroids in human pregnancy urine in relation to the sex of the foetus. *J. Obst. Gyn. Brit. Emp.* **50**, 212.

BUTENANDT A. (1930) Uber das Pregnandiol, einen neuen Sterin-Abkömmling aus Schwangeren-Harn. *Ber. dtsch. Chem. Ges.* **63**, 659.

CASSMER O. (1959) Hormone production of the isolated human placenta. *Acta Endocrinol.* (*Kbh*), Suppl. **45**, .

COLAS A., HEINRICHS LEROY W. & TATUM H.J. (1964) Pettenkofer chromogens in the maternal and fetal circulations. Detection of 3β,16α-dihydroxyandrost-5-en-17-one in umbilical cord blood. *Steroids*, **3**, 417.

COLAS A. & HEINRICHS LEROY W. (1965) Pettenkofer chromogens in the maternal and fetal circulations: anencephalic pregnancies, cesarean sections and tentative identification of 3β,17β-dihydroxyandrost-5-en-16-one in umbilical cord blood. *Steroids*, **5**, 753.

CONRAD S.H., PION R.J. & KITCHIN III J.D. (1967) Pregnenolone sulfate in human pregnancy plasma. *J. clin. Endocr. Metab.* **27**, 114.

CONTRACTOR S.F. & PEARLMAN W.H. (1960) (16-^{3}H)Progesterone metabolism in advanced pregnancy and in oophorectomized-hysterectomized women: urinary ketonic metabolites. *Biochem. J.* **76**, 36.

COYLE M.G., MITCHELL F.L. & RUSSELL C.S. (1956) A report on the chromatographic assay of urinary pregnanediol in pregnancy. *J. Obst. Gynec. Brit. Emp.* **63**, 560.

CRÉPY O., JUDAS O., RULLEAU-MESLIN F. & JAYLE M.F. (1962) Mode de conjugaision des Métabolites de la Progestérone dans les Urines de Femmes Enceintes. *Bull. Soc. Chim. Biol.* **44**, 327.

CUNNINGHAM B. & KUHN H. (1941) Presence of androgens in the placenta. *Proc. Soc. Expt. Biol. Med.* **48**, 314.

DAESSLER C.G. (1964) The glucocorticoid excretion in late pregnancy associated with chronic hypertension and with pre-eclampsia. *Gynaecologia*, **157**, 343.

DAVIS M.E., PLOTZ E.J., LE ROY G.V., GOULD R.G. & WERBIN H. (1956) Urinary steroids after the administration of labeled cholesterol. *Amer. J. Obst. Gynec.* **72**, 740.

DAVIS M.E. & PLOTZ E.J. (1958) Steroid metabolism in human pregnancy. *Amer. J. Obst. Gynec.* **76**, 939.

DAWSON I.M.P., PRYSE-DAVIES J. & SNAPE I.M. (1961) The distribution of six enzyme systems and of lipid in the human and rat adrenal cortex and ACTH, with comments on the distribution in human foetuses and in some natural disease conditions. *J. Path. & Bact.* **81**, 181.

DE COURCY C., BUSH I.E., GRAY C.H. & LUNNON J.B. (1953) A chromatographic investigation of Δ^4-3-ketosteroids and α-ketolic steroids in human urine. *J. Endocrinol.* **9**, 401.

DELL'ACQUA S., MANCUSO S., ERIKSSON G. & DICZFALUSY E. (1966) Metabolism of retrotestosterone and testosterone by midterm human placentas perfused *in situ*. *Biochim. Biophys. Acta*, **130**, 241.

DELL'ACQUA S., MANCUSO S., WIQVIST N., RUSE J.L., SOLOMON S. & DICZFALUSY E. (1967a) Studies on the aromatization of neutral steroids in pregnant women. 5. Metabolism of androst-5-ene-3β,16α,17β-triol in the intact foeto-placental unit at midpregnancy. *Acta Endocrinol.* **55**, 389.

DELL'ACQUA S., MANCUSO S., ERIKSSON G., RUSE J.L., SOLOMON S. & DICZFALUSY E. (1967b) Studies on the aromatization of neutral steroids in pregnant women. 6. Aromatization of 16α-hydroxylated C-19 steroids by midterm placentas perfused *in situ*. *Acta Endocrinol.* **55**, 401.

DE MIQUEL M. & TROEN P. (1966) Metabolism of 17α-hydroxyprogesterone by mid-pregnancy human placentas. *Excerpta Medica Intern. Congr. Series*, **III**, 292.

DEVIS R. (1954) L'élimination des corticoides a cours de la grossesse. *Gynéc. Obstét.* **53**, 57.

DICZFALUSY E. & TROEN P. (1961) Endocrine functions of the human placenta. *Vitamins and Hormones*, **19**, 229.

DICZFALUSY E. & BORELL U. (1961) Influence of oophorectomy on steroid excretion in early pregnancy. *J. clin. Endocr. Metab.* **21**, 1119.

DICZFALUSY E. (1964) Endocrine functions of the human foeto-placental unit. *Fed. Proc.* **23**, 791.

DINGEMANSE E., DE JONGH S.E., KOBER S. & LAQUEUR E. (1930) Ueber Kristallinisches Menformon. *Dtsch. Med. Wschr.* **56**, 301.

DINGEMANSE E., BORCHARDT H. & LACQUEUR E. (1937) LXIX. Capon comb growth-promoting substances ('male hormones') in human urine of males and females of varying ages. *Biochem. J.* **31**, 500.

DIXON W.R. & PENNINGTON G.W. (1966) The isolation and identification of extremely polar unconjugated steroids in human pregnancy urine. *J. Endocrinol.* **34**, 281.

DOBRINER K., LIEBERMAN S., RHOADS C.P. & TAYLOR H.C. (1948) The urinary excretion of ketosteroids in pregnancy. *Obst. & Gynec. Survey*, **3**, 677.

DOE R.P., FERNANDEZ R. & SEAL U.S. (1964) Measurement of corticosteroid-binding globulin in man. *J. clin. Endocr. Metab.* **24**, 1029.

DORFMAN R.I. (1948) Biochemistry of androgens. In *The Hormones*, p. 471. G.Pincus & K.V.Thimann, eds. Academic Press, New York.

EAGLE J.F. (1952) Dehydroepiandrosterone and similar substances in urine of premature infants. *Proc. Soc. Exp. Biol. Med.* **81**, 571.

EASTERLING W.E., Jnr., SIMMER H., DIGNAM W.J., FRANKLAND M.W. & NAFTOLIN F. (1966) Neutral C-19 steroids and steroid sulfates in human pregnancy. II. Dehydroepiandrosterone sulfate, 16α-hydroxydehydroepiandrosterone and 16α-hydroxydehydroepiandrosterone sulfate in maternal and fetal blood of pregnancies with anencephalic and normal fetuses. *Steroids*, **8**, 157.

EBERLEIN W.R. (1965) Steroids and sterols in umbilical cord blood. *J. clin. Endocr. Metab.* **25**, 1101.

FOTHERBY K., COLAS A., ATHERDEN S.M. & MARRIAN G.F. (1957) The isolation of 16α-hydroxydehydroepiandrosterone (3β,16α-dihydroxyandrost-5-en-17-one) from the urine of normal men. *Biochem. J.* **66**, 664.

FOTHERBY K., JAMES F., KAMYAB S., KLOPPER A.I. & WILSON G.R. (1965) Excretion of 6-oxygenated metabolites of progesterone and 5β-pregnane-3α,17α,20α-triol during pregnancy. *J. Endocrinol.* **33**, 133.

FRANCIS F.E., SHEN N.C. & KINSELLA R.A., Jnr. (1960) Enteric excretion of metabolites of steroid hormones in the human. II. Isolation of Δ^5-androsten-3β-ol-17-one from meconium. *J. Biol. Chem.* **235**, 1957.

FRANCIS F.E., SHEN N.C. & KINSELLA R.A., Jnr. (1962) Enteric excretion of metabolites of steroid hormones in the human. III. Isolation of 3α-hydroxy-5β-pregn-16-en-20-one (16-pregnenolone) from meconium. *Biochemistry* (*Wash.*), **1**, 1184.

FRANCIS F.E. & KINSELLA R.A., Jnr. (1966) Enteric excretion of metabolites of steroid hormones in the human subject. IV. Isolation of 5β-pregnane-3α,20α-diol from meconium. *J. clin. Endocr. Metab.* **26**, 128.

FRANCIS F.E. & KINSELLA R.A., Jnr. (1967) Enteric excretion of metabolites of steroid hormones in the human subject. V. Isolation of 5α-pregnane-3α,20α-diol from meconium. *J. clin. Endocr. Metab.* **27**, 211.

FRANTZ A.G., KATZ F.H. & JAILER J.W. (1960) 6β-hydroxycortisol; high levels in human urine in pregnancy and toxemia. *Proc. Soc. Expt. Biol. Med.* **105**, 41.

FUJII K., HOSHINO K. & AOKI I. (1956) Biological studies on gestagen content in human corpus luteum and placenta. *J. Japan Obst. & Gynec. Soc.* **3**, 169.

FUKUSHIMA D.K., SMULOWTIZ M. & WILLIAMS K.I.H. (1961) Δ^5-pregnene-3α,16α,20α-triol and related steroids in adrenocortical carcinoma. *J. Biol. Chem.* **236**, 3147.

FUTTERWEIT W., MCNIVEN N.L. & DORFMAN R.I. (1962) Gas-chromatographic identification of progesterone in human pregnancy plasma. *Biochim. Biophys. Acta*, **71**, 474.

GARDNER L.I. & WALTON R.L. (1954) Plasma 17-ketosteroids of the human fetus: demonstration of concentration gradient between cord and maternal circulations. *Helvet. Paediat. Acta*, **9**, 311.

GIANNOPOULOS G. & SOLOMON S. (1967) Isolation of 15α-hydroxyprogesterone from human pregnancy urine. *Biochemistry*, **6**, 1226.

GOECKE H., WIRZ P. & DANERS H. (1933) Uber das Vorkommen des männlichen Sexual-hormons im Urin von Neugeborenen und in der Placenta. *Arch. Gynäkol.* **153**, 233.

GOLDMAN A.S., YAKOVAC W.C. & BONGIOVANNI A.M. (1966) Development of activity of 3β-hydroxysteroid dehydrogenase in human fetal tissues and in two anencephalic newborns. *J. clin. Endocr. Metab.* **26**, 14.

GUTERMAN H.S. (1953) Progesterone metabolism in the human female: its significance in relation to reproduction. *Recent Progr. Horm. Research*, **8**, 293.

HAFFNER J. (1938) Uber den Progestingehalt in Reifer und in Junger Menschlicher Placenta. *Acta Obst. Gynecol. Scand.* **18**, 125.

HAGOPIAN M., PINCUS G., CARLO J. & ROMANOFF E.B. (1956) Isolation of an unknown substance and 6-ketoprogesterone from perfusates of human placentae. *Endocrinology*, **58**, 387.

HAIN A.M. (1939) Oestrogenic and androgenic substances in advanced pregnancy. *Quart. J. Expt. Physiol.* **29**, 139.

HARTMANN M. & LOCHER F. (1935) Uber Allo-pregnandiol, einen neuen Aokohol aus dem Schwangern harn. *Helv. Chim. Acta*, **18**, 160.

HEARD R.D.H., HOFFMAN M.M. & MACK G.E. (1944) Steroids. VI. The structure of pregnanediol glucuronide from human pregnancy urine. *J. Biol. Chem.* **155**, 607.

HEGNAUER H. (1952) Die Ausscheidung der 17-Ketosteroide im Harn Während der Normalen und Toxischen Schwangerschaft. *Arch. Gynak.* **181**, 659.

HERRMANN W. & SILVERMAN L. (1957) Excretion of pregnane-3α,17α,20α-triol in pregnancy. *J. clin. Endocr. Metab.* **17**, 1482.

HILLMAN D.A., STACHENKO J. & GIROUD C.J.P. (1962) *In vitro* studies of human newborn adrenal cortex. In *The Human Adrenal Cortex*, p. 596. A.R.Currie, T. Symington & J.K.Grant, eds. E. & S.Livingstone Ltd, London.

HIRSCHMANN H., HIRSCHMANN F.B. & ZALA A.P. (1961) Isolation of two new 16α-hydroxysteroids from human pregnancy urine. *J. Biol. Chem.* **236**, 3141.

HORTON R. & TAIT J.F. (1966) Androstenedione production and interconversion rates measured in peripheral blood and studies on the possible site of its conversion to testosterone. *J. Clin. Invest.* **45**, 301.

HUIS IN'T VELD L.G. (1954) L'excrétion des 17-cétostéroides au cours de la grossesse. *Gynéc. Obstét.* **53**, 42.

IKONEN M. & NIEMI M. (1966) Metabolism of progesterone and 17α-hydroxypregnenolone by the foetal human testis *in vitro*. *Nature*, **212**, 716.

ISMAIL A.A.A. & HARKNESS R.A. (1965) The isolation of progesterone from human pregnancy urine. *Biochem. J.* **98**, 15P.

JAFFE R., ERIKSSON G. & DICZFALUSY E. (1965) *In situ* perfusion of the midterm human placenta with cholesterol. *Proc. VI Pan Amer. Congr. Series*, **99**, p. E 182. Excerpta Med. Fdn.

JAFFE R.B. & LEDGER W.J. (1966) *In vivo* steroid biogenesis and metabolism in the human term placenta. I. *In situ* placental perfusion with isotopic pregnenolone. *Steroids*, **8**, 61.

JAFFE R.B. & PETERSON E.P. (1966) *In vivo* steroid biogenesis and metabolism in the human term placenta. 2. *In situ* placental perfusion with cholesterol-7α-^{3}H. *Steroids*, **8**, 695.

JAFFE R.B. (1967) Biogenesis and metabolism of progesterone in the human fetus and placenta. *Clin. Obst. Gynecol.* **10**, 47.

JAYLE M.-F., DESGREZ P., SERPICELLI J. & ROZEG J. (1953) Dosage des corticoides urinaires aprés hydrolyse biologique. *Annales d'Endocrin.* **14**, 877.

JONES K.M., LLOYD-JONES R., RIONDEL A., TAIT J.F., TAIT S.A.S., BULBROOK R.D. & GREENWOOD F.C. (1959) Aldosterone secretion and metabolism in normal men and women and in pregnancy. *Acta Endocrinol.* **30**, 321.

JUNGMANN R.A. & SCHWEPPE J.S. (1967) Biosynthesis and metabolism of neutral steroids by human midterm placenta and fetal liver. *J. clin. Endocr. Metab.* **27**, 1151.

KITCHIN III J.D., PION R.J. & CONRAD S.H. (1967) Metabolism of progesterone by the term human placenta perfused *in situ*. *Steroids*, **9**, 263.

KLEVIT H.D. (1966) Fetal-placental-maternal interrelationships involving steroid hormones. *Pediat. Clin. North Am.* **13**, 59.

KLOPPER A., MICHIE E. & BROWN J.B. (1955) A method for the measurement of pregnanediol in urine. *J. Endocrinol.* **12**, 209.

KLOPPER A.I. & MACNAUGHTON M.C. (1959) The identification of pregnanediol in liquor amnii, bile and foeces. *J. Endocrinol.* **18**, 319.

KLOPPER A. & MICHIE E.A. (1956) The excretion of urinary pregnanediol after the administration of progesterone. *J. Endocrinol.* **13**, 360.

KUMAR D., GOODNO J.A. & BARNES A.C. (1962) Isolation of progesterone from human pregnant myometrium. *Nature*, **195**, 1204.

KYLE T.I. & MARRIAN G.F. (1951) Allopregnane-3α; 20α-diol in the urine of pregnant women. *Biochem. J.* **49**, 80.

LAIDLAW J.C., COHEN M. & GORNALL A.G. (1958) Studies on the origin of aldosterone during pregnancy. *J. Clin. Endocr. Metab.* **18**, 222.

LAMB E., MANCUSO S., DELL'ACQUA S., WIQVIST N. & DICZFALUSY E. (1967) Studies on the metabolism of C-19 steroids in the human foeto-placental unit. I. Neutral metabolites formed from dehydroepiandrosterone and dehydroepiandrosterone sulphate by the placenta at midpregnancy. *Acta Endocrinol.* **55**, 263.

LANMAN J.T. (1953) The fetal zone of the adrenal gland. *Medicine, Baltimore*, **32**, 389.

LANMAN J.T. & SILVERMAN L.M. (1957) *In vitro* steroidogenesis in the human neonatal adrenal gland, including observations on human adult and monkey adrenal glands. *Endocrinology*, **60**, 433.

LIEBERMAN S., DOBRINER K., HILL B.R., FIESER L.F. & RHOADS C.P. (1948) Studies in steroid metabolism. II. Identification and characterization of ketosteroids isolated from urine of healthy and diseased persons. *J. Biol. Chem.* **172**, 263.

LITTLE B., DI MARTINIS J. & NYHOLM B. (1959) The conversion of progesterone to Δ^4-pregnene-20α-ol, 3-one by human placenta *in vitro*. *Acta Endocrinol.* (*Kbh*), **30**, 530.

LITTLE B. & SHAW A. (1960) Conversion of progesterone to 17-alpha-hydroxyprogesterone by human placenta *in vitro*. *Acta Endocrinol.* (*Kbh*), Suppl. **51**, 713.

LITTLE B. & SHAW A. (1961) The conversion of progesterone to 17α-hydroxyprogesterone by human placenta *in vitro*. *Acta Endocrinol.*(*Kbh*), **36**, 455.

LITTLE B., SHAW A. & PURDY R. (1963) The conversion of progesterone to 16α-hydroxypregn-4-ene-3,20-dione and androst-4-ene-3,17-dione by human placenta *in vitro*. *Acta Endocrinol.* (*Kbh*), **43**, 510.

LLOYD C.W., HUGHES E.C., LOBOTSKY J., RIENZO J. & AVERY G.M. (1952) Some hormone studies in normal and toxemic pregnancy. *J. Clin. Invest.* **31**, 1056.

LONGCHAMPT J.E., GUAL C., EHRENSTEIN M. & DORFMAN R.I. (1960) 19-Hydroxy-Δ^4-androstene-3,17-dione; an intermediate in estrogen biosynthesis. *Endocrinology*, **66**, 416.

LURIE A.O., VILLEE C.A. & REID D.E. (1966) Progesterone in the blood. A quantitative method employing gas liquid chromatography. *J. clin. Endocr. Metab.* **26**, 742.

MAGENDANTZ H.G. & RYAN K.J. (1964) Isolation of an estriol precursor, 16α-hydroxydehydroepiandrosterone, from human umbilical sera. *J. clin. Endocr. Metab.* **24**, 1155.

MANCUSO S., DELL'ACQUA S., ERIKSSON G., WIQVIST N. & DICZFALUSY E. (1965) Aromatization of androstenedione and testosterone by the human fetus. *Steroids*, **5**, 183.

MANCUSO S., BENAGIANO G., FROYSA B. & DICZFALUSY E. (1967) Formation of testosterone sulphate by the foetus *in vivo*. *Biochim. Biophys. Acta*, **144**, 183.

MARKER R.E., KAMM O. & MCGREW R.V. (1937) Sterols. IX. Isolation of epi-pregnanol-3-one-20 from human pregnancy urine. *J. Amer. Chem. Soc.* **59**, 616.

MARKER R.E. & KAMM O. (1937) Sterols. XVII. Isolation of pregnanolone from human pregnancy urine. *J. Amer. Chem. Soc.* **59**, 1373.

MARKER R.E. & LAWSON E.J. (1938) Sterols. XLVIII. Isolation of androsterone and pregnanol-3α from human pregnancy urine. *J. Amer. Chem. Soc.* **60**, 2928.

MARKER R.E. & ROHRMANN E. (1939) Sterols. LXX. The steroid content of mares' pregnancy urine. *J. Amer. Chem. Soc.* **61**, 2537.

MARRIAN G.F. (1929) CXVII. The chemistry of oestrin. I. Preparation from urine and separation from an unidentified solid alcohol. *Biochem. J.* **23**, 1090.

MARTIN J.D. & MILLS I.H. (1956) Aldosterone excretion in normal and toxaemic pregnancies. *Brit. Med. J.* **2**, 571.

MCGINTY I.A., MCCULLOUGH N.B. & WOLFER J.G. (1936) Progestin content of human placenta. *Proc. Soc. Expt. Biol. Med.* **34**, 176.

MEIGS R.A. & ENGEL L.L. (1961) The metabolism of andrenocortical steroids by human tissues. *Endocrinology*, **69**, 152.

MIGEON C., KELLER A.R. & HOLMSTROM E.G. (1955) Dehydroepiandrosterone, androsterone and 17-hydroxycorticosteroid levels in maternal and cord plasma in cases of vaginal delivery. *Bull. Johns Hopk. Hosp.* **97**, 415.

MORATO T., LEMUS A.E. & GUAL C. (1965) Efficiency of dehydroepiandrosterone sulphate as an estrogen precursor. *Steroids*, **5** (Suppl. 1), 59.

MORRISON G., MEIGS R.A. & RYAN K.J. (1965) Biosynthesis of progesterone by the human placenta. *Steroids*, **6** (Suppl. 2), 117.

MOSES A.M., LOBOTSKY J. & LLOYD C.W. (1959) The occurrence of pre-eclampsia in a bilaterally adrenalectomized woman. *J. clin. Endocr. Metab.* **19**, 987.

NEHER R. & STARK G. (1961) Nachweis von Corticosteroiden in Menschlicher Placenta und Isolierung von 16α-Hydroxytestosteron. *Experientia*, **17**, 510.

NIEMI M. & BAILLIE A.H. (1965) 3β-Hydroxysteroid dehydrogenase activity in the human fetal adrenal cortex. *Acta Endocrinol.* **48**, 423.

NISSIM J.A. & ROBSON J.M. (1952) The conversion of pregnenolone to a more active progestational substance by incubation with endocrine tissues *in vitro*. *J. Endocrinol.* **8**, 329.

NOALL M.W., SALHANICK H.A., NEHER G.M. & ZARROW M.X. (1953) Method for the isolation of progesterone from human placentae. *J. Biol. Chem.* **201**, 321.

ODELL D. & MARRIAN G.F. (1936) A note on the presence in human pregnancy urine of an acid-hydrolyzable combined form of pregnanediol. *Biochem. J.* **30**, 1533.

OERTEL G.W., WEISS S.P. & EIK-NES K.B. (1959) Determination of progesterone in human blood plasma. *J. clin. Endocr. Metab.* **19**, 213.

OSINKI P.A. (1960) Steroid 11β-ol dehydrogenase in human placenta. *Nature*, **187**, 777.

PALMER R., ERIKSSON G., WIQVIST N. & DICZFALUSY E. (1966a) Studies on the metabolism of C-21 steroids in the human foeto-placental unit. 2. Metabolism of pregnenolone sulphate by midterm placentas perfused *in situ*. *Acta Endocrinol.* (*Kbh*), **52**, 598.

PALMER R., BLAIR J.A., ERIKSSON G. & DICZFALUSY E. (1966b) Studies on the metabolism of C-21 steroids in the human foeto-placental unit. 3. Metabolism of progesterone and 20α- and 20β-dihydroprogesterone by midterm placentas perfused *in situ*. *Acta Endocrinol.* (*Kbh*), **53**, 407.

PARVIAINEN S., SOIVA K. & VARTIAINEN S. (1950) Corticosteroid excretion during pregnancy, especially in toxaemia of late pregnancy. *Acta Obst. Gynec. Scand.* **29**, Suppl. 5.

PATTI A., BONANNO P., FRAWLEY T.F. & STEIN A.A. (1963) Gas-phase chromatography in separation and identification of pregnanediol in urine and blood of pregnant women. *Obst. Gynec.* **21**, 302.

PEARLMAN W.H., PINCUS G. & WERTHESSEN N.T. (1942) The isolation of allo-pregnanol-3β-one-20 from human pregnancy urine. *J. Biol. Chem.* **142**, 649.

PEARLMAN W.H. & CERCEO E. (1952a) The isolation of progesterone from human placenta. *J. Biol. Chem.* **198**, 79.

PEARLMAN W.H. & CERCEO E. (1952b) The isolation of C_{21} steroids from human placenta. *J. Biol. Chem.* **194**, 807.

PEARLMAN W.H. & CERCEO E. (1953) The estimation of saturated and α,β-unsaturated ketonic compounds in placental extracts. *J. Biol. Chem.* **203**, 127.

PEARLMAN W.H., CERCEO E. & THOMAS M. (1954) The conversion of Δ^5-pregnen-3β-ol-20-one to progesterone by homogenates of human placental tissue. *J. Biol. Chem.* **208**, 231.

PEARLMAN W.H. (1957a) A comparative study of (16-^{3}H)-progesterone metabolism in pregnant and non-pregnant women. *Biochem. J.* **65**, 7P.

PEARLMAN W.H. (1957b) (16-^{3}H)Progesterone metabolism in advanced pregnancy and in oophorectomized-hysterectomized women. *Biochem. J.* **67**, 1.

PEARLMAN W.H. & CRÉPY O. (1967) Steroid-protein interaction with particular reference to testosterone-binding by human serum. *J. Biol. Chem.* **242**, 182.

PEARLMAN W.H., CRÉPY O. & MURPHY M. (1967) Testosterone-binding levels in the serum of women during the normal menstrual cycle, pregnancy, and the post-partum period. *J. Clin. Endocr. Metab.* **27**, 1012.

PINCUS G. (1943) New color reaction for certain urinary 17-ketosteroids. *Endocrinology*, **32**, 176.

PINCUS G. & PEARLMAN W.H. (1943) The intermediate metabolism of the sex hormones. *Vitamins and Hormones*, **1**, 293.

PION R., JAFFE R., ERIKSSON G., WIQVIST N. & DICZFALUSY E. (1965) Studies on the metabolism of C-21 steroids in the human foeto-placental unit. I. Formation of α,β-unsaturated 3-ketones in midterm placentas perfused *in situ* with pregnenolone and 17α-hydroxypregnenolone. *Acta Endocrinol. (Kbh)*, **48**, 234.

PION R.J., CONRAD S.H. & WOLF B.J. (1966) Pregnenolone sulfate–an efficient precursor for the placental production of progesterone. *J. clin. Endocr. Metab.* **26**, 225.

PION R.J., JAFFE R.B., WIQVIST N. & DICZFALUSY E. (1967) Formation of dehydroepiandrosterone sulphate by previable human foetuses. *Biochim. Biophys. Acta*, **137**, 584.

PUCK A., SIEVERT C. & MEINECKE F.W. (1953) Quantitativer Nachweis von 17-Ketosteroiden aus dem Mütterlichen Blut und aus dem Nabelschnurblut des Neugeborenen. (Zugleich Untersuchungsreihe zur Bestimmung der Fehlerbreite beim Nachweis von Steronen im Menschlichen Blut.) *Arch. Gynak.* **182**, 414.

RICE B.F., JOHANSON C.A. & STERNBERG W.H. (1966) Formation of steroid hormones from acetate-1-^{14}C by a human fetal testis preparation grown in organ culture. *Steroids*, **7**, 79.

RIESS H. (1952) Über den Nachweis von Männlichen Wirkstoffen im Schwangerenharn und in der Placenta. *Z. Geburtschilfe u. Gynäkol.* **136**, 1.

RINSLER M.G. & RIGBY B. (1957) Function of aldosterone in the metabolism of sodium and water in pregnancy. *Brit. Med. J.* **2**, 966.

RONAN F.F., PARSONS L., NAMIOT R. & WOTIZ H.H. (1960) Studies in steroid metabolism. IX. The excretion of pregnane-3α,17α,20α-triol during pregnancy. *J. clin. Endocr. Metab.* **20**, 355.

RUNNEBAUM B. & ZANDER J. (1962) Progesteron, Δ^4-Pregnen-20α-ol-3-on, Δ^4-Pregnen-20β-ol-3-on und 17α-Hydroxyprogesteron im Plasma der Nabelvene und der Naelarterien. *Klin. Wochschr.* **40**, 453.

RUSE J.L. & SOLOMON S. (1966a) The isolation and origin of urinary 16α-hydroxyprogesterone. *Biochemistry*, **5**, 1072.

RUSE J.L. & SOLOMON S. (1966b) The *in vivo* metabolism of 16α-hydroxyprogesterone. *Biochemistry*, **5**, 1065.

RYAN K.J., MEIGS R. & PETRO Z. (1966) The formation of progesterone by the human placenta. *Amer. J. Obst. Gynec.* **96**, 676.

SALHANICK H.A., NOALL M.W., ZARROW M.X. & SAMUELS L.T. (1952) The isolation of progesterone from human placentae. *Science*, **115**, 708.

SALHANICK H.A., NEAL L.M. & MAHONEY J.P. (1956) Blood content of human placenta. *J. Clin. Endocr. Metab.* **16**, 1120.

SANDBERG A.A., SLAUNWHITE W.R., Jnr. & ANTONIADES H.N. (1957) The binding of steroids and steroid conjugates to human plasma proteins. *Recent Progr. Hormone Res.* **8**, 209.

SANDBERG A.A. & SLAUNWHITE W.R., Jnr. (1959) Transcortin: a corticosteroid binding protein of plasma. II. Levels in various conditions and the effect of estrogens. *J. Clin. Invest.* **38**, 1290.

SANDBERG A.A., ROSENTHAL H., SCHNEIDER S.L. & SLAUNWHITE W.R., Jnr. (1966) Protein-steroid interactions and their role in the transport and metabolism of steroids. In *Steroid Dynamics*, p. 1. G.Pincus, T.Nakao & J.F.Tait, eds. Academic Press, New York.

SEAL U.S. & DOE R.P. (1966) Corticosteroid-binding globulin: biochemistry, physiology, and phylogeny. In *Steroid Dynamics*, p. 63. G.Pincus, T.Nakao & J.F.Tait, eds. Academic Press, New York.

SHEN N.C., KATZMAN M.B., FRANCIS F.E. & KINSELLA R.A., Jnr. (1963) Determination of pregnanolone, pregnanediol, and pregnanetriol in urine. *J. Lab. and Clin. Med.* **61**, 174.

SHIMIZU K., HAYANO M., GUT M. & DORFMAN R.I. (1961) The transformation of 20α-hydroxycholesterol to isocaproic acid and C_{21} steroids. *J. Biol. Chem.* **236**, 695.

SHIMIZU K., SHIMAO S. & TANAKA M. (1965) Conversion *in vitro* of 20α-hydroxycholesterol to 17α,20α-dihydroxycholesterol by human fetal adrenals. *Steroids*, **5** (Suppl. 1), 85.

SHORT R.V. & ETON B. (1959) Progesterone in blood. III. Progesterone in the peripheral blood of pregnant women. *J. Endocrinol.* **18**, 418.

SIITERI P.K. & MACDONALD P.C. (1966) Placental estrogen biosynthesis during human pregnancy. *J. clin. Endocr. Metab.* **26**, 751.

Simmer H.H., Easterling W.E., Jnr., Pion R. & Dignam W.J. (1964) Neutral C-19 steroids and steroid sulfates in human pregnancy. I. Identification of dehydroepiandrosterone sulfate in fetal blood and quantification of this hormone in cord arterial, cord venous and maternal peripheral blood in normal pregnancies at term. *Steroids*, **4**, 125.

Slaunwhite W.R., Jnr. & Sandberg A.A. (1959) Transcortin: a corticosteroid-binding protein of plasma. *J. Clin. Invest.* **38**, 384.

Slaunwhite W.R., Jnr., Karsay M.A., Hollmer A., Sandberg A.A. & Niswander K. (1965) Fetal liver as an endocrine tissue. *Steroids*, **6** (Suppl. 2), 211.

Smith G.V.S. & Kennard J.H. (1937) Progestin and estrin of nineteen placentas from normal and toxemic cases. *Proc. Soc. Expt. Biol. Med.* **36**, 508.

Sobreville L.A., Hagerman D.D. & Villee C.A. (1964) The metabolism of pregnenolone and 17α-hydroxypregnenolone by homogenates of human term placentas. *Biochim. Biophys. Acta*, **93**, 665.

Solomon S., Lenz A.L., Vande Wiele R. & Lieberman S. (1954) Pregnenolone, an intermediate in the biosynthesis of progesterone and the adrenal cortical hormones. *Abstracts, Amer. Chem. Soc.* 126*th Meeting, New York*, p. 29C.

Solomon S., Lanman J.T., Lind J. & Lieberman S. (1958) The biosynthesis of Δ^4-androstenedione and 17α-hydroxyprogesterone from progesterone by surviving human fetal adrenals. *J. Biol. Chem.* **233**, 1084.

Solomon S. (1960) Synthesis of steroids by the placenta. In *The Placenta and Fetal Membranes*, p. 201. C.A.Villee, ed. Williams and Wilkins Co., Baltimore.

Solomon S., Bird C.E., Wilson R., Wiqvist N. & Diczfalusy E. (1964) Progesterone metabolism in the fetal-placental unit. *Excerpta Med. Intern. Congress Series*, **83**, 721.

Solomon S. (1966) Formation and metabolism of neutral steroids in the human placenta and fetus. *J. clin. Endocr. Metab.* **26**, 762.

Solomon S., Bird C.E., Ling W., Iwamiya M. & Young P.C.M. (1967) Formation and metabolism of steroids in the fetus and placenta. *Recent Prog. Horm. Res.* **23**, 297.

Sommerville I.F. & Marrian G.F. (1950) Urinary excretion of pregnanediol in human subjects following the administration of progesterone and of pregnane-3α,20α-diol. *Biochem. J.* **46**, 290.

Stark E., Gyévai A., Szalay K. & Acs Zs. (1965) Hypophyseal-adrenal activity in combined human foetal tissue cultures. *Can. J. Physiol. Pharm.* **43**, 1.

Tait J.F. & Horton R. (1966) The *in vivo* estimation of blood production and interconversion rates of androstenedione and testosterone and the calculation of their secretion rates. In *Steroid Dynamics*, p. 393. G.Pincus, T.Nakao & J.F. Tait, eds. Academic Press, New York.

Tobian L. (1949) Cortical steroid excretion in edema of pregnancy, pre-eclampsia, and essential hypertension. *J. Clin. Endocr. Metab.* **9**, 319.

van Lankeren C. (1936) Erzeugung der Sekretionsphase im Endometrium des Kaninchens (=Corpus Luteum–Hormonwirkung) durch Placentaextrakt. *Arch. Gynäkol.* **160**, 150.

van Leusden H. & Villee C.A. (1965) The *de novo* synthesis of sterols and steroids from acetate by preparations of human term placenta. *Steroids*, **6**, 31.

VENNING E.H. & BROWNE J.S.L. (1936) Isolation of a water soluble pregnanediol complex from human pregnancy urine. *Proc. Soc. Expt. Biol. Med.* **34**, 792.

VENNING E.H. (1938) Further studies on the estimation of sodium pregnanediol glucuronidate in urine. *J. Biol. Chem.* **126**, 595.

VENNING E.H. & BROWNE J.S.L. (1940) A study of the metabolism of crystalline progesterone. *Endocrinology*, **27**, 707.

VENNING E.H. (1946) Adrenal function in pregnancy. *Endocrinology*, **39**, 203.

VENNING E.H. & DYRENFURTH I. (1956) Aldosterone excretion in pregnancy. *J. Clin. Endocr. Metab.* **16**, 426.

VENNING E.H., PRIMROSE T., CALIGARIS L.C.S. & DYRENFURTH I. (1957) Aldosterone excretion in pregnancy. *J. clin. Endocr. Metab.* **17**, 473.

VILLEE D.B., ENGEL L.L. & VILLEE C.A. (1959) Steroid hydroxylation in human fetal adrenals. *Endocrinology*, **65**, 465.

VILLEE D.B., ENGEL L.L., LORING J.M. & VILLEE C.A. (1961) Steroid hydroxylation in human fetal adrenals: formation of 16α-hydroxyprogesterone, 17-hydroxyprogesterone and deoxycorticosterone. *Endocrinology*, **69**, 354.

VILLEE C.A., LORING J.M. & VILLEE D.B. (1962) Synthesis of dehydroepiandrosterone and 16-hydroxypregnenolone. *Excerpta Med. Intern. Congr. Series*, **51**, 143.

VILLEE C.A. & LORING J.M. (1963) 20α-Hydroxysteroid dehydrogenase and 3α-hydroxysteroid dehydrogenase in human fetal liver. *Endocrinology*, **72**, 824.

VILLEE D.B. & VILLEE C.A. (1964) Synthesis of corticosteroids in the fetal-placental unit. *Excerpta Med. Intern. Congr. Series*, **83**, 709.

VILLEE D.B. & DRISCOLL S.G. (1965) Pregnenolone and progesterone metabolism in human adrenals from twin female fetuses. *Endocrinology*, **77**, 602.

VILLEE C.A., LORING J.M. & ROSE M. (1965) Formation and cleavage of steroid sulfates by human fetal adrenals. *Endocrine Soc. Meeting*, *47th*, *New York*. Abstract No. 98.

WARREN J.C. & CHEATUM S.G. (1964) Demonstration of a steroid 17–20 desmolase in the human placenta. *Can. J. Biochem.* **42**, 143.

WHEELER J., FREEMAN S. & CHEN C. (1953) A comparison of the tetrazolium and other methods of steroid estimation applied to urine. *J. Lab. Clin. Med.* **42**, 758.

WILCOX R.B. & ENGEL L.L. (1965) Kinetic studies on the role of 19-hydroxyandrost-4-ene-3,17-dione in estrogen biosynthesis. *Steroids*, **5** (Suppl. 1), 49.

WOOLEVER C.A., GOLDFIEN A. & PAGE E.W. (1961) Studies of the isolated perfused human placenta. II. Progesterone content of perfusates. *Amer. J. Obst. Gynec.* **81**, 1137.

YOUNGLAI E. & SOLOMON S. (1967) The *in vivo* metabolism of 16α-hydroxydehydroisoandrosterone in man. *Biochemistry*, **6**, 2040.

YOUNGLAI E. & SOLOMON S. (1968) The *in vivo* metabolism of 16α-hydroxylated C_{19} steroids in late pregnancy. *Biochemistry* **7**, 1881.

ZANDER J. & SIMMER H. (1954) Die chemische Bestimmung von Progesteron in Organische Substraten. *Klin. Wohnschr.* **32**, 529.

ZANDER J. & VON MÜNSTERMANN A.-M. (1956) Progesteron in Menschlichem Blu undt Geweben. III. Progesteron in der Placenta, in der Uterusschlermhaut und im Fruchtwasser. *Klin. Wschr.* **34**, 944.

ZANDER J., FORBES T.R., VON MÜNSTERMANN A.M. & NEHER R. (1958) Δ^4-3-Keto-pregnene-20α-ol and Δ^4-3-ketopregnene-20β-ol, two naturally occurring metabolites of progesterone. Isolation, identification, biological activity and concentration in human tissues. *J. clin. Endocr. Metab.* **18**, 337.

ZANDER J. (1959) Gestagens in human pregnancy. In *Recent Progress in the Endocrinology of Reproduction:* Proceedings of a Conference, p. 255. C.W.Lloyd, ed. Academic Press, New York.

ZANDER J. (1961) Relationship between progesterone production in the human placenta and the foetus. In *Progesterone and the Defence Mechanism of Pregnancy*, p. 32. G.E.W.Wolstenholme & M.P.Cameron, eds. J. & A.Churchill Ltd, London.

ZANDER J., THIJSSEN J. & VON MÜNSTERMANN A.M. (1962a) Isolation and identification of 16α-hydroxyprogesterone from human corpora lutea and placental blood. *J. clin. Endocr. Metab.* **22**, 861.

ZANDER J., VON MÜNSTERMANN A.M. & RUNNEBAUM B. (1962b) Steroide im Plasma von Menschlichem Plazenta Blut (Nabelschnur-plasma). *Acta Endocrinol.* **41**, 507.

ZANDER J., VON MÜNSTERMANN A.M. & RUNNEBAUM B. (1962c) Nachweis von 6 neuen Steroiden im Plasma von Menschlichem Placenta Blut (Nabelschnurblut). *Klin. Wochschr.* **40**, 436.

ZELEWSKI L. & VILLEE C.A. (1966) The biosynthesis of squalene, lanosterol, and cholesterol by minced human placenta. *Biochemistry*, **5**, 1805.

ZONDEK B. & FINKELSTEIN M. (1952) A neutral fluorogenic substance in human urine and its increased excretion in pregnancy and pseudohermaphroditism. *Acta Endocrinol. (Kbh)*, **11**, 297.

7

Protein Hormones and Hormonal Peptides from the Placenta*

SAM BRODY†

I INTRODUCTION

The placenta occupies a unique position among the endocrine glands. It is a temporary organ with a genetical constitution partly foreign to the mother. It thus constitutes a natural homograft which, however, for a prolonged period of time escapes immunological destruction. During this time it plays a central role in the endocrinology of pregnancy, producing hormones with a profound metabolic influence on the mother, yet it operates with a high degree of autonomy and apparently independently of ordinary homeostatic and regulatory mechanisms in the maternal organism.

The high degree of autonomy displayed by the foeto-placental unit versus the mother requires the presence of built-in autoregulatory mechanisms governing the metabolic processes within this compartment. The physiological significance of the placental protein hormones

* The following abbreviations have been used: ACTH = adrenocorticotrophic hormone; HCG = human chorionic gonadotrophin; HCGP = human chorionic growth hormone-prolactin; (H)FSH = (human) follicle stimulating hormone; HGH = human growth hormone; (H)LH = (human) luteinizing hormone; HMG = human menopausal gonadotrophin; ICSH = interstitial-cell stimulating hormone; MSH = melanocyte stimulating hormone.

† Thanks are due to the Editors-in-chief of *Acta endocrinologica* and *Acta obstetricia et gynecologica scandinavica* and to J. & A.Churchill Ltd, London, and J.B.Lippincott Company, Philadelphia, for generous permission to re-publish some illustrations from earlier publications.

is at present only incompletely understood. Recent findings, however, attribute an important function, at least to HCG, as regards certain processes of intermediary metabolism in the placenta. These results open up an interesting avenue of research as they may provide a missing link as regards the interaction between trophic and steroid hormones in the placenta.

The placental steroid hormones are identical with those produced in the ovary or in the adrenal, although differences in biosynthesis and metabolic pathways may exist. The protein hormones of definite placental origin, on the other hand, although showing resemblance to the corresponding pituitary hormones as regards biological activity, display distinct antigenical and possibly also physico-chemical differences when compared with the hypophyseal substances.

Opinion as to the number of protein hormones and hormonal peptides produced in the placenta has varied considerably over the last ten to fifteen years. Some years ago it was considered that this organ manufactured a rather broad spectrum of such substances, e.g., HCG, ACTH, relaxin, MSH, and vasopressin. To-day a completely different picture emerges. HCG is still on the list but reasonable doubt may be expressed concerning the placental origin of the others. Instead a rather newly discovered factor with growth hormone-like and prolactin-like activities, HCGP, has come into focus. Synthesis by chorionic tissue has been conclusively proven only for HCG and HCGP. Therefore, this chapter will be mainly devoted to a discussion of these two substances. The other hormones of problematic placental origin will only be briefly mentioned in a concluding section.

Quite a few reviews on placental protein hormones have been published over the years. Particularly worthy of mention, apart from the pioneer work so beautifully summarized by Zondek (1935) and Zondek & Sulman (1942), are the excellent surveys by Newton (1938), Thompson (1941), Hamburger (1950, 1957), Loraine (1956, 1957, 1958, 1961), Davis & Plotz (1956), and Diczfalusy & Troen (1961). Although some of these reviews have been published comparatively lately they have in certain respects been outdated by the considerable research activity in this particular segment of endocrinology. The studies on the newly discovered HCGP merit a detailed discussion; other active areas of research include improved methods of extraction and purification, modern data on biochemical and physico-chemical properties, new and fascinating aspects of metabolic function and mechanism of action, and, finally, the application of immunological methods for the detection, assay, and characterization of placental hormones.

Immunoassay methods are nowadays well established procedures in endocrinological research. Although the principles underlying these methods are founded on basic immunological concepts there are a number of specific problems relating to their application in the present context. It would seem that these viewpoints have not been considered in any preceding review. A brief presentation of the general principles involved in the comparatively large number of different serological procedures that have been employed for the placental protein hormones and a systematic analysis of the limitations and possible complications of these procedures are therefore included in this résumé.

In an attempt to formulate a synoptic view on recent progress in this field it was deemed desirable, in view of the considerations briefly mentioned above, to present a comparatively broad panorama of observations bearing on biochemical, biological, antigenical, and clinical properties of the placental protein hormones. Perusal of this information and appraisal of the conceptual and methodological advances over the years will permit re-evaluation of older work in the light of modern contributions and evaluation of recent contributions against a background of established developments and accomplishments. It is the hope of the reviewer that a survey along these lines may provide a proper perspective and a balanced outlook on the achievements of yesterday, on the problems of to-day, and possibly also on the endeavours of to-morrow in this particular area of research.

II HUMAN CHORIONIC GONADOTROPHIN

A CHEMICAL NATURE

I EXTRACTION AND PURIFICATION

a Extraction from normal pregnancy urine

Early attempts to extract the gonadotrophic principle from pregnancy urine were made by means of precipitation with ethanol and subsequent dialysis of the aqueous solution (Zondek 1929a, Evans & Simpson 1929), with uranyl acetate and subsequent extraction with ammonium phosphate (Reiss & Haurowitz 1929), with ammonium sulphate and further purification of the dialysed material by means of tannic acid and barium hydroxide (Dickens 1930), and with phosphotungstic acid from sulpho-salicylic acid-treated urine followed by fractionated ethanol precipitation (Wiesner & Marshall 1931).

The principle of adsorption for extraction and purification of HCG was introduced by Fischer & Ertel (1931) who used kaolin as the adsorbent and dilute ammonia as the eluant. The kaolin method has subsequently been used by, e.g. Scott (1940), Dekanski (1949), and Loraine (1950a). In 1932 Katzman & Doisy introduced their benzoic acid adsorption method. By the addition of acetone the benzoic acid is dissolved and the active material precipitated. This procedure has remained an essential step in a number of subsequent methods. Gurin, Bachman & Wilson (1939, 1940a) have added some significant steps. Because of the occurrence of maximal excretion of the hormone during the first trimester of pregnancy (Browne & Venning 1936; Evans *et al.* 1937) urine collected during this period was used as source material. The crude adsorption product was submitted to differential extraction with ethanol at varying pH values, and further purification was achieved with tannic acid, iodine in potassium iodine, or dialysis, and finally by shaking the water-soluble precipitate with chloroform. The product obtained had a potency of more than 6,000 i.u. per mg. Claesson and co-workers (1948) also used benzoic acid adsorption and ethanol fractionation as initial steps in a preparation procedure, where additional purification of the hormone was achieved by precipitation of impurities with protamine. These investigators claim to have prepared a crystalline HCG possessing a constant specific activity of 6,000 to 8,000 i.u. per mg. The crystallization of the hormone, however, has not been confirmed in other laboratories.

The principle of chromatographic adsorption for extraction and purification of HCG from pregnancy urine was introduced by Katzman and co-workers (1943). Acidified urine from the first months of pregnancy is percolated through a column containing permutit (an artificial aluminosilicate). After washing with water, 76 per cent ethanol, and 76 per cent ethanol containing 10 per cent ammonium acetate, the hormone is eluted with 38 per cent ethanol containing 10 per cent ammonium acetate. The hormone in the eluate is recovered by means of fractional ethanol precipitation. The purest preparations had a potency of 8,500 i.u. per mg. These results were confirmed by Morris (1955), who also found that decalso (a synthetic zeolite) could be substituted for permutit. For a comparison of advantages and disadvantages of these various extraction methods the reader is referred to Loraine (1950a).

For a number of years this purification level of HCG was the ultimate achievement for material from normal pregnancy urine. The publication of Got (1959) and of Got & Bourrillon (1960b) therefore mark a considerable step forward. These investigators describe a complex preparation procedure, integrating a number of earlier purification steps with some additional measures. After adsorption of HCG on benzoic acid it is extracted with a M/15 phosphate buffer at pH 4·8 and then precipitated with 80 per cent acetone. The next step involves fractionation with calcium in 50 per cent ethanol and precipitation in 60 per cent ethanol at pH 1. The active substance is then adsorbed on kaolin at pH 4·5, eluted at pH 11·5, chromatographically adsorbed on a decalso column with 0·05 M acetate buffer at pH 5·5, and eluted by means of 40 per cent ethanol containing 10 per cent ammonium acetate. Final purification is carried out by means of either chromatography on Dowex 2 or zone electrophoresis on starch. The hydrochloric acid-treated resin is suspended in a *tris*-buffer at pH 7·3. Under these conditions inactive impurities are adsorbed on the column. The zone electrophoresis is carried out for 45 to 48 hours at pH 8·6 and +4°C with a potential difference of 400 V and a current of 10–12 mA. The products obtained are claimed to have a specific activity of 11,000 to 12,000 i.u. per mg and the recovery is reported to be approximately 70 per cent.

A small-scale procedure has recently been published by Lytle & Haskell (1964) who, by means of a comparatively simple method, claim to have isolated a highly purified HCG with a specific activity greater than 10,000 i.u. per mg. The urine is treated with benzoic acid, the separated material taken up in phosphate buffer at pH 6, precipitated with ethanol, dissolved in glycine buffer at pH 8·6, and submitted to disc electrophoresis using a current of 5 mA per tube for 35 minutes.

b Extraction from the urine of trophoblastic tumour patients

In contrast to the great difficulties in obtaining highly purified HCG from normal pregnancy urine is the relative ease in preparing highly active hormone preparations from patients with trophoblastic tumours (hydatidiform mole, chorioadenoma destruens, choriocarcinoma). Morris & Morris (unpublished work, 1954, see Morris 1955) isolated material of a specific activity of 12,000 i.u. per mg from a patient with choriocarcinoma, employing a modification of the method of Katzman and associates (1943). Reisfeld & Hertz (1960) extracted HCG from the pooled urine of trophoblastic tumour patients by kaolin adsorption, placed the crude material on a DEAE-cellulose column, and eluted the active substance with gradually increasing concentrations of sodium chloride at pH 8·6. A further 10-fold increase in specific activity was achieved by repeated chromatography on a DEAE-cellulose column and elution by means of a straight-line gradient of sodium chloride at pH 6·0. The last step could be substituted by adsorption of inactive proteins on barium carbonate. The final preparations had a potency of about 15,000 i.u. per mg. Johnsen (1961), finally, obtained a preparation from the urine of patients with hydatidiform moles with a specific activity of 9,100 i.u. per mg by means of a single passage through a permutit column.

2 PURITY

The validity of data on physico-chemical characteristics, biological effects, and antigenical properties of a protein hormone must be critically evaluated against available information on the purity and homogeneity of the preparation used in the laboratory experiment or clinical trial. The complexity of this problem is illustrated by the different requirements for purity that must be fulfilled in different contexts. From a biochemical viewpoint the preparation of a single protein with a characteristic amino acid sequence and specific secondary and tertiary structure is attempted, from a physiological angle the presence of a single biologically active substance is a desideratum, and from an immunological aspect the absence of antigenically active impurities is desirable. Obviously no single criterion of purity may satisfy this broad range of requirements. A number of indices for purity and homogeneity have therefore been used. A realistic appraisal may be based on a combination of data obtained by different methods such as moving-boundary electrophoresis, zone electrophoresis on starch, analytical ultracentrifugation, solubility studies, immunodiffusion, and radiation inactivation.

Pioneer studies were carried out by Gurin and associates (1940b) and Lundgren and co-workers (1942). Their most active preparations (specific activity about 6,000 i.u. per mg) were found to be practically homogeneous with respect to electrical charge and essentially monodisperse in the ultracentrifuge. The material of Claesson and associates (1948) (specific activity 6,000 to 8,000 i.u. per mg) was also reported to be homogeneous as evidenced by means of moving-boundary electrophoresis.

Other investigators, however, employing partly different techniques, have demonstrated inhomogeneity of preparations with similar specific activities. Raacke and co-workers (1954) submitted a number of HCG preparations, assaying 2,000 to 7,000 i.u. per mg, to zone electrophoresis on starch, and invariably observed at least two gonadotrophically active components. Got and associates (1959) and Got & Bourrillon (1960b) by means of immunoelectrophoresis, zone electrophoresis on starch, and moving-boundary electrophoresis examined a preparation at an intermediary stage of purification (specific activity 6,000 to 7,000 i.u. per mg) and clearly demonstrated inhomogeneity of this product and the presence of biologically inactive constituents. Blobel and co-workers (1962) by means of chromatography on Dowex 2 obtained three fractions with similar amino acid composition but with biological activity restricted to the first fraction.

Got (1959), Got and co-workers (1959) and Got & Bourrillon (1960b) have submitted their final preparation of 12,000 i.u. per mg to extensive investigations of homogeneity. On the basis of a large number of physico-chemical and immunological criteria available at present they maintain that their material is homogeneous.

In contrast to these HCG preparations, which have been purified by means of complicated procedures, the highly active material which may easily be recovered from the urine of patients with trophoblastic tumours is grossly inhomogeneous. The preparation of Morris & Morris (unpublished work, 1954, see Morris 1955) assaying 12,000 i.u. per mg was inhomogeneous as shown by sedimentation and solubility studies, and the material of Reisfeld & Hertz (1960) with a specific activity of 15,000 i.u. per mg was heterogeneous as indicated by moving-boundary electrophoresis. The preparation of Johnsen (1961), having a potency of 9,100 i.u. per mg displayed several components when applied to paper chromatography. These findings either favour the interpretation that differences exist between the normal pregnancy and trophoblastic tumour hormone, or invite an attitude of reservation with respect to the claimed purity of the preparations of Got (1959) and of Got & Bourrillon (1960b). In fact, Lunenfeld (1965) by means of ultracentrifugation and immunoelectrophoresis found that an HCG preparation, extracted by Donini (1965) from normal pregnancy urine and assaying 17,000 i.u., was inhomogeneous. It should be mentioned, however, that Wilde & Bagshawe (1965) in a recent publication claim that they have isolated a homogeneous HCG preparation from the urine of patients with trophoblastic tumours. The hormone was purified by means of benzoic acid adsorption, DEAE-cellulose chromatography, Sephadex G-100 chromatography, and DEAE-Sephadex A-50 chromatography. It assayed 10,000 to 15,000 i.u. per mg in the intact rat ventral prostate assay, and was characterized by a single precipitin band when tested immunoelectrophoretically against antisera to crude and purified HCG preparations. Antisera to the highly purified preparation itself had, however, not yet been produced. More complete investigations are awaited with interest.

3 PHYSICO-CHEMICAL PROPERTIES OF HUMAN CHORIONIC GONADOTROPHIN

The original preparation of Gurin and co-workers (1939) with a potency of about 6,000 i.u. per mg was characterized by a number of physico-chemical data by these authors (1940) and by Lundgren and associates (1942). Got & Bourrillon (1960a, c) analysed their preparation having a specific activity of 12,000 i.u. per mg and obtained data differing considerably from those presented by the earlier investigators. Schumacher and associates (1960) and Blobel and associates (1962) have also published data derived from analyses of a commercial preparation with a specific activity of 8,000 i.u. (personal communication). Their results agree rather closely with those of Got & Bourrillon (1960a, c). For more detailed data the reader is referred to Table 7.1.

The original estimates of the molecular weight of HCG of Gurin and co-workers (1940) and of Lundgren and co-workers (1942) were based on sedimentation and diffusion studies and were in the range of 60,000 to 80,000 and 100,000, respectively. Got (1959) and Got & Bourrillon (1960a) by similar methods arrived at 30,000, and Schumacher and associates (1960), also on the basis of sedimentation and diffusion constants, at 25,000. Schumacher and associates (1960) also estimated the molecular weight from the amino acid composition and on the assumption of the carbohydrate moiety amounting to 30 per cent, and then found it to be 12,000 or a multiple thereof.

Some observations relating to these disparate results have been reported. The material of Schumacher and associates (1960), on further purification on Dowex 2, yielded three fractions, the first fraction only being biologically active (Blobel *et al.* 1962). The molecular weight of the first fraction was 57,000, calculated from the sedimentation (2·7) and the diffusion (4·2) constants. After dialysis against calcium ions a considerably higher diffusion constant (7·8) was observed, the sedimentation

TABLE 7.1

Physico-chemical properties of HCG

Specific activity (i.u./mg)	Sedimentation constant	Diffusion constant	Iso-electric point	Electro-phoretic mobility	Partial specific volume	Molecular weight	Reference
6,000–8,000	4·3, 5·4	—	3·2, 3·3	$4{\cdot}85 \times 10^{-5}$ (pH 7·0)	—	60,000–80,000*	Gurin *et al.* (1940b)
6,000–8,000	4·3	4·4	—	—	0·76	100,000*	Lundgren *et al.* (1942)
12,000	2·7	8·2	2·95	$2{\cdot}5 \times 10^{-5}$ (pH 8·6)	0·727	30,000*	Got (1959), Got & Bourrillon (1960b)
8,000‖	2·35, 2·6	7·6 > 11	—	—	—	29,000†	Schumacher *et al.* (1960)
8,000‖	2·6	4·2, 7·8‡	—	—	—	25,000	Blobel *et al.* (1962)
—	—	—	—	—	—	29,000‡	Blobel *et al.* (1962)
—	—	—	—	—	—	57,000§	Blobel *et al.* (1962)

* Calculated from sedimentation and diffusion constants.
† Calculated from light scattering.
‡ After dialysis against calcium ions.
§ After dialysis against EDTA.
‖ Personal communication.

constant remaining unchanged. These findings then indicated a molecular weight of 29,000. The molecular weight of the starting material was 30,000, but after dialysis against the chelating agent EDTA a molecular weight of 57,000 was calculated. The authors conclude that removal of bivalent ions leads to dimerization.

Paul & Odell (1964) and Nydick and associates (1964) have estimated the weight of the active portion of the molecule by means of bioassay and immunoassay of radiation-inactivated material. The molecular weight calculated from the radiation-induced disappearance of biological activity was found to be 27,000 (Paul & Odell 1964) or 30,500 (Nydick *et al.* 1964), whereas that calculated from the radiation-induced loss of serological reactivity was 11,200 (Paul & Odell 1964). These findings were interpreted to demonstrate that the structural unit endowed with immunological activity is considerably smaller than that possessing biological function.

Existing data suggest that the molecular form of HCG is somewhat elongated. Got (1959) and Got & Bourrillon (1960a) found a frictional ratio (f/f_0) of 1·28, which is in good agreement with the value of 1·2 estimated by Schumacher and co-workers (1960). After splitting-off 95 per cent of the sialic acids by treatment with neuraminidase the sedimentation and diffusion data indicate the presence of a nearly spheroid molecule (Blobel *et al.* 1962).

4 BIOCHEMICAL PROPERTIES

HCG is extremely stable in the dry state; in aqueous solutions it may undergo marked loss of biological activity, even when kept in the cold (Gurin *et al.* 1939, Katzman *et al.* 1943). Gurin and associates (1940a) observed a pronounced similarity in the chemical composition of different gonadotrophic preparations in spite of considerable variation in biological potency. This was assumed to be due either to the presence of inactivated hormone, formed in the urine or during the process of preparation, or to the presence of another constituent of similar composition. The importance of this observation has been brought to light in connection with recent immunological studies of HCG in various body fluids and will be discussed in a later section.

In contrast to the repeatedly reported observations on the lability of the hormone in aqueous solution is the finding of Morris & Morris (unpublished work, 1954, see Morris 1955) that their preparation was stable in 0·2 per cent aqueous solution for 18 hours at 0°C from pH 1 to pH 13 and for 8 days at 0°C between pH 3 and pH 11. An explanation of this discrepant finding may be looked for in the fact that the preparation of Morris & Morris was from the urine of a patient with chorionepithelioma. The hormone is stable in glycerol solution, even when treated at 100°C for 1 hour (Gurin *et al.* 1939). A decrease in the rate of inactivation was also noticed in the presence of magnesium chloride, gelatin, and particularly serum protein (Katzman *et al.* 1943).

There is a considerable number of papers dealing with the effects of various inorganic salts, amino acids, chemical compounds, and drugs on the biological activity of HCG. The results of these studies have stimulated the discussion on the chemical nature of HCG. Further contributions to this particular line of research have been made through studies on the effect of pH and temperature on the stability of HCG. For detailed information and references the reader is referred to the works of Fraenkel-Conrat and associates (1940), Bischoff (1940, 1946), Morris (1955), Banik & Chakravarti (1957), Banik (1959), Bourrillon and co-workers (1959), and Got (1959).

The effects of various proteolytic enzymes on the biological integrity of HCG has been studied. Reiss & Haurowitz (1929), demonstrated the inactivating effect of trypsin and papain. This was confirmed by Abramowitz & Hisaw (1939) who also reported that chymotrypsin and ptyalin had the capacity to destroy HCG. The hormone is, however, remarkably resistant to pepsin (Wiesner & Marshall1931). Bourrillon and associates (1959) and Got (1959) have recently revived the interest in these problems. They confirmed earlier results, and added information on the inactivating properties of carboxypeptidase. They also studied the effects of some glucosidolytic enzymes. HCG was slightly attacked by glucosidase and lysozyme, whereas no inactivation could be observed with hyaluronidase.

HCG was thus early recognized to be a protein. Gurin and associates (1939, 1940a) also found that it had a high percentage of carbohydrate, and that it, therefore, was a carbohydrate-polypeptide complex or a glucoprotein. No evidence of separation of the two main constituents could be obtained by shaking aqueous solutions of the hormones with chloroform at a pH range of 5 to 8. The linkage between carbohydrate and protein is therefore a firm one (Gurin *et al.* 1940b).

The nature of the carbohydrate portion of the HCG molecule has been the object of much study. Gurin and co-workers (1940a) found the total amount of carbohydrate to be somewhere between 17·8 per cent and 19·5 per cent and mainly made up by galactose and hexosamine with a molar ratio of 2 : 1. Morris & Morris (unpublished work, 1954, see Morris, 1955) in their admittedly inhomogeneous preparation with a potency of 12,000 i.u. per mg from the urine of a patient with chorionepithelioma found 12·2 per cent galactose and 4·9 per cent hexosamine. Zilliacus & Roos (1951) found the hexosamine to be glucosamine, and Klungsöyr & Stöa (1955), in addition to galactose, could also identify mannose. Got (1959) and Got and co-workers (1960), finally, stated that their preparation with a specific activity of 12,000 i.u. per mg had the following number of residues per molecule: 9 galactose, 9 mannose, 12 glucosamine, 3 galactosamine, and 2 fucose. This corresponds to 11 per cent hexose, 1·2 per cent 6-deoxyhexose, and 8·7 per cent hexosamine.

In 1948 Whitten observed the inactivation of HCG by influenza virus and by the 'receptor destroying enzyme' (RDE obtained from the nutritional medium of Vibrio cholerae). These findings were confirmed by Brossmer & Walter (1948) who, in addition, could demonstrate that this effect was brought about through the action of neuraminidase by splitting off N-acetyl-neuraminic acid (sialic acid). Schumacher and associates (1960) found 6 per cent of sialic acid and concluded that the terminal α-ketosidic sialic acid was of considerable importance for the biological activity of the hormone. Got (1959) and Got and co-workers (1960) found 8·5 per cent of sialic acids, calculated the number of residues per molecule to be 8, and recognized two derivatives, N-acetyl and N-glycolyl sialic acid.

5 NORMAL AND TUMOUR CHORIONIC GONADOTROPHIN—IDENTICAL OR DIFFERENT

It has been generally accepted that the HCG produced in the human placenta is identical to the gonadotrophin synthesized in trophoblastic tumours of the uterus or testis (Zondek 1930b, Twombly & Ferguson 1934, Evans & Simpson 1935, Hamburger 1941, 1958a, b, Evans & Simpson 1950). The occurrence of qualitative differences in the gonadotrophic activity of extracts from the urine of some patients with malignant testicular tumours has been explained by the fact that they excrete a mixture of pituitary and chorionic gonadotrophin (Hamburger 1941, 9158b).

Recently, however, some observations have been reported, which suggest that differences between the normal and tumour chorionic gonadotrophin may, in fact, exist. By means of zone electrophoresis and chromatography followed by paper electrophoresis Reisfeld and associates (1959) demonstrated that the gonadotrophic activity of sera from normal pregnant women was associated with the β- and γ-globulins, whereas the hormone activity of sera from patients with trophoblastic tumours migrated with the α_2- and β-globulins. The results of other investigators on the distribution of HCG in normal pregnancy serum are, however, somewhat at variance with these findings. All activity was found to be located in the β-globulin region (Demol & Fanard 1957, Nagy *et al.* 1961). Demol & Fanard (1957) reported a 50 per cent loss of hormonal activity during their elution procedure with 0·1 N sodium hydroxide from paper electrophoresis strips stained with Amido Black, which may explain their different results. Furthermore, they reported that purified HCG preparations submitted to paper electrophoresis were found in the α_2 and β regions. Similarly, Nagy and co-workers (1961), after addition of a purified HCG preparation to serum and subsequent paper electrophoresis, identified gonadotrophic activity in the bands corresponding to the α_2-, β- and γ-globulins. On the basis of information gleaned from the literature it seems difficult to decide whether various active components represent native forms or denatured products arising during purification and other handling (Spielman & Meyer 1938, Bischoff 1946, Whitten 1953, Raacke *et al.* 1954).

Schwartz & Mantel (1963), by means of a different approach, have also adduced some evidence in favour of the existence of differences between normal and tumour gonadotrophins. The dose-dependent quantal ovarian hyperaemia reaction, elicited by HCG, may be inhibited by pre-injection of HCG-antiserum. After titrating equally active doses of gonadotrophic material from both sources they found that the biological activity of choriocarcinoma gonadotrophin was less inhibited than that of normal pregnancy HCG by equivalent amounts of antiserum. A rather disturbing finding was, however, that the same differential inhibition was observed with antisera produced to gonadotrophic extracts from choriocarcinoma patients.

These results are different from those of Twombly & Ferguson (1934) who demonstrated complete cross-neutralization *in vivo* between tumour gonadotrophin from a patient with a testicular malignancy and antiserum to HCG as well as between HCG and antiserum to tumour gonadotrophin. They are also in contrast to the findings of Midgley and co-workers (1961), who demonstrated that antiserum to HCG neutralized the biological activity of, and showed a common band of identity with, the serum of hamsters bearing transplanted human testicular choriocarcinoma. In principle, Lewis and associates (1964) arrived at the same conclusions. It should be mentioned, however, that the experimental design of Schwartz & Mantel (1963) is strictly quantitative and, therefore, not quite comparable with those of the other investigators.

B BIOLOGICAL PROPERTIES

I GENERAL

Under normal conditions HCG is exclusively produced in the placenta. It is, therefore, a hormone of pregnancy, and its physiological activity may be assumed to be primarily related to metabolic processes of prime importance for the maintenance of gestation. After the discovery of the hormone by Aschheim & Zondek (1927) there was an intense research activity in this field of endocrinology directed towards extraction and purification of HCG and towards the elucidation of its biological properties. In spite of these efforts comparatively little insight into the physiological significance of HCG was gained. As late as in 1944 Levin stated that no clear-cut effects of HCG on mother or foetus had been demonstrated.

In retrospect, this sweeping statement does not seem quite justified. One of the apparently most important physiological effects of HCG, its luteotrophic action, had been suggested several years earlier (Browne & Venning 1938). The demonstration of this function forms a firm basis for attempts to arrive at a more adequate understanding of the endocrinological events that bridge the gap between the luteal phase of the menstrual cycle and the early pregnant state. The hormone apparently plays a key role for the adequate interplay between ovarian and placental function during the first few months of gestation.

The continued secretion of HCG throughout pregnancy and after the time when the corpus luteum has lost its endocrinological importance (Kulseng-Hanssen 1951, Glasser 1952, Tulsky & Koff 1957, Diczfalusy & Borell 1961) has, however, been a puzzling fact, and its physiological significance during the later stages of pregnancy has been difficult to discern. Already at a very early period of pregnancy the placenta assumes a dominant role among the endocrine glands of gestation, adopting the hormonal function of several endocrines and being characterized by a high degree of autonomy. Reciprocal influences and regulatory interrelationships between HCG and the steroidogenic activity of the placenta were early assumed (Smith & Smith 1934, 1937, 1939, 1948). Not until recently, however, has it been possible to remove such assumptions from the realms of speculation and to provide a solid experimental foundation for this interaction in terms of distinct effects of HCG on enzyme activities and hormone metabolism (Troen & Gordon 1958, Troen 1959, 1961, Cédard *et al.* 1961, 1962, 1964, Varangot *et al.* 1965).

The main theme in a large number of investigations dealing with the biological actions of HCG has been the evaluation of the nature of HCG as regards the degree of gonadal influence. In other words, is the hormone a complete gonadotrophic principle, combining the effects of interstitial-cell stimulation and follicle stimulation and thus activating both the endocrine apparatus and the germinative function of the gonad, or is its activity more restricted? The interstitial-cell stimulating properties of HCG have been definitely established. More controversial are the gametokinetic effects, i.e., follicle stimulation in the ovary and spermiogenetic activity in the testis. Such actions have been observed, particularly when large doses of the hormone are administered.

The initial observations of Philipp (1930a, b) on the lack of demonstrable gonadotrophic activity in the pituitary gland of pregnant women has been repeatedly confirmed (Erhardt & Mayes 1930, Vozza 1932, Philipp & Huber 1936, Saxton & Loeb 1937, Witschi & Riley 1940, Bruner 1951). It is probably due to the negative feed-back action of steroids produced by the placenta and will explain the absence of gross contamination of urinary HCG preparations with pituitary gonadotrophic hormones. The interest now centres around the question whether the observed gametokinetic actions are due to small amounts of contaminating pituitary follicle-stimulating hormone in the urinary preparations of HCG or whether they represent an intrinsic property of HCG.

Before going into a more detailed discussion on the biological properties of HCG it should be remembered that a large amount of work has been performed on laboratory animals. HCG is the product of a highly specialized human organ, it is species-specific and a distinctly foreign substance to species other than the human. Its effects in the laboratory animal may possibly be reproduced in the human, in part or completely, but until this has been done caution should be exercised in assuming that actions elicited in the experimental animal would prevail under physiological or pathological conditions in man.

2 EFFECTS ON THE OVARY

At a time when virtually nothing was known about the physiological significance of HCG some characteristic features of the hormone such as its early production in pregnancy and its typical excretion rate at various phases of gestation were held to indicate a particularly active role at a very early stage of implantation. In a number of papers the appearance of HCG in the urine a few days prior to the expected menstrual period has been reported. Thus, it seems to be produced by the ovum almost immediately after fertilization and is secreted into the maternal organism in association with its embedding in the endometrium. Synthesis of HCG may be considered as the result of a highly specialized and impressively rapid process of differentiation with a high degree of priority. The embryo itself has thus far undergone very little growth. Furthermore, the rate of synthesis, after a variable but short lag phase is tremendously accelerated with rapid increase of serum and urinary levels attaining their highest concentration 50 to 70 days after the last menstrual period (for detailed references to the literature the reader is referred to Section G.2).

a Interstitial and theca cell stimulation

In the experimental animal hypertrophy and luteinization of interstitial and theca cells are invariable findings (Evans *et al.* 1932, Leonard 1932, Selye *et al.* 1933, Leonard & Smith 1934a). The data have been summarized and critically discussed by Newton (1938). These effects have also been observed in man as reported in a number of papers (Geist 1933, Geist *et al.* 1941, Westman 1938, Segaloff *et al.* 1951). Some variation in this response has, however, been noted and has been ascribed to the degree of maturity of the follicle at the time of administering the hormone (Westman 1938).

b Gametokinetic properties

It was recognized early that follicle-stimulating properties, originally assumed to be present in HCG, in fact were due to a synergistic action on the ovary by pituitary and placental hormones (Evans *et al.* 1932, Leonard 1932, Leonard & Smith 1934b). The lack of follicle-stimulating activity of HCG, when administered in moderate doses to rodents, was conclusively demonstrated in hypophysectomized animals by Selye and associates (1933), and by Leonard & Smith (1934a). Follicular growth was not induced by HCG under these experimental conditions. Evidence gained in man is more equivocal but partly points in the same direction.

Geist (1933) and Geist and co-workers (1941) were under the impression that HCG caused an arrest in follicular development, and that the follicles ceased to develop beyond the point reached at the time of injection.

A number of reports of dissenting opinions have appeared since, maintaining that extracts of pregnancy urine are also capable of stimulating follicular growth. Whereas some experimental evidence is such as to strongly support this contention, the validity of the results of other investigators may be seriously questioned in the light of established facts discussed above. Thus Anselmino & Hoffmann (1936) concluded that the early pregnancy urine particularly from patients suffering from hyperemesis gravidarum regularly contains gonadotrophic hormone of pituitary origin. Its presence, however, was demonstrated in intact immature rats. Klebanow (1950) maintained that qualitative differences exist with regard to the gonadotrophic effects of extracts from the placenta and decidua, respectively. Preparations from the decidua caused mainly follicle stimulation, whereas the dominating action of the hormone from the placenta was luteinization. Again, intact immature rats and mice were used as test animals. The possibility of FSH release from the pituitary gland of the test animals cannot be excluded under these experimental conditions. Both these studies, however, are interesting with regard to the fact that qualitative differences were noticed in relation to, for example, tissue of origin or stage of pregnancy. More conclusive evidence has been presented by Lyon and associates (1953), who by means of assays on hypophysectomized immature female rats could clearly demonstrate qualitative differences in gonadotrophic actions of urinary extracts from various periods of pregnancy. The urinary concentrates from the earliest period of pregnancy caused only repair and hypertrophy of interstitial tissue. However, urinary extracts from specimens after the 40th day of pregnancy, i.e., when the excretion of HCG has reached high levels, regularly caused stimulation of follicular growth in addition to luteinization.

c Unitary and dualistic concepts

A moot point still is the question whether these various actions are elicited by one single gonadotrophic substance or whether different hormonal principles are involved. With the tacit assumptions, rightly or wrongly, that storage equals production and that no post-mortem degradation of gonadotrophic hormone in the pituitary glands takes place, the repeatedly confirmed lack of pituitary gonadotrophic activity during pregnancy has been adduced in support of the unitary theory. The failure to detect any FSH production in the placenta (Smith & Smith 1937, Diczfalusy 1953, Lyon *et al.* 1953) also favours such a view. On the other hand, reports claiming the successful chemical separation of gametokinetic and luteinizing factors in pregnancy urine have appeared (Vignes *et al.* 1954, Drescher 1954, Drescher & Stange 1955, Crooke *et al.* 1958, Crooke & Butt 1959). The experimental evidence brought forward in favour of the dualistic concept has, however, been criticized (Albert & Derner 1960) both with respect to the assumed efficacy of the separation procedures and the reliability of the assay methods used. To this it may be said that the bioassays of Drescher & Stange (1955) are above criticism but that they are too few and, therefore, cannot be submitted to statistical evaluation.

The work of Albert & Derner (1960) heavily tips the balance towards a unitary view. Evaluation of the quantitative relationship between the simultaneous responses of the ovary and the uterus of the intact rat to various gonadotrophins provides a sensitive and precise method for their biological characterization and distinction (Albert *et al.* 1958; Albert & Kelly 1958). By plotting the actions of HCG on the ovary and on the uterus in absolute coordinates over a range of doses from 0·1 to 30,000 i.u. of HCG, distinct differences in the effects of preparations of human pituitary gonadotrophin were established (Albert & Derner 1960). The inference was that HCG, in addition to its interstitial cell stimulating activity, possesses intrinsic follicle-stimulating properties when given in large amounts. This conclusion is in harmony with that drawn by Hamburger (1933b, 1950) from similar experimental experience. This investigator has also focused the attention on some circumstantial evidence that strongly reduces the likelihood that the experimental effects are caused by contamination with pituitary FSH; the rise in the ovarian weight appears in approximately the same place in the curve, irrespective of hormonal source (pregnancy urine, urine from patients with testicular tumours or chorionepithelioma).

A recent study by Robyn *et al.* (1969) adds some interesting aspects to this discussion. By means of combined biological and immunological methods these authors provided evidence that HCG preparations possessed FSH-like activity which, however, was in several respects dissimilar from the FSH activity of HMG. These results, in principle, support those of Hamburger (1933b) and of Albert & Derner (1960) and indicate that the FSH-like activity of HCG preparations is not due to contamination with FSH of pituitary origin. In additional experiments Robyn *et al.* (1969) found that the FSH-like activity of HCG preparations could be quantitatively neutralized with an anti-HCG serum without completely eliminating their HCG activity. In the view of the authors these data contradict the assumption that the FSH-like activity of HCG is an evenly distributed inherent property of HCG. Among the possible explanations the simplest would be that the FSH-like activity is displayed by a separate hormone different from HCG. The successful separation of FSH and LH factors in pregnancy urine, mentioned in the preceding paragraph, adds credence to this interpretation.

Of some interest in this context is also the demonstration in pregnancy urine of a gonadotrophic substance distinctly different both from gametokinetic and luteinizing factors with respect to mechanism of action. Guyénot (1946), by means of assays on immature female guinea-pigs, distinguished a gonadotrophic principle (principe acmogène) present only during gestation, acting only in the presence of the pituitary gland, and eliciting precocious maturity in this species. The possibility of a hypophysotrophic factor stimulating secretion or release of FSH was discussed. These findings and their interpretation call to mind the clinical case of Siegmund (1932), a six year old girl with a chorioepithelioma and precocious puberty. The relation of the hypothetical hypophysiotrophic principle to the factor G of Lajos and associates (1959) has not been defined. This factor, invariably associated with HCG in the organism and apparently a glycoprotein, could be isolated from HCG by means of chromatographic separation. By itself it had no gonadal effect in intact or hypophysectomized immature rodents but provoked a strong synergistic action with HCG.

d Luteotrophic action

Browne & Venning in 1938 demonstrated a stimulating effect of HCG on the corpus luteum function. This, without doubt, represents one important physiological role of HCG. The excretion of pregnanediol in the urine was used as an index of corpus luteum function. HCG given in relatively small doses caused an increase in the total amount of pregnanediol excreted and a prolongation of the luteal phase for as long as 17 days. Brown and associates (1941) reported rather contradictory findings suggesting that the human ovary is suppressed rather than stimulated by HCG. In 12 patients with normal menstrual cycles, receiving 500 i.u. of HCG daily for 4 to 6 weeks, the majority did not exhibit any significant changes in rhythm, whereas 5 subjects experienced amenorrhoea from 1 to 5 months accompanied by a progressive atrophy of the endometrium. The authors proposed that HCG might even have a gonadotoxic effect. Subsequent work in this field, even by these latter investigators, is more harmonious with the report of Browne & Venning (1938). Thus Brown & Bradbury (1947) and Bradbury and co-workers (1950) found a definite dose dependence with pronounced effects induced by means of daily injections of 5,000 to 20,000 i.u. of the hormone. With these doses the functional activity of the corpus luteum was prolonged, giving rise to a condition of pseudopregnancy with delay of menstruation. On the other hand, HCG failed to induce follicular growth or to stimulate a regressing corpus luteum. The action of HCG was thus limited to a pre-existing, functional corpus luteum. The results of Segaloff and co-workers (1951) also support the concept that HCG in relatively large doses has a luteotrophic action. These investigators confirmed earlier observations on postponed bleeding and pregnancy-like decidual changes in the endometrium and also added some significant findings on HCG-stimulated ovaries. Conspicuous theca-luteinization of many of the follicles and accumulation of theca-lutein cells in and about the scars of atretic follicles were frequent findings.

Experience accumulated from studies on laboratory animals also support the contention of a luteotrophic action of HCG. Thus Hisaw (1944) examined the effects of daily injections of HCG on monkeys. The administration was begun between the 18th and 24th days and continued until the next menstruation. The average length of the experimental cycles was increased to 41·9 days from a normal average of 26·5 days. The prolongation of the functional life of the corpus luteum was associated with histological changes in the corpora lutea comparable with those found during the first month of normal pregnancy and with vascular changes in the endometrium similar to those described in the pregnant uterus of this species. Bryans (1951) completely confirmed these findings and also produced experimental evidence showing that the extension of the length of the luteal phase was associated with the continued presence of progesterone in the blood. Velardo (1959), finally, reported induction of ovulation in adult rats, presumably through a synergistic action with pituitary hormones, and prolongation of the pseudopregnant state.

e Metabolic effects

Comparatively few studies on the effects of HCG on the steroid metabolism in the ovary have been carried out. Rice and associates (1964a), however, when demonstrating that the incubation of slices from human corpus luteum tissue with acetate-1-C^{14} leads to the formation of a large number of labelled steroids, reported that HCG enhances these biosynthetic processes and particularly the formation of progesterone. In additional studies these investigators (Rice *et al.* 1964b) found that normal human ovarian stromal tissue induced the synthesis of radioactive testosterone *in vitro* from acetate-1-C^{14} and that HCG had a stimulating effect also on this metabolic activity.

3 EFFECTS ON THE TESTIS

a Interstitial cell stimulation

The effects of HCG on testicular tissue have been the subject of a large number of studies. In normal male animals hypertrophy of the interstitial tissue and enlargement of the secondary sex organs have been uniformly described after administration of HCG. The stimulation of testicular endocrine activity in terms of the production of male sex hormones was thus an early observation (Collip *et al.* 1933a, b, Smith & Leonard 1934, Evans *et al.* 1934b). In man the interstitial cell stimulating effect of HCG is also pronounced (Maddock & Nelson 1951, 1952).

b Gametokinetic properties

The findings with regard to the response of the seminiferous tubules have been less unanimous. In intact animals all testicular elements may undergo stimulation, which led some investigators to assume a gametokinetic activity of the hormone. Collip and associates (1933a, b), on the basis of experiments on hypophysectomized rats, definitely denied a favourable influence on the seminiferous tubules. Yet, Smith & Leonard (1934), Evans and associates (1934b) and Evans & Simpson (1950) under similar experimental conditions found that HCG caused a considerable increase of testicular weight and maintained spermatogenesis, mating, and fertility. It would seem, however, from the work of Smith & Leonard (1934) that the gametokinetic properties of HCG are dependent on the interval between hypophysectomy and administration of the hormone and the degree of maturity of the animal at the time of operation. Thus, Diczfalusy and co-workers (1950) were unable to detect any stimulating effects of HCG on tubules or germ cells in immature rats hypophysectomized at 22 days of age. The actions of HCG in male laboratory animals have recently been summarized by Noble & Plunkett (1955). It appears safe to conclude that the effects of HCG on testicular tissue are limited to repair and stimulation of the interstitial cells, and that the observed action on the seminiferous tubules is due to a synergistic action between HCG and pituitary gonadotrophins in the intact animal, and is secondary to androgens produced by the stimulated Leydig cells in hypophysectomized animal.

The actions on HCG on the human testis are, in principle, similar to those observed in laboratory animals. Maddock & Nelson (1951, 1952) observed a substantial increase in the number of Leydig cells associated with regressive changes in the seminiferous tubules. The mechanism underlying these changes was assumed to reside in a direct action of HCG on the interstitial cells and an indirect action on the tubular apparatus *via* enhanced oestrogen and androgen secretion and a negative feedback on pituitary FSH secretion. In the light of recent work these changes seem to be transitory and reversible (Glass & Holland 1963; Turner *et al.* 1964).

c Metabolic effects

Parallel with these observations on morphological alterations in the testis induced by HCG certain functional actions have also been noticed. Maddock & Nelson (1951, 1952) found that adult men with functioning testes receiving HCG exhibited an increased rate of urinary 17-ketosteroid excretion. This finding has been repeatedly confirmed (Hibbitt *et al.* 1958, Jayle *et al.* 1959, 1962, Morse *et al.* 1962, Reiss *et al.* 1963). The response was, however, variable, which is probably due to the fact that the rise in excretion is limited to a fraction of the 17-ketosteroids, namely androsterone and aetiocholanolone (Halkerston *et al.* 1957, Jayle *et al.* 1962), whereas rather inconsiderable fluctuations in the excretion rate of dehydroepiandrosterone and of 11-oxy-17-ketosteroids were observed (Jayle *et al.* 1962). It is believed that the testes are the major source of the increased secretion of androgens. This concept is supported by the finding of Eik-Nes and co-workers (1959) that HCG administered to normal human males causes a significant increase in the concentration of plasma androsterone, which is not observed in normal young women. More direct evidence has been produced by Brinck-Johnsen & Eik-Nes (1957) who found increased concentrations of testosterone and androstenedione in spermatic vein blood from dogs following administration of HCG, and by Savard and associates (1961) and Lindner (1961) who have described a considerable rise in the testosterone secretion rate in the spermatic vein of bulls receiving the same treatment. Ibayashi and associates (1965), finally, have observed a definite increase in both testosterone and dehydroepiandrosterone secretion following HCG administration to dogs.

Some insight into the metabolic events underlying these effects has also been gained. Brady (1951) found that *in vitro* biosynthesis by rabbit testicular tissue of testosterone from C^{14}-labelled acetate was markedly accelerated by HCG. Hall & Eik-Nes (1962) found the same effect 1 hour after a single intravenous injection of HCG. A rapid effect of HCG was also found in dogs with an immediate increase in the *in vivo* conversion of 17α-hydroxypregnenolone to 17α-hydroxyprogesterone as well as an increase in testosterone production (Hagen & Eik-Nes 1964). HCG given *in vivo* also enhances the conversion of cholesterol to androstenedione by homogenates of testis from hypophysectomized rats (Hall & Eik-Nes 1963). The response, however, is delayed and the lag phase has been interpreted to indicate that HCG also elicits a non-specific stimulation of the testes. This response would then be similar in nature to the increase in 3β-hydroxysteroid dehydrogenase in the testicular tissue of hypophysectomized rats given HCG (Samuels & Helmreich 1956).

It has long been known that the testis is a major source of oestrogens. Castration causes a drop in the urinary oestrogen level (Scott & Vermeulen 1942) and oestrogens have been recovered from human testicular tissue by Goldzieher & Roberts (1952). Maddock & Nelson (1951, 1952), by means of a bioassay method, noted an increase in the urinary excretion rate from 5 to 16 times pretreatment levels when HCG was given to adult men with functioning testes. This effect was not elicited in men lacking testicular function. These authors also established a relationship between Leydig cell stimulation and increase in oestrogen excretion after administration of HCG. Jayle and associates (1959), by means of a chemical determination procedure, found an approximately 3-fold increase in urinary oestrogen excretion in normal males between 20 and 50 years of age receiving HCG. Separation of the oestrogens into the three standard fractions indicated that HCG elicited an increase of each fraction (Diczfalusy 1957; Jayle *et al.* 1962; Morse *et al.* 1962).

4 EFFECTS ON THE ADRENAL

The question whether HCG has any direct actions on the adrenal is highly controversial. There is experimental evidence both for and against a stimulatory effect on the adrenocortical hormone secretion. Thus, Plate (1952), after injecting relatively large doses of HCG in 2 female castrates and a eunuchoid man with marked testicular atrophy, noticed a rise in the urinary excretion of 17-ketosteroids. Borell (1954), on administration of a large dose of HCG to 17 regularly menstruating women, to one post-menopausal subject, and to 5 ovariectomized patients, reported similar findings. Decio (1955), after studies on a very limited case material, made the same statement, and Birke and co-workers (1954), by means of infrared spectrography, observed a slight tendency to an increase of the urinary excretion of androsterone and aetiocholanolone in 2 orchiectomized patients receiving HCG.

A number of reports of dissenting opinions have been published. Borth and associates (1953) have presented a detailed summary of the earlier literature and also added some of their own observations. In 6 surgically castrated women no effect of HCG on the urinary excretion of oestrone-oestradiol, 17-ketosteroids or corticoids could be observed. Hibbitt and co-workers (1958) compared the response of the urinary 17-hydroxycorticosteroid and 17-ketosteroid levels to the slow intravenous administration of HCG and ACTH to 17 subjects with normal adrenocortical and testicular function. A distinct difference could be noticed. HCG elicited a significant response of the 17-ketosteroid excretion. It was increased already on the first day of infusion, and in some patients remained so for 5 or 6 days after termination of HCG administration. In a few subjects there was also a rise in 17-hydroxycorticosteroid excretion, although the mean level for the whole group was not increased. ACTH, on the other hand, caused a prompt increase in the excretion rate of both types of steroid with a dominance of 17-hydroxycorticosteroids. The levels remained high during the time of infusion, and returned to pretreatment levels immediately after termination. The difference in the patterns of response to the trophic hormones and the failure of HCG to elicit a regular increase in 17-hydroxycorticosteroid excretion was interpreted to indicate either a lack of response or a different response of the adrenals to HCG. The work of Eik-Nes and associates (1959) may also be quoted in support of this opinion. They found an increase in the concentration of plasma androsterone subsequent to administration of HCG to normal human males, whereas the plasma androsterone level remained uninfluenced in normal women. An irregular increase in the level of plasma 17-hydroxycorticosteroids regardless of sex was observed.

Experience gained from experiments on laboratory animals is also controversial. Diczfalusy and associates (1950) in a group of hypophysectomized-gonadectomized male immature rats observed no weight increase of the adrenals after treatment with large doses of HCG, whereas Velardo (1959) observed a slight but statistically significant weight increase of the adrenals both from intact immature and hypophysectomized female rats receiving HCG.

It is difficult to present an interpretation of these disparate results. In any case it seems reasonable to keep in mind two factors of importance which may provide a possible explanation. It is known that administration of oestrogen causes hypertrophy of the adrenal cortex (Tepperman *et al.* 1943), and in any experimental situation involving enhanced oestrogen production indirect stimulation of the adrenal may also occur. This mechanism operates through the release of ACTH and thus postulates the presence of an intact hypophysis. Another explanation to the variable response is the possibility of a stress reaction to the slightly painful injection of HCG as suggested by Eik-Nes and associates (1959). Also in this case the adrenal reaction would be directly elicited by ACTH and the requirement of intact pituitary function is obvious.

5 EFFECTS ON PLACENTAL METABOLISM

Smith & Smith (1934, 1937, 1939, 1948) proposed that metabolic relationships exist between HCG and the steroid metabolism of the human placenta. They had noticed that the precipitous decrease in serum HCG around the 12th week of normal pregnancy was associated with a pronounced increase in the urinary excretion of oestrogens and, furthermore, that the decrease in the excretion of oestrogens immediately before labour was accompanied by an increase of serum HCG. In addition, they had observed an abnormal elevation of serum HCG levels in some patients suffering from toxaemia of pregnancy coinciding with progressively diminishing oestrogen concentrations in the urine. On the basis of these findings and other circumstantial evidence (Smith & Smith 1948) they assumed that HCG had an influence on certain metabolic pathways of oestrogens, and that the abnormal reversed relationship between HCG and oestrogens in some patients with toxaemia was due to deficient utilization of HCG.

It is not until the recent researches of Troen & Gordon (1958) and Troen (1959, 1961) that more precise and experimentally founded information on the metabolic activity of HCG has become available. The experiments were carried out on perfused intact term placentas. Troen & Gordon (1958) could clearly demonstrate that the citrate metabolism remained unimpaired for many hours under these conditions, that oestradiol-17β added to the perfusion fluid had no effect on this metabolism, that the addition of HCG caused a significant increase in citrate disappearance during the whole experimental period (8 hours), and that HCG and oestradiol-17β when added together had a statistically significant effect on the mean hourly utilization of citrate. The hormone-induced enhancement of citrate utilization was completely blocked when the perfusion fluid contained fluoroacetate, indicating that the hormonal action is transmitted through enzymatic pathways.

Another highly interesting metabolic action of HCG has also been demonstrated by Troen (1959, 1961). When C^{14}-labelled oestradiol-17β was added to the perfusion fluid two peaks of radioactivity were obtained, coinciding with the observed distribution of added oestrone and oestradiol as determined by fluorimetry. If HCG was also present in the perfusion fluid, other experimental conditions being equal, the additional conversion of oestradiol to oestriol could also be shown. As oestriol is the quantitatively dominating oestrogen of human pregnancy urine and as its origin during pregnancy is somewhat controversial, this apparent relationship between HCG and oestrogen metabolism may be of considerable importance for our understanding of the physiological significance of HCG in the latter part of pregnancy. Before the newly discovered effects of HCG on citrate and oestrogen metabolism its role in the second half of gestation was completely enigmatic.

Cédard and co-workers (1961, 1962, 1964) have, in principle, confirmed the results of Troen (1959, 1961). They have also noticed a stimulative effect of HCG on the aromatization of neutral and phenolic steroids, and maintain that this effect is achieved through activation of the hydroxylation process (Cédard *et al.* 1964; Varangot *et al.* 1965).

In the light of recent work on the oestrogen metabolism of the foeto-placental unit (Diczfalusy 1966, Jackanicz & Diczfalusy 1968, Reynolds *et al.* 1968) it is wise at present to accept these data with some reservation. In experiments on placentas from mid-pregnancy it has been conclusively shown that the organ lacks the capacity of 16α-hydroxylation and that 16α-hydroxylated intermediates are required as precursors to oestriol. It is probable that the same conditions prevail in the term placenta. It would seem that the substance assumed to be oestriol in the above-mentioned studies is in fact 6α-hydroxyestradiol-17β (Cédard & Knuppen 1965, Alonso & Troen 1966).

Troen (1961) suggests that the demonstration of the biological actions of HCG supports the assumption of autoregulatory processes in placental function. It is well known that the placenta displays a high degree of autonomy in several respects. This refers, *inter alia*, to growth

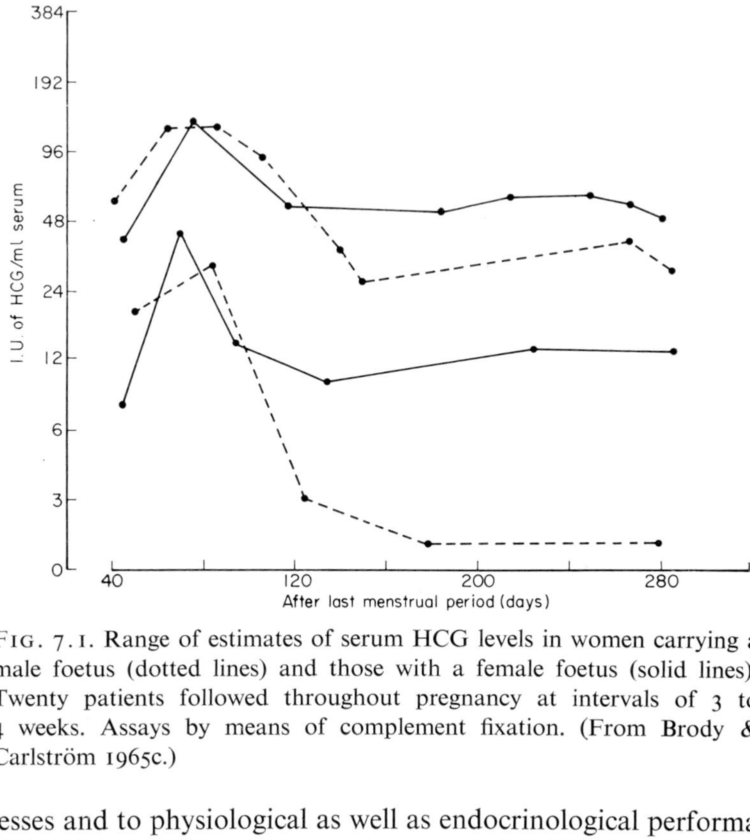

FIG. 7.1. Range of estimates of serum HCG levels in women carrying a male foetus (dotted lines) and those with a female foetus (solid lines). Twenty patients followed throughout pregnancy at intervals of 3 to 4 weeks. Assays by means of complement fixation. (From Brody & Carlström 1965c.)

processes and to physiological as well as endocrinological performance. The latter function is unique among the glands of internal secretion in that the activity of several endocrines are here integrated in one organ. The most obvious example is the production of both gonadotrophic and steroid hormones in the placenta. But even though a high degree of auto-regulatory activity is exercised by the placenta versus the maternal organism, it is possible that the foetus may have a profound influence on placental function. The demonstration of a relation between the sex of the foetus and the maternal HCG level in the last trimester of pregnancy

(Brody & Carlström 1965a, b) favours such an assumption. In women with low HCG values there was a predominance of male foetuses, and in subjects with high levels a preponderance of female foetuses was observed. The difference between the two groups was statistically significant. This finding suggests the possibility of a foetal control mechanism of placental HCG production or an inherent sex-determined difference in metabolic activity as regards this biosynthetic function of the placenta (Fig. 7.1).

C ANTIGENICAL PROPERTIES

I THE THEORY OF ANTIHORMONES

It was an early and repeatedly confirmed observation that prolonged parenteral administration to experimental animals of gonadotrophic hormones gradually diminished and finally extinguished their physiological effects. This sequence of events was demonstrated both with the gonadotrophic hormone from pregnancy urine (Zondek 1930a, 1935, Selye *et al.* 1934a, b) and with pituitary gonadotrophins (Korenchevsky 1930, Collip 1932, McPhail 1933). The refractory state could only be induced by injecting protein hormones into an animal of a heterologous species, whereas the administration of homologous hormone preparations failed to show any decrease in stimulating activity (Smith 1930). An additional important finding was the observation that the condition of unresponsiveness was caused by a humoral factor, and that the inhibitory effect was passively transferable as evidenced by the fact that sera from resistant animals protected test animals from the specific effects of the corresponding hormone (Selye *et al.* 1934a; Bachman *et al.* 1934).

The problem of the nature of the protective substances attracted considerable interest. The first serious attempt to explain these experimental findings and to provide a working hypothesis for further experimentation was done by Collip (1934, 1935) when he formulated his antihormone theory which may be summarized as follows: 'For each hormone there may be an opposite or antagonistic principle. This antagonist is present in the normal subject but may not be detected until it exceeds in amount the hormonal substance with which it is balanced'. Collip and co-workers adduced a number of experimental data which were interpreted to indicate that antigonadotrophic substances were hormones with reverse properties.

2 THE CONCEPT OF A SPECIAL IMMUNE BODY RESPONSE

Twombly (1936), Zondek & Sulman (1937a–e, 1942) and Zondek and co-workers (1938, 1939) in a series of publications arrived at a considerably different conclusion, namely that the antigonadotrophic factor was an immune body. Points of importance in favour of this opinion were the protein nature of all hormones known to produce antihormones, species specificity of the reaction, the globulin nature of the antigonadotrophic principle, the engagement of the reticuloendothelial system in the formation of the inhibitory substance and the necessity to induce its formation on a heterologous species.

One crux remained, however, residing in the fact that the antigonadotrophic factor could only be demonstrated by its inhibitory activity *in vivo* (Selye *et al.* 1934a, b, Bachman *et al.* 1934, Twombly & Ferguson 1934, Twombly 1936, Sulman 1937, Zondek & Sulman 1937a–e, Freud & Uyldert 1947) and not by means of any of the usual serological *in vitro* reactions. Many attempts had been made, but none withstood critical analysis. Precipitating and complement-fixing antibodies had been obtained by immunization with gonadotrophic hormone prepared from pregnancy urine (Bachman 1935, Twombly 1936, van den Ende 1939). Completely unspecific antisera when used in *in vitro* reactions had, however, been prepared as evidenced by the presence of uniform cross reactions of the hyperimmune sera with the gonadotrophic preparation as well as with extracts from male urine (Bachman 1935), by the finding of equally strong reactions with normal male and female sera as with pregnancy sera (Bachman 1935), and by the results of absorption experiments van den Ende 1939). Sulman (1937), using the complement fixation test, concluded that the purified gonadotrophic hormone from pregnancy urine had no *in vitro* antigenical activity. On the basis of these findings and conclusions the theory was, therefore, advanced that the antigonadotrophic factor represented a new type of blood substance closely related to but not identical with the immune bodies (Zondek & Sulman 1942). Thompson (1941) in an authoritative review on antihormones arrived at the same conclusion.

3 THE DEMONSTRATION OF A CONVENTIONAL ANTIBODY RESPONSE

This was the state of matters when Bussard & Grabar (1947, 1948, 1949) in a series of papers presented results of investigations carried out with a view to comparing the *in vivo* inhibitory effect of antigonadotrophic sera with their capacity to precipitate and neutralize the hormone *in vitro*. In contrast to earlier reports (Meyer & Wolfe 1939, van den Ende 1939) they demonstrated the persistence of precipitating antibodies after absorption with nonpregnant sera and urinary specimens, also a certain relation between *in vivo* and *in vitro* effects, and the lack of gonadotrophic activity in the specific precipitate, and the release of such activity from the precipitate after treatment with ethanol. The success was apparently due to the employment of an adjuvant procedure, (aluminium-adsorbed gonadotrophin) and the use of relatively pure hormone preparations. It is difficult, however, to assess the purity of their preparations, as the specific activity is defined in terms of animal units and not in international units. In 1950 Schuyler and co-workers also prepared antisera against HCG that apparently had the capacity to precipitate the hormone. Positive reactions were obtained with HCG preparations as well as with urinary specimens from pregnant women. Quite a few falsely positive reactions, however, were also encountered. Absorption of antisera with non-pregnant urine improved the results. No adjuvant was used in these investigations, and the specific activity of the hormone preparation employed for immunization is not given. The studies of Bussard & Grabar (1947, 1948, 1949) as well as those of Schuyler and co-workers (1950) were carried out with the clearly stated objective of establishing a serological procedure for the detection of HCG in body fluids. The results, however, seem to indicate lack of sufficient accuracy and reliability of the procedures employed.

For a decade attempts to employ serological techniques for the assay of HCG were in abeyance. The break-through occurred in 1960. This year Brody & Carlström (1960) published their results obtained with the complement fixation test, McKean (1960) reported data from experiments performed with the precipitin reaction, and Swierczynska & Samochowiec (1960) as well as Wide & Gemzell (1960) described analyses carried out with the haemagglutination-inhibition reaction. A detailed presentation of the different techniques employed will be given later (Section F.5).

D SITE OF SYNTHESIS

1 TISSUES OF PRODUCTION

HCG was originally assumed to be produced in the hypophysis (Aschheim & Zondek 1927, Zondek & Aschheim 1928). This opinion was early challenged in view of the demonstrated lack of gonadotrophic activity in the pituitary of pregnant women (for references, see Section B. 1). The final proof, required by Zondek, that the excretion of HCG remains unchanged after hypophysectomy has also been presented. The urinary HCG pattern in a hypophysectomized woman was found to be normal throughout pregnancy (Little *et al.* 1958).

There is now indirect as well as direct evidence which conclusively indicates that HCG is synthesized in chorionic tissue. It is found only in tissues and body fluids of normal pregnant women and in patients with hydatidiform mole, chorioadenoma destruens, and choriocarcinoma of the uterus or testis. It is rapidly eliminated from the body after delivery (Johnson *et al.* 1950, Bruner 1951, Albert & Berkson 1951), after spontaneous or therapeutic abortion (Bruner 1951, Brody & Carlström 1962a, Wide 1962), or cure of any of the pathological conditions with trophoblastic tumours.

The beautiful studies of Kido (1937) furnished direct proof of placental production of HCG. Transplantation of chorionic tissue to the anterior chamber of the eye of the rabbit led to growth of the tissue, typical HCG effects on the ovaries of the host, and excretion of HCG in in the urine of the host in larger amounts than could be accounted for by the amount of hormone present in the inoculum. These experiments have been repeated and confirmed (Gurchot *et al.* 1947, Stewart 1951). Gonadotrophic activity of intratesticular implants of human placental tissue in guinea pigs (Grenier & Rebel 1946) and of choriocarcinoma tissue in hamster cheek pouches (Hertz 1959) has also been demonstrated.

The synthesis of HCG by chorionic tissue has also been established in a large number of tissue culture studies. Analyses on cell free supernatant fluid showed the production of HCG as assayed both qualitatively and quantitatively, (Gey *et al.* 1938, Seegar & Gey 1940, Jones *et al.* 1943, Stewart *et al.* 1948, Neuweiler & Herrmann 1953, Soma *et al.* 1961). All investigators found production of HCG in explants of early placental tissue, whereas Stewart and associates (1948) were unable to confirm the finding of Seegar & Gey (1940) and Jones and co-workers (1943) on the synthesis of HCG in tissue cultures from full-term placentas. Specimens cultured from hydatidiform moles were particularly active and could be sustained for long periods of time (Gey *et al.* 1938, Waltz *et al.* 1954).

The role of the foetus in connection with placental HCG production is not quite clear. Sufficient evidence is at hand to indicate that excretion of HCG continues after spontaneous (Brouha & Hinglais 1931, Spielman *et al.* 1933, von Arvay 1934, Zondek 1954, Brody & Carlström 1965a) as well as induced (Cassmer 1959) intrauterine death of the foetus, whenever the whole or parts of the placenta are retained. The presence of HCG in urine may also be detected for several months after termination of abdominal pregnancy, when the foetus is removed but the placenta left *in situ* for resorption. Yet, the foetus may possibly exert a modifying influence on the secretion pattern. This is suggested by the finding of a relation between the sex of the foetus and the serum HCG levels in the latter half of gestation (Brody & Carlström 1965b, c).

2 CELLS OF ORIGIN

There is a general consensus of opinion that HCG is produced in the trophoblastic cells. Some disagreement, however, exists as to whether the hormone is produced in the cytotrophoblast (Langhans cells) or in the syncytiotrophoblast of the chorionic villi, or possibly also in the cytotrophoblast of the cell columns and the trophoblastic shell. The results of some investigations indicate the possibility that HCG may be produced at all these sites. In addition, evidence has been presented showing that the amnion epithelium may also be a locus of HCG synthesis.

Attempts to trace the cellular localization of HCG, which has in the majority of reports been tacitly assumed to equal the site of production, have been made with various techniques, such as comparative histological examination of HCG-producing tissues and assay of the urinary excretion level of the hormone, comparative tissue culture studies and analyses of HCG production *in vitro*, histochemical methods, and in the last few years immunohistochemical procedures. Until recently, the current concept favoured the idea that HCG is produced in the Langhans cells. Lately, however, findings have been made, *inter alia*, with the fluorescent antibody technique, that cast some doubt on this assumption. These studies rather indicate the syncytiotrophoblast to be the site of synthesis. In addition, some evidence has been presented based on ultra-structure studies compatible with the interpretation that these cells are differentiated Langhans cells and, in contrast to these latter cells, endowed with the capacity of considerable protein synthesis.

a Evidence in favour of HCG production in the Langhans cells

Already in 1938 Gey and co-workers suggested an association between the vigorous growth in tissue culture of cells resembling Langhans cells and the *in vitro* synthesis of HCG. These studies were extended and confirmed (Jones *et al.* 1943; Stewart *et al.* 1948; Stewart 1951). The results of Tenney & Parker (1939) on the rough correspondence between the amount of HCG found and the amount of trophoblastic cells in the placenta or mole were interpreted to suggest that actively proliferating cytotrophoblast was more important in the production of HCG than the derivative syncytium (Wislocki & Bennett 1943). Furthermore, some histochemical evidence has been presented pointing in the same direction. Most investigations with this technique are based on attempts to demonstrate the carbohydrate moiety of the hormone. The periodic-acid Schiff (PAS) staining method, elaborated by McManus (1946) and Hotchkiss (1948), has been used for the visualization of polysacharides. After removal of glycogen by pre-treatment with diastase and of acid mucopolysacharides by the use of hyaluronidase (Asboe-Hansen 1951) the PAS reaction may reveal the presence of the carbohydrate fraction of the hormone with greater certainty. Zilliacus (1953) and Botella-Llusia and co-workers (1957) found PAS-positive material in the Langhans cells of enzyme-treated placentas from early pregnancies. Weber (1963), apparently not employing enzymatic pre-treatment, also reported a positive PAS reaction in these cells of early placentas, no such reaction being elicited in corresponding cells of term placentas. Finally, results have been obtained by means of immunofluorescent staining which have also been adduced in support of the opinion that HCG is synthesized in the Langhans cells (Thiede & Choate 1963). Treatment of sections of quick-frozen placental tissue with HCG-antisera and subsequent staining by means of fluorescein-conjugated anti-rabbit γ-globulin, (indirect immunofluorescent staining, see Section F. 5), gave a positive fluorescence in the Langhans cells of immature placentas, and to a lesser degree also in those of term placentas.

b Evidence in favour of HCG production in the syncytiotrophoblastic layer

In 1944 Baker and associates on the basis of histochemical findings assumed that HCG is produced in the syncytial layer of the chorionic villi. A more or less positive PAS reaction in these cells without (Pali & Lajos 1952) and after enzyme pre-treatment (Zilliacus 1953, Botella-Llusia *et al.* 1957, McKay *et al.* 1958, Wislocki & Padycula 1961, Szontágh & Traub 1962, Dallenbach-Hellweg & Nette 1963), has also been presented in favour of such an interpretation. Furthermore, in tissue culture studies on cells obtained ftom trypsinized villi of mostly early placentas, Soma and associates (1961) found a relation between the number of giant multinuclear cells and the amount of HCG in the nutritive medium. The most suggestive findings indicating that HCG is synthesized in the syncytial cells have, however, been obtained by means of immunohistochemical techniques (Midgley & Pierce 1962, Leznoff & Davis 1963, Thiede & Choate 1963). Midgley & Pierce (1962) used fluorescein-labelled HCG-antisera, (direct immunofluorescent staining, see Section F.5), whereas the other groups used the indirect method. Midgley & Pierce (1962) found positive fluorescence in the syncytiotrophoblastic cells of immature placentas, hydatidiform mole, chorioadenoma destruens, and choriocarcinoma, whereas no stainable HCG was detected in term placentas. Leznoff & Davis (1963) noticed a bright fluorescence in the cytoplasm of the syncytial cells of the chorionic villi in all sections of placentas of less than 14 weeks gestation, but also in the corresponding cells of several term placentas. In choriocarcinomas specific fluorescence was seen in the syncytial giant cells. Thiede & Choate (1963) reported an intense fluorescence in the cytoplasm of the syncytium of all villi of early and of a majority of term placentas.

c Evidence in favour of HCG production in the cytotrophoblastic cells of the basal plate and the placental septa

Wislocki (1951), on the basis of the presence in the basal cytotrophoblast at term of strongly PAS positive, diastase-resistant cytoplasmic components, assumed that HCG could be synthesized in these cells during the last part of pregnancy. Similar results were also obtained by Thomsen (1958), Thomsen & Willemsen (1956), Lewin (1960), Weber (1963), and Dallenbach-Hellweg & Nette (1963). Thiede & Choate (1963) with indirect immunofluorescent staining found positive fluorescence in the cytotrophoblast of the cell columns and of the anchoring villi.

d Evidence in favour of HCG production in the foetal membranes

Stamm & Riotton (1958) found PAS positive material in the chorial cell layer from normal pregnancies and therefore assumed that these cells took part in the synthesis of HCG. Weber (1963) also reported positive PAS reaction in cytotrophoblasts of the chorion laeve. Thiede & Choate

(1963) with their immunohistological technique described an intense fluorescence in the epithelium of the amnion investing the foetal surface of the placenta as well as that adjacent to the chorion.

e Critical discussion

As is obvious from this review of the literature it seems at present very difficult to point out a particular cell which may be exclusively responsible for the synthesis of HCG. A number of objections may be raised against the various techniques employed. Thus, it has been maintained that the identification of the Langhans cells in tissue culture is rendered extremely difficult due to loss of cytologic characteristics under such conditions (Neuweiler & Herrmann 1953, Waltz *et al.* 1954). On the assumption that this opinion is correct, stress should be laid on the association between giant multinuclear cells in the tissue culture and HCG production *in vitro* (Soma *et al.* 1961). Considerable doubt as to the validity of conclusions based on histochemical findings has also been raised. Aside from the problem of the specificity of these reactions, it may be questioned whether enough HCG is present in the cells to account for droplet staining. Diczfalusy (1953) found a maximum of about 500 i.u. of HCG per g. wet weight of placenta in the peak period. In the light of the reported specific activity of HCG being in the range of 12,000 i.u. per mg (Got 1951) this would mean the presence of approximately 40 μg per g wet tissue at most and in the majority of placentas the concentration of hormone would be much less. This amount would hardly be detectable by histochemical means.

The introduction of immunohistological methods has definitely tipped the scale to the advantage of the syncytiotrophoblastic cells as the main site of synthesis of HCG. Midgley & Pierce (1962) were able to observe positive fluorescence only in the syncytial layer, and furthermore only in early placentas. Leznoff & Davis (1963) confirmed this cellular localization of the fluorescence, but could also, apparently due to the higher sensitivity of the indirect fluorescent antibody technique, report positive fluorescence in term placentas. Thiede & Choate (1963) also confirmed the findings of Midgley & Pierce (1962) but, in addition, also found some fluorescence in the cytotrophoblast. This discrepant result may possibly be understood in the light of the recent electron microscopical findings of Midgley & Pierce (1962) which strongly support the view that syncytiotrophoblast is derived by differentiation from cytotrophoblast. The former cells have a cytoplasm which is highly organized with a well-developed endoplasmic reticulum forming dilated ribonucleoprotein-containing cisternas. These structures are known to be associated with protein synthesis. On the other hand, the cytoplasmic arrangement in the cytotrophoblast is characterized by the presence of ribosomes in dispersed form, which has been interpreted to indicate the production of structural protein and thus typical for a very immature cell type. The findings of Thiede & Choate (1963) may then tentatively be interpreted to indicate that the production of HCG in the cytotrophoblast may start somewhat before the transition of these cells into syncytial cells takes place.

E METABOLISM AND EXCRETION

Relatively little is known about the metabolism of HCG and its exact fate in the human organism, particularly during pregnancy, is still a matter of conjecture. Zondek & Sulman (1945) have summarized earlier investigations on these problems and also added some observations of their own. In experiments on rats they found that after the administration of a large amount of HCG only 50 per cent of the dose could be recovered from the body of the animal after an hour, and after 24 hours, when stimulation of the target organ sets in, only a small fraction, (about 10 per cent), of the hormone can be recovered. The rate of inactivation thus follows a logarithmic curve. The urinary excretion of the injected HCG amounts, on an average, to approximately 5 to 10 per cent of the injected dose.

This picture was derived from experiments on non-primate animals. Due to the heterologous character of the injected hormone some doubt was expressed as to the significance of these findings as regards human beings (Johnson *et al.* 1950). These investigators examined the rate of disappearance of HCG from serum and urine *post partum*. After 12 hours no positive reactions were seen in serum, whereas the extinction point of the bioassay procedure on urine was reached first after 36 hours. These differences in the rate of elimination of HCG from blood and urine have also been noticed with immunological techniques (Brody & Carlström 1965a), although a somewhat longer persistence of the hormone in the body was seen in this study. The higher sensitivity of the immunoassay procedures used may explain the discrepancy. It would seem, however, that the rate of elimination of HCG from blood follows a logarithmic function in the human being (Brody & Carlström, unpublished results).

Johnson and co-workers (1950) found that no more than 5·8 per cent of the serum gonadotrophin was eliminated by the kidneys, which is at variance with earlier as well as later reports indicating values between 20 per cent to about 100 per cent (Friedman & Weinstein 1937, Bradbury & Brown 1948, Lloyd *et al.* 1949, Knorr 1961). One possible explanation of these divergent results may be that the findings of Johnson and associates (1950) are based on studies on pregnant women and that the metabolism of HCG is altered during gestation. The nature of the extrarenal disposal of HCG is entirely unknown.

A number of investigators have estimated the renal clearance of HCG in normal and abnormal pregnancy (Gastineau *et al.* 1949, Loraine 1950b, Johnson *et al.* 1950). In all these studies the clearance rate was found to be less than 1 ml per minute and essentially constant throughout pregnancy. The conclusion is therefore warranted (Loraine 1958) that variations in the HCG concentration throughout pregnancy rather reflect changes in the rate of production and destruction of the hormone than alterations in the rate of renal excretion.

F METHODS OF DETERMINATION

1 GENERAL

Repeated attempts have been made to devise a chemical method for the determination of HCG, but no such procedure is available at present. This situation is partly due to lack of chemical or physico-chemical techniques capable of recognizing minute amounts of a specific protein in the presence of large quantities of other proteins, and partly to the inadequacy of existing methods to distinguish a protein in concentrations such as HCG occurs in under physiological conditions.

The assay of HCG, therefore, has to be based on well-defined and easily measurable activities of the hormone. A great number of its biological actions have formed the basis for an equally large number of bioassay procedures. These methods, when carried out under strictly standardized conditions, require a considerable set of animals and are, therefore, expensive and time-consuming. These circumstances, *inter alia*, have made it desirable to find other techniques for measurement. Such methods, taking advantage of the antigenic properties of HCG, have now been devised.

A number of reviews have been devoted to the principles which should govern biological determination methods for HCG and to the problems associated with the application of different assay procedures. Particular mention should be made of the excellent contributions by Emmens (1939), Thayer (1946), Loraine (1950a, 1956, 1957, 1958, 1961), Hamburger (1950, 1957), Borth (1952), Diczfalusy (1953, 1954), and Diczfalusy & Loraine (1955). No similar review dealing with the principles and practice of the various immunological methods now in use for the detection and assay of HCG has yet appeared.

2 PRINCIPLES OF ASSAY

a Criteria of validity

Quantitative bioassays or immunoassays should yield unbiased estimates of potency and of the limits within which the estimate falls at a given level of probability. Certain conditions pertaining to, *inter alia*, dose-response relationship and experimental design must be established to permit the extraction of statistically valid and meaningful data. These requirements as well as the special type of statistics necessary for the evaluation of the assay results have been authoritatively dealt with by Emmens (1948, 1950), Bliss (1952), Finney (1952), Gaddum (1953a, b), Diczfalusy (1954), and Borth and associates (1957a).

The characteristic standards set up for the relation between dose and response are regression and linearity. Regression indicates increase or decrease of the effect metameter with change of dose. The slope should be relatively steep, the magnitude of the variation around the line small, and the variance constant at all levels of response. Linearity implies that the relationship between log dose and response is satisfied by a straight line. When comparing the potency of 2 preparations it is necessary that they have similar biological or serological activity. This is indicated by the parallel course of the dose-response curves. The 2 preparations should always be assayed simultaneously in order to avoid the introduction of errors due to variation in sensitivity of the test animals or of the serological system.

b Criteria of reliability

A complete set of standard characteristics for analytical procedures has been formulated by Borth (1952). Among these the criteria of reliability are the most important, including the factors of sensitivity, specificity, accuracy, and precision. Short definitions will be given here to facilitate the further discussion.

Sensitivity indicates the minimum detectable amount of a substance or of a biological or serological activity, significantly different from zero. Specificity refers to the power of a given method to discriminate exclusively the substance or the activity under study. In instances where a comparative analysis between a purified product of the substance and the pure chemical entity is not possible, it is necessary to resort to circumstantial rather than absolute evidence. Accuracy is defined as the capacity of a method to measure the true value, which may be estimated by means of recovery experiments. Precision, finally, denotes the reproducibility of the analytical results and may be calculated by statistical evaluation of the variation of individual measurements.

Whereas estimates of sensitivity, specificity, and accuracy may be used for direct comparison of methods this is not invariably the case with different estimates of precision. The introduction by Gaddum (1933) of an index of precision (λ) therefore served a very useful purpose. It is the value s/b, where s indicates the standard deviation of the response and b symbolizes the slope of the regression line. This quantity is absolute in the sense that it is uninfluenced by experimental design and dose unit and may be used for direct comparison of the precision of various methods. Loraine (1958) has suggested the following classification of assays according to their degree of precision: $\lambda = 0{\cdot}2$ indicates a very precise method; $\lambda = 0{\cdot}2$–$0{\cdot}3$ is an acceptable degree of precision; $\lambda = 0{\cdot}3$ or greater may be considered unsatisfactory. Other objective expressions for precision are the term L, expressing the ratio b/s (Woolf 1953), and the term g, an estimate of the significance of the regression coefficient (Finney 1952). In common use is also the calculation of the fiducial limits of error. It is an accurate interval, at a stated level of probability, within which the true value is found. For exact formulas of computation the reader is referred to Finney (1952), Diczfalusy (1954), and Borth and associates (1957).

c *Criteria of practicability*

This concept is based on the factors of speed, cost, and skill required to carry out the test (Borth 1952). These characteristics are of importance when considering, e.g., the clinical applicability of a method. It is obvious, however, that easy performance and rapidity must be critically balanced against insufficient reliability and that an overall estimation of the method is required.

3 INTERNATIONAL STANDARD PREPARATIONS

Activity measurements of HCG are comparative. It was early recognized that assays, even carried out under rigidly standardized conditions, showed considerable variation between different colonies of animals and on different occasions within the same colony. Thus, in a comparative study it was found that the amount of a certain preparation of HCG, required to give a 100 per cent increase in ovarian weight varied from 3 to 50 μg (Emmens 1939). Moreover, highly variable amounts were necessary to elicit a number of biological actions used as indices of response (D'Amour & D'Amour 1940, Sealy & Sondern 1940). It is now accepted that activity measurements of HCG should be carried out simultaneously with a standard preparation. To achieve uniformity the first International Standard for HCG was set up in 1939 under the auspices of the League of Nations. By definition the International Unit is the gonadotrophic activity displayed by 0·1 mg of the standard preparation.

In the Memorandum (League of Nations 1939) it was explicitly stated that the International Standard should be exclusively used as a reference preparation for activity measurements of pregnancy urine. The criteria to be fulfilled for its use as a standard of reference also for assays on serum have, however, been discussed in some detail by Diczfalusy (1953).

Due to shortage of the first International Standard it has now been replaced. Under the supervision of the National Institute for Medical Research, London, a collaborative assay was carried out of a material which was compared with the first International Standard. The International Unit of HCG is now defined as the activity contained in 0·001279 mg. of the second International Standard (Bangham & Grab 1964).

Unfortunately, data are still published with reference to home-made animal units of HCG. There is no excuse any more for such unscientific presentation of results. They make all comparative work meaningless.

4 BIOASSAY PROCEDURES

a Qualitative tests

Qualitative tests serve the purpose of aiding in the diagnosis of pregnancy. They exist in great number and have been devised with emphasis on rapid and easy performance. It does not seem indicated, however, to give a detailed account here on the biological pregnancy reactions which now seem to have been outdated by the modern serological tests. Therefore the reader interested in this subject is referred to Loraine (1958) and Hon (1961) for references and discussion of practical problems.

b Quantitative bioassays

This field will also be very briefly discussed here. A plethora of information on the considerable literature that has been published over the years is found in a large number of reviews (for references see section F.1).

The assays are of 2 main types:

1. Quantal methods based on qualitative responses. The end-point is a positive or negative reaction. Examples of this type of assay are the formation of corpora lutea in the immature rat or mouse, vaginal cornification in the immature or adult rat, ovarian hyperaemia in the immature rat, and expulsion of spermatozoa in amphibia.

2. Quantitative methods based on graded responses. These assays are usually carried out on the intact, immature rat. The following indices of response are in common use: increase in ovarian weight, uterine weight, total prostatic weight, seminal vesicle weight, and weight of the total accessory reproductive organs.

The bioassays may also be conveniently classified into those depending on a primary or a secondary response. Primary-response assays are based on measurable actions of HCG exerted directly on the ovary or testis, whereas secondary response methods depend on effects elicited through the stimulation of gonadal hormone secretion by HCG.

Table 7.2 gives a summary of some relevant data for the most extensively used procedures for quantitative bioassay of HCG. Among the primary-response assays the graded ovarian-weight method suffers from lack of precision and sensitivity. The other two primary-response tests mentioned in the table, namely the ovarian hyperaemia and the spermiation techniques, are quantal. This in itself causes some disadvantages; the statistical calculations are more complicated and twice the number of observations are required for any given degree of precision as compared with a graded-response assay (Gaddum 1933, 1953a). The spermiation test is rapid and precise, but relatively insensitive. The ovarian hyperaemia test is extremely rapid and results can be obtained after only 4 hours. The specificity, on the other hand, may be questionable. It appears that adrenocortical hormones (cortisone and hydrocortisone) may affect the response of the ovary (Payne 1951, Smith 1955, Behrman & Niemann 1955b) which may also be enhanced by a pituitary synergist (Fried & Rakoff 1950), or inhibited by a serum factor (Albert 1948).

TABLE 7.2

Bioassay of HCG

Index of response	Indices of precision	*L*	References	Comments
Ovarian weight (rat)	0·319*	3·13*	Sealy & Sondern (1940)	Inaccurate, insensitive
Ovarian weight (rat)	0·240	4·16	Diczfalusy & Loraine (1955)	
Ovarian hyperaemia (rat)	0·450*	2·22*	Albert & Berkson (1951)	Extremely rapid, sensitive, questionable specificity
Ovarian hyperaemia (rat)	0·123	8·13	Borth *et al.* (1957)	
Expulsion of spermatozoa (toad)	0·120–0·176*	8·33–5·68*	Wohlzogen (1953)	Rapid, relatively insensitive, seasonal variations
Uterine weight (rat)	0·329*	3·06*	Delfs (1941)	Sensitive, unspecific when applied directly to plasma, serum, or pregnancy urine
Uterine weight (rat)	0·240†	4·18†	Sealy & Sondern (1940)	
Uterine weight (rat)	0·149*	6·70*	Dorfman & Rubin (1947)	
Uterine weight (rat)	0·086	11·63	Diczfalusy & Loraine (1955)	
Vaginal cornification (vitamin B-deficient rats)	0·115*	8·70*	Heard & Winton (1939)	Sensitive, unspecific in the presence of oestrogens
Vaginal cornification (rat)	0·276	3·62	Loraine (1950)	
Prostatic weight (rat)	0·139	7·19	Loraine (1950)	Sensitive, suitable for direct assays on plasma, serum, pregnancy urine, and tissues
Prostatic weight (rat)	0·108	9·26	Diczfalusy & Loraine (1955)	
Prostatic weight (rat)	0·100	10·00	Loraine (1956)	
Prostatic weight (hypophysectomized rat)	0·184	5·43	Diczfalusy & Loraine (1955)	

TABLE 7.2 (*continued*)

Index of response	Indices of precision	L	References	Comments
Seminal vesicle weight (rat)	0·200*	5·00*	Watts & Adair (1943)	Sensitive, somewhat less precise than the prostatic weight assay, otherwise same advantages
Seminal vesicle weight (rat)	0·195	5·13	Loraine (1950)	
Seminal vesicle weight (rat)	0·143	7·00	Diczfalusy & Loraine (1955)	
Seminal vesicle weight (hypophysectomized rat)	0·128	7·81	Diczfalusy & Loraine (1955)	
Total accessory reproductive organs (rat)	0·210	4·76	Diczfalusy (1953)	Precision and other advantages about the same as for the weight assay
Total accessory reproductive organs (rat)	0·105	9·52	Diczfalusy (1954)	
Total accessory reproductive organs (rat)	0·109	9·18	Diczfalusy & Loraine (1955)	

* Adapted from Diczfalusy (1954).
† Adapted from Loraine (1956).

Furthermore, attention must be paid to the effect of serum, some dilution being necessary for precise and accurate results. In undiluted serum an underestimation of HCG is liable to occur (Borth *et al.* 1957b). The strain of animals appears to be of great importance, the test being satisfactory and precise in the hands of Borth and associates (1957b), but less satisfactory in the experience of, e.g., Loraine (1956, 1958).

Among the secondary-response assays included in Table 7.2 the vaginal cornification test is a quantal assay and, therefore, *a priori* less satisfactory. It is sensitive and may be made fairly precise (Heard & Winton 1939), but it is unsuitable in the presence of oestrogens which have to be removed prior to assay. The oestrogens are also an interfering factor in the uterine weight assay. In addition, inaccurate results are obtained with this method when HCG in serum is being tested (Maddock & Leach 1952, Diczfalusy & Loraine 1955), the augmentation observed apparently being due to prolonged absorption from the site of application (Maddock & Leach 1952).

The weight increase of the accessory reproductive organs appears to be a precise and accurate index of response. Loraine (1950, 1956) favours the prostatic weight assay, whereas Diczfalusy (1954) has demonstrated the suitability of the weight of the total accessory reproductive organs as a measure of activity. The seminal vesicle weight assay has a slightly lesser degree of precision (Loraine 1950, Diczfalusy & Loraine 1955). These methods do not require the removal of oestrogens, and they may with advantage be directly applied to the estimation of serum HCG.

c Problems of specificity

None of the bioassay procedures is strictly and absolutely specific for HCG. In principle, all the reactions may be elicited by ICSH. This has, however, little significance in practical work, as the level of ICSH in the urine or in serum is considerably below the sensitivity threshold of the tests. Some consideration of this possible factor of disturbance has been given by, *inter alia*, Albert & Berkson (1951) in connection with the rat ovarian hyperaemia reaction as a test for HCG. A number of other hormones may also under special conditions interfere with some of the assays. FSH, for example, may influence the uterine weight reaction, which, in fact, has been used for the assay of this hormone. HCG, in contrast to FSH, does not affect ovarian weight until considerable amounts are administered, and Delfs (1941) therefore recommends routine examination of the ovaries as a check. The possible interference of adrenal steroids with the rat ovarian hyperaemia reaction has been touched upon earlier, and the augmenting effect in some assays of serum when used as a vehicle for HCG has been mentioned. For more detailed information on the particular problems of specificity the reader is referred to Diczfalusy (1953).

d Sensitivity

The sensitivity threshold for various bioassay procedures varies considerably. The rat ovarian hyperaemia reaction, the uterine weight test, and the vaginal cornification method are among the most sensitive assays showing positive response with amounts of HCG of about 0·25 i.u. (D'Amour & D'Amour 1940, Sealy & Sondern 1940, Delfs 1941, Albert

& Berkson 1950, Borth *et al.* 1957b). The sensitivity inherent in the techniques depending on the weight increase of the male accessory reproductive organs is slightly less, a noticeable reaction being elicited by 1 i.u. (D'Amour & D'Amour 1940, Sealy & Sondern 1940). The ovarian weight increase reaction is comparatively insensitive as a test for HCG (D'Amour & D'Amour 1940, Sealy & Sondern 1940), and the spermiation test in frogs and toads apparently the most insensitive. To illustrate this fact it may be mentioned that the ED_{50} (50 per cent of the animals showing positive reaction) is 23·4 i.u. in the male toad *Bufo marinus* (Hon & Morris 1956), whereas it is only 0·4 i.u. in the rat ovarian hyperaemia reaction (Borth *et al.* 1957b).

Considerable seasonal variation in sensitivity has also been noticed in all bioassay procedures, where this factor has been examined (Loraine 1950, Diczfalusy 1953, Hon & Morris 1956).

5 IMMUNOASSAY PROCEDURES

a Antigenicity

Antigenicity refers to the capacity of a substance to elicit the formation of antibody and to the ability of this substance to react with the antibody in a manner which can be observed. A certain minimal size of the chemical component is required, antigens usually having a molecular weight of 10,000 or greater. Even smaller molecules such as clupein, insulin, and glucagon, have, however, been found to be antigenic, and the lower molecular weight limit is, therefore, uncertain. Of paramount importance is the size of the surface area which is indicated by the fact that non-antigenic small molecules may become antigenic after adsorption onto inert particles.

Distinct physico-chemical units, apparently constituted by 4 or 5 amino acid or monosaccharide residues, create the structural basis of antigenic activity. These antigenic or determinant sites do not seem to form a simple regular repetitive sequence on the molecular surface area but rather a complicated mosaic.

b Preparation of antiserum

HCG probably has a molecular weight of about 30,000 (see Section A.3) and, therefore, fulfills one important requirement for antigenicity. Another condition for efficient antibody production, namely taxonomic distance between antigen donor and recipient, has also been satisfied.

Rabbits have almost exclusively been used for these experiments. In view of the repeated earlier failures to demonstrate *in vitro* antigenicity of the hormone it may, however, be definitely considered a weak antigen.

Rapid elimination and excretion of a substance reduces its antigenic properties. Adjuvants have been used in such situations in order to increase the antibody response. These substances, in principle adsorbents or emulsions, are usually nonantigenic themselves, and probably exercise their effect through prolongation of the exposure of the antigen to the antibody-forming cells. Thus, Bussard & Grabar (1947) used aluminium salts, Dodin (1959) employed HCG-coated erythrocytes, and Brody & Carlström (1960) used Freund adjuvant (1947, 1951) to enhance antibody production. Freund adjuvant is a water-in-oil emulsion (incomplete Freund adjuvant) and the effect may be increased by the addition of mycobacteria (complete Freund adjuvant). The intensification of the antibody response is probably brought about by inciting local inflammation and by retarding absorption, destruction, and elimination of the antigen. Brody & Carlström (1961) compared the effects of incomplete and complete Freund adjuvant on the complement-fixing HCG-antibody titer, and also studied the relative importance of different routes of antigen administration and variation in dosage. The following scheme will yield a high-titer antiserum (Brody & Carlström 1961): 10 to 20 ml of HCG-adjuvant mixture (12,500 i.u.) containing mycobacteria is given at 4 sites subcutaneously and intramuscularly. This is repeated twice at intervals of 3 weeks. A booster injection of HCG in saline (3,000 i.u.) is given intravenously 4 to 6 weeks after the last inoculation. Blood is withdrawn by cardiac puncture 1 week after the booster injection.

c Antigen-antibody reactions employed for the detection and assay of HCG

1 *Complement fixation.* The complement fixation test was devised by Bordet & Gengou in 1901. This reaction for the detection of antigen or antibody is based on the fact that complement combines with antigen-antibody complexes even when these complexes do not form visible aggregates. Complement is a unifying term for a group of components, largely protein in nature, present in fresh blood serum. Guinea-pig serum is ordinarily used as the source of complement. The chemical nature of the complement components is only poorly understood, although their reaction dynamics have been extensively studied (Mayer 1964). The complement factors react with an antigen-antibody complex

in a particular order, one step of interaction requiring the participation of Ca^{++} and another the presence of Mg^{++} ions.

In principle, a known amount of complement is added to a mixture of a soluble or particulate antigen and its antiserum. After complement fixation is completed in the test system, an indicator system is added to

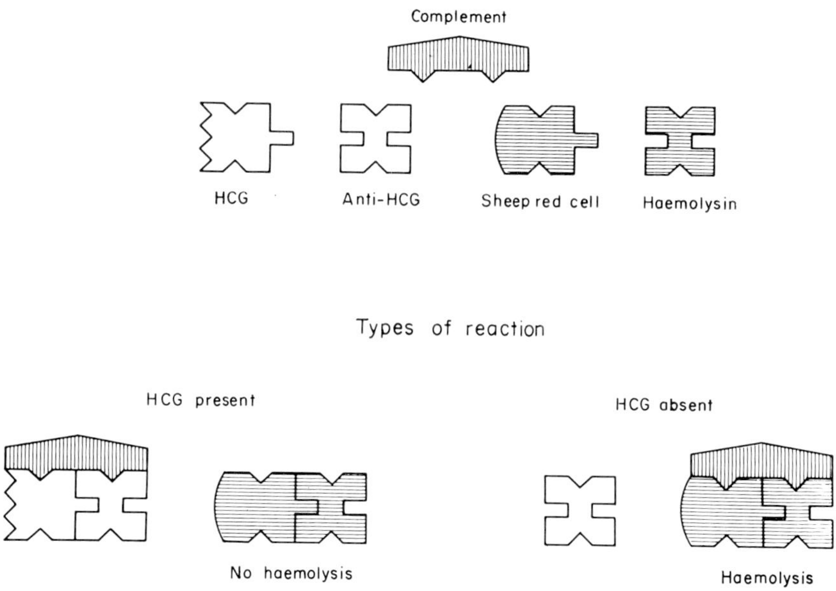

FIG. 7.2. Schematic representation of principle for complement fixation.

determine the amount of non-fixed complement. The indicator system usually consists of sheep erythrocytes and specific haemolysin. The degree of haemolysis is inversely proportional to the amount of complement fixed. As, in general, all reagents are used in constant amounts except one, the unknown, of which varying dilutions are employed, the degree of haemolysis will be a measure of the amount of the unknown involved in the test system. The sensitivity of the method is directly related to measurable changes in the concentration of nonfixed complement, which thus constitutes the limiting factor in this system. The sensitivity of the test is determined by the capacity of the indicator system to discriminate minute changes in complement fixed. The complement may be used at a concentration which is critical in relation to the amount of sensitized red blood cells to be added. In this case fixation may be recognized in a quantal fashion (Fulton & Dumbell 1949) or is in certain modifications quantitatively measurable (Stein & Ngu 1950) upon addition of the indicator system. The complement may also be added in great excess, in which case the amount of non-fixed complement is assayed by back-titration against the indicator system (Mayer *et al.* 1948). The principle of complement fixation is schematically illustrated in Fig. 7.2.

The complement fixation test for the serological determination of

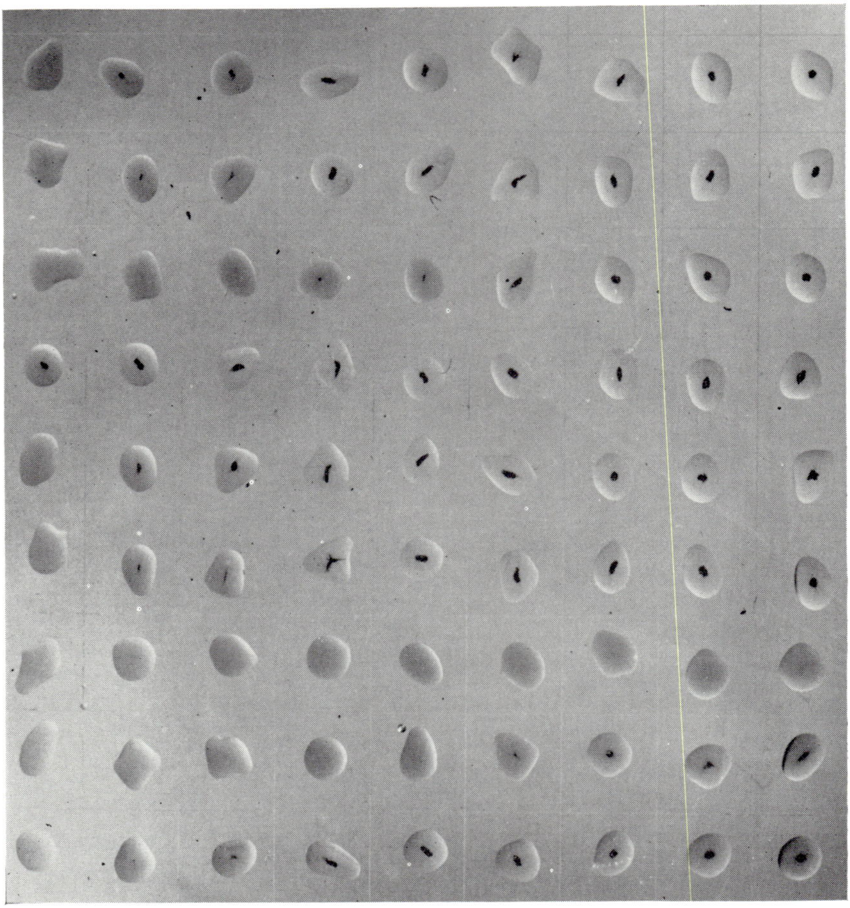

FIG. 7.3. Reaction patterns in the micro-modification procedure of complement fixation used for estimation of HCG. Different serum samples in vertical arrangement assayed at 1·26-fold serial dilution steps. Haemolysis = negative reaction; no haemolysis (dot formation) = positive reaction.

HCG was introduced by Brody & Carlström (1960), and its application has been described in detail (Brody & Carlström 1961, 1962a, b, c). Figure 7.3 illustrates the reaction patterns in the micro-modification employed.

2 *Precipitation.* The precipitation reaction refers to the formation of non-soluble antigen-antibody aggregates. A requirement for this reaction to occur, as is also the case for complement fixation, is that antigen and antibody exist in optimal or immunologically equivalent proportions. Antigen-antibody aggregation is less pronounced, and under extreme conditions completely absent, in the regions of antigen or antibody excess. For the HCG-anti-HCG system this has been demonstrated in the complement fixation test by Brody & Carlström (1961) and in the precipitation reaction by Keele and co-workers (1962). The zone phenomena may probably be explained by a disproportion of available reactive groupings on antigen and antibody, respectively. Thus, a certain amount of antigen, constituting an excess with a particular antiserum dilution in the conventional precipitation reaction, may be found to react with its antibody when adsorbed onto an inert particle, all other conditions being equal. The explanation is probably that some of the antigenic radicals have now been oriented towards the adsorptive surface and made unavailable to the antibody.

The precipitation reaction may be carried out by simple mixture of the reactants. It may also be applied as the interfacial or ring test. This test is usually performed in small test tubes or capillary tubes in such a fashion that mixing does not occur. The antiserum, as a rule, constitutes the bottom layer and the antigen solution is carefully layered on top.

The precipitation reaction for the successful assay of HCG has been used by McKean (1960) in the form of an interfacial test. This is a quantal reaction, quick and easy, but unfortunately lacking in sufficient sensitivity. The quantitative aspects of this technique have been studied by Keele and co-workers (1962).

3 *Immunodiffusion.* Immunodiffusion refers to a precipitation reaction which takes place in a supporting medium through which one or both reactants are diffused towards the other. In this serological system advantage is being taken–within reasonable limits–of automatic adjustment to optimal proportions between antigen and antibody. In the zone where this occurs the reactants form visible bands of precipitation. The main advantage inherent in this technique is its capacity to detect more than one antigen-antibody system. It is characterized by a very high resolving

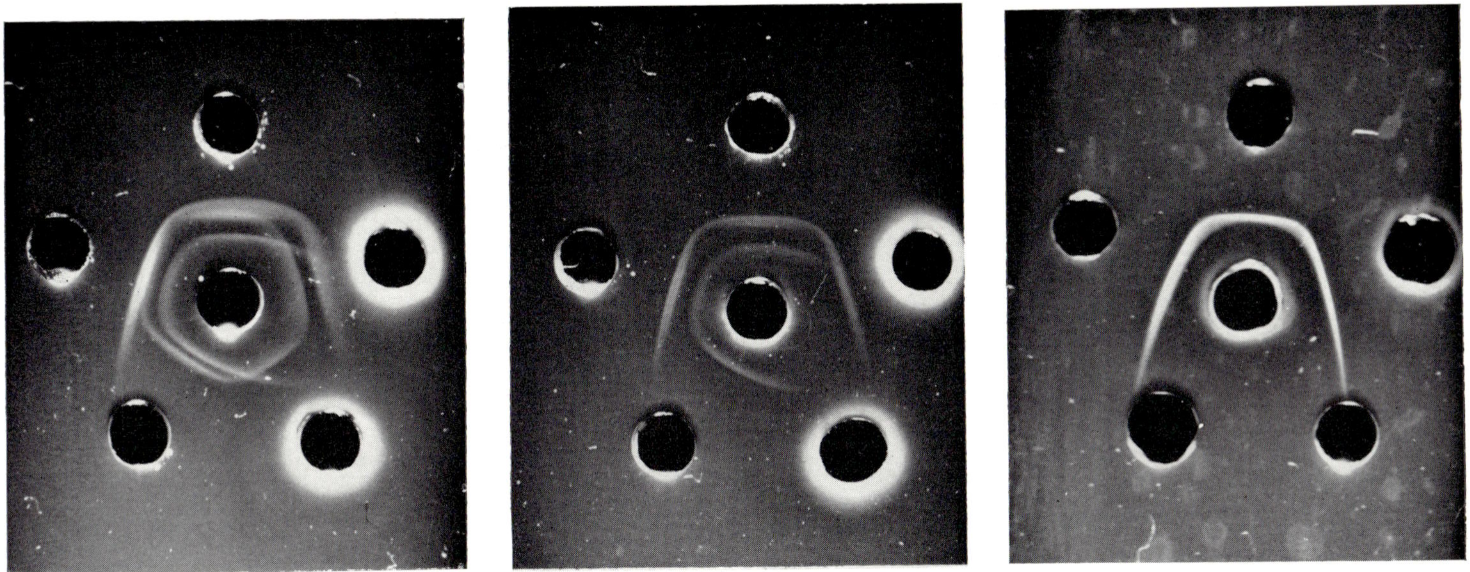
(a) (b) (c)

FIG. 7.4. Double diffusion in 2 dimensions (Ouchterlony plate technique) of HCG from various sources and antiserum to HCG. Central well = antiserum; top well = commercial HCG preparation (Gonadex, Leo, Sweden); right superior well = pregnancy serum; right inferior well = nonpregnant serum; left inferior well = nonpregnant urine; left superior well = pregnancy urine. (a) = untreated antiserum; (b) = saturated antiserum; (c) = absorbed antiserum. For explanation see text Section F.5.d. (From Brody & Carlström 1963.)

power which, in addition to its great versatility and elegant simplicity, has made it an indispensable analytical tool for specificity studies of immune systems.

Three gel diffusion procedures are widely used. One of them, the tube method developed by Oudin (1952), represents single diffusion in one dimension. A solution of antigen is layered over an agar-gelled antiserum in a tube. The antigen diffuses into the gel and produces one or several bands of precipitate. The methods of Oakley & Fulthorpe (1953), and of Preer (1956) are also one-dimensional. The antiserum is placed at the bottom of a tube and a layer of agar is placed directly above the antiserum and allowed to solidify; subsequently the antigen solution is placed on top of the agar layer. In this technique both reactants diffuse, neither remains at a constant concentration during the test, and planes of precipitate are formed at points of equivalence of antigen and antibody.

The technique of double diffusion in two dimensions was devised by Ouchterlony & Elek independently in 1948. Agar is poured on a glass plate and wells at a convenient distance from each other are cut in the agar. Antigen and antibody, poured into adjacent wells, diffuse towards each other and form more or less sharp bands at the zone of optimal concentration. The number of bands indicates the minimum number of antigen-antibody systems. Each precipitation line is considered to represent a distinct antigen-antibody complex, although under certain conditions a single system may give rise to several bands. This technique is particularly suitable for the study of complex antigen-antibody systems (Fig. 7.4).

Ouchterlony (1953) distinguished 3 principal types of reaction when in a 3-basin arrangement related antigens in adjacent wells are allowed to diffuse against an antiserum poured into the central well. Fusion of the precipitate lines is recognized as a reaction of identity and indicates serological identity of the antigens. When the precipitate lines intersect the pattern is referred to as a reaction of nonidentity. This is interpreted as indicating complete lack of serological relation between the 2 antigens. The 3rd type of reaction is characterized by spur formation which denotes that the antigens share certain antigenic determinants.

Immunoelectrophoresis involves electrophoretic separation of one of the reactants, usually the antigen, followed by specific precipitation by double gel diffusion (Grabar & Williams 1955). Agar is most frequently used for the supporting medium. The reservoir for the reactant to be separated by electrophoresis is usually cut in the centre of the agar strip

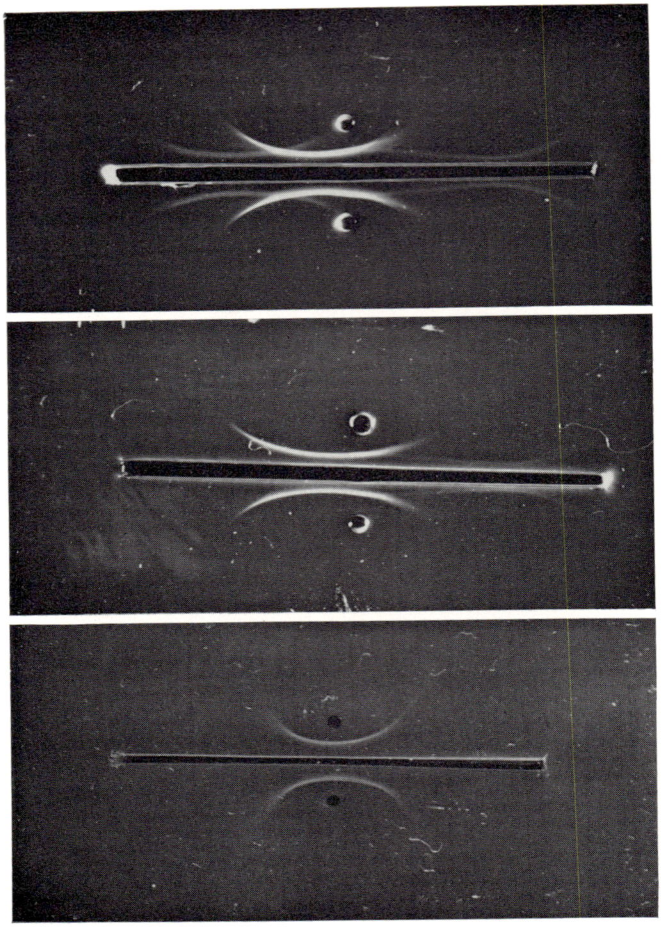

FIG. 7.5. Immunoelectrophoresis according to Scheidegger (1955) of a commercial HCG preparation (Gonadex, Leo, Sweden). Longitudinal basin filled with antiserum to HCG. Catode to the right. (a) = untreated antiserum; (b) = saturated antiserum; (c) = absorbed antiserum. (From Brody & Carlström 1963.)

to allow for electro-osmotic movement. After electrophoresis troughs are cut in the agar parallel with the line of migration of the antigen and filled with the antiserum. The antibody diffuses at right angles from the longitudinal trough meeting the radially diffusing antigenic components. Precipitate bands appear in the form of arcs about the separated antigenic spots. Immunoelectrophoresis is an analytical procedure allowing the identification and characterization of very complex antigen-antibody mixtures. The micro-method of Scheidegger (1955) constitutes an ingenious and commonly adopted modification of the original procedure (Fig. 7.5).

Immunodiffusion methods have been used extensively in the study of the HCG-anti-HCG system. With the double diffusion method of Ouchterlony the heterogeneity of antisera prepared by immunization with commercial HCG preparations has been clearly demonstrated (for references see Section F.5.d). Furthermore, with this method the effect of different procedures for restricting the specificity of an antiserum could be checked (Brody & Carlström 1963). These results have been confirmed by immunoelectrophoretic analyses (Brody & Carlström 1963) which have also shown a mobility of serum HCG coinciding with that of the β-globulins (Midgley *et al.* 1961). These results corroborate the findings of Demol & Fanard (1957) obtained with other methods. A somewhat different electrophoretic mobility was reported by Lunenfeld and associates (1962), namely that the hormone appeared in the α_5 and α_2 regions as well as, with some preparations, in the β-globulin region. The latter investigators examined urinary HCG preparations, and a change in structure during extraction and purification may explain the observed differences. Both in the work of Midgley and co-workers (1961) and of Lunenfeld and associates (1962) the immunoelectrophoretic distinction of the hormone was corroborated by simultaneous simple electrophoresis and subsequent bioassay of eluates of agar segments. There was good agreement between the localization of antigenical and biological activity.

4 *Agglutination inhibition.* This reaction is based on the observation that erythrocytes or other particles may be used to adsorb proteins. The system is a sensitive indicator for the presence of antibody reacting with the protein. Furthermore, the interaction between antiserum and antigen may be inhibited by the addition of homologous or cross-reacting antigen. This assay is quantal, and the end-point determined by serial dilution of the antigen. A schematic illustration of the reaction is given in Fig. 7.6.

A technique for coupling proteins to erythrocytes was originally described by Pressman and associates (1942), who used a *bis*-diazotized benzidine. The finding of Boyden (1951) that soluble antigens can be adsorbed on tannic acid-treated erythrocytes was a major advance. Agglutination of the antigen-coated erythrocytes is conveniently visualized by the appearance of a smooth carpet of cells in round-bottomed test-tubes. When coated red blood cells are mixed with antiserum and homologous antigen the antibody displays preferential reactivity with the soluble antigen which, when present in sufficient amount, prevents agglutination. The visible effect is the formation of a dark ring or of a small discrete button of cells at the bottom of the tube.

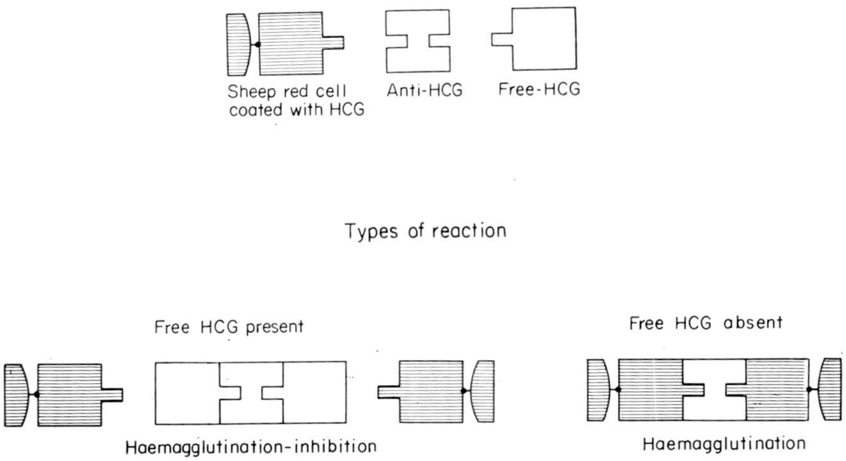

FIG. 7.6. Schematic representation of principle for agglutination-inhibition.

The relative fragility of the red cell has necessitated the introduction of special procedures to overcome this disadvantage. Treatment of the erythrocytes with formaldehyde (Flick 1948, Weinbach 1958, 1959) or pyruvic aldehyde (Ling 1961) was found to be suitable. Weinbach (1959) demonstrated that treatment with formaldehyde and tannic acid yielded an inert, stable particle with excellent adsorptive capacity. Even in this state the particles can be used only for a limited period, which, however, can be considerably prolonged by freeze-drying (Weinbach 1959). These principles have been adopted by Wide & Gemzell (1960) in their haemagglutination-inhibition reaction for the assay of HCG (Fig. 7.7).

Some of the disadvantages inherent in the red cell when used as an inert carrier of antigens may be avoided by the employment of the latex particle. This is a styrene monomer polymerized so that it forms a colloidal suspension in water. The particle, which is negatively charged, spherical in form, and with a diameter of 0·8 to 1·1 μ, was introduced into serological work by Singer & Plotz (1956). The latex agglutination inhibition reaction for the serological determination of HCG has been used by, e.g., Robbins and associates (1962).

In principle, the inert particle is sensitized with the antigen added to the suspension at an optimal concentration, which is highly variable for different proteins. The highest dilution of the homologous antiserum, which causes a complete agglutination pattern of a certain amount of particles, is the titre of the antiserum. With fixed amounts of coated particles and of antiserum, and with appropriate control of pH and ionic

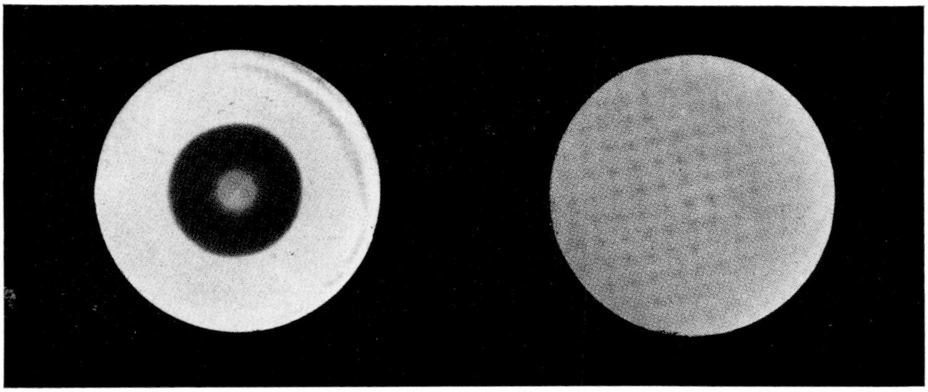

FIG. 7.7. Reaction patterns in the test tube modification of haemagglutination-inhibition used for the assay of HCG. Mat formation (a) = negative reaction; dot formation (b) = positive reaction.

environment the agglutination will be inhibited by a certain minimum amount of antigen. The sensitivity of the method is directly related to the titre of the antibody, which thus constitutes the limiting factor in this system.

5 *Radioimmunoassay*. This very elegant technique for the assay of antigen is based on a series of observations of Berson and associates (1956). Firstly, by means of paper electrophoresis and paper chromatography they found that labelled insulin (insulin-I_{131}), when bound to its antibody, migrates as a single peak away from the starting line, whereas unbound insulin remains at the point of origin. Secondly, it was assumed that the law of mass action is applicable for the reaction between antigen and antibody, and that the binding of labelled antigen to its antibody is comparatively inhibited in the presence of unlabelled antigen. The ratio of bound and free labelled antigen will consequently be reduced in the

presence of non-radioactive antigens which will displace some of the labelled from the antigen-antibody complex, the ratio being inversely proportional to the amount of unlabelled antigen. Bound labelled antigen may, in principle, be separated from the free fraction by means of paper electrophoresis or chromatoelectrophoresis (Berson *et al.* 1956, Berson & Yalow 1957, 1958).

Certain modifications as to the fractionation of free and bound labelled antigen have been presented. Grodsky & Forsham (1960) introduced the method of preferential precipitation of bound insulin with sodium sulfite and Hales & Randle (1963) made use of the known fact that the antigen-antibody complex may be precipitated by addition of anti-γ-globulin serum and collected by means of filtration on cellulose acetate membranes.

Radioimmunoassay of HCG has been used by Paul & Odell (1964) and Wilde and associates (1965). It provides a very sensitive method, and should, in principle, be applicable to the assay of HCG in both serum and urine, and can be used in a graded fashion.

6 *Fluorescent antibodies.* This method permits the detection of antibodies by direct microscopical examination and renders possible the identification and localization of antigens in micro-organisms and tissues. It, therefore, provides a new dimension in histochemistry. It was introduced in 1941 by Coons and co-workers and is based on the visualization of antibodies which have been labelled by coupling with fluorescent dyes.

In principle, this technique may be employed in 2 different ways. Direct staining of fixed tissue sections by exposure to the fluorescent antibody followed by washing to remove excess of antibody has been used; this requires great care in the interpretation of the microscopic picture due to widespread unspecific fluorescence. The validity of the conclusions may be increased by including the inhibition reaction; treatment of the sections with unlabelled homologous antibody prior to their exposure to the labelled antibody should prevent specific fluorescence. The indirect fluorescent antibody staining, the other procedure, like the inhibition reaction is a 2-stage procedure. After treatment of a tissue section with unlabelled homologous antibody and removal of excess antibody, the section is exposed to a labelled antibody against the homologous antigen; if the latter has become fixed to certain tissue structures by union with its antigen, the attachment of the labelled antibody to the reaction complex will be visible by the appearance of specific fluorescence.

The fluorescent antibody technique has been used rather extensively, both in its direct and indirect application, in attempts to trace the cellular origin and localization of HCG (Midgley & Pierce 1962; Leznoff & Davis 1963, Thiede & Choate 1963). The results, on the whole, favour the view that HCG is mainly synthesized in the syncytial layer, which contradicts the conventional opinion that the Langhans cell is the site of origin (see Section D.2).

d Problems of specificity

Specificity refers to the capacity of a method to detect and estimate one substance or one factor exclusively. Both as regards the bioassay and immunoassay of such relatively complicated chemical constituents as HCG it seems useful to make a clear distinction between specificity of the reaction *per se* and its specificity when applied to the assay of the substance in purified form or in body fluids. Certain *a priori* conditions inherent in the reaction may make it impossible to achieve absolute specificity. For example, this type of specificity may be invalidated by the occurence of cross-reactions (see below) between substances, or by the fact that they elicit a similar or identical biological response. Yet the assay procedure may be rendered specific (relative specificity) under certain conditions and with special precautions taken. In this section certain factors which may affect both absolute and relative specificity will be discussed.

1 *Cross-reactions.* It is usually understood that the reaction between antigen and antibody is specific. This is an oversimplification and requires qualification.

An antigen may be assumed to engender the production of a series of distinct antibodies, each with specific affinity for a particular reactive grouping on the surface of the antigen molecule. The capacity of various determinant sites to elicit the formation of antibody is apparently subject to considerable variation with differences as to, e.g., intensity of stimulation and time of appearance. The antigen-antibody reaction must be considered to represent the sum total of the union between the antigen and the family of antibodies.

It is obvious that the small part of an antigen, which constitutes an active radical, may exist in different body constituents from completely unrelated sources. The substances then will share one or several antigenic determinants, and in consequence will cross-react with antisera produced against any of the antigenically related antigens. Specificity still exists at the level of determinant sites but not at the molecular level.

Cross-reactions between HCG-antisera and several gonadotrophic hormones have been demonstrated. Thus, Brody & Carlström (1961) found a weak cross-reaction with an HMG preparation. Isersky and associates (1963) reported that antiserum to HCG neutralizes biological HCG activity, and also neutralizes that follicle-stimulating activity which is contained in HCG and HMG preparations. Furthermore, this group has reported that antiserum to HMG neutralizes the follicle-stimulating activity of both HMG and HCG preparations. Fulthorpe and co-workers (1963) found that considerable cross-agglutination occurs when erythrocytes are coated with HMG and tested with HCG-antiserum. McGarry & Beck (1964) claimed that antiserum to purified HFSH can react with large quantities of HCG. Saxena & Henneman (1964) demonstrated that antisera to FSH neutralized the biological activity of HMG as well as HCG.

Wide and co-workers (1961) reported that the reaction between HCG and its homologous antiserum is inhibited by HLH. A large number of authors have demonstrated that antiserum to HCG is able to neutralize the biological activity of HLH (Wide *et al.* 1961, Wide 1962, Goss & Taymor 1962, Taymor *et al.* 1963, Isersky *et al.* 1963, Paul & Ross 1964, Goss & Lewis 1964). Immunoelectrophoresis of HCG and HLH with anti-HCG after thermal and chemical treatment of the antigens has shown the presence of a common antigen (Shahani & Rao 1964). All these findings, however, are equivocal and may be explained either as being due to contamination of the HCG preparation with HLH or, in fact, by cross-reaction between the hormones. Goss & Lewis (1964) have added some significant observations indicating cross-reaction. They found that antiserum to HLH inactivates the biological activity of HCG and, furthermore, that HCG and HLH, when reacted in agar with both homologous and heterologous antisera, share a major antigenic component.

2 *Immunologically active impurities.* The production of HCG-antisera is usually achieved by means of immunization with commercial hormone preparations with activities of less than 5,000 i.u. per mg. In view of the fact that preparations with considerably higher specific activity have been produced (Morris & Morris, unpublished work, see Morris 1955, Got 1959, Got & Bourrillon 1960b, Johnsen 1961, Wilde & Bagshawe 1965, Donini 1965) it is obvious that the commercial products are rather impure. It was soon recognized that these impurities were antigenically active, and that antisera prepared by immunization with such a mixture of antigens contained separate antibodies for several antigenic

components (Brody & Carlström 1960, 1961, 1962a, b, 1963, Rao & Shahani 1961, Midgley *et al.* 1961, Wide 1962, Keele *et al.* 1962, Kiistala *et al.* 1962, Kaivola *et al.* 1962, 1963, Fulthorpe *et al.* 1963, Hamashige & Arquilla 1963, 1964, Goss 1964, Carlsson 1964). It is known that minute traces of contaminating antigen may induce the formation of a disproportionately large amount of antibody, a tendency that will be further enhanced by incorporation of the antigen into an efficient adjuvant.

The occurrence of unspecific antigen-antibody reactions may seriously disturb the specificity of an immunoassay method for HCG. That this, in fact, may take place with quite a few antisera and that precautions have to be taken to trace and, if necessary, to eliminate their effects has been emphasized (Brody & Carlström 1960, 1961, 1962a, b, c, 1963, Carlström & Brody 1962, Kiistala *et al.* 1962, Kaivola *et al.* 1962, 1963, Wide 1962, Carlsson 1964). The distinction of different antigen-antibody systems, the distribution of various antigens in the HCG preparation, urine and serum, and the elucidation of their serological relationships have been achieved by means of immunodiffusion studies, including 2-dimensional double diffusion in agar as well as immunoelectrophoresis (Brody & Carlström 1961, 1962b, 1963, Carlström & Brody 1962).

In principle, 2 different methods have been employed for the elimination of interfering antibodies (Brody & Carlström 1960, 1961, 1962a, b, 1963). One of these has been referred to as a saturation procedure and is dependent on the existence of zones of non-reactivity between antigen and antibody when either constituent is present in excess (see Section 5.c). The HCG preparation contains comparatively small amounts of an unspecific antigen common to the preparation, urine, and serum. It stimulates the production of a low-titer antibody. The addition to the antiserum of nonpregnant serum containing considerable quantities of the homologous antigen will, therefore, prevent the reaction of this unspecific antigen-antibody system. Such saturated antisera are specific when employed for the assay of HCG in human serum with the complement fixation test. The titer of the specific antibody remains unchanged.

The other method is a conventional serological technique. The unspecified antibodies are absorbed with the antigens producing them. Urine from a man or a nonpregnant woman may be used. Absorbed antisera may be employed for the assay of HCG in urine and serum. We have, however, pointed out that such absorption causes a reduction of the specific titer (Brody & Carlström 1962), probably due to cross-reaction with HMG. To avoid this effect Goss (1964) has used lyophilized urinary extract from children. The patterns obtained in double immunodiffusion in 2 dimensions and in immunoelectrophoresis before and after application of these 2 procedures are seen in Figs. 7.4 and 7.5.

3 *Extraneous influences on antigen-antibody reactions.* A number of factors of unspecific nature may seriously invalidate the results of immunoassays. Thus, in the presence of anticomplementary factors complement may be fixed unspecifically and simulate an antigen-antibody union. These effects can and should be routinely checked with control tests (Brody & Carlström 1960, 1961, 1962a). The problem is of no practical importance when proper technique is used.

The agglutination inhibition tests may yield completely erroneous values when assays are performed on human sera, particularly at low dilutions. The distorted results are due to the presence of non-specific inhibitors in serum. The nature of such inhibitory factors has been studied by, e.g., Grumbach & Kaplan (1962), who also attempted to remove them by various means. It would seem unwise to apply the agglutination inhibition methods directly to the assay of HCG in serum. Extraction of the hormone is, therefore, necessary before this reaction is carried out (Mishell *et al.* 1963).

e Sensitivity of immunoassays

There is great variation with regard to the sensitivity level of various immunoassay techniques. Immunodiffusion methods are comparatively insensitive. Among these reactions the Preer test (1956) is claimed to be among the most sensitive. The minimum amount of HCG that is distinguished by means of this technique is approximately 90 i.u. (Keele *et al.* 1962). Somewhat more satisfactory results have been obtained with the precipitation reactions. With the quantitative precipitation reaction the minimum detectable amount of HCG can be reduced to about 28 i.u. (Keele *et al.* 1962), and with the interfacial precipitation procedure to about 8 i.u. per ml. (McKean 1960).

Considerably better results have been achieved with other serological methods. With the complement fixation test the lower limit is 0·1 to 0·5 i.u. of HCG per ml (Brody & Carlström 1961), and with the haemagglutination-inhibition reaction the sensitivity threshold has been claimed to be around 0·02 to 0·04 i.u. per ml (Wide & Gemzell 1962). It would appear that these differences are due to variation in antiserum titer. When the same antiserum was used as a reactant in both methods the sensitivity was equal for the 2 procedures (Brody & Carlström 1965a). According to Wilde and associates (1965) it is possible to detect concentrations of 0·06 i.u. per ml by means of their radioimmunoassay, which accordingly does not differ essentially from the minimum amount of HCG detectable by means of complement fixation or haemagglutination-inhibition.

f Precision of immunoassays

The complement fixation method for the measurement of HCG in the modification of Fulton & Dumbell (1949) is a quantal assay. Its precision, when used for the quantitative estimation of HCG in serum, has been evaluated in simultaneous duplicate determinations of standard and unknown samples (Brody & Carlström 1961). The 95 per cent confidence limits for a mean value is obviously dependent on the dilution factor and the number of determinations performed in the assay. With 1·26-fold serial dilutions these confidence limits, expressed as a percentage of the mean value of duplicate analyses, are −20 per cent and +25 per cent (Brody & Carlström 1961).

The haemagglutination-inhibition reaction is also a quantal assay. Its precision in the quantitative determination of HCG has been studied by Wide (1962). With 1·26-fold serial dilution steps and a quadruplicate arrangement of the assay the fiducial limits of error of estimated value ($P=0·05$) were 84 per cent to 118 per cent.

In contrast to the haemagglutination-inhibition reaction it is possible to carry out the complement fixation test in a graded fashion. The end-point in this modification of the test is not read as haemolysis or no haemolysis; rather the degree of haemolysis is measured spectrophotometrically. With this technique a number of 4-point assays of standard and unknown have been carried out. The results have been analysed according to Borth and associates (1957) and the method has been found to be characterized by a very high index of precision: the weighted mean λ is 0·032 and the weighted mean L is 31·01 (Brody 1966). This compares very satisfactorily with the indices of precision for various bioassay techniques (see Table 7.2).

6 COMPARISON BETWEEN BIOASSAYS AND IMMUNOASSAYS

The relationship between biological and serological activity of HCG has received considerable attention within the last few years. A number of comparative assays have been carried out, and the agreement between the results obtained with the different principles of measurement has varied considerably. Borth and associates (1964) have tabulated some data of their own and of other investigators on the correlation between bioassay and immunoassay estimates of the concentration of HCG in urine; r^2 (the square of the correlation coefficient) ranged from 0·99 to 0·02.

Wide (1962) performed parallel bioassays and immunoassays on urine samples from normal pregnant women throughout pregnancy, from patients with chorionepithelioma, and on commercial HCG preparations. The weight increase of the accessory reproductive organs in hypophysectomized or intact immature rats was used as bioassay and a haemagglutination-inhibition reaction as immunoassay. The indices of discrimination, i.e., the ratio of biological and serological activity, were always lower than unity in the urine samples. The biological activity was only a small fraction of the serological activity, particularly in mid-pregnancy. For the commercial HCG preparations, on the other hand, the index of discrimination was almost 1·00. Wide (1962) explained the discrepancies observed in the urine samples as possibly due to the presence of biologically inactive but serologically active HCG. In principle, the same results were obtained by Hobson & Wide (1964), where the same interpretation was put forward. Toaff and associates (1965), using parallel quantitative spermiation tests in frogs and a quantitative haemagglutination-inhibition reaction on urine samples from normal pregnant women, were unable to find any correlation between immunological and biological activity ($r = 0·14$). The conclusion was that a different spectrum of urinary constituents was measured by immunoassay as compared with bioassay.

These experiences have, in some quarters, (and rightly so), provoked an attitude of scepticism about the validity of results obtained by means of quantitative immunoassay of HCG. It should be emphasized, however, that the comparative analyses have so far been carried out only on urine and only with one of the existing serological methods.

Probably there are several explanations for the disparate findings. Some of the antigenically active impurities of the HCG preparations used for the preparation of antisera are common to serum and urine but others are only found in the urine (Brody & Carlström 1962c, 1963). The urinary contaminants seem to dominate the picture qualitatively. The precise nature of these contaminants is not known, and it may well be that some of them are typical for pregnancy urine. If this be so, their elimination by means of conventional absorption procedures is likely to be unsuccessful. Furthermore, there is a certain risk of some loss of biological activity of HCG in the urinary tract although antigenical activity may remain intact. That this is possible is supported by the finding of Twombly (1936) that hormone preparations completely lacking biological activity still retain the capacity to elicit neutralizing antibodies to the hormone. In addition, there is good evidence that the structural unit possessing biological function is considerably larger than the unit displaying antigenical activity (Paul & Odell 1964, Nydick *et al.* 1964) and that the biological unit is, therefore, more vulnerable to adverse environmental conditions than the antigenical one with possible fragmentation of the biologically active molecule into smaller sub-units lacking biological but still possessing serological activity. Even if this may occur it is, however, difficult to understand why a preferential destruction of biological activity would take place in mid-pregnancy as claimed by Wide (1962).

For several such reasons serum appears to be more suitable for the purpose of specific quantitative immunoassay of HCG. In order to test the validity of this reasoning a collaborative investigation between several centres on the comparative bioassay and immunoassay of HCG in serum was undertaken (Bell and associates 1967). The bioassays were carried out by means of the total prostatic weight in intact immature rats (RP) and ovarian hyperaemia in intact immature rats (OH), the immunoassays by means of the complement fixation test (CF). Samples were collected at each centre according to a particular scheme and aliquots sent to the other participating laboratories. All stages of pregnancy were examined in a total of 90 samples. No systematic differences between biological and serological activities were noticed in the different trimesters of pregnancy. The mean ratio of results (index of discrimination) for any 2 methods were calculated. They were for RP/CF 0·9–1·3, for OH/CF 1·8–3·8, and for OH/RP 1·7–2·9 (range of means for different groups of samples distributed according to place of collection). There is thus good agreement between RP and CF but a less satisfactory comparison between OH and CF or OH and RP. The reason for the discrepancy between RP and CF on one hand and OH on the other is not quite clear at the moment. It is certainly possible that the discussion on the specificity of the RP and OH tests in Section F.4 might have some bearing on the problem. It should be pointed out, however, that the variation in ratios between individual samples was considerable in all the comparisons. In part this variation may be caused by the transport of samples between the laboratories and the impact of physico-chemical influences on the biological activity of HCG (cf. the preceding paragraph): in part it may also be due to differences in sensitivity and precision between the different methods used (cf. Table 7.2 and Sections F.4 and F.5). The results of Lau & Jones (1965) may be adduced in support of the first-mentioned explanation. In a comparison between assays of HCG in serum by means of CF and the Delfs bioassay carried out in the same laboratory the values obtained showed an almost exact agreement.

G CONCENTRATION IN TISSUES AND BODY FLUIDS IN NORMAL AND ABNORMAL PREGNANCY

I CONCENTRATION IN HCG-PRODUCING TISSUES

a Placenta

The first systematic study on the HCG concentration in placental tissue with methods of defined accuracy and precision and with the results expressed in international units was undertaken by Diczfalusy (1953). Two different methods were used, namely one depending on the increased weight of the accessory reproductive organs in immature male rats and the other based on the formation of corpora lutea in immature mice. There was good agreement between the results obtained with the 2 methods. The highest concentration of the hormone occurred during the 2nd and 3rd lunar month with an abrupt decrease thereafter to relatively constant values throughout pregnancy. During the peak period the highest values were around 500 i.u. per g wet tissue, and after the 4th lunar month below 20 i.u. per g wet tissue.

Loraine & Matthew (1953) also examined the HCG concentration in placental tissue. Specimens both from normal and abnormal pregnancy were investigated by means of the prostate weight method in intact immature rats. The study, however, was limited to the last 10 weeks of pregnancy. In normal placentas the range ($P=0{\cdot}95$) was 2·39 to 7·73 i.u. per g wet weight. In moderate and severe pre-eclamptic toxaemia and in diabetic pregnancy the HCG concentration was usually significantly higher. The range in these cases was 1·92 to 14·39 i.u. per g wet weight.

b Trophoblastic tumours

Diczfalusy and associates (1958) analysed the HCG concentration in 14 hydatidiform moles using the weight increase of the male accessory reproductive organs as criterion of response. When plotting the HCG concentrations expressed as i.u. per g wet weight of the hydatidiform moles against their respective menstrual age they were all found to fall above the upper limit of the 95 per cent fiducial range of a large number of estimates on normal placental tissue obtained throughout pregnancy. Hobson (1955) has also examined mole tissue from a number of patients using the male *Xenopus laevis* as test animals. The results in this study were expressed in i.u. per g dry weight and are therefore not comparable to those of Diczfalusy and associates (1958). In a later study Hobson (1958) reinvestigated this problem and in 8 hydatidiform moles found concentrations of HCG ranging from 72 to 3,049 i.u. per g wet weight. The conclusion drawn by the author is that the HCG concentration in the pathological tissue at all stages of pregnancy is higher than in normal placental tissue of corresponding gestational age.

2 CONCENTRATION IN SERUM AND URINE

a Normal pregnancy

Time of appearance. The fertilized ovum apparently synthesizes HCG at a very early state, and positive reactions have been obtained as early as 10 days after conception or about 5 days before the date on which the first missed period was due (Hamburger 1933a, Browne & Venning 1936, Tenney & Parker 1937, Jones *et al.* 1944, Smith *et al.* 1951, Lyon *et al.* 1953, Brown *et al.* 1958). Measurable amounts of HCG are thus excreted at the time of implantation of the conceptus.

General pattern. According to Zondek (1935) the concentration of HCG in the urine increases rapidly during the first months of pregnancy, declining gradually during the last trimester and rapidly after parturition. Browne & Venning (1936) and Evans and associates (1937) demonstrated what is now considered the classical gonadotrophin excretion pattern during pregnancy, i.e., the invariable occurrence of the early peak phenomenon. There is a sharp rise in HCG concentration to a peak between the 50th and 60th day after the last menstrual period, followed by an initially rapid and thereafter more gradual decline of the HCG levels. This pattern has been repeatedly confirmed both for serum and urine (Boycott & Rowlands 1938, Rakoff 1939).

Levels during pregnancy. Quite a few studies on the HCG levels in serum and in the urine throughout pregnancy have been carried out and the values expressed in international units. A wide array of assay procedures have, however, been used and the results have differed considerably.

The HCG concentration in serum has been estimated with bioassay techniques by Jones and associates (1944), Wilson and associates (1949), Albert & Berkson (1951), Haskins & Sherman (1952), Behrman & Niemann (1955a), and Loraine (1957), and with immunoassay methods by Brody & Carlström (1962a) and Mishell and co-workers (1963). Some data from these papers have been summarized in Table 7.3. The first-trimester peak usually occurs between 60 and 80 days, after which there is a sharp decline to low level values. In most studies a small but rather consistent secondary rise is observed in the last trimester. The significance of this second-peak phenomenon is obscure, and it occurs with both male and female foetuses (Brody & Carlström 1965b). The highest HCG levels have been reported with the uterine weight and the ovarian hyperaemia reactions and with the haemagglutination-inhibition test. The estimates obtained by means of the male frog test, the prostatic

TABLE 7.3

HCG in blood

Method of assay	Maximum level (i.u. per ml)	Occurrence of second peak	Reference
Uterine weight (rat)	600	+	Jones and associates (1944)
Ovarian hyperaemia (rat)	250	+	Wilson and associates (1949)
Ovarian hyperaemia (rat)	600	−	Albert & Berkson (1951)
Male frog (*Rana pipiens*)	120	+	Haskins & Sherman (1952)
Ovarian hyperaemia (rat)	500	+	Behrman & Niemann (1955a)
Prostatic weight (rat)	100	−	Loraine (1957)
Complement fixation	200	+	Brody & Carlström (1962)
Haemagglutination-inhibition	500	−	Mishell and associates (1963)

weight reaction, and the complement-fixation technique indicate a considerably lower range of HCG levels (see Table 7.3).

Investigators using the 3 last-mentioned techniques report similar levels in the first trimester of pregnancy. Considerable differences between bioassay and immunoassay levels have, however, been observed in the last trimester. Loraine (1957) found that at this period the concentration was between 4 and 11 i.u. per ml ($P = 0{\cdot}99$) and suggested that readings consistently outside this range should be regarded as abnormal.

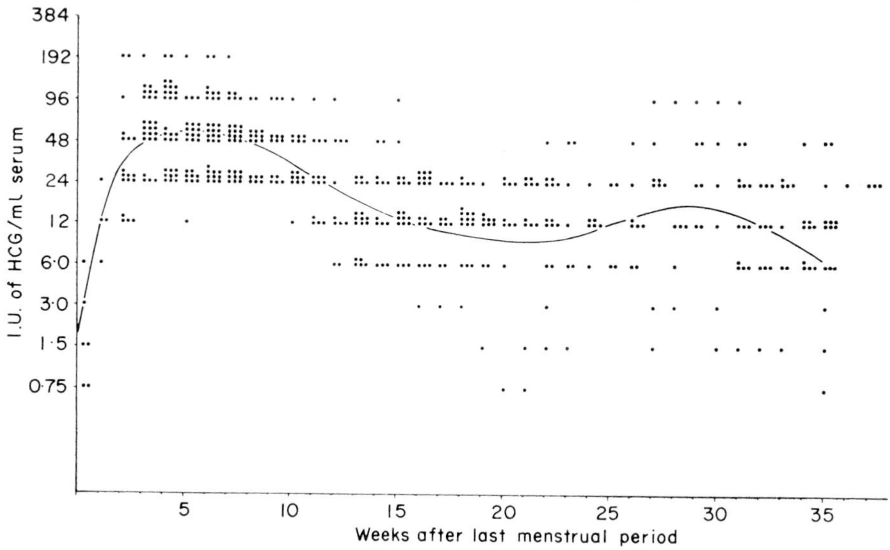

FIG. 7.8. Serum HCG levels in normal pregnancy. Analyses on single specimens from 474 subjects. Twofold serial dilution steps. Assays by means of complement fixation. Solid line indicates mean values. (From Brody & Carlström 1962a.)

Brody & Carlström (1962, 1965b, c), on the other hand, using the complement fixation test found a scatter of estimates between 0·75 and 96 i.u. per ml in completely normal subjects (Fig. 7.8). The reason for these discordant findings is not clear at present.

The HCG levels in the urine throughout pregnancy have been reported in international units by Wilson and associates (1949), Loraine (1950a), Albert & Berkson (1951), Hon & Morris (1956), and Borth and associates (1959) using bioassay procedures, and by Wide (1962) and Carlsson (1964) by means of the haemagglutination-inhibition reaction. On the whole, there is during normal pregnancy a satisfactory quantitative agreement between serum and urinary levels (Loraine 1950b).

b Multiple pregnancy

Jones and associates (1944) performed serial HCG analyses on serum in 2 twin pregnancies. One of the patients showed abnormally high HCG values maintained throughout pregnancy, whereas the other case had definitely elevated levels in mid-pregnancy, later falling to within the normal range. Borth and associates (1959) have also performed a longitudinal study on a patient with a twin pregnancy and in addition to other investigations also considered the urinary gonadotrophin excretion. From the time of the peak until delivery all values were above or at the upper limit of the normal range. Haskins & Sherman (1952) and Behrman & Niemann (1955b) have reported single abnormally elevated levels in cases of twin pregnancy. As has been pointed out by Delfs (1957) these findings assume clinical significance in patients where the picture is such that a trophoblastic tumour may be suspected.

c Toxaemia of pregnancy and diabetic pregnancy

A number of papers have been published on the results of analyses of HCG in blood and urine from patients with these complications. Smith & Smith (1934, 1939, 1948) had noticed higher serum levels in the majority of such cases as compared with normally pregnant women. This finding, however, could not be completely confirmed by Loraine & Matthew (1950). These investigators observed significantly increased urinary and serum concentrations only in patients suffering from severe pre-eclamptic toxaemia.

Loraine & Matthew (1954) also examined the serum HCG levels and the urinary excretion rate in a number of pregnant women with diabetes mellitus. They found abnormally high values in 33 per cent out of 52 patients. This is a considerably smaller figure than that presented by White (1952) who recorded pathologically increased serum concentrations in 91 per cent of the cases.

According to Loraine & Matthew (1950, 1954) analyses of HCG carry little or no clinical significance in these complications of pregnancy. For a detailed survey of the literature and an authoritative discussion of these problems the reader is referred to Loraine (1956, 1958).

d Abortion

Rakoff (1940) indicated the value of quantitative HCG determinations on serum as a diagnostic procedure for the demonstration of intrauterine foetal death. The application of this finding for the assessment of the viability of the pregnancy in cases of threatened abortion has been made by a number of investigators, employing various bioassay techniques for the estimation of HCG both in serum (Delfs & Jones 1948, Delfs 1957, Vermelin *et al.* 1957) and in the urine (Szejnberg & Rabau 1950, Rabau & Szejnberg 1955, Hon & Morris 1955, 1956, Zondek & Goldberg 1957).

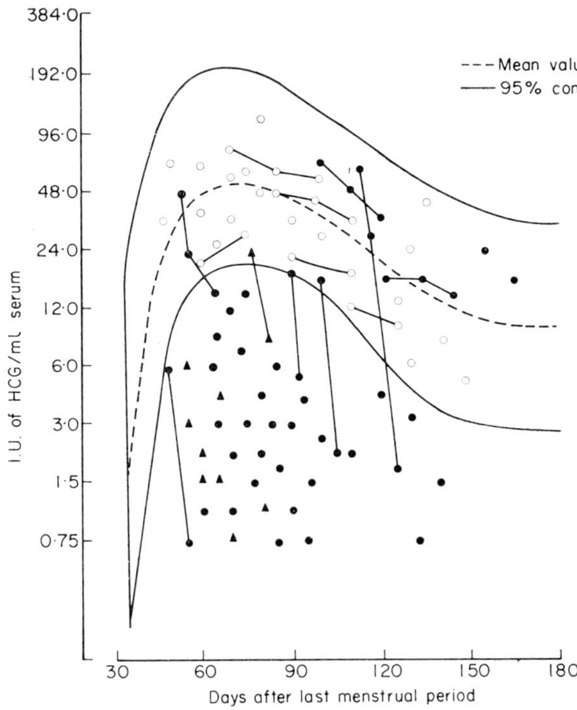

FIG. 7.9. Serum HCG levels in disturbed pregnancy. Open dots = threatened abortion; black dots = inevitable or incomplete abortion; triangles = ectopic pregnancy. Assays by means of complement fixation at 1·26-fold serial dilution steps. Solid lines indicate 95 per cent confidence limits for the range of estimates in normal pregnancy. (From Brody & Carlström 1965a.)

These investigators showed that subnormal HCG levels were usually associated with abortion. On the other hand, normal levels were seen in quite a few unsuccessful pregnancies. The questionable specificity and relatively low degree of precision inherent in the bioassay techniques used in these studies may in part explain the equivocal results.

Brody & Carlström (1962a), by means of the complement-fixation technique, analysed the HCG concentration of serum in patients with clinical evidence of threatened abortion. Reduction of HCG levels below the normal range was invariably associated with abortion. Normal HCG values usually indicated a favourable outcome of the pregnancy. In a minority of cases abortion occurred in spite of normal HCG levels. These abortions took place in the second half of pregnancy with the expulsion of foetuses longer than 25 cm. It was tentatively suggested that the aetiological mechanism in these cases differed from that obtaining in patients in whom a compromised placental function in early pregnancy may be assumed. Furthermore, it was emphasized that the low HCG levels which occur in quite a few normal pregnancies during the latter half of pregnancy restrict the value of these analyses to the first 4 or 5 months of gestation. The considerable prognostic value of serum HCG estimations in disturbed pregnancies during this period has been confirm- on a larger case material (Brody & Carlström 1965a). Figure 7.9 illustrates these findings.

e Hydatidiform mole

Zondek (1929a) reported that the urinary concentration of HCG in patients with hydatidiform mole was 2 to 3 times higher than in normal pregnancy. Zondek (1942) repeated his work, and also recommended analyses of cerebro-spinal fluid for safer diagnosis. Hamburger (1944) has collected the results of quantitative HCG analyses in the urine from a comparatively large case material. His conclusions were that patients with this complication generally show a higher urinary excretion of HCG than normal patients but that the levels both in normal and abnormal conditions are so scattered and the overlap so great that it is impossible to base a safe diagnosis on hormonal analyses. This opinion has been repeatedly endorsed (Hobson 1955, 1958, Hamburger 1958a).

Delfs (1957), however, on the basis of a careful analysis on the diagnostic value of HCG levels in serum, concluded that such analyses are of considerable importance in cases with a suspected trophoblastic tumour. She pointed out the necessity of relating the individual value to the normal range of estimates at the actual time of pregnancy and also emphasized the necessity to correlate laboratory data with clinical information. With due regard to these considerations all patients with hydatidiform mole showed abnormally elevated serum HCG concentrations. Delfs (1957) also stresses the importance of negative reactions in cases where difficulties exist among pathologists as to the malignant character of material obtained from curettage. Repeated negative reactions justify conservative handling.

These findings lend point to the discussion on the merits of serum HCG assays versus urinary analyses. Delfs (1957) has emphasized the superiority of serum assays and has provided experimental evidence to support this opinion. Brody & Carlström (1962b) have also stressed this view and demonstrated its validity in, e.g., predicting the outcome of pregnancy in patients with threatened abortion (Brody & Carlström 1962a, 1965a). From a technical point of view, immunoassays on serum are also preferable to those on urine. The reader interested in these problems is referred to Brody & Carlström (1965c).

f Choriocarcinoma of the uterus

The common association of this condition with a high urinary excretion of HCG was also recognized by Zondek (1929a). In this paper and in later work (Zondek 1935, 1937) the usefulness of quantitative HCG analyses for the detection and diagnosis of this highly malignant tumour is discussed. The height of the HCG level is not reliable as an index of the seriousness of the condition. In about 50 per cent of the cases this tumour appears after a hydatidiform mole and may be diagnosed early by the persistence of HCG in blood or urine. Repeated assays of HCG must, therefore, be routinely performed in every patient after the expulsion of a hydatidiform mole. Rising levels or the detection of HCG in the body fluids after more than 4 to 6 weeks following evacuation of the uterus necessitates a complete follow-up of the patient (Hamburger 1944), including curettage, pelvic angiography, and pulmonary x-ray. Delfs (1957) and Hobson (1959) have performed serial HCG assays in serum and urine, respectively, after surgical treatment of choriocarcinoma and chorioadenoma destruens, and consider these analyses a valuable prognostic aid. Hertz and associates (1958) and Brewer and coworkers (1964) have also used the gonadotrophin titers as a major guide in the clinical evaluation of patients with trophoblastic tumours of the uterus submitted to chemotherapy.

g Choriocarcinoma of the testis

The capacity of this highly malignant tumour to produce gonadotrophic hormone, sometimes in considerable amounts, has been long known through the report of Zondek (1935). Hamburger (1941) has devoted considerable interest to the qualitative analysis of the excreted hormonal product, and by means of simultaneous estimation of the ovarian and uterine response in infantile rats has been able to differentiate between patients excreting HCG, FSH or both, either in a sequential fashion, or simultaneously. The subject of gonadotrophic hormone excretion in different types of malignant testicular tumours has also been considered by Furuhjelm (1941) and was subsequently reviewed by Twombly (1944). He also pointed out the relation between HCG excretion and the occurence of radio-resistance with consequent poor prognosis. An additional important contribution on the endocrinological complexities encountered in testicular tumour-bearing men has been made by Hamburger (1958b), dealing with the correlation between morphology of the tumour and the excretion pattern of gonadotrophins and steroids. Hobson (1965), finally, has shown that the excretion of HCG may on occasion be very high in men with choriocarcinoma, and, furthermore, emphasized the diagnostic value of HCG excretion in testicular tumours of questionable nature. As this investigator correctly points out the classification of a testicular tumour as a seminoma needs correction when excretion of HCG is demonstrated. Hobson (1965) also reports the poor prognosis in men with testicular tumours who excrete HCG.

H ADMINISTRATION OF HCG

I DIAGNOSTIC ASPECTS

The stimulative actions of HCG on the endocrine apparatus of the ovary as well as the testis have been suggested as a means of evaluating the endocrine function of the gonads. Thus, Jayle and co-workers (1959) have proposed the administration of 20,000 i.u. of HCG given in 2 doses on day 3 and day 6 after the ovulation-induced rise in temperature as a test of luteal function. The excretion of oestrogens and pregnanediol is used as a measure of the functional capacity of the ovary at this phase of the menstrual cycle. Jayle and associates (1961) have subsequently introduced a more refined test of luteal function by means of simultaneous administration of HCG and dexamethasone and subsequent analysis of the urinary excretion of 17-oxosteroids, 17,21-hydroxy-20-oxosteroids, pregnanediol, pregnanetriol, and the 3 standard oestrogens. The authors maintain that this method permits the characterization of different anomalies of corpus luteum function.

The determination of changes in oestrogen excretion produced by a standard dose of HCG was suggested as a test of the functional capacity of the testis or, more specifically, of the Leydig cells (Maddock & Nelson 1952). Considerable interest in this problem has been devoted by Jayle and co-workers (1959, 1962), who in addition to the output of oestrogens also measured the urinary excretion of 17-oxosteroids as an index of testicular function. Some modifications of this test were recommended by Huis in't Veld and co-workers (1961) and by Morse and associates (1962). A somewhat different approach to this problem was proposed by Eik-Nes and co-workers (1959), who suggested that analysis of the plasma androsterone concentration after administration of HCG might serve as a clinical test of testicular function in man.

2 THERAPEUTIC CONSIDERATIONS

a Cryptorchidism

The value of HCG therapy versus surgical treatment in cases of cryptorchidism was claimed by Schapiro as early as 1931. In the course of time, however, its real effect has been questioned. It is now well-known that in the large majority of patients a spontaneous descent of the testicles may occur at any time up to puberty. This finding, together with the fact that undescended testicles do not predispose to malignant degeneration, make a conservative attitude to surgery during childhood understandable (Nowakowski 1959, Johnsen 1962). A more active line with early hormonal treatment has, on the other hand, been advocated by Knorr (1963). The possibility of improving fertility by means of such therapy cannot be excluded.

b Hypogonadism in the male

It is useless to treat primary hypogonadism with gonadotrophic hormones. Secondary hypogonadism, on the other hand, constitutes one of the main indications for HCG therapy in the male. Its effect is mainly dependent on the integrity of various testicular elements. In almost all cases there is stimulation of Leydig cell activity with production of androgens and, particularly in patients with idiopathic eunuchoidism, an improvement of secondary sex organ development (Heller & Nelson 1948, Nowakowski 1959). On the other hand, restitution of fertility will be related to the state of the seminiferous tubules at the beginning of treatment. In cases of delayed puberty the administration of HCG may have spectacular effects in this respect due to secondary androgen stimulation of a well-developed tubular apparatus. In hypogonadal eunuchoids, however, with failure on the part of the seminiferous tubules it is more logical to give, in addition to HCG, a hormonal preparation with the capacity of stimulating gametogenic tissue in a direct fashion, e.g., a human menopausal gonadotrophin preparation. Such trials are under way (Apostolakis & Voigt 1965) and the results are awaited with great interest.

c Oligospermia

Administration of HCG has assumed some significance in the treatment of oligospermia in patients with an apparently normal endocrine testicular function and normal urinary excretion rates of gonadotrophins. This condition up to now has proved to be relatively resistant to therapy, which is also illustrated by the large number of therapeutic regimes. The rate of success for the various types of treatment is in the order of 15 per cent. Glass & Holland (1963) treated such patients with large doses of HCG and reported positive results in more than 50 per cent of the cases. These authors emphasize the variable aetiological background of this functional deficiency, e.g., viral infections, severe allergic reactions, and hepatic insufficiency. It is highly probable that therapeutic success will be largely dependent on the establishment of diagnostic criteria for selecting the proper candidates for this treatment. Such diagnostic criteria do not exist at present.

d Hypogonadism in the female

Only secondary hypogonadism is amenable to therapy with gonadotrophic hormones as is the case in the male. HCG has been used for many years, either concurrently with, or subsequent to, anterior pituitary extracts from different animals or pregnant mare serum gonadotrophin in attempts to induce ovulation in women suffering from pituitary disorders or hypothalamic amenorrhoea (Mazer & Ravetz 1941, Rydberg 1943, Hamblen & Davis 1945). The results have been variable and, in particular, it has been difficult to produce repeated ovulation by means of this type of therapy. The main reason for the failures may be assumed to be due to species specificity of the gonadotrophic hormones and the formation of antibodies neutralizing their biological actions.

The logical conclusion of these considerations was drawn by van Wagenen & Simpson (1957) and Simpson & van Wagenen (1958), who were successful in inducing repeated ovulations in the rhesus monkey by means of an FSH preparation obtained from the pituitaries of the same species. In women this principle was first employed by Gemzell and associates (1958) and somewhat later by Buxton & Herrmann (1961). Successful results, in a number of patients leading to pregnancy, have been achieved with sequential therapy including human pituitary FSH and HCG. Reviews of these problems have been presented by Kotz & Herrmann (1961) and by Gemzell (1962).

A severe obstacle to the common use of this therapeutic regimen has been the scarcity of available human pituitary FSH. Therefore, from a practical point of view, the replacement of such preparations by HMG marks an interesting development (Lunenfeld *et al.* 1962, Rosemberg *et al.* 1963, Vande Wiele & Turksoy 1965).

III HUMAN CHORIONIC GROWTH HORMONE-PROLACTIN

A GENERAL

Extracts have been prepared from the human placenta displaying both growth hormone-like and prolactin-like activities. The 2 activities will here be discussed in the same section with reference to the well-founded opinion of Kaplan & Grumbach (1964) that the bioassay data of the partially purified preparations do not yet provide definitive information as to the endocrinological nature of the substance. It may well be that the two main biological actions are displayed by separate hormonal entities. Some results presented by Josimovich & MacLaren (1962) would suggest such a possibility, as the growth hormone potency during the purification process increased until the final step, at which somatotropic and lactogenic activity were largely separated. On the other hand, this finding may be explained by the inactivation of certain structural groups responsible for growth-promoting activity intrinsic in a molecule that also possesses lactogenic properties. The claim that highly purified HGH itself displays lactogenic action may, by analogy, be adduced in support of such an interpretation (Ferguson & Wallace 1961, Chadwick *et al.* 1961), even if the validity of this argument is lessened in the light of the differential precipitation studies of Wilhelmi (1961), in view of the results of Brauman and associates (1964), and particularly with regard to the report of Apostolakis (1965) on a highly potent pituitary prolactin fraction. Until further experimental evidence is brought forward on the placental factor the question as to its possible unimolecular or multiple molecular nature will remain unsettled. In this review the name suggested by Kaplan & Grumbach (1964), namely human chorionic growth hormone-prolactin (HCGP) will be used.

Ehrhardt (1936) was the first to report the presence of prolactin-like activity in the human placenta. The urinary excretion during pregnancy of a substance with similar action was reported by Coppedge & Segaloff (1951). Ito & Higashi (1961) and Higashi (1961, 1962) presented a procedure for the extraction and purification of a placental substance with lactogenic properties, and Josimowich & MacLaren (1962) independently described a method to isolate a protein from the same source with similar properties, present also in retroplacental as well as in peripheral blood at term, and being immunochemically related to, yet not identical with, human pituitary growth hormone.

Fukushima (1961) prepared an extract from the human placenta and maternal blood which exhibited somatotropic effects, e.g., potent stimulation of tibial growth in hypophysectomized rats. Any information on possible lactogenic properties of this substance was not given. Circumstantial evidence suggesting the placenta as a possible source of a growth hormone-like factor had been brought forward some years earlier by Gemzell and associates (1955) when, by means of the tibial growth test, they demonstrated an increased growth activity in retroplacental blood.

B CHEMICAL NATURE

I EXTRACTION AND PURIFICATION

A number of methods for the extraction and purification of the growth hormone-prolactin from the human placenta have been published within the last few years. The methods of Ito & Higashi (1961), Higashi (1961, 1962), and Fukushima (1961) are mainly based on differential extraction at various pH values and ammonium sulphate concentrations as well as precipitation in acetone and/or ethanol. Josimovich & MacLaren (1962) also included chromatography on an Amberlite CG-50 column, Cohen and associates (1964) employed a DEAE-cellulose column followed by Sephadex G-75 filtration, and Friesen (1965a) used Sephadex G-100. Friesen (1965b) subsequently published a method leading to considerably higher yields of active material by employing, as starting material, Fraction VII, a by-product of the extraction of γ-globulin from human placentas. Turtle *et al.* (1966) have isolated HCGP of high specific activity by a modification of the method reported by Cohen and associates (1964) Precipitation at pH 5 prior to gel filtration consistently removed 36 per cent of protein with minimal loss of HCGP activity. Florini and co-workers (1966), finally, have devised procedures for large-scale production of approximately 70 per cent pure material and for further purification of this material by gel filtration on Sephadex G-100.

2 PURITY

Fairly pure preparations have been obtained. Detailed data will be found in the paper of Cohen and associates (1964). The homogeneity of their placental preparation was obviously greater than that of the Raben HGH. Yet, some impurities were present. By means of vertical starch gel descending electrophoresis slight contamination with serum proteins, mainly albumin, was observed. Florini *et al.* (1966) reported that their most highly purified product appeared homogeneous by most of the criteria employed by the authors. However, moving boundary electrophoresis and starch gel electrophoresis revealed the presence of small amounts of contaminating material.

3 BIOCHEMICAL AND PHYSICO-CHEMICAL PROPERTIES

The placental material is a protein with a maximum absorption in the ultraviolet region at 278 mμ and with a minimum at 257 mμ (Friesen 1965a). The tyrosine/tryptophan ratio is reported to be between 3·0 and 3·5, and the $E_{1\,\text{cm}}^{1\,\text{per cent}}$ is 9·43, and the amino acid composition very similar to that of HGH (Friesen 1965a). Florini *et al.* (1966) reported that elemental analysis of their highly purified material revealed the presence of 49·22 per cent carbon, 7·39 per cent hydrogen, 15·15 per cent nitrogen, 1·16 per cent sulphur and 24·50 per cent oxygen. The results suggest that the protein does not contain any significant amounts of carbohydrate or lipid. Analysis of the amino acid content gave results which were consistent with those obtained by Friesen (1965a). Immunoelectrophoretic analysis indicates that the placental hormone has a faster-moving anodal component than HGH (Kaplan & Grumbach 1964). Friesen (1965a) also claims that differences exist as to electrophoretic mobility between the somatotropic substance from the placenta and HGH.

On the basis of its elution volume from Sephadex G-100 a molecular weight of 30,000 has been calculated (Friesen 1965a). This is at variance with the estimates of Higashi (1962) based on the sedimentation constants of 2 active placental preparations. He claims that the molecular weights of the 2 active components with slightly different biological action were 45,000 and 80,000, respectively. Florini and associates (1966) also determined the molecular weight of their highly purified material in the ultracentrifuge and found it to be 38,000. Ultracentrifugal analysis of the same material in 5 M guanidine hydrochloride showed a single peak with a molecular weight of 18,600. On the basis of their findings the authors conclude that HCGP is a dimer constituted by 2 peptide chains of equimolecular weight.

C BIOLOGICAL PROPERTIES

The biological properties of HCGP have been studied extensively in animals. In man a rather limited number of observations have been published up to the present time.

Fukushima (1961) found that extracts prepared from early human placentas had a considerable activity in the tibial test, whereas preparations from term placentas were inactive in this respect. Kaplan & Grumbach (1964), however, reported growth hormone-like activity also in extracts from term placentas, although the effects were admittedly comparatively weak. Tibial growth and *in vivo* uptake of radioactive sulphate by costal cartilage were used as indices of response. Friesen (1965a) also observed that extracts from term placentas possessed somatotropic action. The effect was tested on the weight change of hypophysectomized male rats. The results, however, were variable; some batches being completely inactive, although no significant variations between the different preparations were observed by means of starch gel electrophoresis. Florini and associates (1966) have also contributed to the controversial issue of the growth-promoting activity of HCGP. These authors consistently observed a somatotropic effect provided that sufficiently high doses were given. They also demonstrated a dose-dependent stimulation of growth in hypophysectomized or intact rats and in intact mice.

Prolactin-like activity of placental extracts as evidenced in the pigeon crop sac assay has been repeatedly reported (Ito & Higashi 1961, Josimovich & MacLaren 1962; Kaplan & Grumbach 1964, Friesen 1965b, Florini *et al.* 1966). Stimulation of lactation in pseudo-pregnant or virgin rabbits by means of such extracts has also been shown (Josimovich & MacLaren 1962, Friesen 1965b).

Among other effects elicited by this placental substance may be mentioned its luteotropic action (Josimovich *et al.* 1963, Florini *et al.*

1966). Furthermore, it has been found capable of increasing the circulating ketone bodies in fasted rats and of stimulating the incorporation of labelled glucose into fat (Friesen 1965a). Riggi and associates (1966) found a significant rise of plasma free fatty acid concentration in fasted rabbits or monkeys following the intramuscular injection of a single dose of HCGP. They also observed that this factor caused hyperglycemia, hypertriglyceridemia and an elevation of plasma free fatty acids when given daily to rabbits for 25 days. These results are highly interesting in view of the diabetogenic effect of pregnancy.

Comparatively little is known concerning the effects of HCGP in man. Beck & Daughaday (1967), however, have studied the acute metabolic effects and disposition of this substance in 5-hour and 12-hour infusions of physiological doses of a highly purified preparation. The mean plasma half-life, metabolic pool size, and turnover rate of HCGP were similar to those previously calculated for HGH. From their data the authors concluded that the secretion rate of HCGP is in the range of 290 mg daily. After 12-hour infusions the glucose tolerance was decreased in the majority of test subjects despite an increased insulin response. On the other hand there were no significant changes in the mean blood glucose, plasma insulin, and free fatty acid concentrations in fasting subjects before and after HCGP administration.

It is obvious that a substance with so many activities would provoke much speculation concerning its possible physiological significance. Its lactogenic and somatotropic effects appear to have been firmly established. Its stimulative activity on body growth seems attributable to a true protein anabolic effect. Riggi and associates (1966) conclude that the hormone possesses biological properties closely resembling those displayed by HGH. Josimovich and Atwood (1964) have found that HCGP potentiates HGH in the tibial test, and these investigators also propose a synergistic action between HGH and HCGP. This view is supported by the results of Florini and co-workers (1966) who demonstrated the potentiation of HGH by HCGP on body weight gains in hypophysectomized immature male rats. Kaplan & Grumbach (1964) have implied that HCGP might be the trigger of metabolic changes serving the manifold demands of the maternal and foetal organisms during the course of pregnancy. This seems to be a fruitful hypothesis; it opens up a large number of avenues of research and invites experimental verification. Highly interesting contributions according to this general line of thought have since been made in studies on the glycolipometabolic changes produced by HCGP. Riggi and associates (1966) discuss the possibility that HCGP might act as a diabetogenic factor in pregnancy, thereby increasing the availability of glucose to the foetus with maintenance of elevated plasma lipid concentrations in the maternal circulation. Beck & Daughaday (1967) further strengthen this view by demonstrating decreased carbohydrate tolerance and impaired peripheral glucose utilization coinciding with increased plasma insulin responses to glucose. The suggestion that HCGP might act as an insulin antagonist is supported directly by the demonstrated metabolic effects induced by HCGP and indirectly by the parallel increases in the plasma levels of insulin and HCGP during pregnancy (Spellacy & Goetz 1963, Spellacy *et al.* 1965a, b, Beck *et al.* 1965, Spellacy *et al.* 1967).

D ANTIGENICAL PROPERTIES

Josimovich & MacLaren (1962) were the first to report an immunological relationship between a substance which they had extracted from the human placenta and HGH. By means of the double diffusion technique of Ouchterlony they found a reaction of partial identity between HGH on the one hand and the placental extract and retroplacental as well as peripheral term serum on the other. The demonstration of these antigenical properties intrinsic in a substance of placental origin has opened up a new segment in the endocrinology of gestation and has triggered an impressive research activity in this field. In fact, the cross-reactivity between the placental protein and HGH is so far the one consistent finding attributable to this new factor (Josimovich & MacLaren 1962, Josimovich *et al.* 1963, Josimovich & Atwood 1964, Kaplan & Grumbach 1964, Grumbach & Kaplan 1965), which apparently possesses considerably more elusive biological properties.

Kaplan & Grumbach (1964), after absorption of anti-HGH serum with the placental protein, failed to elicit any reaction by means of immunoelectrophoresis between the antiserum and placental homogenate, whereas a precipitin band of unaltered electrophoretic mobility appeared with HGH. As could be inferred from these as well as from the earlier results some antigenic determinants are common to the 2 factors; others, however, are specific for HGH. These distinct differences have stimulated considerable speculation as to possible relationships between antigenical structure and biological function. Josimovich & MacLaren (1962) proposed that HGH had one or more antigenical groups in excess of those inherent in the placental factor, and that these antigenically reactive groups were in some way associated with structural sub-units of the molecule engaged in its somatotropic activity. However, as pointed out above, several investigators have observed growth hormone-like properties of placental extracts cross-reacting with HGH (Kaplan & Grumbach 1964, Grumbach & Kaplan 1965, Friesen 1965). Josimovich and associates (1963) also discuss another possible interpretation of their experimental results, namely that antiserum to HGH is, in fact, constituted by antibodies to 2 different but up to recently inseparable entities, namely HGH and a pituitary prolactin. Although Josimovich and co-workers more or less reject this explanation it would seem rather plausible in the opinion of the reviewer. In fact, Josimovich & MacLaren (1962) have themselves achieved some separation of a somatotropic and lactogenic factor (see above). Furthermore, Greenwood and associates (1964) have presented some data, which suggest the occurrence of increased concentrations of HGH both in the foetal and maternal organisms and, in addition, the appearance in the later stages of pregnancy of a substance showing antigenical similarity to but not identity with HGH.

It could be argued that some of the biological effects, particularly the luteotropic activity, claimed to be elicited by HCGP, might in fact be displayed by contaminating HCG. The HCGP preparations, however, seem to be free from HCG. This has been demonstrated by immunological means as the two substances apparently lack any serological relationship (Josimovich *et al.* 1963, Kaplan & Grumbach 1964).

E SITE OF SYNTHESIS

Conclusive evidence has been brought forward that HCGP is synthesized in placental tissue. Such a statement is based on circumstantial findings as well as direct proof.

I TISSUE OF PRODUCTION

With some rare exceptions, possibly due to analytical errors, HCGP has only been found during pregnancy. It is cleared from the circulation within a day or two after parturition (Greenwood *et al.* 1964, Kaplan & Grumbach 1965). Comparatively large amounts of the substance have been found in the blood and in the placenta of a patient who had been hypophysectomized 12 weeks prior to delivery (Josimovich & Atwood 1964). HCGP has also been recovered from the trophoblast of a blighted ovum and from a hydatidiform mole which indicates that the substance may be produced even in the absence of a foetus (Josimovich & Atwood 1964).

Conclusive evidence that placental tissue actually synthesizes HCGP has been brought forward by Grumbach & Kaplan (1965). Fragments from 2 first trimester placentas and 1 term placenta were established in tissue culture. The supernatant nutrient media from the explants of chorionic villi contained detectable HCGP for between 43 and 136 days.

2 CELLS OF ORIGIN

Sciarra and associates (1963) have used the fluorescent antibody technique, both in its direct and indirect application, in attempts to localize HCGP within placental tissue. A number of steps were taken to ensure the specificity of the reaction. In all instances specific fluorescence was localized to the cytoplasm of the syncytiotrophoblastic layer of the chorionic villi, whereas no specific fluorescence was observed within the cytotrophoblastic cells. The earliest placental specimen examined was from the 12th week of pregnancy.

F ASSAY PROCEDURES AND BODY FLUID LEVELS

1 BIOASSAY

The bioassay methods used for the detection of HCGP are those which have been generally employed for the demonstration of somatropic, lactogenic, and luteotropic activity. Thus, somatotropic properties of HCGP have been inferred from positive effects in assays based on the ability to promote widening of the tibial epiphyseal cartilage of hypophysectomized immature rats (Greenspan *et al.* 1949) or to stimulate the *in vivo* uptake of radioactive sulphate by costal cartilage in the hypophysectomized rat (Collins & Baker 1961). Lactogenic effects have been deduced from its ability to cause growth of the crop-sac of pigeons (Riddle & Bates 1939 and a number of subsequent modifications), and luteotropic action has been assumed in view of its capacity to maintain a decidual reaction in pseudo-pregnant, hypophysectomized rats (Josimovich *et al.* 1963).

All these methods may be considered qualitative or only roughly semi-quantitative. For more precise and accurate estimations of HCGP in tissues and body fluids it has, therefore, been necessary to resort to immunoassay procedures.

2 IMMUNOASSAY

Greenwood and associates (1964) have employed a radio-immunoelectrophoretic method using HGH-I^{131} and antiserum to HGH and determined the fraction of antiserum-bound labelled hormone by means of electrophoresis and radioactivity measurements. A standard reference curve was obtained with various concentrations of unlabelled HGH. The slope of this curve was calculated and may be considered as characteristic for the specific immunological reaction between HGH and anti-HGH provided that the hormone preparation is sufficiently pure in relation to the sensitivity of the assay procedure.

Inhibition curves parallel to that of the standard curve were obtained with plasma samples from non-pregnant subjects and from patients with acromegaly. Serial assays on blood from a pregnant woman showed that criteria for parallelism were fulfilled at 8 weeks. An estimate of 20 μg of HGH per ml was obtained, a value which is considerably higher than that found in non-pregnant women (1 to 6 μg per ml). Later in pregnancy, however, a reduced slope was found, invalidating the HGH determinations in plasma by means of this method. The inference was that in addition to HGH there appeared during the second and third trimester another substance, showing antigenic determinants with HGH, but not being identical with it. This cross-reacting substance, apparently similar to that contained in the preparations of Ito & Higashi (1961), Fukushima (1961) Josimovich & MacLaren (1962), Kaplan & Grumbach (1964), and Friesen (1965), was found by Greenwood and associates (1964) in extracts of human placenta, in plasma throughout pregnancy from about the 8th week, and in retroplacental maternal blood, but not in umbilical cord blood or in the amniotic fluid. It had disappeared from maternal blood within 2 to 8 days *post partum*. The growth hormone levels in the foetus were considerably increased, approximately 50 μg per ml, and in the amniotic fluid more than double this concentration was found.

Kaplan & Grumbach (1965) have also used a radioimmunoassay procedure, but with somewhat different reactants. They employed HCGP-I^{131} and antiserum prepared against a highly purified HCGP. For the separation of bound and free labelled hormone they applied the method of Berson & Yalow (1958). With this procedure no reaction was observed with a HGH preparation at concentrations of 0·05 to 10·0 μg per ml, with serum from normal adults or children, or with samples from patients with active acromegaly, thus indicating a high degree of specificity of this technique for the assay of the placental factor.

These investigators found low levels of HCGP at 56 days after the last menstrual period (0·53 μg per ml) with a sharp rise up to more than 20 μg per ml at the end of pregnancy. The 24-hour urinary excretion rate also showed a marked increase during gestation with values around 100 μg towards the end. Only insignificant amounts of this hormone were present in foetal blood, the maternal serum concentrations being about 50 to 200 times higher. In a small number of amniotic fluid analyses the levels ranged from 2·0 to 11·1 μg of HCGP per ml.

Josimovich & Atwood (1964) have reported a somewhat different urinary excretion pattern of HCGP during pregnancy. They used the Ouchterlony 3-basin double diffusion technique, and their results are, therefore, only roughly quantitative. However, these investigators found a 24- to 320-fold greater amount HCGP in the urine at 6 to 8 weeks' of pregnancy than at term.

Yen and associates (1965) have employed a different approach to this problem. They made use of a haemagglutination inhibition procedure with HGH-coated erythrocytes and antiserum to HGH. The sensitivity was considerably increased by pre-incubation of the hormone to be assayed with the HGH-antiserum for 12 hours at 5°C, and the specificity and accuracy improved by means of an extraction procedure of HGH from serum. With this extraction procedure no HCGP could be recovered from a serum sample to which 1 mg of the purified substance had been added. Furthermore, the slopes of the inhibition curves obtained with the HGH standard and extracts from maternal and foetal sera were parallel. This procedure thus measures the HGH concentration during pregnancy apparently without HCGP being an interfering factor.

Yen and associates (1965) found a normal range of 1 to 6 μg HGH per ml of serum. In maternal serum during pregnancy slightly elevated levels were observed with a mean around 10 μg per ml. In foetal blood the concentrations were still higher with a mean of 19·9 μg in umbilical arterial blood and 13·1 μg in umbilical venous blood. The difference was statistically significant. This latter finding apparently indicates active production of HGH in the pituitary gland of the foetus.

These studies suggest the complexity of the problem. They indicate that the maternal organism, particularly towards the end of pregnancy, is flooded with a substance which displays both somatotropic and lactogenic properties although of comparatively weak potency, which shares some antigenic determinants with HGH, and which to some extent is also found in the amniotic fluid, but almost not at all within the foetus. On the other hand, a substance immunologically identical to HGH, has been demonstrated in substantial amounts in foetal blood, whereas the maternal blood levels are only slightly elevated. This picture emerges from the reports quoted above and is also substantiated by experimental data provided by Grumbach & Kaplan (1965). The findings certainly raise a number of questions, so far completely unanswered, among which the most fascinating are the physiological significance of these endocrinologically active substances and the problem of their transplacental passage.

IV OTHER PROTEIN HORMONES OR HORMONAL PEPTIDES

A GENERAL

A number of other protein hormones have been assumed to be produced in the placenta. The experimental evidence brought forward to support these assumptions is, however, very tenuous. The conclusions have largely been based on circumstantial findings or incomplete verification. Actual proof has not yet been produced in any instance. Thus the occurrence of higher concentrations of these substances in the placenta than in other tissues or body fluids has not been demonstrated and the conclusive criterion, i.e., their demonstration in the culture medium of chorionic cells propagated in tissue culture, has not been established. On the other hand it does not seem permissible to disregard the human placenta as a potential source of a considerably larger spectrum of protein hormones than HCG and HCGP, particularly as some results have been forthcoming that might be interpreted to indicate certain qualitative differences between the activities of the placental extracts and the corresponding hypophysial factors. Thus ACTH and MSH, isolated from chorionic tissue, have been found to display dose-response curves different from those of pituitary ACTH and MSH (Yamamoto & Morioka 1956, Karkun & Sen 1963). Furthermore, it has been claimed that pituitary MSH causes darkening of the entire body of hypophysectomized frogs whereas pregnancy urine, pregnancy serum, and placental extracts induces expansion of the melanocytes only in the hind part of the body (Stolte *et al.* 1952, 1953). In view of the existence of certain definite differences between HCGP and the corresponding pituitary factor(s), both with respect to biological potency and, even more, as regards antigenical activity, it seems legitimate to speculate on the possible role of the human placenta as a source of a full set of protein hormones similar to, but not identical with those produced in the hypophysis. Their detection and characterization may be difficult with biological methods but could possibly be achieved by means of serological techniques, as has been the case with HCGP.

B ADRENOCORTICOTROPHIC HORMONE

Jailer & Knowlton (1950) reported a decrease in ascorbic acid in the adrenals of newborn or hypophysectomized rats after injecting extracts from human placenta. This finding was subsequently confirmed in a large number of papers (the reader is referred to Diczfalusy & Troen (1961) for a detailed survey of the literature). Assali & Hamermesz (1954) claimed that extracts from chorionic tissue displayed higher ACTH activity than preparations from intervillous blood. Schwers & Fanard (1958), on the other hand, maintained that all the ACTH activity was derived from the blood and that almost none was present in the placenta.

It is probable that the serum ACTH levels are increased during pregnancy but at present the role of the placenta in this context remains obscure. The finding of Little and associates (1958) has been taken as an argument against any significant extra-pituitary production of ACTH during pregnancy (Diczfalusy & Troen 1961). Little and co-workers (1958) gave a detailed report on a patient who was hypophysectomized during the 26th week of pregnancy. For the next 6 weeks she received 75 mg cortisone daily, which was then abruptly discontinued. After 48 hours clinical signs of acute adrenal insufficiency appeared. It is true that this might suggest the absence of any more considerable formation of ACTH in the placenta. The possibility still exists, however, that the placenta produces an ACTH-like substance that only to a very small degree may take over the function of pituitary ACTH.

C MELANOCYTE-STIMULATING HORMONE

It is an ancient observation that pregnancy is associated with increased dermal and mucosal pigmentation at certain preferential sites. Konsuloff (1934) reported the urinary excretion during gestation of a substance capable of eliciting darkening of the skin of hypophysectomized frogs. Elevated serum levels of MSH have been found by Shizume & Lerner

(1954). The latter investigators claimed that the urinary excretion of this hormone showed an increase towards the end of pregnancy and that pre-pregnant levels were attained within 5 days *post partum*. Dahlberg (1960) has presented a detailed survey of the literature in this field, a critical examination of the analytical methods, and his own results on the urinary excretion of MSH in non-pregnant and pregnant women. An increased excretion rate during pregnancy was noted with considerable individual fluctuations and without any statistically significant differences between the various months of gestation.

The presence of MSH hormone in placental extracts has been claimed by several investigators (Sulman & Bergmann 1953, Eschbach 1959). A critical attitude to this opinion is, however, taken by Karkun & Sen (1963). It is true that they were also able to isolate MSH activity from the placenta, but the potency of the extracts was rather small. These authors also point out the interfering action of ACTH when present in the extracts, as this hormone also provokes melanophore changes in amphibian skin. It may therefore be concluded that additional studies are necessary to establish a more conclusive view on the possible MSH-synthesizing activity of the human placenta.

D THYROID-STIMULATING HORMONE

A number of changes occur in the maternal organism during pregnancy that may be caused by increased synthesis of TSH. Akasu and co-workers (1955) isolated a substance from the human placenta with TSH-like properties when tested on guinea-pigs. Philipp (1955) also suggested that chorionic tissue was a site of production of TSH. Ueda and associates (1964), however, were not able to support this opinion. Extracts of human placentae obtained at normal deliveries and caesarean sections consistently showed a lower TSH activity than that displayed by human sera from pregnant as well as non-pregnant patients.

E RELAXIN

Relaxin, a hormone of pregnancy causing relaxation of the symphysis of the guinea-pig, was reported to be present in the blood of pregnant women by Pommerenke (1934) and by Abramson and co-workers (1937). Zarrow and associates (1955) performed a quantitative study and found 0·2 guinea-pig units per ml in the first trimester and 2 units per ml in the last few weeks of pregnancy. In the placenta they found a range from 0·5 to 4·0 units per g. Dallenbach & Dallenbach-Hellweg (1964) carried out a serological investigation on the role of the placenta as a potential source of this hormone. They used the fluorescent antibody technique both in its direct and indirect form. Positive fluorescence was noticed in the basal trophoblastic cells but also in the decidual cells. These investigators concluded that it was highly probable that relaxin was not only stored but also formed at the two sites exhibiting positive fluorescence.

It is difficult to evaluate the validity of these results. Dallenbach & Dallenbach-Hellweg (1964) do not in their paper state the source of the antigen used for preparation of the antisera. Furthermore, their antisera were apparently heterogeneous in the Ouchterlony plate, which invalidates the specificity of the fluorescent antibody reaction. No information on the necessary removal of unspecific antibodies is given.

F OXYTOCIN AND VASOPRESSIN

A number of reports indicate the presence of these highly active peptides in the human placenta (the reader is referred to Diczfalusy & Troen (1961) for references to the literature). The evidence, however, is not conclusive and further research is necessary. The catabolic activity of placental tissue with respect to these hormones seems more definitely established. Enzymes capable of inactivating oxytocin as well as vasopressin have been found in the human placenta (Hawker 1956, Hooper & Jessup 1959). It is possible that these enzymes are produced in chorionic tissue. This area of research has been reviewed by Caldeyro-Barcia (1960).

REFERENCES

ABRAMOWITZ A.A. & HISAW F.L. (1939) The effects of proteolytic enzymes on purified gonadotropic hormones. *Endocrinology*, **25**, 633.

ABRAMSON D., HURWITT E. & LESNICK G. (1937) Relaxin in human serum as a test for pregnancy. *Surg. Gynec. Obstet.* **65**, 335.

AKASU F., KAWAHARA S., OHKI H., HARANO M. & TEJIMA Y. (1955) Thyroid stimulating hormone extracted from human placenta. *Endocr. Japon.* **2**, 297.

ALBERT A. (1948) A clinical bio-assay for chorionic gonadotropin. *J. clin. Endocr.* **8**, 619.

ALBERT A. & BERKSON J. (1951) A clinical bioassay for chorionic gonadotropin. *J. clin. Endocr.* **11**, 805.

ALBERT A. & DERNER I. (1960) Studies on the biologic characterization of human gonadotropins. VI. Nature and number of gonadotropins in human pregnancy urine. *J. clin. Endocr.* **20**, 1225.

ALBERT A. & KELLY S. (1958) Studies on the biologic characterization of human gonadotropins. II. Comparison of human pituitary gonadotropin (urine) and human chorionic gonadotropin (urine). *J. clin. Endocr.* **18**, 1067.

ALBERT A., KELLY S. & KOBI J. (1958) Studies on the biologic characterization o human gonadotropins. I. Human pituitary gonadotropin from urine of normal men, and postmenopausal and castrated women. *J. clin. Endocr.* **18**, 843.

ALONSO C. & TROEN P. (1966) Perfusion studies of the human placenta. V. Metabolism of [^{3}H] estrone [^{35}S] sulfate and [^{14}C] estradiol-17β at mid-pregnancy. *Biochemistry* **5**, 337.

ANDERSEN F. (1938) Lesions of the fetuses of rats after treatment of the mothers with gonadotropic hormones. *Acta path. microbiol. scand.*, Suppl. **37**, 60.

ANSELMINO K.J. & HOFFMANN F. (1936) Über die Ausscheidung von hypophysär gebildeten, gonadotropen Hormonen in der normalen Schwangerschaft und bei den Schwangerschaftstoxikosen. *Z. Geburtsh. Gynäk.* **114**, 52.

APOSTOLAKIS M. (1965) Lack of high growth hormone activity in highly active human pituitary prolactin extracts. *Proc. 2nd Internat. Congr. Endocr., London* 1964, part II, p. 1257. Excerpta Medica Foundation, Internat. Congr. Ser. No. 83.

APOSTOLAKIS M. & VOIGT K.-D. (1965) *Gonadotropine.* Georg Thieme Verlag, Stuttgart.

ARVAY A.V. (1934) Beiträge zur innersekretorischen Funktion der Plazenta bzw. des Chorion. *Endokrinologie*, **14**, 309.

ASBOE-HANSEN G. (1951) *Om Bindevaevets Mucinøse Substanser.* Dissertation. Copenhagen.

ASCHHEIM S. & ZONDEK B. (1927) Hypophysenvorderlappenhormon und Ovarialhormon im Harn von Schwangeren. *Klin. Wschr.* **6**, 1322.

ASSALI N.S. & HAMERMESZ J. (1954) Adrenocorticotropic substances from human placenta. *Endocrinology*, **55**, 561.

BACHMAN C. (1935) Immunologic studies of anti-gonadotropic sera. *Proc. Soc. exp Biol. (N.Y.)*, **32**, 851.

BACHMAN C., COLLIP J.B. & SELYE H. (1934) Anti-gonadotropic substances. *Proc. Soc. exp. Biol. (N.Y.)*, **32**, 544.

BAKER B.L., HOOK S.J. & SEVERINGHAUS A.E. (1944) The cytological structure of the human chorionic villus and decidua parietalis. *Amer. J. Anat.* **74**, 291.

BANGHAM D.R. & GRAB B. (1964) The Second International Standard for chorionic gonadotrophin. *Bull. Wld Hlth Org.* **31**, 111.

BANIK U.K. (1959) Effect of pH and temperature on the stability of human chorionic gonadotrophin. *Ann. Biochem. exp. Med.* **19**, 5.

BANIK U.K. & CHAKRAVARTI H.S. (1957) Inactivation of human chorionic gonadotrophin by addition of drugs. *Ann. Biochem. exp. Med.* **17**, 63.

BECK P. & DAUGHADAY W.H. (1967) Human placental lactogen: studies of its acute metabolic effects and disposition in normal man. *J. clin. Invest.* **46**, 103.

Beck P., Parker M.L. & Daughaday W.H. (1965) Radioimmunologic measurement of human placental lactogen in plasma by a double antibody method during normal and diabetic pregnancies. *J. clin. Endocr.* **25**, 1457.

Behrman S.J. & Niemann P. (1955a) Serum gonadotrophins in normal and abnormal pregnancy. I. Quantitative and qualitative analysis. *Fertil. and Steril.* **6**, 236.

Behrman S.J. & Niemann P. (1955b) Serum gonadotrophins in normal and abnormal pregnancy. II. Function and action of chorionic gonadotrophin hormones. *Fertil and Steril.* **6**, 415.

Bell E.T., Borth R., Brody S., Carlström G. & Menzi A. (1967) Comparison of bioassay and immunoassay. Read by Borth in *Recent Research on Gonadotrophic Hormones. Proceedings of Fifth Gonadotrophin Club Meeting Edinburgh*, 1966, p. 77. E.T.Bell & J.A.Loraine, eds. Livingstone, Edinburgh and London.

Berson S. A. & Yalow R. S. (1957) Ethanol fractionation of plasma and electrophoretic identification of insulin-binding antibody. *J. clin. Invest.* **36**, 642.

Berson S.A. & Yalow R.A. (1958) Isotopic tracers in the study of diabetes. *Advanc. biol. med. Phys.* **5**, 349.

Berson S.A., Yalow R.S., Bauman A., Rothschild A. & Newerly K. (1956) Insulin-I^{131} metabolism in human subjects. Demonstration of insulin binding globulin in the circulation of insulin treated subjects. *J. clin. Invest.* **35**, 170.

Birke G., Franksson C. & Plantin L.-O. (1954) On the excretion of androgens in carcinoma of the prostate. *Acta endocr. (Kbh.)* **15**, Suppl. 17.

Bischoff F. (1940) The action of cysteine or cyanide upon gonadotropic extracts. *J. biol. Chem.* **134**, 641.

Bischoff F. (1946) The temperature coefficient for the denaturation of chorionic and mare serum gonadotropins in aqueous and in urea solutions. *J. biol. Chem.* **165**, 399.

Bliss C.I. (1952) *The Statistics of Bioassay.* Academic Press, New York.

Blobel R., Uhlig H. & Schumacher G. (1962) Biochemical studies with human chorionic gonadotrophin (HCG). *Acta endocr. (Kbh.)*, Suppl. **67**, 72.

Bordet J. & Gengou O. (1901) Sur l'existence de substances sensibilisatrices dans la plupart des serums anti-microbiens. *Ann. Inst. Pasteur*, **15**, 289.

Borell U. (1954) The effect of large doses of human chorionic gonadotrophin on the excretion of neutral 17-ketosteroids in women. *Acta endocr. (Kbh.)*, **17**, 13.

Borth R. (1952) The chromatographic method for the determination of urinary pregnanediol. In *Steroid Metabolism and Estimation.* Ciba Foundation Colloquia on Endocrinology, vol. **2**, p. 45. G.E.W.Wolstenholme, ed. Churchill, London.

Borth R., Gsell M. & de Watteville H. (1953) Urinary steroids and vaginal smear in ovariectomized women treated with chorionic gonadotrophin. *Acta endocr. (Kbh.)*, **14**, 316.

Borth R., Diczfalusy E. & Heinrichs H.D. (1957a) Grundlagen der statistischen Auswertung biologischer Bestimmungen. *Arch. Gynäk.* **188**, 497.

Borth R., Lunenfeld B. & de Watteville H. (1957b) Effect of serum used as vehicle on the quantal assay of human chorionic gonadotrophin by the ovarian hyperaemia response in rats. *Acta endocr. (Kbh.)*, **24**, 119.

Borth R., Lunenfeld B., Stamm O. & de Watteville H. (1959) Gonadotrophin and steroid excretion in a case of twin pregnancy. *Acta obstet. gynec. scand.* **38**, 417.

BORTH R., FERIN M. & MENZI A. (1964) Comparison of bioassay and immunoassay of human chorionic gonadotrophin in urine. Paper presented at the 2nd International Congress of Endocrinology, London.

BOTELLA-LLUSIA J., NOGALES F. & DURAN J.M. (1957) Über den Nachweis der Glykoproteine im menschlichen Trophoblast. *Arch. Gynäk.* **188**, 269.

BOURRILLON R., GOT R. & MARCY R. (1959) Stabilité de la gonadotrophine choriale humaine sous l'effet d'agents chimiques. *Bull. Soc. Chim. biol. (Paris)*, **41**, 345.

BOYCOTT M. & ROWLANDS I.W. (1938) The biological nature and quantitative variation of the gonadotropic activity of pregnant women's serum. *Br. med. J.* i, 1097.

BOYDEN S.V. (1951) The adsorption of proteins on erythrocytes treated with tannic acid and subsequent hemagglutination by antiprotein sera. *J. exp. Med.* **93**, 107.

BRADBURY J.T. & BROWN W.E. (1948) Absorption and excretion of chorionic gonadotropin administered intramuscularly in women. *J. clin. Endocr.* **8**, 1037.

BRADBURY J.T., BROWN W.E. & GRAY L.A. (1950) Maintenance of the corpus luteum and physiologic actions of progesterone. *Recent Progress in Hormone Res.* **5**, 151.

BRADY R.O. (1951) Biosynthesis of radioactive testosterone *in vitro*. *J. biol. Chem.* **193**, 145.

BRAUMAN J., BRAUMAN H. & PASTEELS J.L. (1964) Immunoassay of growth hormone in cultures of human hypophysis by the method of complement fixation: comparison of the growth hormone secretion and the prolactin activity. *Nature*, **202**, 1116.

BREWER J.J., GERBIE A.B., DOLKART R.E., SKOM J.H., NAGLE R.G. & TOROK E.E. (1964) Chemotherapy in trophoblastic diseases. *Amer. J. Obstet. Gynec.* **90**, 566.

BRINCK-JOHNSEN T. & EIK-NES K. (1957) Effect of human chorionic gonadotropin on the secretion of testosterone and 4-androstene-3,17-dione by the canine testis. *Endocrinology*, **61**, 676.

BRODY S. (1966) Immunoassay of human chorionic gonadotrophin. Methodological and statistical aspects of a graded-response procedure based on complement fixation. *Acta endocr. (Kbh.)*, **52**, 113.

BRODY S. & CARLSTRÖM G. (1960) Estimation of human chorionic gonadotrophin in biological fluids by complement fixation. *Lancet*, ii, 99.

BRODY S. & CARLSTRÖM G. (1961) Studies on the determination of human chorionic gonadotrophin by complement fixation. *Scand. J. clin. Lab. Invest.* **13**, 683.

BRODY S. & CARLSTRÖM G. (1962a) Immunoassay of human chorionic gonadotropin in normal and pathologic pregnancy. *J. clin. Endocr.* **22**, 564.

BRODY S. & CARLSTRÖM G. (1962b) Immunoassay of human chorionic gonadotrophin – methodological and clinical aspects. *Acta endocr. (Kbh.)*, Suppl. **67**, 19.

BRODY S. & CARLSTRÖM G. (1962c) Determination of human chorionic gonadotropin in biological fluids by complement fixation. In *Immunoassay of Hormones*. Ciba Foundation Colloquia of Endocrinology **14**, 329. G.E.W.Wolstenholme & M.P.Cameron, eds. Churchill, London.

BRODY S. & CARLSTRÖM G. (1963) The problem of specificity in serologic determination of human chorionic gonadotrophin. *Acta endocr. (Kbh.)*, **42**, 485.

BRODY S. & CARLSTRÖM G. (1965a) Human chorionic gonadotropin in abnormal pregnancy. Serum and urinary findings using various immunoassay techniques. *Acta obstet. gynec. scand.* **44**, 32.

BRODY S. & CARLSTRÖM G. (1965b) Human chorionic gonadotropin pattern in serum and its relation to the sex of the fetus. *J. clin. Endocr.* **25**, 792.

BRODY S. & CARLSTRÖM G. (1965c) Problems associated with the quantitative immunoassay of human chorionic gonadotropin. In *Gonadotrophins. Physicochemical and Immunological Properties.* Ciba Foundation Study Group No. 22, p. 70. G.E.W.Wolstenholme & J.Knight, eds. Churchill, London.

BROSSMER R. & WALTER K. (1958) Enzymatische Abspaltung von Lactaminsäure und Inaktivierung von Choriongonadotropin-präparaten. *Klin. Wschr*, **36**, 925.

BROUHA L. & HINGLAIS H. (1931) Le diagnostic de la grossesse par la réaction de Brouha-Hinglais-Simonnet. *Gynéc. et Obstét.* **24**, 42.

BROWN J.B., KLOPPER A. & LORAINE J.A. (1958) The urinary excretion of oestrogens, pregnanediol and gonadotrophins during the menstrual cycle. *J. Endocr.* **17**, 401.

BROWN W.E. & BRADBURY J.T. (1947) A study of the physiological action of human chorionic hormone. The production of pseudopregnancy in women by chorionic hormone. *Amer. J. Obstet. Gynec.* **53**, 749.

BROWN W.E., BRADBURY J.T. & METZGER I. (1941) Are the anterior pituitary-like substances gonadotropic? A clinical evaluation in the woman. *Amer. J. Obstet. Gynec.* **41**, 582.

BROWNE J.S.L. & VENNING E.M. (1936) Excretion of gonadotropic substances in the urine during pregnancy. *Lancet*, **231**, 1507.

BROWNE J.S.L. & VENNING E.H. (1938) The effect of intramuscular injection of gonadotropic substances on the corpus luteum phase of the human. *Amer. J. Physiol.* **123**, 26.

BRUNER J.A. (1951) Distribution of chorionic gonadotropin in mother and fetus at various stages of pregnancy. *J. clin. Endocr.* **11**, 360.

BRYANS F.E. (1951) Progesterone of the blood in the menstrual cycle of the monkey. *Endocrinology*, **48**, 733.

BUSSARD A. (1949) Le problème des antihormones examiné à la lumière des resultats de l'étude expérimentale des sérums antigonadotropes. *Bull. l'Assoc. Diplomés de Microbiologie*, **34**, 8.

BUSSARD A. & GRABAR P. (1947) Activité physiologique et immunochimique des sérums antigonadotropes. *Bull. Soc. Chim. biol.* **29**, 195.

BUSSARD A. & GRABAR P. (1948) Preuve théorique de la possibilité de réaliser un diagnostic immunochimique de la grossesse. *Ann. Inst. Pasteur*, **75**, 14.

BUXTON C.L. & HERRMANN W. (1961) Induction of ovulation in the human with human gonadotrophins. *Amer. J. Obstet. Gynec.* **81**, 584.

CALDEYRO-BARCIA R. (1960) Oxytocin in pregnancy and labour. *Acta endocr.* (*Kbh.*), Suppl. **50**, 41.

CARLSSON M.G. (1964) The use of haemagglutination inhibition reaction for qualitative and quantitative determinations of HCG in normal and pathological pregnancies. *Acta endocr.* (*Kbh.*), **46**, 142.

CARLSTRÖM G. & BRODY S. (1962) Determination of human chorionic gonadotrophin by complement fixation. *Acta path. microbiol. Scand. Suppl.* **154**, 237.

DORFMAN R.I. & RUBIN B.L. (1947) Studies on the bioassay of hormones. The assay of chorionic gonadotrophin from human pregnancy urine and serum. *Endocrinology*, **41**, 456.

DRESCHER J. (1954) Die Isolierung der Follikelstimulierenden Verbindung aus dem Choriongonadotropin. *Acta endocr.* (*Kbh.*), **15**, 325.

DRESCHER J. and STANGE H.-H. (1955) Vergleichende Untersuchungen über die Wirkung der isolierten Follikel-stimulierenden Verbindung aus Chorion- und hypophysären Gonadotropinen auf Ovarien hypophysektomierter, infantiler Ratten. *Acta endocr.* (*Kbh.*), **19**, 289.

EHRHARDT K. (1936) Über das Laktationshormon des Hypophysenvorderlappens. *Münch. med. Wschr.* **83**, 1163.

EHRHARDT K. & MAYES B.T. (1930) Beitrag zum Hormongehalt des menschlichen und tierischen Hypophysenvorderlappens. *Zbl. Gynäk.* **54**, 2949.

EIK-NES K.B., OERTEL G.W., NIMER R. & TYLER F.H. (1959) Effect of human chorionic gonadotropin on plasma concentrations of 17-hydroxycorticosteroids, dehydroepiandrosterone and androsterone in man. *J. clin. Endocr.* **19**, 1405.

ELEK S.D. (1948). Recognition of toxicogenic bacterial strains *in vitro*. *Br. med. J.* **1**, 493.

EMMENS C.W. (1939) Analysis of the assays carried out in various laboratories on the contributions offered towards the international standard preparation of the gonadotrophic substance of urine of pregnancy. *Bull. Hlth. Org.* **8**, 862.

EMMENS C.W. (1948) *Principles of Biological Assay*. Chapman & Hall, London.

EMMENS C.W. (1950) Statistical methods. In *Hormone Assay*, p. 1. C.W.Emmens, ed.

ESCHBACH J. (1959) Contribution à l'étude de l'hormone mélanotrope présente dans des extraits placentaires anormaux (moles et chorioépithéliomas). *Bull. Féd. Soc. Gynéc. d'Obstét. Franc.* **11**, 188.

EVANS H.M. & SIMPSON M.E. (1929) Impairment of the birth mechanism due to hormones from the anterior hypophysis. *Proc. Soc. exp. Biol.* (*N.Y.*), **26**, 595.

EVANS H.M. & SIMPSON M.E. (1935) Similarity of the urinary gonadotropic hormone occurring in some cases of testicular neoplasm with that found in the urine of pregnancy. *Anat. Rec.* **61**, Suppl. p. 16.

EVANS H.M. & SIMPSON M.E. (1950) Physiology of the gonadotrophins. In *The Hormones. Physiology, Chemistry and Applications*. Volume II, p. 351. G.Pincus & K.V.Thimann, eds. Academic Press, New York.

EVANS H.M., MEYER K. & SIMPSON M. (1932) Relation of prolan to the anterior hypophyseal hormones. *Amer. J. Physiol.* **100**, 141.

EVANS H.M., PENCHARZ R.I. & SIMPSON M.E. (1934a) The repair of the reproductive system of hypophysectomized female rats by combinations of an hypophyseal extract (synergist) with pregnancy-prolan. *Endocrinology*, **18**, 601.

EVANS H.M., PENCHARZ R.I. & SIMPSON M.E. (1934b) Maintenance and repair of the reproductive system of hypophysectomized male rats by hypophyseal synergist, pregnancy-prolan and combinations thereof. *Endocrinology*, **18**, 607.

EVANS H.M., KOHLS C.L. & WONDER D.H. (1937) Gonadotropic hormone in the blood and urine of early pregnancy. *J. Amer. med. Ass.* **108**, 287.

FERGUSON K.A. & WALLACE A.L. (1961) Prolactin activity of human growth hormone. *Nature, Lond.* **190**, 632.

FINNEY D.J. (1952) *Statistical Methods in Biological Assay*. Charles Griffin, London.

FISCHER F.G. & ERTEL L. (1931) Zur Kenntnis der Hypophysen-vorderlappen-Hormone aus Schwangerenharn. *Hoppe-Seylers Z. Physiol. Chem.* **202**, 83.

FLICK J.A. (1948) Use of formalin-treated red cells for the study of influenza. A virus hemagglutinizing activity. *Proc. Soc. exp. Biol. (N.Y.)*, **68**, 448.

FLORINI J.R., TONELLI G., BREUER C.B., COPPOLA J., RINGLER I. & BELL P.H. (1966). Characterization and biological effects of a purified placental protein (human). *Endocrinology*, **79**, 692.

FRAENKEL CONRAT H.L., SIMPSON M.E. & EVANS H.M. (1940) The effect of thiol compounds on gonadotrophins. *Science*, **91**, 363.

FREUD J. & UYLDERT I.E. (1947) Antigonadotrophic activity in male rats. *J. Endocr.* **5**, 59.

FREUND J. (1947) Some aspects of active immunization. *Ann. Rev. Microbiol.* **1**, 291.

FREUND J. (1951) The effect of paraffin oil and mycobacteria on antibody formation and sensitization. *Amer. J. clin. Path.* **21**, 645.

FRIED P.H. & RAKOFF A.E. (1950) Improvement of the rat ovary hyperemia test for pregnancy by adding a pituitary synergist. *J. clin. Endocr.* **10**, 423.

FRIEDMAN M.H. & WEINSTEIN G.L. (1937) The excretion of gonadotropin by normal human males after the ingestion and injection of extracts of pregnancy urine. *Endocrinology*, **21**, 489.

FRIESEN H. (1965a) Purification of a placental factor with immunological and chemical similarity to human growth hormone. *Endocrinology*, **76**, 369.

FRIESEN H. (1965b) Further purification and characterization of a placental protein with immunological similarity to human growth hormone. *Nature*, **208**, 1214.

FUKUSHIMA M. (1961) Studies on somatotropic hormone secretion in gynecology and obstetrics. *Tohoku J. exp. Med.* **74**, 161.

FULTHORPE A.J., PARKE J.A.C., TOVEY J.E. & MONCKTON J.C. (1963) Pregnancy diagnosis by a one-stage passive haemagglutination inhibition method. *Br. med. J.* **1**, 1049.

FULTON F. & DUMBELL J.R. (1949) The serological comparison of strains of influenza virus. *J. gen. Microbiol.* **3**, 97.

FURUHJELM M. (1941) Excretion of gonadotropic hormones in cases of tumour of testis. *Nord. Med.* **11**, 2603.

GADDUM J.H. (1933) Reports on biological standards. III. Methods of biological assay depending on a quantal response. *Spec. Rep. Ser. Med. Res. Coun., Lond.* **183**, 1.

GADDUM J.H. (1953a) Bioassays and mathematics. *Pharmacol. Rev.* **5**, 87.

GADDUM J.H. (1953b) Simplified mathematics for bioassays. *J. Pharm. Pharmacol.* **6**, 345.

GASTINEAU C.F., ALBERT A. & RANDALL L.M. (1949) Renal clearance of chorionic gonadotropic hormone in pregnancy, in neoplasm of testis and in hydatidiform mole. *J. clin. Endocr.* **9**, 615.

GEIST S.H. (1933) Reaction of the mature human ovary to Antuitrin-S. *Amer. J. Obstet. Gynec.* **26**, 588.

GEIST S.H., GAINES J.A. & SALMON U.J. (1941) The effect of gonadotropins upon the human ovary. *Amer. J. Obstet. Gynec.* **42**, 619.

GEMZELL C.A. (1962) Induction of ovulation with human pituitary gonadotrophins. *Fertil. and Steril.* **13**, 153.

GEMZELL C.A., HEIJKENSKJÖLD F. & STRÖM L. (1955) Method for demonstrating growth hormone activity in human plasma. *J. clin. Endocr.* **15**, 537.

GEMZELL C.A., DICZFALUSY E. & TILLINGER G. (1958) Clinical effect of human pituitary follicle-stimulating hormone (FSH). *J. clin. Endocr.* **18**, 1333.

GEY G.O., SEEGAR G.E. & HELLMAN L.M. (1938) The production of a gonadotrophic substance (Prolan) by placental cells in tissue culture. *Science*, **88**, 306.

GLASS S.J. & HOLLAND H.M. (1963) Treatment of oligospermia with large doses of human chorionic gonadotropin. *Fertil. and Steril.* **14**, 500.

GLASSER J.W.H. (1952) Early removal of the corpus luteum of pregnancy. *Bull. Margaret Hague Maternity Hosp.* **5**, 112.

GOLDZIEHER J.W. & ROBERTS I.S. (1952) Identification of estrogen in the human testis. *J. clin. Endocr.* **12**, 143.

GOSS D.A. (1964) Preparatory adsorption of antisera to urinary gonadotropins with an extract of pediatric urine (Peduex). *J. clin. Endocr.* **24**, 408.

GOSS D.A. & LEWIS J., Jnr. (1964) Immunologic differentiation of luteinizing hormone and human chorionic gonadotropin in compounds of high purity. *Endocrinology*, **74**, 83.

GOSS D.A. & TAYMOR M.L. (1962) Measurement of LH activity by latex-HCG agglutination inhibition. *Endocrinology*, **71**, 321.

GOT R. (1959) Gonadotropine choriale humaine. Isolement et caractérisation. *Thèse de Sciences, Paris.*

GOT R. & BOURRILLON R. (1960a) Nouvelles données physiques sur la gonadotropine choriale humaine. *Biochim. biophys. Acta*, **39**, 241.

GOT R. P & BOURRILLON R. (1960b) Nouvelle méthode de purification de la gonadotropine choriale humaine. *Biochim. biophys. Acta*, **42**, 505.

GOT R. & BOURRILLON R. (1960c) Critères de pureté de la gonadotropine choriale humaine. *Bull. Soc. Chim. biol. (Paris)*, **42**, 31.

GOT R., LEVY G. & BOURRILLON R. (1959) Analyse immunoeléctrophorétique de la gonadotropine choriale humaine. *Experientia (Basel)*, **15**, 480.

GRABAR P. & WILLIAMS C.A., Jnr. (1955) Méthode immunoélectrophorétique d'analyse de mélanges de substances antigéniques. *Biochim. biophys. Acta*, **17**, 67.

GREENSPAN F.S., LI C.H., SIMPSON M.E. & EVANS H.M. (1949) Bioassay of hypophyseal growth hormone; tibia test. *Endocrinology*. **45**, 455.

GREENWOOD F.C., HUNTER W.M. & KLOPPER A. (1964) Assay of human growth hormone in pregnancy, at parturition and in lactation. Detection of a growth-hormone-like substance from the placenta. *Br. med. J.* i, 22.

GRENIER J. & REBEL A. (1956) Recherches, par la méthode de la greffe intra-testiculaire, sur l'activité gonadotrope du placenta humain. *C.R. Soc. Biol. (Paris)*, **150**, 987.

GRODSKY G.M. & FORSHAM P.H. (1960) An immunochemical assay of total extractable insulin in man. *J. clin. Invest.* **39**, 1070.

Grumbach M.M. & Kaplan S.L. (1962) Immunochemical studies on human growth hormone: a consideration of the human growth hormone-anti-human growth hormone system and its application to the assay of growth hormone. In *Immunoassay of Hormones.* Ciba Foundation Colloquia on Endocrinology, **14**, 63. G.E.W.Wolstenholme & M.P.Cameron, eds. Churchill, London.

Grumbach M.M. & Kaplan S.L. (1965) *In vivo* and *in vitro* evidence of the synthesis and secretion of chorionic 'growth hormone-prolactin' by the human placenta: its purification, immunoassay and distinction from human pituitary growth hormone. *Proc. 2nd Internat. Congr. Endocr., London* 1964, part I, p. 691. Excerpta Medica Foundation, Internat. Congr. Ser. No. 83.

Gurchot C., Krebs E.T., Jnr. & Krebs E.T. (1947) Growth of human trophoblast in eye of rabbit. Its relationship to the origin of cancer. *Surg. Gynec. Obstet.* **84**, 301.

Gurin S., Bachman C. & Wilson D.W. (1939) The gonadotropic hormone of urine of pregnancy. I. A simple method of extraction and purification. *J. biol. Chem.* **128**, 525.

Gurin S., Bachman C. & Wilson D.W. (1940a) The gonadotropic hormone of urine of pregnancy. II. Chemical studies of preparations having high biological activity. *J. biol. Chem.* **133**, 467.

Gurin S., Bachman C. & Wilson D.W. (1940b) The gonadotropic hormone of pregnancy. III. Evidence of purity obtained by studies of electrophoresis and sedimentation. *J. biol. Chem.* **133**, 477.

Gusdon J.P. & Yen S.S.C. (1967) *In vitro* biosynthesis of human placental lactogen (HPL) by placental tissue. *Obstet. Gynec.* **30**, 635.

Guyénot E. (1946) Les deux actions gonadotropes de l'urine de femme enceinte. I. Variations indépendantes des seuils acmogène et crinogène. *Rev. suisse Zool.* **53**, Suppl. 1.

Hagen A.A. & Eik-Nes K.B. (1964) Conversion of 17α-hydroxypregnenolone to 17α-hydroxyprogesterone by the canine testis *in vivo. Biochim. biophys. Acta*, **86**, 372.

Hales C.N. & Randle P.J. (1963) Immunoassay of insulin with insulin-antibody precipitate. *Biochem. J.* **88**, 137.

Halkerston I.D.K., Hillman J., Palmer D., Reiss M. & Rundle A. (1957) The influence of chorionic gonadotrophin on the steroid metabolism of sexually retarded men. *J. Endocr.* **16**, 156.

Hall P.F. & Eik-Nes K.B. (1962) The action of gonadotropic hormones upon rabbit testis *in vitro. Biochim. biophys. Acta*, **63**, 411.

Hall P.F. & Eik-Nes K.B. (1963) The influence of gonadotropins *in vivo* upon the biosynthesis of androgens by homogenate of rat testis. *Biochim. biophys. Acta*, **71**, 438.

Hamashige S. & Arquilla E.R. (1963) Immunological studies with a commercial preparation of human chorionic gonadotropin. *J. clin. Invest.* **42**, 546.

Hamashige S. & Arquilla E.R. (1964) Immunologic and biologic study of human chorionic gonadotropin. *J. clin. Invest.* **43**, 1163.

Hamblen E.C. & Davis C.D. (1945) Treatment of hypo-ovarianism by the sequential and cyclic administration of equine and chorionic gonadotropins–so called one-two cyclic gonadotropic therapy. *Amer. J. Obstet. Gynec.* **50**, 137.

HAMBURGER C. (1933a) Om nogle Hypofyseforlaphormonanalyser i de første Stadier af en Graviditet. *Ugeskr. Laeg.* **95**, 284.

HAMBURGER C. (1933b) Studies on gonadotropic hormones from the hypophysis and chorionic tissue with special reference to their differences. *Thesis. Acta path. microbiol. Scand.* Suppl. **17**, .

HAMBURGER C. (1941) On the nature of gonadotrophin in cases of malignant tumours of the testis. *Acta path. microbiol. Scand.* **18**, 457.

HAMBURGER C. (1944) Contribution to the hormonal diagnosis of hydatidiform mole and chorionepithelioma, based on 76 cases with hormonal analyses. *Acta obstet. gynec. Scand.* **24**, 45.

HAMBURGER C. (1950) Gonadotropins. In *Hormone assay*, p. 173. C.W.Emmens, ed. Academic Press, New York.

HAMBURGER C. (1957) The assay of gonadotropic hormones. A survey. *Acta endocr. (Kbh.)*, Suppl. **31**, 59.

HAMBURGER C. (1958a) Gonadotrophins in cases of hydatidiform mole and chorion-epithelioma of the uterus. In *Hormone Production in Endocrine Tumours.* Ciba Foundation Colloquia on Endocrinology, **12**, 190. G.E.W.Wolstenholme & M. O'Connor, eds. Churchill, London.

HAMBURGER C. (1958b) Gonadotrophins, androgens and oestrogens in cases of malignant tumours of the testis. In *Hormone Production in Endocrine Tumours.* Ciba Foundation Colloquia on Endocrinology, **12**, 200. G.E.W.Wolstenholme & M.O'Connor, eds. Churchill, London.

HASKINS A.L. & SHERMAN A.I. (1952) The quantitative assay of serum chorionic gonadotropin in pregnancy, using the modified frog technique. *J. clin. Endocr.* **12**, 385.

HAWKER R.W. (1956) Inactivation of antidiuretic hormone and oxytocin during pregnancy. *Quart. J. exp. Physiol.* **41**, 301.

HEARD R.D.H. & WINTON S.S. (1939) Use of the dietary anoestrus adult rat for the assay of the oestrus-inducing gonadotrophic substance. *J. Physiol.* **96**, 248.

HELLER C.G. & NELSON W.O. (1948) Classification of male hypogonadism and a discussion of the pathologic physiology, diagnosis and treatment. *J. clin. Endocr.* **8**, 345.

HERTZ R. (1959) Choriocarcinoma of women maintained in serial passage in hamster and rat. *Proc. Soc. exp. Biol. (N.Y.)*, **102**, 77.

HERTZ R., BERGENSTAL D.M., LIPSETT M.B., PRICE E.B. & HILBISH T.F. (1958) Chemotherapy of choriocarcinoma and related trophoblastic tumours in women. *J. Amer. med. Ass.* **168**, 845.

HIBBITT L.L., STARNES W.R. & HILL S.R. (1958) Studies in man on testicular and adrenal response to adrenocorticotropin and human chorionic gonadotropin. *J. clin. Endocr.* **18**, 1315.

HIGASHI K. (1961) Studies on the prolactin-like substance in human placenta. III. *Endocr. Japon.* **8**, 288.

HIGASHI K. (1962) Studies on the prolactin-like substance in human placenta. IV. *Endocr. Japon.* **9**, 1.

HISAW F.L. (1944) The placental gonadotrophin and luteal function in monkeys (*Macaea mulatta*). *Yale J. Biol. Med.* **17**, 119.

HOBSON B.M. (1955) The excretion of chorionic gonadotrophin in normal pregnancy and in women with hydatidiform mole. *J. Obstet. Gynaec. Brit. Emp.* **62**, 354.

HOBSON B.M. (1958) Further observations on the excretion of chorionic gonadotrophin by women with hydatidiform mole. *J. Obstet. Gynaec. Brit. Emp.* **65**, 253.

HOBSON B.M. (1959) The excretion of chorionic gonadotrophin by women with chorioadenoma and choriocarcinoma. *J. Obstet. Gynaec. Brit. Emp.* **66**, 282.

HOBSON B.M. (1965) The excretion of chorionic gonadotrophin by men with testicular tumours. *Acta endocr.* (*Kbh.*), **49**, 337.

HOBSON B. & WIDE L. (1964) The immunological and biological activity of human chorionic gonadotrophin in urine. *Acta endocr.* (*Kbh.*), **46**, 632.

HON E.H. (1961) *A Manual of Pregnancy Testing*. Little, Brown & Company, Boston, Mass.

HON E.H. & MORRIS J.MCL. (1955) Gonadotrophin titers in disturbed pregnancies. *Surg. Gynec. Obstet.* **101**, 59.

HON E.H. & MORRIS J.MCL. (1956) Further experience with the toad method of testing for chorionic gonadotropin in normal and in disturbed pregnancy. *J. clin. Endocr.* **16**, 1354.

HOOPER K.C. & JESSUP D.C. (1959) The distribution of enzymes destroying oxytocin and vasopressin in human placentae. *J. Physiol.* **146**, 539.

HOTCHKISS R.D. (1948) A microchemical reaction resulting in the staining of polysaccharide structures in fixed tissue preparations. *Arch. Biochem.* **16**, 131.

HUIS IN'T VELD L.G., LOUWERENS B. & VAN DER SPEK P.A.F. (1961) Administration of chorionic gonadotrophin as a test of the endocrine function of the testis. *Acta endocr.* (*Kbh.*), **37**, 208.

IBAYASHI H., NAKAMURA M., UCHIKAWA T., MURAKAWA S., YOSHIDA S., NAKAO K. & OKINAKA S. (1965) C_{19} steroids in canine spermatic venous blood following gonadotropin administration. *Endocrinology*, **76**, 347.

ISERSKY C., LUNENFELD B. & SHELESNYAK M.V. (1963) Immunologic studies on gonadotropins. II. Biological assessment of the antigenic nature of the follicle-stimulating principle in human chorionic gonadotropin preparations. *J. clin. Endocr.* **23**, 54.

ITO Y. & HIGASHI K. (1961) Studies on the prolactin-like substance in human placenta. II. *Endocr. Japon.* **8**, 279.

JACKANICZ T.M. & DICZFALUSY E. (1968) Absence of 16α-hydroxylating activity in the human midterm placenta. *Steroids* **11**, 877.

JAILER J.W. & KNOWLTON A.I. (1950) Stimulated adrenocortical activity during pregnancy in addisonian patient. *J. clin. Invest.* **29**, 1430.

JAYLE M.F., SCHOLLER R. & VEYRIN-FORRER F. (1959) Phénolstéroides urinaires. II. Applications cliniques. *Acta endocr.* (*Kbh.*), **4**, 401.

JAYLE M.F., VEYRIN-FORRER F., GELLER S. & MÈGE F. (1961) Classification biochimique des insuffîcances lutéales à l'aide d'une nouvelle épreuve d'exploration dynamique du corps jaune. *Gynéc. et Obstét.* **60**, 381.

JAYLE M.F., SCHOLLER R., SFIKAKIS A. & HÉRON M. (1962) Excrétion des phénolstéroides et des 17-cétostéroides après administration de gonadotropinies chorioniques à des hommes. *Clin. chim. Acta*, **7**, 212.

JOHNSEN S. (1961) Critical note on claims of isolation of so-called pure gonadotropins from human urine. In *Human Pituitary Gonadotrophins*, p. 186. A. Albert, ed. Charles C.Thomas, Springfield.

JOHNSEN S.G. (1962) The management of male hypogonadism. *Acta endocr. (Kbh.)*, Suppl. **40**, 66.

JOHNSON C.E., ALBERT A. & WILSON R.B. (1950) Renal and extrarenal disposal of chorionic gonadotropin in the immediate postpartum period. *J. clin. Endocr.* **10**, 371.

JONES G.E.S., GEY G.O. & GEY M.K. (1943) Hormone production by placental cells maintained in continuous culture. *Bull. Johns Hopkins Hosp.* **72**, 26.

JONES G.E.S., DELFS E. & STRAN H.M. (1944) Chorionic gonadotropin and pregnanediol values in normal pregnancy. *Bull. Johns Hopkins Hosp.* **75**, 359.

JOSIMOVICH J.B. & ATWOOD B.L. (1964) Human placental lactogen (HPL), a trophoblastic hormone synergizing with chorionic gonadotropin and potentiating the anabolic effect of pituitary growth hormone. *Amer. J. Obstet. Gynec.* **88**, 867.

JOSIMOVICH J.B. & MACLAREN J.A. (1962) Presence in the human placenta and term serum of a highly lactogenic substance immunologically related to pituitary growth hormone. *Endocrinology*, **71**, 209.

JOSIMOVICH J.B., ATWOOD B.L. & GOSS D.A. (1963) Luteotrophic, immunologic and electrophoretic properties of human placental lactogen. *Endocrinology*, **73**, 410.

JUNGCK E.C. & BROWN W.E. (1952) Human pituitary gonadotropin for clinical use: preparation and lack of antihormone formation. *Fertil. and Steril.* **3**, 224.

KAIVOLA S., KIISTALA U. & AXELSON E. (1962) Studies on a serological pregnancy test. II. *Ann. Med. exp. Fenn.* **40**, 419.

KAIVOLA S., KIISTALA U. & AXELSON E. (1963) Studies on a serological pregnancy test. III. *Acta endocr. (Kbh.)*, **42**, 395.

KAPLAN S.L. & GRUMBACH M.M. (1964) Studies of a human and simian placental hormone with growth hormone-like and prolactin-like activities. *J. clin. Endocr.* **24**, 80.

KAPLAN S.L. & GRUMBACH M.M. (1965) Immunoassay for human chorionic 'growth hormone-prolactin' in serum and urine. *Science*, **147**, 751.

KARKUN J.N. & SEN D.P. (1963) Studies on the melanophore-expanding substance from human placenta. *Ann. Biochem. exp. Med.* **23**, 81.

KATZMAN P.A. & DOISY E.A. (1932) Preparation of extracts of the anterior pituitary-like substance of urine of pregnancy. *J. biol. Chem.* **98**, 739.

KATZMAN P.A., GODFRID M., CAIN C.K. & DOISY E.A. (1943) The preparation of chorionic gonadotropin by chromatographic adsorption. *J. biol. Chem.* **148**, 501.

KEELE D.K., REMPLE J., BEAN J. & WEBSTER J. (1962) Immunologic reactions to human chorionic gonadotropin. *J. clin. Endocr.* **22**, 287.

KIDO I. (1937) Die menschliche Placenta als Produktionsstätte des sogenannten Hypophysenvorderlappenhormons. *Zbl. Gynäk.* **61**, 1551.

KIISTALA U., KAIVOLA S. & AXELSON E. (1962) Studies on a serological pregnancy test. I. *Ann. Med. exp. Fenn.* **40**, 414.

KLEBANOW D. (1950) Qualitative and quantitative Unterschiede im Prolangehalt von Plazenta und Decidua graviditatis. *Zbl. Gynäk.* **72**, 977.

KLUNGSÖYR L. & STÖA K.F. (1955) The chemical nature of human chorionic gonadotrophin. *Acta endocr.* (*Kbh.*), **18**, 288.

KNORR D. (1961) Über die Ausscheidung von parenteral zugeführtem humanen Choriongonadotropin (HCG). *Klin. Wschr.* **39**, 128.

KNORR D. (1963) Die Wirkung von Choriongonadotropin auf den Steroidhormon-Stoffwechsel des Kindes. *Acta endocr.* (*Kbh.*), Suppl. **44**, 84.

KONSULOFF S. (1934) Schnelldiagnose der Schwangerschaft durch die Melanophorenreaktion. *Klin. Wschr.* **13**, 776.

KORENCHEVSKY V. (1930) Influence of hypophysis on metabolism, growth and sexual organs of male rats and rabbits; influence of extracts of hypophysis on body weight, weight of fat, of sexual organs and of endocrine organs of rats. *Biochem. J.* **24**, 383.

KOTZ H.L. & HERRMANN W. (1961) A review of the endocrine induction of human ovulation. *Fertil. and Steril.* **12**, 375.

KULSENG-HANSSEN K. (1951) Maintenance of early pregnancy despite extirpation of three corpora lutea. *Acta obstet. gynec. Scand.* **30**, 420.

LAJOS L., NAGY D. & GÁTI I. (1959) Gonadotrophins in pregnancy. *Gynaecologia* (*Basel*), **148**, 59.

LANDAU R.L. & LAVES M.L. (1959) Urinary pregnanetriol of testicular origin. *J. clin. Endocr.* **19**, 1959.

LAU L.H. & JONES G.S. (1965) Immunoassay of serum-human chorionic gonadotropin by quantative complement fixation and its comparison with the Delfs bioassay and two International Standard preparations. *Amer. J. Obstet. Gynec.* **92**, 483.

LEAGUE OF NATIONS (1939) Memorandum on the international standard for the gonadotrophic substance of human urine of pregnancy (chorionic gonadotrophin). *Bull. Hlth. Org.* **8**, 884.

LEONARD S.L. (1932) Increased stimulation of immature rat ovaries by combined injections of prolan and hypophyseal sex hormone. *Proc. Soc. exp. Biol.* (*N.Y.*), **30**, 403.

LEONARD S.L. & SMITH P.E. (1934a) Responses of the reproductive system of hypophysectomized rats to injections of pregnancy-urine extracts. II. The female. *Anat. Rec.* **58**, 175.

LEONARD S.L. & SMITH P.E. (1934b) The hypophyseal-like qualities of the gonadotropic principle found in the urine of certain individuals. *Amer. J. Physiol.* **108**, 22.

LEVIN L. (1944) The physiology of the gonadotrophic substances of blood, urine and non-hypophyseal tissues. In *The Chemistry and Physiology of Hormones*, p. 162. F.R.Moulton, ed. Publication of the American Association for the Advancement of Science, Washington.

LEWIN E. (1960) Histochemische Untersuchungen an Plazenten von Extrauteringraviditäten. *Gynaecologia* (*Basel*), **149**, 184.

LEWIS J., Jnr., DRAY S., GENUTH S. & SCHWARTZ H.S. (1964) Demonstration of immunological similarities of human pregnancy gonadotropin and choriocarcinoma gonadotropin with antisera prepared in rabbits and monkeys. *J. clin. Endocr.* **24**, 197.

LEZNOFF A. & DAVIS B.A. (1963) The cytological localization of human chorionic gonadotropin. *Canad. J. Biochem.* **41**, 2517.

LINDNER H.R. (1961) Androgens and related compounds in the spermatic vein blood of domestic animals. I. Neutral steroids secreted by the bull testis. *J. Endocr.* **23**, 139.

LING N.R. (1961) The attachment of proteins to aldehyde-tanned cells. *Brit. J. Haemat.* **7**, 299.

LITTLE B., SMITH O.W., JESSIMAN A.G., SELENKOW H.A., VAN'T HOFF W., EGLIN J.M. & MOORE F.D. (1958) Hypophysectomy during pregnancy in a patient with cancer of the breast: case report with hormone studies. *J. clin. Endocr.* **18**, 425.

LLOYD C.W., HUGHES E.C., EVA M.L. & LOBOTSKY J. (1949) The urinary excretion of chorionic gonadotrophin by human females following parenteral administration of aqueous or beeswax solutions. *J. clin. Endocr.* **9**, 268.

LORAINE J.A. (1950a) The estimation of chorionic gonadotrophin in the urine of pregnant women. *J. Endocr.* **6**, 319.

LORAINE J.A. (1950b) Renal clearance of chorionic gonadotrophin in normal and pathological pregnancy. *Quart. J. exp. Physiol.* **36**, 11.

LORAINE J.A. (1956) Bioassay of pituitary and placental gonadotropins in relation to clinical problems in man. *Vitam. and Horm.* **14**, 305.

LORAINE J.A. (1957) Some general principles in the bioassay of anterior pituitary and placental hormones in blood with special reference to clinical problems. In *Hormones in Blood.* Ciba Foundation Colloquia on Endocrinology, **11**, 19. G.E.W.Wolstenholme & E.C.P.Millar, eds. Churchill, London.

LORAINE J.A. (1958) *The Clinical Application of Hormone Assay.* Livingstone, Edinburgh and London.

LORAINE J.A. (1961) Human chorionic gonadotrophin (HCG). In *Hormones in Blood*, p. 285. C.H.Gray & A.L.Bacharach, eds. Academic Press, London and New York.

LORAINE J.A. & MATTHEW G.D. (1950) Chorionic gonadotrophin in toxaemias of pregnancy. *J. Obstet. Gynaec. Brit. Emp.* **57**, 542.

LORAINE J.A. & MATTHEW G.D. (1953) The placental concentration of chorionic gonadotrophin in normal and abnormal pregnancy. *J. Obstet. Gynaec. Brit. Emp.* **60**, 640.

LORAINE J.A. & MATTHEW G.D. (1954) Le Diabète, **2**, 43. Quoted from Loraine (1956).

LORAINE J.A. & SCHMIDT-ELMENDORFF H. (1963) Human gonadotrophins. In *Modern Trends in Human Reproductive Physiology*–1, p. 18. H.M.Carey, ed. Butterworths, London.

LUNENFELD B. (1965) Contribution to the discussion. In *Gonadotropins. Physico-chemical and Immunological Properties.* Ciba Foundation Study Group No. 22, p. 59. G.E.W.Wolstenholme & J.Knight, eds. Churchill, London.

LUNENFELD B., RABAU E., HARELL-STEINBERG A. & SZEJNBERG A. (1957) Effect of injection medium on quantal assay of chorionic gonadotrophin in male toads. *Acta endocr.* (*Kbh.*), **24**, 113.

LUNENFELD B., ISERSKY C. & SHELESNYAK M.C. (1962) Immunologic studies on gonadotropins. I. Immunogenic properties and immunologic characterization of human chorionic gonadotropin preparations (HCG) and their homologous antisera. *J. clin. Endocr.* **22**, 555.

LUNDGREN H.P., GURIN S., BACHMAN C. & WILSON D.W. (1942) The gonadotropic hormone of urine of pregnancy. IV. *J. biol. Chem.* **142**, 367.

LUNENFELD B., RABAU E., SULOMIVICI S. & ESHKOL A. (1963) Treatment of amenorrhoea by gonadotropic substances from women's urine. *Harefuah*, **64**, 289.

LYON R.A., SIMPSON M.E. & EVANS H.M. (1953) Quantitative changes in urinary gonadotrophins in human pregnancy during the period of rapid increase in hormone titer. *Endocrinology*, **53**, 674.

LYTLE I.M. & HASKELL J.G. (1964) Human chorionic gonadotropin: Isolation by disk electrophoresis. *Amer. J. Obstet. Gynec.* **89**, 156.

MADDOCK W.O. & LEACH R.B. (1952) Tenfold increase in biological activity of chorionic gonadotrophin when mixed with plasma thereby allowing its measurement in the plasma of men receiving the hormone. *J. Lab. clin. Med.* **40**, 923.

MADDOCK W.O. & NELSON W.O. (1951) Increased estrogen excretion due to stimulation of Leydig cells in adult men receiving chorionic gonadotropin. *J. clin. Endocr.* **11**, 769.

MADDOCK W.O. & NELSON W.O. (1952) The effects of chorionic gonadotropin in adult men: increased estrogen and 17-ketosteroid excretion, gynecomastia, Leydig cell stimulation and seminiferous tubule damage. *J. clin. Endocr.* **12**, 985.

MADDOCK W.O., TOKUYAMA I. & LEACH R.B. (1953) Augmentation of human chorionic gonadotrophin by plasma and other non-hormonal substances. *Proc. Soc. exp. Biol. (N.Y.)*, **84**, 352.

MAYER M.M. (1964) Complement and complement fixation. In *Kabat and Mayer's Experimental Immunochemistry*, 2nd ed., 2nd print. Charles C.Thomas, Springfield, Ill.

MAYER M.M., OSLER A.G., BIER O.G. & HEIDELBERGER M. (1948) Quantitative studies of complement fixation; method. *J. Immunol.* **59**, 195.

MAZER C. & RAVETZ E. (1941) The effect of combined administration of chorionic gonadotrophin and the pituitary synergist on the human ovary. *Amer. J. Obstet. Gynec.* **41**, 474.

McGARRY E.E. & BECK J.C. (1964) Some studies with antisera to human FSH. *Fertil. and Steril.* **14**, 558.

McKAY D.G., HERTIG A.T., ADAMS E.C. & RICHARDSON M.V. (1958) Histochemical observations on the human placenta. *Obstet. and Gynec.* **12**, 1.

McKEAN C. (1960) Preparation and use of antisera to human chorionic gonadotrophin. *Amer. J. Obstet. Gynec.* **80**. 596.

McMANUS J.F.A. (1946) Histological demonstration of mucin after periodic acid. *Nature*, **158**, 202.

McPHAIL M.K. (1933) The effect on the reproductive organs of the rat of prolonged treatment with ovary-stimulating substances. *J. Physiol.* **80**, 105.

MEYER R.K. & WOLFE H.R. (1939) Gonadotropic inhibitory substance and precipitins in blood of monkeys receiving gonadotropic hormone preparations. *J. Immunol.* **37**, 91.

MIDGLEY A.R., Jnr. & PIERCE G.B., Jnr. (1962) Immunohistochemical localization of human chorionic gonadotropin. *J. exp. Med.* **115**, 289.

MIDGLEY A.R., Jnr., PIERCE G.B., Jnr. & WEIGLE W.O. (1961) Immunobiological identification of human chorionic gonadotropin. *Proc. Soc. exp. Biol. (N.Y.)*, **108**, 85.

MISHELL D.R., Jnr., WIDE L. & GEMZELL C.A. (1963) Immunologic determination of human chorionic gonadotrophin in serum. *J. clin. Endocr.* **23**, 125.

MORRIS C.J.O.R. (1955) Chemistry of the gonadotrophins. *Brit. med. Bull.* **11**, 101.

MORSE W.I., CLARK A.F., MACLEOD S.C., ERNST W.A. & GOSSE C.L. (1962) Urine estrogen responses to human chorionic gonadotropin in young, old and hypogonadal men. *J. clin. Endocr.* **22**, 678.

NAGY D., GÁTI I. & KELLER G. (1961) Transport of chorionic gonadotrophin (HCG) in blood. *Acta endocr. (Kbh.)*, **36**, 438.

NEUWEILER W. & HERRMANN U. (1953) Über die hormonale Tätigkeit der explantierten menschlichen Placenta. *Gynaecologia (Basel)*, **135**, 219.

NEWTON W.H. (1938) Hormones and the placenta. *Physiol. Rev.* **18**, 419.

NOBLE R.L. & PLUNKETT E.R. (1955) Biology of the gonadotropins. *Brit. med. Bull.* **11**, 98.

NOWAKOWSKI H. (1959) Der Hypogonadismus im Knaben- und Mannesalter. *Ergebn. inn. Med. Kinderheilk.* **12**, 219.

NYDICK M., BERRY R.J. & ODELL W. (1964) Molecular weight of human chorionic gonadotropin as estimated by means of radiation inactivation of biologic activity. *J. clin. Endocr.* **24**, 1049.

OAKLEY C.L. & FULTHORPE A.J. (1953) Antigenic analysis by diffusion. *J. Path. Bact.* **65**, 49.

OUCHTERLONY Ö. (1948) *In vitro* method for testing toxin-producing capacity of diphtheria bacteria. *Acta path. microbiol. Scand.* **25**, 186.

OUCHTERLONY Ö. (1953) Antigen-antibody reactions in gels. IV. Types of reactions in coordinated systems of diffusion. *Acta path. microbiol. Scand.* **32**, 231.

OUDIN J. (1952) Specific precipitation in gels and its application to immunochemical analysis. In *Methods in Medical Research*, p. 335. A.C.Corcoran, ed. Year Book Publishers, Chicago.

PALI K. & LAJOS L. (1952) Histochemische Untersuchungen der innersekretorischen Tätigkeit der Hypophyse und der Placenta. *Gynaecologia (Basel)*, **133**, 37.

PAUL W.E. & ODELL W.D. (1964) Radiation inactivation of the immunological and biological activities of human chorionic gonadotropin. *Nature, Lond.* **203**, 979.

PAUL W.E. & ROSS G.T. (1964) Immunologic cross-reaction between human chorionic gonadotropin and human pituitary gonadotropin. *Endocrinology*, **75**, 352.

PAYNE R.W. (1951) Relationship of pituitary and adrenal cortex to ovarian hyperemia reaction in the rat. *Proc. Soc. exp. Biol. (N.Y.)*, **77**, 242.

PHILIPP E. (1930a) Hypophysenvorderlappen und Placenta. *Zbl. Gynäk.* **54**, 450.

PHILIPP E. (1930b) Die Bildungsstätte des 'Hypophysenvorderlappenhormons' in der Gravidität. *Zbl. Gynäk.* **54**, 1858.

PHILIPP E. (1955) Die hormonale Wirkung der Plazenta. *Dtsch. med. Wschr.* **80**, 243.

PHILIPP E. & HUBER H. (1936) Die hormonale Rolle der Decidua. *Zbl. Gynäk.* **60**, 2706.

PLATE W.P. (1952) The stimulating effect of chorionic gonadotrophin on the adrenal cortex. *Acta endocr.* (*Kbh.*), **11**, 119.

POMMERENKE W.T. (1934) Experimental ligamentous relaxation in the guinea pig pelvis. *Amer. J. Obstet. Gynec.* **27**, 708.

PREER J.R. (1956) A quantitative study of a technique of double diffusion in agar. *J. Immunol.* **77**, 54.

PRESSMAN D., CAMPBELL D.H. & PAULING L. (1942) The agglutination of intact azo-erythrocytes by antisera, homologous to the attached groups. *J. Immunol.* **44**, 101.

RAACKE I.D., LI C.H. & LOSTROH A. (1957) Zone electrophoresis on starch of human chorionic gonadotrophin and its separation into two active components. *Acta endocr.* (*Kbh.*), **17**, 366.

RABAU E. & SZEJNBERG L. (1955) Value of quantitative human chorionic gonadotropin estimation by frog test method in pathological pregnancies. *Gynaecologia* (*Basel*), **139**, 158.

RAKOFF A.E. (1939) Studies on the concentrations of estrogenic and gonadotropic hormones in the serum of pregnant women. *Amer. J. Obstet. Gynec.* **38**, 371.

RAKOFF A.E. (1940) The hormonal diagnosis of intra-uterine fetal death. The value of quantitative serum prolan determinations as a diagnostic procedure. *Pennsylvania med. J.* **43**, 669.

RAO S.S. & SHAHANI S.K. (1961) The antigenicity of human chorionic gonadotrophin. *Immunology*, **4**, 1.

REISFELD R.A., BERGENSTAL D.M. & HERTZ R. (1959) Distribution of gonadotropic hormone activity in the serum proteins of normal pregnant women and patients. *Arch. Biochem. Biophys.* **81**, 456.

REISFELD R.A. & HERTZ R. (1960) Purification of chorionic gonadotropin from the urine of patients with trophoblastic tumours. *Biochim. biophys. Acta*, **43**, 540.

REISS M. & HAUROWITZ F. (1929) Zur Chemie des Hypophysenvorderlappen-Sexualhormons. *Z. ges. exp. Med.* **68**, 371.

REISS M., HILLMAN J. & DAVIS R.H. (1963) Effect of prolonged treatment with human chorionic gonadotropin on the endogenous steroid hormone metabolism of physically and mentally retarded boys. *J. clin. Endocr.* **23**, 11.

REYNOLDS J.W., MANCUSO S., WIQVIST N. & DICZFALUSY E. (1968) Studies on the aromatisation of neutral steroids in pregnant women. *Acta endocr.* (*Kbh.*) **58**, 377.

RICE B.F., HAMMERSTEIN J. & SAVARD K. (1964a) Steroid hormone formation in the human ovary: II. Action of gonadotropins *in vitro* in the corpus luteum. *J. clin. Endocr.* **24**, 606.

RICE B.F., HAMMERSTEIN J. & SAVARD K. (1964b) Steroid hormone formation in the human ovary: III. Action of gonadotropins on testosterone synthesis by normal ovarian stromal tissue. *Steroids*, **4**, 199.

RIDDLE O. & BATES R.W. (1939) In *Sex and Internal Secretion*, 2nd ed. E.Allan, C.H.Dauforth & E.Doisy, eds. Williams & Wilkins, Baltimore.

RIGGI S.J., BOSHART C.R., BELL P.H. & RINGLER I. (1966) Some effects of purified placental protein (human) on lipid carbohydrate metabolism. *Endocrinology*, **79**, 709.

ROBBINS J.L., HILL G.A., CARLE B.N., CARLQUIST J.H. & MARCUS S. (1962) Latex agglutination reactions between human chorionic gonadotropin and rabbit antibody. *Proc. Soc. exp. Biol. (N.Y.)*, **109**, 321.

ROBYN C., PETRUSZ P. & DICZFALUSY E. (1969) Follicle stimulating hormone-like activity in human chorionic gonadotrophin preparations. *Acta endocr. (Kbh.)* **60**, 137.

ROSA P. (1958) La fonction endocrine. In *Le Placenta Humain*, p. 481. J.Snoeck, ed. Masson, Paris.

ROSEMBERG E., COLEMAN J., DEMANY M. & GARCIA C.R. (1963) Clinical effect of human urinary postmenopausal gonadotropin. *J. clin. Endocr.* **23**, 181.

ROSENFELD S.S., LAPAN B. & BARON H. (1941) Effects of human pregnancy serum on parturition in the rat. *Endocrinology*, **29**, 276.

RYDBERG E. (1943) The use of the gonadotropic hormones in the therapy and their dosage. *Acta obstet. gynec. Scand.* **23**, 555.

SAMUELS L.T. & HELMREICH M.L. (1956) Influence of chorionic gonadotrophin on the 3β-ol dehydrogenase activity of testes and adrenals. *Endocrinology*, **58**, 435.

SAVARD K., MASON N.R., INGRAM J.T. & GASSNER F.X. (1961) The androgens of bovine spermatic venous blood. *Endocrinology*, **69**, 324.

SAXENA B.B. & HENNEMAN P.H. (1964) Immunologic studies with human pituitary follicle-stimulating hormone. *J. clin. Endocr.* **24**, 1271.

SAXTON J. & LOEB L. (1937) Thyroid stimulating and gonadotropic hormones of the human anterior pituitary gland at different ages and in pregnant and lactating women. *Anat. Rec.* **69**, 261.

SCHAPIRO B. (1931) Ist der Kryptoschismus chirurgisch oder hormonal zu behandeln? *Dtsch. med. Wschr.* **57**, 718.

SCHEIDEGGER J.J. (1955) Une micro-méthode de l'immuno-électrophorèses. *Int. Arch. Allergy*, **7**, 103.

SCHUMACHER G., UHLIG H., BLOBEL R., MOHR E. & SCHLUMBERGER H.D. (1960) Physikalisch-chemische und biochemische Untersuchungen über Chorion-gonadotropin. *Naturwissenschaften*, **47**, 517.

SCHUYLER L.H., ANDERSON K., SASLAW S. & ERICKSON C.C. (1950) A serologic study of chorionic gonadotrophin. *Proc. Soc. exp. Biol. (N.Y.)*, **75**, 517.

SCHWARTZ H.S. & MANTEL N. (1963) Evidence for a variant of gonadotropin in choriocarcinoma. *Cancer Res.* **23**, 1724.

SCHWERS J. & FANARD A. (1958) La fonction endocrine. In *Le Placenta Humain*, p. 612. J. Snoeck, ed. Masson, Paris.

SCIARRA J.J., KAPLAN S.L. & GRUMBACH M.M. (1963) Localization of anti-human growth hormone serum within the human placenta: Evidence for a human chorionic 'growth hormone-prolactin'. *Nature, Lond.* **199**, 1005.

SCOTT L.D. (1940) Concentration and detoxification of human urine for biological pregnancy diagnosis. *Br. J. exp. Path.* **21**, 320.

SCOTT W.W. & VERMEULEN C. (1942) Studies on prostatic cancer. V. Excretion of 17-ketosteroids, estrogens and gonadotropins before and after castration. *J. clin. Endocr.* **2**, 450.

SEALY J.L. & SONDERN C.W. (1940) The comparative action of graded doses of international standard gonadotropic substance (chorionic gonadotrophin) on normal infantile male and female rats. *Endocrinology*, **26**, 813.

SEEGAR G.E. & GEY G.O. (1940) The production of hormones by human placental cells in continuous tissue culture. *Amer. J. Physiol.* **129**, P459.

SEGAL S.J. (1957) Response of weaver finch to chorionic gonadotrophin and hypophysial luteinizing hormone. *Science*, **126**, 1242.

SEGALOFF A., STERNBERG W.H. & GASKILL C.J. (1951) Effects of luteotropic doses of chorionic gonadotropin in women. *J. clin. Endocr.* **11**, 936.

SELYE H., COLLIP J.B. & THOMSON D.L. (1933) On the effect of the anterior pituitary-like hormone on the ovary of the hypophysectomized rat. *Endocrinology*, **17**, 494.

SELYE H., COLLIP J.B. & THOMSON D.L. (1934a) Loss of sensitivity to anterior pituitary-like hormone of pregnancy urine. *Proc. Soc. exp. Biol. (N.Y.)*, **31**, 487.

SELYE H., BACHMAN C., THOMSON D.L. & COLLIP J.B. (1934b) Further studies on loss of sensitivity to anterior pituitary-like hormone of pregnancy urine. *Proc. Soc. exp. Biol. (N.Y.)*, **31**, 1113.

SHAHANI S.K. & RAO S.S. (1964) Immunochemical and biological similarity between human luteinizing hormone and one of the antigenic components of human chorionic gonadotrophin. *Acta endocr. (Kbh.)*, **46**, 317.

SHIZUME K. & LERNER A.B. (1954) Determination of melanocyte-stimulating hormone in urine and blood. *J. clin. Endocr.* **14**, 1491.

SIEGMUND H. (1932) Pubertas praecox als Folge chorionepitheliomatöser Wucherungen. *Arch. Gynäk.* **149**, 498.

SIMPSON M.E. & VAN WAGENEN G. (1958) Experimental induction of ovulation in the Macaque monkey. *Fertil. and Steril.* **9**, 386.

SINGER J.M. & PLOTZ C.M. (1956) The latex-fixation test. I. Application to the serologic diagnosis of rheumatoid arthritis. *Amer. J. Med.* **21**, 888.

SMITH E.K. (1955) Interrelationships of anterior pituitary and adrenal cortex in the rat ovarian hyperemia reaction. *Endocrinology*, **56**, 567.

SMITH G.V. & SMITH O.W. (1934) Excessive gonad-stimulating hormone and subnormal amounts of oestrin in the toxaemias of late pregnancy. *Amer. J. Physiol.* **107**, 128.

SMITH G.V. & SMITH O.W. (1939) The anterior pituitary-like hormone in late pregnancy toxemia. *Amer. J. Obstet. Gynec.* **38**, 618.

SMITH G.V. & SMITH O.W. (1948) Internal secretions and toxemia of late pregnancy. *Physiol. Rev.* **28**, 1.

SMITH O.W. & SMITH G.V. (1937) Prolan and estrin in the serum and urine of diabetic and non-diabetic women during pregnancy, with especial reference to late pregnancy toxemia. *Amer. J. Obstet. Gynec.* **33**, 365.

SMITH P.E. (1930) Hypophysectomy and a replacement therapy in the rat. *Amer. J. Anat.* **45**, 205.

SMITH P.E. & LEONARD S.L. (1934) Responses of the reproductive system of hypophysectomized and normal rats to injections of pregnancy-urine extracts. I. The male. *Anat. Rec.* **58**, 145.

SMITH R.A., ALBERT A. & RANDALL L.M. (1951) Chorionic gonadotropin in the blood and urine during early pregnancy. *Amer. J. Obstet. Gynec.* **61**, 514.

SOMA H., EHRMANN R.L. & HERTIG A.T. (1961) Human trophoblast in tissue culture. *Obstet. and Gynec.* **18**, 704.

SPELLACY W.N. & GOETZ F.C. (1963) Plasma insulin in normal late pregnancy. *New Engl. J. Med.* **268**, 988.

SPELLACY W.N., GOETZ F.C., GREENBERG B.Z. & ELLS J. (1965a) Plasma insulin in normal 'early' pregnancy. *Obstet. Gynec.* **25**, 862.

SPELLACY W.N., GOETZ F.C., GREENBERG B.Z. & ELLS J. (1965b) Plasma insulin in normal midpregnancy. *Amer. J. Obstet. Gynec.* **92**, 11.

SPELLACY W.N., COHEN W.D. & CARLSON K.L. (1967) Human placental lactogen levels as a measure of placental function. *Amer. J. Obstet. Gynec.* **97**, 560.

SPIELMAN F., GOLDBERGER M.A. & FRANK R.T. (1933) Hormone diagnosis of viability of pregnancy. *J. Amer. med. Ass.* **101**, 266.

SPIELMAN M.A. & MEYER R.K. (1938) Electrophoresis of prolan. *Proc. Soc. exp. Biol. (N.Y.)*, **37**, 623.

STAMM O. & RIOTTON G. (1958) Ein Beitrag zur funktionellen Morphologie der Eihäute. *Geburtsh. u. Frauenheilk.* **18**, 310.

STEIN G.J. & NGU D.V. (1950) Quantitative complement fixation test: titration of luetic sera by unit of 50 per cent hemolysis. *J. Immunol.* **65**, 17.

STEWART H.L., Jnr. (1951) Hormone secretion by human placenta grown in the eyes of rabbits. *Amer. J. Obstet. Gynec.* **61**, 990.

STEWART H.L., Jnr., SANO M. & MONTGOMERY T.L. (1948) Hormone secretion by human placenta grown in tissue culture. *J. clin. Endocr.* **8**, 175.

STOLTE L.A.M., BAKKER J.H.J., VERBOOM E. & DAUVILLIER P.W. (1952) Mechanism of Konsuloff test and identity of melanophore hormone. *Ned. T. Geneesk.* **96**, 2068.

STOLTE L.A.M., BAKKER J.H.J., VERBOOM E. & DAUVILLIER P.W. (1953) Mechanism of pregnancy reaction of Konsuloff; identity of melanophore hormone. *Ned. T. Geneesk.* **97**, 21.

SULMAN F. (1937) Does the gonadotropic hormone induce antibodies or anti-hormones? *J. exp. Med.* **65**, 1.

SULMAN F.G. & BERGMANN F. (1953) Adrenocorticotrophic activity of placental extracts. *J. Obstet. Gynaec. Brit. Emp.* **60**, 123.

SWIERCZYNSKA Z. & SAMOCHOWIEC E. (1960) Serologic detection of chorion gonadotropin in urine. Its value in the diagnosis of pregnancy. *Polski Tyg. Lek.* **15**, 1217.

SZEJNBERG L. & RABAU E. (1950) Pregnancy tests on male batrachia native to Israel and their use in normal and disturbed pregnancy. *Gynaecologia (Basel)*, **130**, 221.

SZONTÁGH F.E. & TRAUB A. (1962) Zur Histochemie des Trophoblasten. *Z. Geburtsh. Gynäk.* **159**, 68.

TAYMOR M.L., GOSS D.A. & BUYTENDORP A. (1963) Immunologic cross-reaction between luteinizing hormone and human chorionic gonadotropin. *Fertil. and steril.* **14**, 603.

TENNEY B. & PARKER F. (1937) Some observations on the gonadotrophic hormones of pregnancy. *Endocrinology*, **21**, 687.

TENNEY B. & PARKER F. (1939) Hydatidiform mole and chorionepithelioma. *New Engl. J. Med.* **221**, 598.

TEPPERMAN J., ENGEL F.L. & LONG C.N.H. (1943) Review of adrenal cortical hypertrophy. *Endocrinology*, **32**, 373.

THAYER S.A. (1946) Methods of bioassay of animal hormones. *Vitam. and Horm.* **4**, 311.

THIEDE H.A. & CHOATE J.W. (1963) Chorionic gonadotropin localization in the human placenta by immunofluorescent staining. II. Demonstration of HCG in the trophoblast and amnion epithelium of immature and mature placentas. *Obstet. and Gynec.* **22**, 433.

THIEDE H.A., CHOATE J.W. & BINDSCHADLER D.D. (1963) Chorionic gonadotropin localization in the human placenta by immunofluorescent staining. I. Production and characterization of anti-human chorionic gonadotropin. *Obstet. and Gynec.* **22**, 310.

THOMPSON K.W. (1941) Antihormones. *Physiol. Rev.* **21**, 588.

THOMSEN K. (1958) Studien zur Histochemie der Placenta. *Geburtsh. u. Frauenheilk.* **18**, 354.

THOMSEN K. & WILLEMSEN R. (1959) Histochemische Untersuchungen über die Produktionsorte der Choriongonadotropine. *Acta endocr.* (*Kbh.*), **30**, 161.

TOAFF R., AYALON D., LUNENFELD B. & ESHKOL A. (1965) Immuno-titrations and qualitative bioassays of pregnancy urine. *J. Obstet. Gynaec. Brit. Emp.* **72**, 236.

TROEN P. (1959) Perfusion studies of the human placenta. In *Recent Progress in Endocrinology of Reproduction*, p. 299. C.W.Lloyd, ed. Academic Press Inc., New York.

TROEN P. (1961) Perfusion studies of the human placenta. II. Metabolism of C^{14}-17β-estradiol with and without added human chorionic gonadotropin. *J. clin. Endocr.* **21**, 895.

TROEN P. & GORDON E.E. (1958) Perfusion studies of the human placenta. I. Effect of estradiol and human chorionic gonadotropin on citric acid metabolism. *J. clin. Invest.* **37**, 1516.

TULSKY A.S. & KOFF A.K. (1957) Some observations on the role of the corpus luteum in early human pregnancy. *Fertil. and Steril.* **8**, 118.

TURNER H.H., ZANARTU J.A. & NELSON W.O. (1964) Effect of chorionic gonadotropin therapy on fertility in males with scrotal testes. *Fertil. and Steril.* **15**, 24.

TURTLE J.R., BECK P. & DAUGHADAY W.H. (1966) Purification of human placental lactogen. *Endocrinology*, **79**, 187.

TWOMBLY G.H. (1936) Studies on the nature of antigonadotropic substances. *Endocrinology*, **20**, 311.

TWOMBLY G.H. (1944) The relationship of hormones to testicular tumors. *Surgery*, **16**, 181.

TWOMBLY G.H. & FERGUSON R.S. (1934) Protective substances in sera of animals injected with anterior pituitary-like hormone of teratoma testis urine. *Proc. Soc. exp. Biol.* (*N.Y.*), **32**, 69.

TYLER E.T. & SINGHER H.O. (1956) Male infertility–status of treatment, prevention and current research. *J. Amer. med. Ass.* **160**, 91.

UEDA Y., MOCHIZUKI M., KISHIMOTO Y., WASHIO T., MIZUSAWA S. & ISHIGAMI O. (1964) Thyrotropin in placenta and fetus. *Endocr. Japon.* **11**, 67.

VANDE WIELE R.L. & TURKSOY R.N. (1965) Treatment of amenorrhoea and of anovulation with human menopausal and chorionic gonadotropins. *J. clin. Endocr.* **25**, 369.

VAN DEN ENDE M. (1939) Precipitins in antigonadotrophic sera. *J. Endocr.* **1**, 156.

VAN WAGENEN G. & SIMPSON M.E. (1957) Induction of multiple ovulation in the rhesus monkey (*Macaca mulatta*). *Endocrinology*, **61**, 316.

VARANGOT J., CEDARD L. & YANNOTTI S. (1965) Perfusion of the human placenta *in vitro*. Study of the biosynthesis of estrogens. *Amer. J. Obstet. Gynec.* **92**, 534.

VELARDO J.T. (1959) Hormonal actions of chorionic gonadotropin. *Ann. N.Y. Acad. Sci.* **80**, 65.

VERMELIN H., RIBON M. & RIBON C. (1957) Intéret et limites d'interprétation du dosage de prolan dans les avortements. *Bull. Féd. Soc. Gynec. Obstet. Franc.* **9**, 210.

VIGNES P., ROBEY M. & SIMONNET H. (1954) Recherches sur le dosage des gonadotrophines. I. Separation par chromatographie de deux principes gonadotropes dans l'urine de femme enceinte. *Bull. Soc. Chim. biol.* (*Paris*), **36**, 1163.

VOZZA F. (1932) Über die Herkunft der sogenamten Hypophysenvorderlappenhormone in der Schwangerschaft. *Z. Geburtsh. Gynäk.* **102**, 468.

WALTZ H.K., TULLNER W.W., EVANS V.J., HERTZ R. & EARLE W.R. (1954) Gonadotrophic hormone secretion from hydatid mole grown in tissue culture. *J. nat. Cancer Inst.* **14**, 1173.

WATTS R.M. & ADAIR F.L. (1943) Excretion of estrogen and gonadotropin in late pregnancy. *Amer. J. Obstet. Gynec.* **46**, 183.

WEBER J. (1963) Histochemical studies of the production of gonadotrophin in the placenta and foetal membranes. *Acta obstet. gynec. Scand.*, Suppl. **42**, 6 82.

WEINBACH R. (1958) Die Verwandbarkeit formolbehandelter Erythrocyten als Antigen träger in der indirekten Haemagglutination. I. Mitteilung. *Schweiz. Z. allg. Path.* **21**, 1043.

WEINBACH R. (1959) Die Verwendbarkeit formolbehandelter Erythrocyten als Antigenträger in der indirekten Haemagglutination. II. Mitteilung. *Schweiz. Z. allg. Path.* **22**, 1.

WESTMAN A. (1938) Über den Luteinisierungseffekt des gonadotropen Chorionhormons auf die Ovarien der Frau. *Acta path. microbiol. Scand.*, Suppl. **37**, 560.

WHITE P. (1952) Pregnancy complicating diabetes. In *Treatment of Diabetes Mellitus*, p. 676. E.P.Joslin, ed. 9th ed. Kimpton, London.

WHITTEN W.K. (1948) Inactivation of gonadotrophins. II. Inactivation of pituitary and chorionic gonadotrophins by influenza virus and receptor-destroying enzyme. *Aust. J. sci. Res.* B, **1**, 388.

WHITTEN W.K. (1953) Inactivation of gonadotrophins. IV. The effect of periodate ions and 'blood-group enzyme' on the biological activity of chorionic gonadotrophin. *Aust. J. biol. Sci.* **6**, 300.

WIDE L. (1962) An immunological method for the assay of human chorionic gonadotrophin. *Acta endocr.* (*Kbh.*), Suppl. **41**, 70.

WIDE L. & GEMZELL C.A. (1960) An immunological pregnancy test. *Acta endocr.* (*Kbh.*), **35**, 261.

WIDE L. & GEMZELL C.A. (1962) Determination of gonadotropins in urine by a haemagglutination inhibition reaction. In *Immunoassay of Hormones.* Ciba Foundation Colloquia on Endocrinology, **14**, 296. G.E.W.Wolstenholme & M.P.Cameron, eds. Churchill, London.

WIDE L., ROOS P. & GEMZELL C. (1961) Immunological determination of human pituitary luteinizing hormone (LH). *Acta endocr.* (*Kbh.*), **37**, 445.

WIESNER B.P. & MARSHALL P.G. (1931) The gonadotropic hormones. I. The preparation and properties of extracts of anterior lobe, placenta, and pregnancy urine. *Quart. J. exp. Physiol.* **21**, 147.

WILDE C.E. & BAGSHAWE K.D. (1965) The purification of chorionic gonadotropin. In *Gonadotropins. Physicochemical and Immunological Properties.* Ciba Foundation Study Group No. 22, p. 46. G.E.W.Wolstenholme & J.Knight, eds. Churchill, London.

WILDE C.E., ORR A.H. & BAGSHAWE K.D. (1965) A radioimmunoassay of human chorionic gonadotrophin. *Nature, Lond.* **205**, 191.

WILHELMI A.E. (1961) Fractionation of human pituitary glands. *Canad. J. Biochem.* **39**, 1659.

WILSON R.B., ALBERT A. & RANDALL L.M. (1949) Quantitative studies on the production, destruction, and elimination of chorionic gonadotropin in normal pregnancy. *Amer. J. Obstet. Gynec.* **58**, 960.

WISLOCKI G.B. (1951) The histology and cytochemistry of the basal plate and septa placentae of the normal placenta delivered at full term. *Anat. Rec.* **109**, 359.

WISLOCKI G.B. & BENNETT H.E. (1943) The histology and cytology of the human and monkey placenta, with special reference to the trophoblast. *Amer. J. Anat.* **73**, 335.

WISLOCKI G.B. & PADYCULA H.A. (1961) Histochemistry and electron microscopy of the placenta. In *Sex and Internal Secretion*, p. 883. W.C.Young, ed. Williams & Wilkins Co., Baltimore.

WITSCHI E. & RILEY G.M. (1940) Quantitative studies on the hormones of human pituitaries. *Endocrinology*, **26**, 565.

WOOLF B. (1953) *Pharmacol. Rev.* **5**, 87. Quoted from Gaddum (1953a).

YAMAMOTO M. & MARIOKA T. (1956) Studies on the human placental ACTH-like substances. II. Column chromatography. *J. Pharm. Soc. Jap.* **76**, 1038.

YEN S.S.C., PEARSON O.H. & STRATMAN S. (1965) Growth hormone levels in maternal and cord blood. *J. clin. Endocr.* **25**, 655.

ZARROW M.X., HOLMSTRÖM E.G. & SALHANICK H.A. (1955) The concentration of relaxin in the blood serum of normal pregnant women. *Endocrinology*, **15**, 22.

ZILLIACUS H. (1953) Polysaccharide structures in normal chorionic villi, hydatidiform mole and chorionepithelioma with special reference to chorionic gonadotropic hormone. *Gynaecologia* (*Basel*), **135**, 161.

ZILLIACUS H. & ROOS B.-E. (1951) Paper partition chromatography of sugars from chorionic gonadotrophic hormone. *Acta endocr.* (*Kbh.*), **6**, 147.

ZONDEK B. (1929a) Weitere Untersuchungen zur Darstellung, Biologie und Klinik des Hypophysenvorderlappenhormons (Prolan). *Zbl. Gynäk.* **53**, 834.

ZONDEK B. (1929b) Hypophysenvorderlappen und Schwangerschaft. *Endokrinologie*, **5**, 425.

ZONDEK B. (1930a) Hypophysenvorderlappen. *Arch. Gynäk.* **144**, 133.

ZONDEK B. (1930b) Versuch einer biologischen (hormonalen) Diagnostik beim malignen Hodentumor. *Chirurg*, **2**, 1072.

ZONDEK B. (1935) *Hormone des Ovariums und des Hypophysenvorderlappens*, 2nd ed. Julius Springer, Vienna.

ZONDEK B. (1937) Gonadotropic hormone in the diagnosis of chorionepithelioma. *J. Amer. med. Ass.* **108**, 607.

ZONDEK B. (1942) The importance of increased production and excretion of gonadotropic hormone for diagnosis of hydatidiform mole. *J. Obstet. Gynaec. Brit. Emp.* **49**, 397.

ZONDEK B. (1954) Some problems related to ovarian function and to pregnancy. *Recent Progr. Hormone Res.* **10**, 395.

ZONDEK B. & ASCHHEIM S. (1928) Das Hormon des Hypophysenvorderlappens. Darstellung chemische Eigenschaften, biologische Wirkungen. *Klin. Wschr.* **7**, 831.

ZONDEK B. & GOLDBERG S. (1957) Placental function and foetal death. I. Urinary gonadotrophin titration test in early pregnancy. II. Urinary oestriol excretion test in advanced pregnancy. *J. Obstet. Gynaec. Brit. Emp.* **64**, 1.

ZONDEK B. & SULMAN F. (1937a) The antigonadotropic factor. Origin and preparation. *Proc. Soc. exp. Biol. (N.Y.)*, **36**, 708.

ZONDEK B. & SULMAN F. (1937b) The antigonadotropic factor. Species specificity and organ specificity. *Proc. Soc. exp. Biol. (N.Y.)*, **36**, 712.

ZONDEK B. & SULMAN F. (1937c) Some properties of the antigonadotropic factor. *Proc. Soc. exp. Biol. (N.Y.)*, **37**, 193.

ZONDEK B. & SULMAN F. (1937d) Mechanism of prolan-antiprolan-reaction in simultaneous and unsimultaneous application of both active principles. *Proc. Soc. exp. Biol. (N.Y.)*, **37**, 198.

ZONDEK B. & SULMAN F. (1937e) The antigonadotropic factor. Reversibility of the prolan-antiprolan effect. *Proc. Soc. exp. Biol. (N.Y.)*, **37**, 343.

ZONDEK B. & SULMAN F. (1942) *The Antigonadotropic Factor*. Williams & Wilkins, Baltimore.

ZONDEK B. & SULMAN F. (1945) The mechanism of action and metabolism of gonadotropic hormones in the organism. *Vitam. and Horm.* **3**, 297.

ZONDEK B., SULMAN F. & HOCHMAN A. (1938) The preparation of concentrated antigonadotropic factor (antiprolan). *Biochem. J.* **32**, 1891.

ZONDEK B., SULMAN F. & HOCHMAN A. (1939) The antigonadotropic factor. The quantitative aspects of the prolan-antiprolan reaction. *Proc. Soc. exp. Biol. (N.Y.)*, **40**, 96.

8
Enzymology of the Placenta

DWAIN D. HAGERMAN*

One of the tenets of modern biochemistry is that the structure and function of any tissue are the end result of the activity of the enzymes contained in that tissue. These enzymes are a protein expression of genetic information contained in and transmitted by deoxyribonucleic acid, with modifications introduced by the processes of cellular differentiation. From this proposition we deduce that a complete and detailed understanding of the enzyme constituents of any tissue should lead directly to a complete and detailed understanding of the structure and function of that tissue. Moreover, the description of the enzyme complement of a given tissue is now as essential a part of the characterization of the tissue as previously has been the histologic description of the tissue. No complete description of the enzyme complement of any tissue exists; perhaps more is known about the enzymes of *Escherichia coli* than those of any other living thing, and in the higher forms there seems to be little doubt that rat liver is the most extensively characterized organ as far as enzymes are concerned. This chapter describes the present state of knowledge of the enzymology of a specific organ, the placenta.

The enzymes of the placenta are of two kinds. First, there are those catalysts that are essential for the continued existence of the cells of the organ. Presumably this constellation of enzymes is very similar in cells of all kinds. Second, the placenta contains in addition enzymes which provide the catalytic capabilities for the performance of the various specialized

* The investigations of the author are supported in part by NIH Research Grants No. AM 11846, National Institute of Arthritis and Metabolic Diseases, and No. HD 00781, National Institute of Child Health and Human Development, United States Department of Health, Education and Welfare.

functions of the tissue. It is the existence of this kind of enzymic specialization that distinguishes organ from organ and tissue from tissue.

A description of the enzymes of the placenta is important to biologists and clinicians who are primarily interested in the functional capabilities of the placenta and its diseases, but in addition the placental enzymes have an inherent interest of their own to the enzymologist, because this organ is the most conveniently available human tissue for the study of human enzymes as such. A comparison of the detailed chemical characteristics of human enzymes with those of the same enzymes from other species is of great interest, but unfortunately only a small number of enzymes isolated from human tissues have so far been characterized with sufficient precision to permit detailed comparison with the same enzymes isolated from the tissues of other species. For example, human liver alcohol dehydrogenase has been highly purified and thoroughly characterized (von Wartburg *et al.* 1964). The human liver enzyme is structurally very similar to the corresponding horse liver enzyme, but there are significant functional differences between the two protein molecules. Likewise, Nisselbaum & Bodansky (1961a, 1961b, 1963) prepared crystalline human heart lactate dehydrogenase in an electrophoretically and ultracentrifugally homogeneous state and showed that it is immunochemically distinct from the human liver enzyme, but did not make direct comparisons with the enzymes from other species. On the basis of further experiments with the enzyme from human brain, these authors concluded that 'in a single species the lactic dehydrogenase variants possessing the same electrophoretic, chromatographic and immunological characteristics are identical, regardless of their tissue of origin' (Nisselbaum *et al.* 1964). The evidence available for the human placenta lactate dehydrogenase does not contradict this conclusion (Wiggert & Villee 1964, van Bogaert, di Peretti & Villee 1967). From these examples of inter-organ similarity of enzymes in one species and of inter-specific differences in enzymes from the same tissue of different species, it is clear that further study of highly purified enzymes from the readily available human placenta is warranted for comparative purposes.

Interest in the enzymes of the placenta has recently increased, perhaps in part as a result of the general increase of interest in enzymology. This increased research activity is reflected in the literature. When Page & Glendenning (1955) tabulated the known enzymes of the human placenta the list contained 45 entries. A similar tabulation made late in 1963 gave a total of 63 reasonably well characterized enzymes that had been detected in the placenta (Hagerman 1964). The survey of the literature completed early in 1968 for the preparation of this chapter disclosed more than a score of additional descriptions of characterized enzymes of the placenta, making a total of more than 85 enzymes. These figures refer to enzymes detected or investigated directly, and do not include those whose existence has been inferred from histochemical or metabolic studies. The total may be compared with the approximately 800–1,000 different enzymes that have been described from all sources (Dixon & Webb 1964).

METHODS OF INVESTIGATION

A variety of methods may be utilized in the identification, isolation and characterization of these protein molecules. The customary method of detection of an enzyme is the measurement of its catalytic activity as evidenced by the conversion of a single substrate to a single, well-defined product. This method of detection is completely unambiguous if the substrate is pure and the product is well characterized chemically, provided that no spontaneous reaction occurs which might convert the substrate to the product in the absence of the enzyme. In practice, control analyses with inactivated enzymes are used to satisfy the latter criterion. The recent widespread use of radioactively labeled substrates with very high specific activity has made careful chemical characterization of the enzyme reaction product vitally important in enzyme assays dependent upon radioactivity measurements. This consideration is of particular importance with enzymes which catalyse the interconversion of steroids, and several procedures have been devised to ensure radiochemical purity of isolated material presumed to be products of enzyme reactions. Such direct chemical or radiochemical enzyme assays may usually be conducted on simple homogenates of tissues in which the only preparation of the material is the rupturing of the cell membranes so that no cellular permeability barriers exist to prevent access of the substrate to the enzyme. However, simple homogenates frequently show relatively low enzyme activities and it may be necessary to concentrate the enzyme before studies can be continued.

Fractionation of the cell organelles often follows homogenization of the tissue. The fractionation may be achieved by differential centrifugation in isotonic sucrose or potassium chloride, by adjustment of ionic strength, pH or metal ion composition of the suspending medium, or by the more precise method of density gradient centrifugation. The fractions obtained from these procedures are usually found to have the enzyme of interest concentrated in one particular type of cell constituent, and the removal by the same procedures of large amounts of inactive protein frequently considerably simplifies the problems of enzyme assay. If upon cell fractionation the enzyme is found to be in the soluble fraction of the tissue, further purification can be attempted without complication; but if the enzyme under study is found to be in one of the particulate constituents of the cell it is essential to free the enzyme into a soluble state before it can be further purified. A great variety of empirical procedures have been devised for the solubilization of enzymes from cell particulates and in most instances the ingenuity and patience of the investigator determines whether or not a given enzyme can be obtained in solution. Having obtained a soluble protein, techniques for further purification of the material are reasonably well standardized.

Fractionation is attempted on the basis of size, shape, solubility, charge distribution and of other kinds of interactions of the enzyme molecules with other molecules, particular use being made of column chromatography, gel filtration, countercurrent distribution, electrophoresis, salting out, density gradient separation and so on. When such separations are performed in a quantitative manner the separation procedures themselves provide evidence as to the homogeneity of the resulting product. The ultimate objective is the isolation of a protein preparation that is possibly crystalline but certainly homogeneous with respect to size, shape, charge distribution, chemistry and amino acid sequence. Measurements of these properties of protein molecules are for the most part theoretically simple but technically demanding, often requiring highly complex instrumentation.

The assay of purified enzymes is fundamentally a kinetic analysis of the reaction catalysed by the enzyme in which one measures under optimal conditions of pH, temperature, ionic strength, etc., the initial rate of the reaction. A concentration of substrate sufficient to give zero order kinetics (in which the reaction velocity is virtually independent of substrate concentration) is used, and an amount of activity proportional to the amount of protein analysed must be found. A practical point is that the very large number of determinations of activity needed during the extensive chemical manipulations required for the purification of most enzymes makes it highly desirable that the enzyme assay be technically simple and rapid. A direct spectrophotometric determination of the disappearance of substrate or appearance of product is frequently the most useful; colorimetric analyses for the determination of disappearance of substrate or appearance of product over a short period of incubation are less convenient but entirely feasible; radiochemical enzyme assays in which the product of the reaction must be rigorously purified before determination of the enzyme activity can be considered to have been achieved make the purification of an enzyme slow and laborious.

When the purified enzyme has been obtained it is ordinarily characterized in detail with regard to the kinetics of the reaction catalysed, including the effects of substrate and product concentration, activators and inhibitors, the effect of pH, the substrate specificity of the enzyme, the equilibrium point and energetics of the reaction, etc.; with respect to the amino acid analysis of the protein; and with respect to the primary, secondary, tertiary and quaternary structure of the protein. It has recently become apparent that the quaternary, or sub-unit, structure of many enzymes is important in the regulation of the catalytic activities of the protein molecule. As a result, a detailed understanding of the factors involved in maintaining or modulating these aspects of structure is essential to a complete understanding of the functions of the molecule. Many enzymes contain prosthetic groups of relatively small molecular weight, and some contain metal ions that are essential to catalytic activity. These substances must be identified. A complete chemical characterization of the active site is desirable so that the chemical mechanism by which the enzyme catalyzes the reaction can be completely understood.

In addition to the direct methods of enzyme characterization, considerable information about the enzyme constituents of a tissue can sometimes be obtained by purely inferential methods. For example, one may study *in vivo* the overall metabolism from ingestion to excretion of a given chemical compound. From the changes which take place during metabolism, one can deduce the kinds of enzymes which must be involved. Similar investigations can be done by organ perfusion or in slices or minces of tissues. Under these circumstances a given substrate is usually incorporated into a variety of products and all of them should be characterized. It is unfortunately difficult in such experiments to determine the relative activities of the many enzymes that are involved in the conversion of the original material administered to the products isolated. Whenever intact cells are used experimentally the problem of the permeability of the cell membrane to the substrate used also arises, so that it is not possible to infer from a negative experiment with whole cells that a given enzyme is absent from the tissue. It may be only that the substrate did not have access to the enzyme under the conditions of the experiment. However, if the overall metabolic pathways of interest are known from studies of other organisms or tissues, then relatively simple experiments with intact cells can provide strong presumptive evidence of the existence of a considerable number of enzymes. For example, from the fact that placenta slices readily convert glucose to carbon dioxide (Villee 1953) one can infer that the tissue probably contains all of the enzymes of the glycolytic pathway and all of the enzymes and cofactors involved in the final oxidative pathway, the electron transmitter system. Such a conclusion is not absolutely certain, for it might be that an entirely new pathway for metabolism could exist in any given specific instance. In point of fact the human placenta does contain the enzymes of these pathways.

For an adequate understanding of the enzymatic organization of any tissue both types of study mentioned above are essential. The direct methods of enzyme assay measure the *capabilities* of the tissue constituents in disorganized cells. If such homogenates are fully saturated with cofactors and no inhibition is present, one can measure the maximal rate of metabolism of a given substrate to a given product. Except for cases of direct activation or inhibition of specific enzymes such an homogenate is free from metabolic control. The *actualities* of metabolism are more precisely reflected by experiments with intact cells. Isolated tissues *in vitro* are of course free from any metabolic controls derived from other tissues present in an intact animal. Isolated tissue studies provide the only feasible method for measuring with any degree of accuracy the magnitude of alternative pathways of metabolism although such studies are fraught with many complications of recycling, pool size, and so forth. Such studies are also probably the ultimate arbiter of the physiologic relevance of any postulated metabolic control mechanism.

Possibilities for correlation between enzyme content and structural details of the tissue have been illustrated in a review by Wynn (1965), and modern data on the chemical composition of the human placenta are given by Winick *et al.* (1967).

PLACENTAL ENZYMES

The summary of available information about the enzymes that have been detected in the placenta which follows was prepared with the aid of references obtained from earlier works on the subject (Page & Glendenning 1955, Kyank 1958, Velardo & Rosa 1963, Hafez 1964, Hagerman 1964) and those found in a re-examination of the entire literature. The discussion is organized according to the classification proposed by the Commission on Enzymes of the International Union of Biochemistry (Report, 1961; Recommendations, 1964). This classification is based upon the nature of the chemical reaction catalysed by the enzymes instead of the older and less rational practice of classification of enzymes according to their substrate specificity. According to the classification used the 6 major groups of enzymes are: oxidoreductases, transferases, hydrolases, lyases, isomerases and ligases. The enzymes are listed by their trivial names, and are of human origin unless otherwise specified. An attempt has been made to describe only those enzymes whose identity has been reasonably well established. Except for β-hydroxybutyrate dehydrogenase and α-glycerophosphate dehydrogenase (Boss & Craig 1962), no enzymes have been detected in placenta by histochemical techniques that have not also been shown to be present by other methods (Padykula 1958, Lobel *et al.* 1962, Wachstein *et al.* 1963, Curzen 1964).

Alcohol (*ethanol*) *dehydrogenase* linked to NAD is present in the soluble fraction of human placenta but has not been purified (Hagerman, unpublished).

Polyol dehydrogenase with specificity for NADP has been purified 55-fold from the soluble portion of bovine placenta. The enzyme has a broad pH optimum and prefers propanediol and glycerol as substrates (Velle & Engel 1964). It does not attack ethanol but does react slowly with sorbitol as substrate and may therefore be similar or identical to the NADP specific enzyme described below.

Sorbitol dehydrogenase was found to be present in human placenta in connection with an investigation of fructose production by the organ (Roux *et al.* 1959). These authors demonstrated the conversion of sorbitol to fructose, and their results have been confirmed and extended in experiments with extracts of the tissue (Ritter & Leuthardt 1963) When fortified with NAD such extracts convert glucose to sorbitol, the NAD presumably being reduced by other reactions occurring in the extracts. When NAD is replaced by NADP, sorbitol is oxidized to fructose. Whether there are two enzymes with limited substrate and cofactor specificity involved in these reactions or whether a single rather nonspecific hexitol dehydrogenase catalyzes both reactions is unknown.

In the sheep placenta (which produces large amounts of fructose from glucose), Britton *et al.* have shown that sorbitol is an intermediate in fructose synthesis 1967). These authors formulate their results in terms of two enzymes, an aldose reductase and a sorbitol dehydrogenase, although the existence of the latter enzyme in this tissue had earlier been denied by others. Isolation of these enzyme activities might serve to clarify this reaction sequence.

Lactate dehydrogenase is a soluble enzyme in placenta and exists in the same 5 isozymic forms as those found in other human tissues. Types III, IV and V are somewhat more predominant in placenta than in other tissues (Wiggert & Villee 1964) and it is these components which are increased in the serum during labor (Meade & Rosalki 1963, Hawkins & Whyley 1966). The latter observations confirm an earlier proposal that the placenta is responsible for the increase in the serum concentration of the enzyme observed during labor (Hagerman & Wellington 1959). The tissue concentration of this NAD-linked enzyme is not altered by the presence of placental pathology (Stark & Oweis 1963). More recent studies done by polyacrylamide gel electrophoresis demonstrate not only the preponderance of the anodic enzymes already mentioned but also two additional intermediate electrophoretically separable bands with lactate dehydrogenase activity. At 17 weeks of gestation only the 3 most rapidly migrating enzymes are detectable in placenta extracts. Chorion and amnion both contain all 5 of the isozymes (van Bogaert, di Perretti & Villee 1967).

Malate dehydrogenase from human placenta is NAD linked and exists in two isozymic forms. The proportion of the more anodic fraction upon electrophoresis is somewhat greater in placenta than in other human tissues (Wiggert & Villee 1964). The concentration of serum malate dehydrogenase increases during labor which may reflect release of the placental enzyme (Meade & Rosalki 1963), but the tissue concentration of the enzyme is not elevated by placental pathology (Stark & Oweis 1963).

Isocitrate dehydrogenase is another placental enzyme that is apparently released into the blood during labor in the human (Meade & Rosalki 1963). The soluble placental enzyme is specific for NADP and decarboxylates added oxalosuccinate (Villee & Gordon 1955). Partial purification of the enzyme has been achieved but its properties have not been studied in any detail (Hagerman, unpublished).

Phosphogluconate dehydrogenase is present in extracts of human term placenta at nearly as high a concentration as in erythrocytes (Chieffi *et al.* 1963a). The enzyme is specific for NADPH (Hagerman, unpublished).

Glucose-6-phosphate dehydrogenase is present in high concentration in extracts of human term placenta (Chieffi *et al.* 1963a), and has been partially purified from this source (Betz & Warren 1965). The purified enzyme is stabilized by glycerol, NADP and NADPH, and estimates of its Michaelis constants are $1{\cdot}75 \times 10^{-4}$ M for glucose-6-phosphate and $2{\cdot}5 \times 10^{-5}$ M for NADP. The latter value is about 10-fold greater than the constant for the enzyme from other sources and if it can be verified by measurements upon more nearly homogeneous samples of enzyme another example of interspecific variations of enzyme properties will have been provided. The partially purified placenta enzyme is inhibited *in vitro* by a variety of steroid hormones when they are added in rather high concentrations but it seems unlikely that these inhibitory effects are of any physiologic importance in the intact animal.

Hydroxysteroid dehydrogenases. The 17β-estradiol dehydrogenase from human placenta is perhaps the most extensively studied placenta enzyme. It was detected by Ryan & Engel (1953) and considerably purified by Langer & Engel (1958). The soluble preparations studied by the latter authors utilized either NAD or NADP as the hydrogen acceptor, showed a broad pH optimum which was higher when the reaction was measured in the forward (dehydrogenation) direction, and utilized 17β-estradiol and 3-O-methyl-17β-estradiol most effectively as substrates. Langer *et al.* (1959) showed that the enzyme would attack a wide variety of 17β-hydroxysteroids, and the authors inferred from their specificity studies that the substrates were probably attached to the enzyme by hydrophobic bonding and other weak forces to the rear (α) surface of the steroid. Their kinetic measurements gave small Michaelis constants for both substrate and co-substrate, suggesting that these components of the reaction system were rather tightly associated with the enzyme. Tight binding of substrate and co-substrate appears to be a general characteristic of steroid metabolizing enzymes. The enzyme was investigated further by Jarabak *et al.* (1962) who achieved a purification of greater than 3,000-fold from the original homogenate with high yield. Their procedure depended upon stabilization of the enzyme with glycerol which permitted a vigorous and effective heat denaturation step, followed by salt fractionation and column chromatography. The purified enzyme prepared by this procedure utilizes both NAD and NADP as co-substrates and it will dehydrogenate a wide variety of

17β-hydroxysteroids (Adams *et al.* 1962). The protein is homogeneous upon ion exchange chromatography and stabilized solution electrophoresis but no information upon its ultracentrifugal homogeneity, amino acid composition or sequence is yet available. The highly purified enzyme will dehydrogenate 17β-estradiol-17αD at about 35–40 per cent of the rate observed with the non-deuterated steroid with either NAD or NADP as co-substrate. Although the reaction velocity is decreased by introduction of the deuterium (isotope effect) the Michaelis constant for the steroid is not altered (Adams *et al.* 1965). Since the deuterium is on the same side of the molecule as was postulated for the binding by Langer & Engel, the active site of the enzyme must be quite spacious to permit entry of the larger deuterium atom. The kinetics of the enzyme suggest an ordered Bi-Bi mechanism with the steroid binding first (Warren & Crist 1967). The enzyme activity is widespread, being detectable in the placentas of the mare, ewe, cat, bitch, ferret, rat, rabbit, pig and guinea-pig (Dollefeld & Breuer 1966; Ferguson & Christie 1967; Christie 1968). A similar enzyme specific for 17α-estradiol is found in sheep and cow placenta (Ainsworth & Ryan 1966).

Evidence for the existence of two separable protein moieties with 17β-estradiol dehydrogenase activity from placenta, one utilizing NAD and the other NADP as co-substrate, has been presented (Hagerman & Villee 1959). Kellogg & Glenner (1960) published photomicrographs which showed the NAD linked activity to be present in both the syncytiotrophoblast and perivascular stroma while the NADP linked enzyme was found only in the stroma. In contrast Kleiner *et al.* (1962) found the NADP enzyme only in the syncytiotrophoblast. Recently two other histochemical investigations of this problem have been reported in which the original observations of Kellogg & Glenner are confirmed and extended (Koide & Mitsudo 1965; Mitsudo & Koide 1966). Perfusion studies make it clear that this enzyme is important in the metabolism of estrogens during pregnancy (Cedard *et al.* 1961; cf. chapter by Diczfalusy in this book). These dehydrogenase activities catalyse a substrate-mediated transhydrogenation reaction by which hydrogen may be transferred from one pyridine nucleotide to another as a result of alternate oxidation and reduction at position 17 of the steroid molecule (Talalay & Williams-Ashman 1958; Crist & Warren 1966), and this reaction accounts for about half of the estrogen dependent transhydrogenation catalysed by crude extracts of human term placenta (Hagerman & Villee 1965). The total transhydrogenation activity of placental extracts is said to be *increased* in a variety of pathological states of the organ (Pulkkinen & Willman (1967)). Preparations of 'native' estradiol dehydrogenase from human term placenta exhibit a concentration dependent reversible trimerization and it has been shown that the monomeric units of the enzyme catalyze steroid dehydrogenation while the trimer does not (Hagerman 1966).

The existence of 20α-hydroxysteroid dehydrogenase activity in the soluble fraction of human term placenta was demonstrated by Little *et al.* (1959). The enzyme does not reduce the 20-ketone group of 17α-hydroxyprogesterone caproate (Wiener *et al.* 1961) and from studies of a more highly purified preparation of the enzyme it would appear to be identical to the 17β-hydroxysteroid dehydrogenase described above (Purdy *et al.* 1964). Another 20-ketone reductase has been described as being localized in the microsomal fraction of placenta but it is not known whether this is a distinct enzyme (Meigs & Engel 1961). The isomeric 20β-dihydrosteroids are not oxidized by placenta (Palmer *et al.* 1966).

The presence of a 6β-hydroxysteroid dehydrogenase in placenta can be inferred from the perfusion results of Hagopian *et al.* (1956), and an 11β-hydroxysteroid dehydrogenase has been investigated in crude homogenates of human placenta by Osinski (1960). The latter enzyme utilizes a variety of 11-oxygenated steroids as substrates, will accept either NAD or NADP as co-substrate with the latter showing greater activity, and appears to be concentrated in the cell membrane. The reaction was shown to be reversible, as expected, but the enzyme has not been purified. A similar activity was found in placental microsomes (Meigs & Engel 1961).

Microsomal preparations from term human placenta also catalyse an oxidation of 3α-hydroxysteroids and the cofactor may be either of the pyridine nucleotides (Meigs & Engel 1961). The same enzyme may participate in the conversion of corticosteroids to their tetrahydro derivatives described by Venning & Sybulski (1962), and might contribute to the production of pregnanediol by the tissue, which has been shown to contain the steroid (Cagnazzo *et al.* 1962). The microsomes do not contain any Δ^4-reductase activity (Meigs & Engel 1961) but this enzyme is present in whole homogenates (Venning & Sybulski 1962) so that evidence for the existence in placenta of all of the enzymes required to convert progesterone to pregnanediol is available. This evidence provides an example of the fact that the mere existence of the necessary enzymes in a tissue does not prove that they form an active metabolic pathway of the organ, since in this instance perfusion studies indicate that progesterone is not reduced to pregnanediol to any significant extent by placenta (Palmer *et al.* 1966). A similar 3α-reductase is present in the rat placenta (Howard 1968).

Considerable information is available about the 3β-hydroxysteroid dehydrogenase-Δ^5 to Δ^4-isomerase complex in placenta. The complex was originally shown to be present in rat placenta by Samuels *et al.* (1950) and in human placenta by Nissim & Robson (1952). The conclusion of the latter authors was based on bioassay data and it has been confirmed by chemical methods by Pearlman *et al.* (1954) and by Sobrevilla *et al.* (1964) in placenta homogenates and by perfusion studies (Pion *et al.* 1965). The reaction is rapid (Pion *et al.* 1966; Jaffe & Ledger 1966). Koide & Torres (1965) provide evidence that the enzyme is in a particulate fraction of the tissue, mitochondria or microsomes or both. In the rat placenta the enzyme or enzymes reaches a maximum activity histochemically about two-thirds of the way through gestation (Deane *et al.* 1962). The enzyme accepts a wide variety of substrates (Baillie *et al.* 1965) and has been shown to be present in the placentas of man, mouse, rat (cf. Deane & Rubin 1965), rabbit (Howard 1968) and bat (Fonda & Peyre 1965), but was not detected histochemically in the ferret placenta (Galil & Deane 1966). Using a bacterial source it has been possible to highly purify and crystallize an enzyme which catalyses only the isomerization (Kawahara *et al.* 1962) and chemical evidence obtained with enzyme preparations from the adrenal suggest that these reactions are distinct in mammalian tissues also (cf. Ewald *et al.* 1964). The investigations are complicated by the fact that the isomerization proceeds at an appreciable rate non-enzymatically but presumably there are separate enzymes for the two reactions in the placenta (Baulieu *et al.* 1963; Venning & Sybulski 1962). Koide & Torres (1966) have described a placental isomerase preparation free of dehydrogenase activity, and further evidence for the existence of separate enzymes for the two reactions comes from the comparative studies of Bloch & Newman (1966). They showed that dehydroepiandrosterone is converted to Δ^4-androstenedione by the placentas of cat, dog, cow, pig, rat and human, but that in the guinea-pig and armadillo androst-5-ene-3β-diol was the major product. It has been suggested that different steroids containing the Δ^5-3β-hydroxy configuration may be oxidized and isomerized by different enzymes or pairs of enzymes

(Villee, personal communication), but none of these postulated enzymes have been isolated.

Human placenta was reported to contain enzymatic activities for the interconversion of 16-keto and 16-hydroxy phenolic steroids (Ryan 1960), but this activity was not detected by Dahm & Breuer (1966).

Xanthine oxidase is absent from human placenta (Hayashi *et al.* 1964).

Succinate dehydrogenase has been known for many years to be present in placenta. The evidence for this consists of increased oxygen consumption by the tissue resulting from the addition of the substrate to minces of tissue (Tesauro, 1935). The enzyme has not been purified, but is inhibited by malonate (Hosoya & Kawada 1958).

3-*Ketosteroid* Δ^4-*dehydrogenase* activity is present in placenta (Venning & Sybulski 1962) and Loke (1964) has shown that the enzyme occurs in the soluble fraction of the tissue. When NAD plus ATP are supplied as cofactors with testosterone as substrate, the products are the 5α- and 5β-androstanediones.

Glutamate dehydrogenase of human term placenta is a mitochondrial enzyme with many of the characteristics of the animal liver enzyme. The placental enzyme has been purified to the point of being more than 600 times as active as a simple placental homogenate but was not obtained in a homogeneous state. The purified enzyme will accept either NAD or NADP as co-substrate, the activity with the latter being about one-third that with the former nucleotide, and the kinetic constants of the placenta enzyme are similar to those of the liver enzyme (Gaull *et al.* 1960). NAD^+ activates the enzyme but $NADP^+$ does not and estrone, estradiol and progesterone inhibit the $NADP^+$-linked activity at steroid concentrations which are not dissimilar to those found *in vivo* (Peterson & Warren 1966).

Monoamine oxidase in placenta homogenates has been measured by the Warburg technique of measurement of oxygen consumption in the presence of suitable amine substrates. The enzyme is inhibited by ephedrine, as are the analogous enzymes from other tissues, and tyramine, tryptamine, isoamylamine and butylamine are decreasingly effective as substrates in that order (Luschinsky & Singher 1948). Two groups of investigators have found decreased activity of the enzyme in placentas from patients with toxemia (Sandler & Coveny 1962; de Maria 1964) but another group found no change (Lindberg & Westling 1962). It may be that the patients were selected by somewhat different criteria in these various studies, but it seems unlikely that the enzyme deficiency (if it exists) is related causally to the disease (cf. Klinge *et al.* 1964).

Diamine oxidase (*histaminase*) has been studied in slices of placenta by measurement of disappearance of biological activity (Swanberg 1950). The activity was shown to increase rapidly during the first half of pregnancy and thereafter to remain fairly constant. The enzyme is concentrated in the decidual portion of the placenta. Lindahl (1960) measured the activity of the enzyme in placenta by a manometric method and Lindberg (1963) showed that ^{14}C-histamine is metabolized mainly to imidazole-acetic acid. This enzyme activity was more carefully examined by Kapeller-Adler (1965) who was able to achieve a 120-fold purification of the protein. The product was homogeneous on Sephadex G-200, and upon cellulose acetate electrophoresis at pH 8·6 the single band of protein migrated at a velocity similar to that of the α_2-globulins. The properties of the purified enzyme are rather different from those of the purified hog kidney histaminase and resemble more closely those of pea seedling diamine oxidase (cf. Smith 1967). Perfusion studies show release of the enzyme from placenta over long periods of time which may reflect net synthesis of the enzyme (Southern *et al.* 1966).

Pyridine nucleotide transhydrogenase has been measured in human term placenta mitochondria and its properties appear to be similar to the corresponding mitochondrial enzyme in other tissues (Hagerman & Villee 1961). The soluble fraction of human term placentas contains at least two distinguishable transhydrogenating systems, all of which react more rapidly in the presence of minute quantities of natural estrogens. One of these reactions is a substrate mediated transhydrogenation, catalysed by the 17β-estradiol dehydrogenase described above (Jarabak *et al.* 1962). Activation of this system is achieved only by steroids possessing the 17β-hydroxy or 17-carbonyl group and of these compounds the natural estrogens are the most potent (Adams *et al.* 1962; Hecker & Farthofer-Boeckh 1963). As mentioned before, the estradiol dehydrogenase can exist as either a monomer or a trimer. The trimeric form of the enzyme does not catalyse estradiol dehydrogenation but can promote the transfer of hydrogen from NADPH to NAD (Hagerman 1966). Another transhydrogenating system present in the soluble fraction is a specific pyridine nucleotide transhydrogenase that is activated by a variety of both natural and synthetic estrogens (Hagerman & Villee 1965). The activators may or may not be 17β-hydroxysteroids

(Hagerman & Villee 1961). A preparative scale separation of this enzymatic activity from the estradiol dehydrogenase has been achieved (Karavolas & Engel 1966). Possible inter-relationships among the protein moieties responsible for these transhydrogenations have not yet been fully explored. A similar transhydrogenase has been partially purified from rat placenta which contains negligible amounts of 17β-hydroxysteroid dehydrogenase. The rat enzyme, like the human enzyme, is activated equally well by diethylstilbestrol and 17β-estradiol, and somewhat less effectively by testosterone and hexestrol (Shirasu 1964).

NADPH cytochrome c reductase is present in placenta microsome preparations but has not been purified or studied in detail (Hagerman *et al.* 1966). It is inhibited by the drug clomiphene citrate.

NADH and NADPH diaphorases are both present in all placentas examined histochemically for these enzyme activities (Boss & Craig 1962) and the NAD linked enzyme can be purified by the Straub procedure (Hagerman, unpublished). It appears to be a lipoamide dehydrogenase.

Cytochrome oxidase activity of placenta slices has been measured by means of oxygen uptake in the Warburg apparatus. The oxygen consumption of the tissue is increased 8 times over the control values by the addition of hydroquinone, in accordance with the properties of the purified enzyme (James *et al.* 1948).

Catalase was reported to be present in washed minced preparations of placenta, but in this very early work the presence of the enzyme may have been due to contamination of the tissue preparation with blood (Löb & Higuchi 1909).

Steroid hydroxylases are present in placenta and as far as is known require both NADPH and molecular oxygen as do other enzymes of this class. The soluble fraction of human term placenta hydroxylates progesterone at both the 16α- and 17α-positions (Little & Shaw 1961; Little *et al.* 1963) and testosterone at the 16α-position (Loke 1964). Similar reactions were *not* observed when progesterone was perfused at midpregnancy (Palmer *et al.* 1966). Evidence for a 21-hydroxylase is contained in the metabolic investigations reported by Roversi & Polvani (1963). Likewise, hydroxylation at position 6β of progesterone has been demonstrated (Berliner & Salhanick 1956; Palmer *et al.* 1966; Kitchin *et al.* 1967). The 19-*nor* compound, estr-4-ene-3, 17-dione, is hydroxylated at position C-1 (Townsley & Brodie, 1966).

Hydroxylation of estrone, estradiol and estriol at C-2 is catalysed by placenta (Lucis, 1965) and the enzyme is microsomal (Fishman 1967). Perfusion experiments with estrone or estradiol demonstrated 6α-hydroxylation of these phenolic substrates both at term (Cedard & Knuppen 1965) and at 5 to 6 months gestation (Alonso & Troen 1966). Some investigators have reported 16α-hydroxylation of estrone or estradiol by term placentas studied by perfusion (Troen 1961; Cedard *et al.* 1962) but these observations were not confirmed in homogenate experiments reported by Slaunwhite *et al.* 1965). The latter authors did find, however, that at 3 to 5 months of gestation the placenta will convert estrone to both 16α- and 16β-hydroxyestrone and thence to estriol and 16-epiestriol. Taken together, and assuming that the products isolated were correctly identified despite the very tiny amounts produced in all of these experiments, it seems probable that there is a relatively non-specific 16-hydroxylase with a preference for C-21 steroids present in placentas early in gestation and that the activity of this postulated enzyme decreases nearly to the vanishing point by the end of gestation. Other hydroxylases whose substrates and products have not been identified are present in placenta (Dixon & Pennington 1965), and further experimental work on this subject is clearly desirable.

Hydroxylation at position 19 of neutral C-19 steroids is almost certainly a step in the normal sequence of reactions leading to aromatization, despite the fact that the 19-*nor* steroids are only slowly aromatized. Longchampt *et al.* (1960) demonstrated the presence of this enzyme in placenta microsomes and the kinetic studies of Wilcox & Engel (1965a) confirm the importance of the enzyme. Unfortunately, no satisfactory method for the solubilization of any of these microsomal mixed function oxidases has been reported, which has made detailed investigations of the nature of the hydroxylation capabilities of placenta most difficult.

Imidazole methyltransferase was detected in an investigation of histamine metabolism in placenta. The enzyme requires S-adenosyl methionine as a methyl donor but its substrate specificity and other properties are unknown (Lindahl 1960; Lindberg 1963).

Estrogen methyltransferase activity is present in placenta (Lucis 1965; cf. Troen 1961). The enzyme appears to be quite specific for 2-hydroxy phenolic steroids.

Ornithine carbamoyltransferase is one of the few enzymes that has been specifically searched for in placenta and not detected (Bastide *et al.* 1963).

Transketolase, an enzyme of the pentose phosphate pathway of carbohydrate metabolism, has been measured in both human term placenta and in rat placenta at various stages of pregnancy. The enzyme in the rat is somewhat more active early in pregnancy (Chieffi & Mangiarotti 1962).

Transaldolase, another enzyme of the pentose phosphate pathway, has an activity in human and rat placenta parallel to transketolase (Chieffi & Mangiarotti 1962). Neither of these enzymes has been purified from the tissue.

Choline acetyltransferase is present in the placentas of man and monkeys, but is not present in the placentas of the mongoose, lemur, horse, cow, sheep, goat, pig, hamster, rabbit, guinea-pig or rat (Hebb & Ratkovic 1962). The activity of the enzyme in the human organ increases from early gestation until 24 weeks and then decreases rapidly to somewhat less than one-third the maximum at term. At 24 weeks it is more active in placenta than in any other vertebrate tissue (Bull *et al.* 1961). The enzyme has been partially purified from extracts of placenta acetone powders and has a molecular weight of 59,000 by sucrose density gradient centrifugation analysis (Bull *et al.* 1964). Preparations of the enzyme made from placentas obtained at mid-gestation had a Michaelis constant for choline of $2{\cdot}5 \times 10^{-3}$M (Hemsworth & Morris 1964). The equilibrium constant is given as $5{\cdot}1 \times 10^{3}$ and a mechanism of catalysis involving an acetylated enzyme as intermediate has been proposed (Schuberth 1966; Morris 1966).

Carnitine palmityltransferase has been identified in human placenta, where it is primarily found in the mitochondria. The enzyme is believed to be involved in the regulation of the rate of fatty acid oxidation (Norum 1966).

Acyl glycerophosphorylcholine acyltransferase, the enzyme which completes the synthesis of lecithin, has been demonstrated in human placenta by means of radioactive tracer experiments (Robertson & Sprecher 1966).

UDP-glucuronyltransferase with estriol as acceptor may be present in small amounts in placenta although the perfusion studies which provide the evidence for this possibility gave only a small yield of the estriol conjugates and the authors considered their identification of the reaction product only tentative (Troen *et al.* 1966).

Methionine adenosyltransferase, the enzyme which catalyses the synthesis of S-adenosylmethionine from ATP and methionine has been detected in extracts of human term placenta (Lindahl 1960).

Thiaminase catalysing a destruction of the vitamin by an unknown chemical reaction is present in human placenta (da Cunha & Azevedo 1956).

Aspartate aminotransferase and alanine aminotransferase (*glutamic-oxaloacetic and glutamic-pyruvic transaminases*) are both present in the human placenta at low levels of activity. The range of variation in activity from one placenta to another is wide and there is no difference in the activity of pathological as compared to normal placentas (da Cunha & Azevedo 1961; Stark & Oweiss 1963). Opinion is divided as to whether the elevated serum activity that appears during pregnancy originates from the placenta, but it seems likely that the enzymes are not released from the placenta into the bloodstream until active labor begins (Stark & Oweiss 1963; Meade & Rosalki 1963). Recombination of the purified placental aspartate aminotransferase apoenzyme with pyridoxal phosphate is inhibited by estrogen sulfates (Pulkkinen & Willman 1966).

Tyrosine aminotransferase is also present in the rat placenta at an activity of about one-tenth that of the maternal liver. The human placenta appears not to have been examined for the presence of the enzyme (Guettner & Goetze 1964).

Hexokinase activity capable of nonspecific conversion of a variety of hexoses into their 6-phosphates is present in the placentas of all species examined (human, monkey, rat and guinea-pig) but in contrast to the enzyme in most tissues this placenta enzyme did not phosphorylate fructuse (Walker *et al.* 1967). No evidence was obtained by these authors for the presence of a specific placental *glucokinase* in any of the species examined, although it has been reported that placenta slices respond to insulin addition *in vitro* with an increased rate of glucose uptake (Villee 1953) Insulin is said to be without effect on glucose metabolism in the sheep and goat placenta (Battaglia 1961).

Fructokinase, the enzyme which phosphorylates fructose to give fructose-6-phosphate, is present in homogenates of human term placenta and is competitively inhibited by glucose (Chieffi & Mangiarotti 1963b). Since the enzyme has not been purified, it cannot be stated with certainty that the observed reaction is not catalysed by hexokinase rather than a specific fructokinase, but because of the general similarity between the enzymes of the placenta and the liver, it seems reasonable to suppose that placenta does contain a specific fructokinase.

Phosphofructokinase activity has been detected in extracts of human placenta (Chieffi & Mangiorotti 1963a).

Glycerokinase could not be detected in rat placenta (Theil 1966).

NAD kinase at low levels of activity is present in the soluble fraction of human term placenta (Hagerman & Villee, unpublished).

Creatine kinase was described as being present in homogenates of human term placenta on the basis of the usual measurement of the reaction in the reverse (creatine producing) direction (Bastide *et al.* 1962).

Adenylate kinase is found in the microsomal fraction of human placenta homogenates and has a pH optimum of about 7·7. It is not affected by azide, is inhibited by citrate and activated by cysteine (Cerletti & Zichella 1960).

Phosphoglucomutase is present in the soluble fraction of human term placentas and is said to be more active in normal than in pathological placentas (Mangiarotti & Chieffi 1963; Ricciardi *et al.* 1963).

Ribonuclease (which is included among the transferases because of its catalysis of intramolecular transfer of phosphate during hydrolysis) is more active in the human placenta early in gestation than later (Brody 1953, 1957).

Aryl sulphotransferase (*sulfokinase*) is present in human and guinea-pig placenta because perfusion of these organs with any of the 3 classic estrogens, estrone, estradiol or estriol, gives rise to the corresponding sulphates (Levitz *et al.* 1960; Troen *et al.* 1962; Troen *et al.* 1966). Bovine placenta contains much more sulfokinase activity than is present in the human tissue. Since the bovine enzyme will sulfurylate dehydroepiandrosterone and testosterone as well as estrone the enzyme is either rather nonspecific or there are present both alkyl and aryl sulfokinases (Holcenberg & Rosen, 1965).

Carboxylesterase activity is present in small amounts in homogenates of blood free human term placenta as measured by the ability of these preparations to hydrolyze benzoylarginine ethyl ester (Bastide *et al.* 1963).

Lipase activity toward glycerol tributyrate can be detected in glycerol extracts of fresh human placenta at all stages of gestation. The activity is inhibited by sodium arsanilate and cocaine, but not by quinine or strychnine (Abe 1930). When triacetin or olive oil is the substrate the pH optimum is 7–7·5, and the enzyme activity is inhibited by heavy metal ions (Ogino 1956). Histochemical studies of the enzyme utilizing sorbitol esters of palmitic or stearic acid as substrate showed that the activity was present in the syncytiotrophoblast at all stages of gestation (Leonardi & Rigano 1960).

Lipoprotein lipase (‘*clearing factor lipase*’) activity is present in both rat and human placenta. In the rat the amount of activity in the placenta is similar to that in the rat heart and is considerably less than that in rat epididymal adipose tissue. The human placenta is less active than the rat placenta (Mallow & Alousi 1965).

Phospholipase A and Lysophospholipase are present in rat placenta acetone powders and homogenates respectively but at much lower levels of activity than in either maternal or fetal liver (Winkler 1964).

Acetylesterase activity is also present in human term placenta as evidenced by the capacity of the tissue to hydrolyze 19-*nor*-17α-ethynyl-17β-acetoxy-androst-4-en-3-one (norethindrone acetate) when the compound is incubated *in vitro* with homogenates of placenta (Betz & Warren 1963). Presumably this reaction is catalysed by a different enzyme than the lipase mentioned above or the acetylcholinesterase described below (Perrotta & Lewis 1958, Cedard *et al.* 1964).

Acetylcholinesterase is present in human placenta that has been carefully freed of blood (Navratil 1939, Perotta & Lewis 1958), and its presence is of special interest since the placenta is free of nerve elements (Torda 1942). The enzyme is a true cholinesterase, for Ord & Thompson (1950) showed that homogenates act upon both acetyl-β-methylcholine and acetylcholine but not upon benzoylcholine. The enzyme is inhibited by diisopropylphosphofluoridate, and the inhibition constants and kinetics are similar to those of the brain enzyme.

Alkaline phosphatase was studied in placenta breis by Busse as early as 1936. He used β-glycerophosphate as substrate and demonstrated an optimum for the activity at pH 9·4, with a secondary optimum at pH 5·4, which is probably the result of the presence of a second enzyme in the tissue. The enzyme is activated by magnesium and inhibited by cysteine. The enzyme is stable to acetone powder preparation and can be purified by alcohol precipitation. It is remarkably stable to heat denaturation, fully resisting treatment at 70°C for 30 minutes when heated in the presence of magnesium ion (Neale *et al.* 1965). The enzyme was reported to be present mainly in the soluble plus microsomal fraction of human placenta (Stark & Jung 1955) and was later localized in the microsomal fraction by Ahmed & King (1959). The activity of the enzyme is said to be lower in pathological placentas than in normal specimens (Humke 1963) and decreases rapidly in cases of postmaturity. However, Jeacock *et al.* (1963) found no difference in activity between placentas from normal and abnormal pregnancies except for a slight increase in the last few weeks of gestation in severe toxemia. These same authors describe a steady increase in the activity of the enzyme from the second month of gestation to term, and a similar increase is reported by Sharov (1963). The increased activity of alkaline phosphatase in the serum of pregnant women was said to be due to the appearance of electrophoretically distinguishable isozymes identical to those of the placenta (Boyer 1961), but this result was not confirmed in an independent investigation (Meade & Rosalki 1963). Further studies of the electrophoretic behavior of the human placenta enzyme indicate that the inheritance of the enzyme is under the control of 3 autosomal allelic genes that are inherited so as to give a typical Hardy-Weinburg population distribution of the 6 possible phenotypes (Robson & Harris 1965). The pattern of inheritance deduced from population studies was confirmed in a small number of cases of twins.

Ahmed & King (1960a) applied a standard procedure for the purification of the enzyme to placenta tissue and by making appropriate modifications were able to prepare an electrophoretically homogeneous material with a specific activity at least as high as the best preparations obtainable from other tissues. The maximal velocity for this preparation was similar for β-glycerophosphate and phenylphosphate, in contrast to the situation with the intestinal enzyme which hydrolyzes phenylphosphate more rapidly. The Michaelis constants of the placenta enzyme are also different from those of the intestinal enzyme. The pH optimum of the purified placenta enzyme is 10·2 when phenylphosphate is the substrate and 9·8 when β-glycerophosphate is used. The enzyme has an absorption maximum in the ultra-violet region at 278 mμ, it contains no carbohydrate, and amino acid analysis shows that proline, arginine and histidine are absent. Magnesium ion activates the enzyme, which hydrolyses a wide variety of monophosphates but not diethyl- or diphenylphosphate, inorganic metaphosphate or pyrophosphate. The enzyme is also activated less efficiently by cobalt and manganese ions, while nickel, calcium, cadmium, zinc and beryllium all inhibit. The enzyme is also inhibited by cyanide, iodide, arsenate, and formaldehyde (Ahmed & King 1960b). As is the case with many phosphatases, the placenta enzyme will catalyse group transfer as well as hydrolytic reactions (Georgatsos 1967).

Restudy of the possible clinical significance of the blood concentrations of the specific placental isozyme has given promising correlations (Messer 1967) but identification of the desired enzyme activity in blood is not a simple procedure even in the light of the detailed knowledge of the properties of the enzyme that is now available (Dymling 1966, Fishman *et al.* 1968).

Acid phosphatase is a soluble enzyme (Ahmed & King 1959, cf. Stark & Jung 1955) and decreases in activity as pregnancy advances (Jeacock *et al.* 1963). Ma & Chen (1965) demonstrated that the specific activity of both acid and alkaline phosphatases (units of enzyme activity per mg of protein nitrogen) is lower in hydatidiform mole than in normal placenta. DiPietro & Zengerle (1967) have shown that this activity is due to at least 3 distinct isozymes of molecular weight greater than 200,000, 105,000 and 35,000 respectively. The high molecular weight enzyme is probably lysosomal and is characterized by tartrate inhibition, while the 105,000 enzyme is more sensitive to *p*-chloromercuribenzoate. Both of these isozymes appear to be typical acid phosphatases. In contrast, the small enzyme does not rapidly hydrolyse customary phosphatase substrates, is stimulated by purines and is inhibited by pyridoxine-5-phosphate. The true substrate for the third isozyme probably has not yet been identified.

Glucose-6-phosphatase has recently been identified with pyrophosphatase activity in liver (Nordlie & Arion 1964, Arion & Nordlie 1964, Stetten 1964, Stetten & Taft 1964) and it may be assumed that the same is true for placenta although the assumption remains to be proved. The activity of a placental enzyme which will hydrolyse glucose-6-phosphate increases proportionally to the weight of the organ as gestation proceeds (Carter & Weber 1966). *Inorganic pyrophosphatase* activity is localized in the microsomal fraction of placenta homogenates (Cerletti & Zichella 1960) and is activated by magnesium and cysteine but inhibited by zinc, copper and mercury ions (Hsü 1958). The glucose-6-phosphatase activity is likewise present in the microsomal fraction of the tissue (Ahmed & King 1959) and its activity is reportedly higher in pathological placentas (Ricciardi *et al.* 1963). Since slices of human placenta do not secrete glucose into the incubation medium after the 14th week of pregnancy (Villee 1953) the physiologic role of this enzyme activity is debatable (cf. DiPietro *et al.* 1967, Walker *et al.* 1967). Such slices do, however, secrete small amounts of fructose even at term, and it has been suggested that this activity of the tissue may be due to this enzyme or another phosphatase acting non-specifically upon fructose-6-phosphate (Roux *et al.* 1959, Ritter & Leuthardt 1963).

Phosphodiesterase activity is present in human placenta, for as a result of the combined action of this enzyme and a phosphomonoesterase the tissue can hydrolyse *bis*-phenylphosphate and release inorganic phosphate (da Cunha 1937).

Deoxyribonuclease activity has been measured in placenta (Brody 1953).

Arylsulphatase activity in the placenta probably explains the conversion of estrone sulfate, estradiol sulfate and estriol sulfate to the corresponding free estrogens in perfusion experiments with human placenta (Mikhail *et al.* 1963, Diczfalusy *et al.* 1963, Haynes *et al.* 1964, Schwers & Govaerts-Videtzky 1964, Goebelsmann *et al.* 1966a, 1966b). These enzyme activities are present in the human placenta prior to the 10th week of gestation (Schwers & Rodesch 1964, Alonso & Troen 1966). It is unknown whether the enzyme or enzymes responsible for the hydrolysis of the estrogen sulfates are identical to those which catalyse the hydrolysis of 2-hydroxy-5-nitrocatechol sulfate and *p*-hydroxycatechol sulfate. A fraction which specifically splits the former of these synthetic substrates can be extracted from acetone powders of placenta, while the activity toward the latter compound remains in the residue after such an extraction. The soluble enzyme preparation with activity toward 2-hydroxy-5-nitrocatechol sulfate has a double pH optimum at pH 5·0 and 6·0, and these observations indicate the presence of at least 3 and perhaps more arylsulphatases in placenta (Gniot & Dzialoszynski 1964, Kuczynski *et al.* 1964). A partial separation of these activities has been reported (Gniot 1966). The enzyme responsible for the hydrolysis of estriol sulfate is found primarily in the microsomal fraction (Pulkkinen & Paunio 1963, French & Warren 1966). The activity could not be brought into solution but on the basis of kinetic properties, stability and pH optima it would appear that there are at least 3 different lipid-membrane bound enzymes present in the microsomal fraction (French & Warren 1967, Pasqualini *et al.* 1967). One of these is the aryl sulfatase which hydrolyses the 3-o-sulfates of the estrogens.

Rat placenta homogenates hydrolyse estrone sulfate at an appreciable rate, but do not attack estradiol 17-sulfate (Zuckerman & Hagerman unpublished).

Sterol sulfatase activity toward dehydroepiandrosterone sulfate has been detected in homogenates of human 20 week and term placentas

(Warren & Timberlake 1962, French & Warren 1965, Warren & French 1965), which confirms the observations of Pulkkinen (1961) with other 3β-hydroxysteroids. The latter author found that steroids with either the 5α-reduced or Δ^5-configuration can serve as substrates, and could find no 3α-hydroxysteroid sulfatase activity in placenta. The latter activity, as well as a steroid 21-sulfatase, has been detected in small amounts (Pasqualini *et al.* 1967). As in the rat, human placenta sulfatase does not act on estradiol-17β-sulfate (French & Warren 1966). Mid-gestation human placenta will also hydrolyse Δ^5-pregnenolone sulfate (Palmer *et al.* 1966). The reaction is very rapid (Pion *et al.* 1966). Presumably this enzyme (or enzymes) participates in the rapid conversion of dehydroepiandrosterone sulfate to estrogens in the pregnant woman (Baulieu & Dray 1963, Siiteri & MacDonald 1963). The enzyme is microsomal (Morato *et al.* 1965) and has a Michaelis constant for dehydroepiandrosterone sulfate of about 4×10^{-5} M (French & Warren 1965, 1967).

Lysozyme (or *muraminidase*) was shown to be present in the placenta in somewhat higher concentration early in pregnancy than at term (Prudden *et al.* 1949) and the enzyme has been purified from extracts of term placenta by Petit *et al.* (1963). Their purified preparations were homogeneous upon chromatography on carboxymethyl cellulose and had a molecular weight of 15,000. The amino acid composition of the enzyme was determined but sequence analysis has not yet been reported. The enzyme is clearly distinct in composition from those obtained from other organisms.

Glycoside hydrolases for a variety of di- and polysaccharides have been reported to be present in human placenta but the experiments upon which these results are based were unfortunately performed in such a way as to make the results inconclusive by modern standards of enzyme identification (Löb & Higuchi 1909, Maeda 1923, Dellapiane 1926, Abe 1931). Bulmer (1965) has presented histochemical evidence for the presence of β-galactosidase in rat placenta, and some experiments by Zoch (1965) again suggest that human placenta contains enzymes which can hydrolyse maltose, glycogen or starch directly to oligo- or monosaccharides.

β-Glucuronidase is active in human term placenta (Fishman & Anlyan 1947, Conte 1965) and from histochemical studies in the rat placenta, Bulmer (1962, 1965) concluded that the activity of the enzyme falls as gestation proceeds, there being more in the fetal placenta than in

the maternal placenta at all stages of gestation. It has been suggested that reversal of the hydrolytic reaction catalysed by this enzyme might be a significant route of formation of steroid and other conjugates with glucuronic acid, but the position of the equilibrium is such that this mechanism seems unlikely under physiologic conditions. Under special conditions *in vitro* it is possible to demonstrate glucuronosyl transfer reactions catalysed by the enzyme, and these experiments indicate that in the hydrolytic reaction the enzyme serves as a transferase with water as the acceptor. Estriol 3-glucosiduronate is not hydrolysed in perfusion experiments done at mid-pregnancy in the human (Goebelsmann *et al.* 1966a, 1966b), nor does term rat placenta hydrolyse estriol 16-glucosiduronate (Zuckerman & Hagerman unpublished).

Leucine aminopeptidase is present in both syncytiotrophoblast and cytotrophoblast in the human placenta (Kleiner *et al.* 1962) but in the rat placenta histochemical localization places the greatest degree of activity in the basal decidual cells (Hopsu *et al.* 1961). In the human the activity of the enzyme in serum increases as pregnancy advances, and it has been suggested that determinations of serum leucine aminopeptidase activity may be useful in the differential diagnosis between hydatidiform mole or choriocarcinoma and pregnancy after 25 weeks gestation (Lewis 1962), a hypothesis which assumes that the enzyme is normally released into the blood stream from the placenta and is decreased in amount in the diseased tissues (cf. Zsolnai *et al.* 1964). This enzyme activity persists in tissue culture, while histaminase gradually disappears (Ayavou *et al.* 1966).

Carboxypeptidase or protaminase activity is stated to be present in human placenta without citation of experimental details (Page & Glendenning 1955).

Glycyl-glycine, glycyl-leucine and glycyl-proline dipeptidase are present in human placenta (Vescia & Fidanza 1948, Zoch 1965).

Renin, the enzyme responsible for the conversion of angiotensinogen into angiotensin, was detected in the rabbit placenta with the aid of biological methods in amounts similar to those found in the nonpregnant uterus (Gross *et al.* 1964). Human amniotic fluid and umbilical cord blood also contain the activity and the placenta may provide the enzyme that appears in increased blood concentration during pregnancy (Brown *et al.* 1963, Brown *et al.* 1964).

Peptidase activities of a poorly defined character and acting upon a variety of substrates have also been described to be present in the placenta. Freinkel & Goodner (1960) described an enzyme in the soluble fraction of human placenta which degrades insulin, and Hooper (1960) achieved a solubilization of vasopressinase activity from the particulate fraction of placenta by the use of a cholate-trypsin treatment. Similarly, Page (1946) found that placenta contains an enzyme activity, presumably a peptidase, that destroys oxytocin, and the activity was localized to the soluble fraction of the tissue (Hooper & Jessup 1959). It is inhibited by di-isopropylphosphofluoridate (Hooper 1959). A protein with thromboplastic, and therefore enzymic, activity has been isolated from placenta and characterized as a lipoprotein (Chargaff 1945). The older references of Maeda (1923), Arinstein (1926) and Abe (1932) also presents the results of experiments on peptidases in placenta, from which it may be concluded that the tissues contain a considerable variety of these enzymes, none of which have been purified or adequately investigated by modern methods.

Glutaminase was demonstrated to be present in placenta by Luschinsky (1951), who found that crude homogenates of the tissue readily converted glutamine to ammonia and glutamic acid. The enzyme is activated by phosphate ion and has a pH optimum of 9. The activity of the enzyme falls to half its original value between 8 and 40 weeks gestation in the human.

Urease is not present in human placenta (Wehefritz & Gierhake 1928).

Arginase activity has been reported to be present in placenta (Maeda 1923, Wehefritz & Gierhake 1928, Tarantino & Pasquinelli 1947).

Guanase activity is present in homogenates of human term placenta but *adenine deaminase* activity is absent (Hayashi *et al.* 1964, Hayashi & Olmsted 1965, Hayashi 1965). *Adenosine deaminase* activity is present but *guanosine deaminase* is absent. The complex metabolic pathways of purine and pyrimidine bases, nucleosides and nucleotides in placenta should be investigated further with more highly purified enzyme preparations (cf. Mangoni *et al.* 1964).

Inorganic pyrophosphatase has already been considered under the heading *glucose-6-phosphatase*.

ATPase (yielding AMP and pyrophosphate) is found in the microsomal fraction of human placenta (Cerletti & Zichella 1960). Its pH optimum is 8·2 and the enzyme is activated by low concentrations of magnesium. The enzyme is said to be localized to the surface microvilli and the syncitial pinocytotic vesicles (Lister 1966).

Acylphosphatase activity has been reported to be present in placenta (Guerritore & Dellapiane 1955).

Nucleotide pyrophosphatase activity toward FAD is present in placenta as assayed by the disappearance of FAD upon incubation with saline extracts of placenta. Residual FAD was measured with *apo-d*-amino acid oxidase; the hydrolytic activity is maximal at pH 7·2 (Comline & Whatley 1948). This enzyme is probably responsible for the conversion of FAD to FMN investigated by Lust *et al.* (1954) as a possible mechanism for the placental transport of the vitamin.

Malonyl-CoA-decarboxylase was shown to be present in human placenta in investigations of malonate metabolism by the tissue, but the enzyme has not been characterized (Hoysoya & Kawada 1958).

Hydroxytryptophan decarboxylase activity is present in human placenta in small amounts and its concentration is not altered by toxemia of pregnancy (Klinge *et al.* 1964).

Sterol 20-22 *lyase* (*desmolase*) was solubilized by buffer extraction of an acetone powder of placenta mitochondria. The enzyme converts cholesterol to pregnenolone in the presence of NADPH and oxygen (Morrison *et al.* 1965, Ryan *et al.* 1966). It may be presumed that 20α,22-dihydroxycholesterol is an intermediate in the reaction, and partial purification of the enzyme confirms the earlier report of Solomon (1960) that cholesterol is converted to pregnenolone and progesterone by perfused human placenta.

Steroid 17-20 *lyase* (*desmolase*) activity is present in small amounts in the placenta, as demonstrated by the conversion of progesterone to androst-4-ene-3,17-dione found by Little *et al.* (1963) and by Warren & Cheatum (1964). (But cf. Sobrevilla *et al.* 1964.) *In situ* perfusion studies at midgestation showed no conversion of pregnenolone, 17-hydroxypregnenolone or progesterone to either C-19 or C-18 steroids (Pion *et al.* 1965, Jaffe *et al.* 1963), so that the metabolic pathway made possible by this enzyme appears to be a very minor one. This enzymatic differentiation of the tissue accounts for the net production of progesterone by placenta. The enzyme is also absent from the placentas of sheep, cow, horse, sow and rabbit (Ainsworth & Ryan 1966).

DOPA decarboxylase is not present in placenta (Page 1945).

Fumarase activity has been shown to be present in extracts of placenta, and its presence is confirmed by the known metabolic capabilities of the tissue (da Cunha & Jacobsohn 1936).

Aconitase is very active in soluble preparations from human term placenta but has not been purified from the tissue (Villee & Gordon 1955).

Histidine ammonia-lyase (*histidase*) is not present in placenta (Page & Glendenning 1955).

Tyrosine deiodinase was not detected in slices of human term placenta by Yamazaki *et al.* (1960), but more recently it was reported that incubation of homogenates of the tissue with thyroxine gave rise to iodine and 3,3′,5′-tri-iodothyronine (Louros *et al.* 1964).

Ribulose-5-phosphate epimerase and Ribose-5-phosphate isomerase are both confined to the soluble fraction of human term placenta, and together with other enzymes already described complete the system required for metabolism of glucose by way of the pentose phosphate or monophosphate shunt pathway (Chieffi *et al.* 1963b).

Steroid-Δ^5 *to* Δ^4*-isomerase* has been considered under the heading *hydroxysteroid dehydrogenases.*

Malonyl-CoA synthetase is an active enzyme in human placenta but it has not been extensively purified (Hosoya & Kawada 1958).

Steroid aromatizing system, capable of converting certain C-19 steroids to the corresponding phenolic estrogens, was shown to be present in placental slices by Meyer (1955), and the system was studied in some detail by Ryan (1959a, 1959b) and others (Gual *et al.* 1962, cf. Dorfman *et al.* 1962, Knuppen & Breuer 1963, Cedard *et al.* 1964). The complex is widespread in the animal kingdom, being present in the placentas of sheep, cow, horse and sow as well as in the human. It was not detectable in rabbit or guinea-pig placentas (Ainsworth & Ryan 1966), but the armadillo placenta will aromatize 16α-hydroxy-dehydroepiandrosterone to estriol (Brinck-Johnsen *et al.* 1967). The complex is confined to the microsomal fraction of the human term placenta but has not yet been brought into solution so that detailed dissection of the several reactions involved can be done. The substrate specificity of the system has been extensively examined. To be a substrate a steroid must be unsaturated in ring A or B of the steroid molecule, with Δ^4-unsaturation a customary requirement. (Dehydroepiandrosterone is aromatized *in vitro* but is almost certainly first oxidized to the Δ^4-3-ketone.) Androsta-5,7-diene-3β-ol-17-one gives rise to the corresponding estra-5,7,9-triene-3β-ol-17-one or -3β,17β-diol), a reaction which has organic mechanism implications as well as suggesting the pathway of equilin and equilenin synthesis. Hydroxy substitution of C-7 (α or β) does not prevent aromatization. Axial substituents at C-11 slow the reaction, and

19-nor compounds are slowly converted. The presence of rings C and D is required, although compounds with a 5-membered ring B are acted upon. Substitutions at 11α- or 9α- do not interfere with the activity of the enzyme, but C-21 hydroxysteroids are inert. The oxidized compounds 19-hydroxyandrostenedione, 19-hydroxydehydroepiandrosterone and 19-oxoandrostenedione, as well as 19-carboxyandrostenedione, are readily aromatized, 19-hydroxylated compounds being among the best substrates. The C-18 compounds 19-*nor*-testosterone and 19-*nor*-androstenedione are poor substrates (Hayano *et al.* 1960, Morato *et al.* 1961, Cedard *et al.* 1963, Varangot *et al.* 1965, Wilcox & Engel 1965b, dell'Acqua *et al.* 1965, Starka & Breuer 1966).

In the non-pregnant woman, dehydroepiandrosterone sulfate is not a precursor of estrogens but in pregnancy this ester is converted to estriol without entering the body pool of estrone plus estradiol (Siiteri & MacDonald 1963, Warren & Timberlake 1964, MacDonald & Siiteri 1965). When the sulfate, labelled in both the alcoholic and acid portions of the molecule, was incubated with microsomes from term placenta the ester proved to be a better precursor of estrone than either dehydroepiandrosterone itself or androstenedione (Morato *et al.* 1965). From the radioactivity ratios in the substrate and in dehydroepiandrosterone, androstenedione and estrone isolated from incubation mixtures, these same authors concluded that the most likely sequence of reactions was: dehydroepiandrosterone sulfate → 19-hydroxydehydroepiandrosterone sulfate → 19-hydroxydehydroepiandrosterone → 19-hydroxyandrostenedione → estrone.

The corresponding reaction in micro-organisms has been shown to proceed via the introduction of a double bond in ring A (Δ^1), but in the placental system the mechanism appears to involve a primary hydroxylation of the C-10 methyl group to give the 19-hydroxy compound (Longchampt *et al.* 1960, Morato *et al.* 1961, O'Kelly & Grant 1967). Since the 19-oxo derivative is a better substrate than the 19-hydroxy compound, Morato *et al.* concluded that it too is an intermediate. Experimentally, aromatization of testosterone, androstenedione or 19-hydroxyandrostenedione gives formaldehyde and formic acid (Breuer & Grill 1961, Axelrod *et al.* 1965), the former of these authors claiming that formaldehyde is the major product while the latter found chiefly formate. The 1-β-hydrogen is eliminated preferentially in the final step of aromatization (Morato *et al.* 1962, Townsley *et al.* 1966). Dorfman (1962) has concluded that there is a single enzyme responsible for the aromatization of both the 19-hydroxy and 19-oxo compounds. According to Hollander (1962) addition of the postulated intermediate, 19-hydroxyandrostenedione, inhibits the overall reaction but does not trap any radioactivity from labelled testosterone in the overall reaction, from which it was concluded that the 19-hydroxy compound is not an obligatory intermediate in the reaction. The kinetic studies of Wilcox & Engel (1965a) however, show clearly that the 19-hydroxy compound is an intermediate and that the initial hydroxylation is the rate limiting step in the overall sequence when androstenedione is the substrate. How the enzyme system achieves the aromatization of the 19-*nor* compounds is not at all clear if one accepts the postulate of a single enzyme complex for the whole of the aromatization sequence. The problem of determining the chemical mechanisms of the reactions will probably not be solved until the enzyme(s) have been brought into solution.

Aromatization by placental preparations is inhibited by SU 4885 (Metapyrone) which presumably reflects inhibition of the 19-hydroxylation (Giles & Griffiths 1964). Aromatization is accelerated by Clomid (Smith & Day 1963) and the mechanism of this effect appears to be an inhibition of the NADPH disposal systems present in the preparation (Hagerman, Smith & Day 1966).

The *in vitro* aromatization experiments done with cell-free preparations have been fully confirmed by *in vitro* and *in vivo* perfusion experiments (Cedard *et al.* 1963, Bolté *et al.* 1964a, 1964b, 1964c, 1964d). From the early experiments of Ryan (1959b) it was clear that estriol could be formed as a result of aromatization of precursors that had previously been 16-hydroxylated, and the more recent perfusion experiments have verified this conclusion. The results suggest that the large amounts of estriol produced in pregnancy are the result of 16-hydroxylation of neutral steroids in the fetus with subsequent placental aromatization, although direct 16-hydroxylation of estrone by the fetus has not been excluded. The major pathway appears to be from dehydroepiandrosterone sulfate through the corresponding 16α-hydroxy compound rather than via androst-5-ene-3β,16α,17β-triol. That is, the ring D ketols are preferred as substrates for aromatization over the vicinal glycols. The 17β-hydroxysteroid dehydrogenase does not readily accept 16-hydroxy compounds, so that the 2 pathways remain relatively distinct (Kirschner *et al.* 1966, Lamb *et al.* 1966, dell'Acqua *et al.* 1967a, 1967b). Despite some reports of estriol formation in placenta preparations, and despite the demonstrated capability of the placenta to hydroxylate progesterone

(Little *et al.* 1963), it is now clear that the placenta does not convert significant amounts of either estrone or estradiol to estriol by 16-hydroxylation.

Early in pregnancy the corpus luteum contributes substantially to estrogen synthesis (Wu *et al.* 1967) although the placenta appears to be competent to perform its part of the task from early in gestation (Cedard *et al.* 1966). At mid-pregnancy the fetal liver not only performs the hydroxylation vital to estriol synthesis but also has an inherent capability for both aromatization and interconversion of hydroxy and keto steroids (Benagiano *et al.* 1967). The entire subject of steroid metabolism in the fetoplacental unit has been reviewed (Diczfalusy *et al.* 1961, Zander 1963) and is discussed again elsewhere in this book.

Starka *et al.* (1965) have shown that the placenta of the horse can aromatize C-19 steroids but no equilin or equilenin was produced when Δ^4-steroids were used as substrates. Ring B unsaturated substrates give the unsaturated estrogens (Starka *et al.* 1966a). It may be inferred from the report of Vinson & Jones (1964) that the mouse placenta contains a steroid aromatizing system.

OTHER ENZYMES

Some mention of investigations of overall metabolic pathways in placenta is desirable (cf. Villee 1962). The early studies (Hellman *et al.* 1950) of oxygen consumption as a measure of total human placenta metabolism have been extended by a number of investigators (Villee 1953a, Friedman *et al.* 1962) and consistently show a gradual decline in oxygen consumption by tissue slices as the tissue ages. When considered in groups, the placentas from toxemic patients show a somewhat lower oxygen consumption but the difference is not sufficiently great to be seen in individual cases (Friedman *et al.* 1962). Experimentally induced toxemia also leads to a decrease in oxygen consumption in rat placentas (Goldstein *et al.* 1964). Placental mitochondria carry out oxidative phosphorylation (Villee & Hagerman 1961, Schreiner & Villee 1965), although the P/O ratios observed experimentally are rather low. The experimental work is complicated by the presence of an active ATPase. Careful measurements in the pregnant sheep show that a substantial portion of the oxygen consumed by the uterus and its contents is reduced by the placenta and fetal membranes (Campbell *et al.* 1966).

As already mentioned, the fact that placenta can convert glucose to lactic acid (Villee 1953) implies that all of the enzymes of the glycolytic pathway are present and those that have been studied in cell-free or purified preparations have been noted above. The early experiments have been confirmed by Hayakawa (1964) and by di Bella *et al.* (1966). Valuable comparative measurements of the activities of several enzymes have been reported by Danesino *et al.* (1961) and by Lapan & Friedman (1965). The human placenta appears to contain the enzymes required for the synthesis of hexosamines (Jozwik *et al.* (1967) and presumably the products of these reactions are utilized in the synthesis of chorionic gonadotrophin.

Measurements by Beaconsfield *et al.* (1964) (cf. Ginsburg & Jeacock 1964b) showed that human placenta contains an active 'shunt' or pentose-phosphate pathway of carbohydrate metabolism early in gestation and that its magnitude decreases as gestation proceeds. Whether the observed decrease is the *result* of decreased rates of biosynthesis, as the authors of this work conclude, or is the *cause* of decreased biosynthesis or is simply one of many time dependent variables observable in placental development cannot be settled until more information is available concerning the integrated mechanisms of control of placental metabolism. The addition of adrenaline to placenta slices increases the rate of lactate formation from glucose in both normal and diabetic placentas (Ginsburg & Jeacock 1964a, 1964c, 1966).

Protein synthesis occurs in human placenta (Dancis *et al.* 1957, Komine 1960, Joel *et al.* 1961, Sybulski & Tremblay 1967) and the rate of incorporation of glycine into placental protein decreases as gestation proceeds (Goetze *et al.* 1964, Mori 1965, Mori & Iso 1965). The addition of triiodothyronine to homogenates of human placenta is said to increase the rate of incorporation of amino acids into protein (Quinto *et al.* 1964). Matthaei & Schoeck (1967) have isolated the components of the synthesizing system (ribosomes, 'pH 5 enzymes', transfer RNA and supernatant factors) from human placenta. With these materials they have shown that 27 of the 64 codons are identical in the human and *E. coli*, with another 13 probably identical.

Very little is known about the enzymes of RNA and DNA synthesis in placenta (Joel *et al.* 1961, Beaconsfield *et al.* 1964), although an RNA fraction with template activity for protein synthesis has been isolated from placental nuclei (Silverstein & Bondy 1966).

Human term placenta contains all of the enzymes necessary for the synthesis of fatty acids and triglycerides (Roux & Villee 1960, Hosoya *et al.* 1960, Kleine 1967). Winkler (1963) has examined the incorporation of radioactive inorganic phosphate into placenta phospholipids. The specific activity of the various fractions decreases in the order lecithin, lysolecithin, and sphingomyelin. The rate of lecithin turnover increases 40-fold from gestational day 16 to 22 in the rat placenta which probably reflects vigorous synthesis of membranous portions of the cells, as does the rapid conversion of lysolecithin to lecithin and triglyceride (Eisenberg *et al.* 1967). Conversion of acetate to cholesterol has also been demonstrated both in perfused placenta (Levitz *et al.* 1962) and in tissue minces (van Leusden & Villee 1965). The reaction sequence in placenta appears to follow that known for other cholesterol synthesizing tissues (Zelewski & Villee 1966, Villee *et al.* 1966).

The placenta is commonly said to 'protect' the fetus, the implication of such a statement presumably being that the protection resides in the barrier aspect of the placenta which may restrain access of noxious substances to the placenta. Because of the great permeability of the organ such protection is not great. Recently, some biochemical aspects of possible placental protection have been discovered. Juchau *et al.* (1968) have demonstrated that smoking in pregnant women causes an apparent induction of placental enzymes capable of hydroxylation of 3,4-benzpyrene. These reactions are of the type that have been called detoxifying and might be postulated to be protective for the fetus.

Some miscellaneous reports on the composition of the placenta are of interest to the student of placental enzymes. The mouse placenta contains increasing amounts of 5-hydroxytryptamine as pregnancy advances (Robson & Senior 1964). The human placenta contains appreciable quantities of all classes of lipids containing both saturated and unsaturated fatty acids (Porcellate *et al.* 1959, Neil *et al.* 1961, Eberhagen 1963, Ichikawa & Yamada 1964), as well as a variety of organic acids (Hosoya *et al.* 1961). Both ethanolamine phosphate and choline phosphate have been isolated in appreciable amounts from goat placenta (Neil *et al.* 1961). These same compounds, in addition to glycerophosphoryl ethanolamine and glycerophosphoryl choline, have also been detected in human placenta (Porcellate *et al.* 1959). They presumably serve as precursors of the phospholipids and their biosynthetic intermediates identified by Nelson *et al.* (1967).

FETAL ENZYMES

By the time the embryos of most forms have grown to a size sufficient for enzyme investigations most of the processes of differentiation that result in the appearance of new enzyme activities have already taken place. As a result the changes that have been observed experimentally in fetal tissues as a function of gestational age are for the most part purely quantitative. This situation results primarily from the fact that a central core of enzymes is required for the maintenance of life in any type of cells. This core includes the energy producing systems of glycolysis, the tricarboxylic acid cycle and the triglyceride oxidizing complex, and the electron transmitter system coupled with oxidative phosphorylation. In a sense ancillary to these, but nonetheless essential to growth of the cell, are the synthetic systems for the manufacture of carbohydrate polymers, for lipids, for proteins, and for the nucleic acid information storage, transmission and translation devices. None of these enzymes would be expected to suddenly appear or disappear during normal development. (In the process of final specialization for function exceptions to this generalization may be found, as for example in erythrocytes and cornified epithelial cells.) The remaining enzymes, those responsible for the specialized functions of cells, might appear or disappear during embryonic development. If the function of these specialized cells is essential to the fetus, and if that function cannot be served by supplying or removing something from the fetal circulation via the transport capabilities of the placenta to the maternal circulation, then the placenta might be required to provide the enzyme capability in question. A very few possible examples of such substitution by placental enzymes for essential fetal functions are known.

Prior to about the 14th week of gestation in the human the placenta can secrete glucose while the fetal liver cannot; thereafter the placenta loses this ability while the fetal liver acquires it. These facts suggest that the placenta substitutes for the fetal liver in this function early in gestation (Villee 1953c). However, it is known that the placenta is rather freely permeable (by facilitated diffusion) to glucose at all stages of gestation (Hagerman & Villee 1960) so that there does not seem to be any real need for the placenta to secrete glucose at any time in fetal development. And in several species, liver glucose 6-phosphatase does not appear until the time of parturition (cf. Dawkins 1963), without correlation with the amount of this enzyme in the placenta.

Rat placenta contains transaminases with an activity about one tenth that of the maternal liver, while the fetal liver is still less active during gestation in this species (Guettner & Goetze 1964) and it might be suggested that here again the placenta is doing something for the fetus that it cannot do for itself. There seems to be no real reason to believe, however, that the maternal liver is not fully capable of performing all of the transamination required during growth of the fetus, with concurrent transport of the reaction products to the fetus via the blood.

Very early in gestation, prior to tissue and organ differentiation in the fetus, the situation is probably quite different and the trophoblast may well perform vital functions of nourishment for the fetal cells, but unfortunately no experimental evidence on this point is yet available. A useful discussion of recent investigations of the metabolism of fetal liver is available (Whipple & Sterling 1963).

PLACENTAL-FETAL RELATIONSHIPS

Possible substitution of placental enzymes for undeveloped capabilities of the fetus has been mentioned above and is an important although relatively unexplored part of this subject. The most important placental-fetal relationship is undoubtedly the establishment and maintenance of physical separation between the maternal and fetal portions of the organism. This separation is essential for immunologic reasons and may have other uses to both fetus and mother. To provide the immunologic separation the placenta must prevent the transfer of any appreciable amount of protein from mother to fetus or vice versa, while at the same time permitting ready access of the fetus to the maternal supply of nutrients. From this point of view, the older concept of the placenta as simply a semi-permeable membrane of large physical area has considerable utility, and the enzyme complement of the tissue represents merely the mechanism for the establishment and maintenance of the membrane. The consequences of failure of the barrier are well known to the clinician.

In addition the placenta has assumed various endocrinologic responsibilities in the course of evolution. It synthesizes and secretes chorionic gonadotrophin early in gestation in order to maintain the corpus luteum of pregnancy. It synthesizes another peptide hormone, placental lactogen, which has both lactogenic and somatotrophic hormone-like activities. Later in gestation it synthesizes and secretes progesterone which is an essential hormone for the maintenance of pregnancy (although the reasons for this essentiality remain obscure). In addition it utilizes C-19 steroids produced by both the mother and fetus for the production of prodigious amounts of estrogenic hormones which are found in the total organism at this time. Although the major portion of the estrogens made in pregnancy results from aromatization in the placenta of C-19 precursors supplied to the organ by both the mother and the fetus, it has recently been shown that the fetus alone can carry out this reaction, producing both estrone and estradiol from either androstenedione or testosterone (Mancuso *et al.* 1965). The fetal liver vigorously conjugates estrone and estradiol (Schwers *et al.* 1965, Zuckerman & Hagerman unpublished) and in addition can convert one or both of these estrogens to estriol (Engel *et al.* 1958, 1962). The fetal liver also conjugates estriol to form a sulfate and a sulfoglucosiduronate (Diczfalusy *et al.* 1964). The experiments of Emerman *et al.* (1965) show that estrone sulfate can be converted to estradiol sulfate without hydrolysis of the ester, a finding that implies that the 17β-hydroxysteroid dehydrogenase involved does not possess stringent structural specificity with regard to ring A of the molecule.

The distribution of the enzymes of steroid metabolism between the placenta and the fetus which defines the capabilities and interrelationships of the functional 'feto-placental unit' was examined in a group of internally consistent experiments under the same conditions by Jungmann & Schweppe (1967). A tabular summary of the locations of the physiologically most important of these enzymes is shown in Table 8.1. A consideration of the enzyme distribution and the blood concentrations of the steroids involved (Colás *et al.* 1964, Klausner & Ryan 1964, Magendantz & Ryan 1964, Simmer *et al.* 1964, Colás & Heinrichs 1965) leads to the conclusion that there is a complex steroid hormone relation-

TABLE 8·1

Relative feto-placental distribution of steroid metabolizing enzymes at mid-pregnancy

Enzyme	Placenta	Fetal Liver
Δ^5-3β-Hydroxysteroid dehydrogenase and Δ^5-isomerase	++	0
17α-Hydroxylase	0	+
C-21-Side-chain cleavage system	0	0
16α-Hydroxylase	0	+++
Aromatizing system	+++	+

The magnitude of enzyme activity indicated is an estimate of the probable physiologic importance of the enzyme. The major side-chain cleavage activity is in the fetal adrenal.

ship between mother, placenta and fetus that is discussed in detail elsewhere in this book (cf. Diczfalusy & Troen 1961, Diczfalusy *et al.* 1965).

Control of the rates of enzymic processes depends upon both the *amount* of the enzyme present in the cell and the *activity* of the enzyme (as a function of substrate concentration, presence of activators or inhibitors, pH, etc.) at a given time. Control of enzyme amount is a relatively slow process and proceeds via the genetic-protein synthesizing machinery, while effects of the environment of the enzyme upon its activity provides a means of rapid alterations in the rates of metabolic processes. The tissue distribution of enzymes already mentioned is an example of control via enzyme amount; recent experiments by Wiener & Allen (1967) show how activity of an enzyme might be controlled in the placenta. These authors found that concentrations of 20α-dihydroprogesterone similar to those present in the placenta significantly inhibited the conversion of pregnenolone to progesterone by the tissue. This observation could be an example of end-product (feedback) inhibition which might be important in the regulation of steroid biosynthesis. Many other such controls undoubtedly await discovery in the placenta.

PROBLEMS IN PLACENTAL ENZYMOLOGY

The first task of the enzymologist when he examines any tissue is to determine what enzymes are present. This portion of the enzymic investigation of the placenta is now well begun, although there are many known enzymes which have not been examined in the placenta. For example, the pathways for the synthesis of purines and pyrimidines and their conversion into polyphosphates have not been carefully examined in the placenta, and the whole class of ligases has been neglected. The next major problem for enzyme investigations of this tissue is the preparation and characterization of the enzymes known to exist in the placenta. This undertaking will be interesting in its own right as an exercise in pure enzymology but the comparative, mechanistic, physiologic and pathologic information to be gained from such studies should not be overlooked. Some instances in which seeming changes in enzymic activity are specifically associated with pathologic processes have already been mentioned; another example may be seen in the biochemical studies of diabetic placentas (Hagerman 1964, Ginsburg & Jeacock 1966). Unfortunately, none of this work has progressed to the point where the information available is very useful to the clinician.

After the chemistry of the isolated and purified components of the tissue has been defined, the task of resynthesis of this information to give a complete understanding of the functioning of the intact cell arises. It is becoming increasingly clear that the microscopic organization of the interior of the cell is vitally important both in controlling the direction of chemical pathways and in the regulation of the rates of such reactions. Such organization is most clearly seen thus far in the electron transmitter system and in the organization of the ribosome for protein synthesis, but it would seem unlikely that even the enzymes which experimentally are found in the cytosol, or 'soluble fraction', by most procedures actually exist in the cell in a simple homogeneous single phase solution. Instead, these enzymes may be constrained by the gel properties of the cell in such a way that substrates can progress in an orderly fashion through the metabolic pathways such as those of glycolysis. New techniques of examination of cellular structure, perhaps involving histochemical examination at the electron microscopic level of resolution, will be required to examine this hypothesis.

Another major task is to delineate the enzymic characteristics of the very early embryo and of its placenta. Here the primary need is for improved microtechniques of tissue preparation and enzyme assay. Perhaps the methods of tissue culture of specific cell lines will be useful in this regard (cf. Soma *et al.* 1961, Starka *et al.* 1966b; etc.). When the data are available, the rewards should be great in advancing an understanding of the process of differentiation. And when the basic outline of the course of events has been laid out, it may then be possible to investigate with the same tools the mechanisms which control this poorly understood process. Of special interest in this connection is the clinical problem of choriocarcinoma. A detailed biochemical study of the failure of growth control in an organ which early in gestation grows at a very rapid pace and then quite suddenly ceases growth and is discarded might provide a critical test case for the validity of the currently widely discussed suggestion of a virus etiology of carcinoma.

REFERENCES

ABE M. (1930) Investigation of placental ferments in various stages of pregnancy. *Jap. J. Obst. Gynecol.* **13**, 301.

ABE M. (1931) Investigation of placental ferments in various stages of pregnancy. *Jap. J. Obst. Gynecol.* **14**, 514.

ABE M. (1932) Investigation of placental ferments in various stages of pregnancy. *Jap. J. Obst. Gynecol.* **15**, 44.

ADAMS J.A., JARABAK J. & TALALAY P. (1962) The steroid specificity of the 17β-hydroxysteroid dehydrogenase of human placenta. *J. Biol. Chem.* **237**, 3069.

ADAMS J.A., JACOBSON H.I., LEVY H.R. & TALALAY P. (1965) The estrogenic activity and enzymatic oxidation of 17β-estradiol-17αD. *Steroids*, Suppl. **1**, 75.

AHMED Z. & KING E.J. (1959) Placental phosphatases. *Biochim. Biophys. Acta*, **34**, 313.

AHMED Z. & KING E.J. (1960a) Purification of placental alkaline phosphatase. *Biochim. Biophys. Acta*, **40**, 320.

AHMED Z. & KING E.J. (1960b) Kinetics of placental alkaline phosphatase. *Biochim. Biophys. Acta*, **45**, 581.

AHMED Z. & REIS J.L. (1958) The activation and inhibition of 5-nucleotidase. *Biochem. J.* **69**, 386.

AINSWORTH L. & RYAN K.J. (1966) Steroid hormone transformation by endocrine organs from pregnant mammals. I. Estrogen biosynthesis by mammalian placental preparations *in vitro*. *Endocrinology*, **79**, 875.

ALONSO C. & TROEN P. (1966) Perfusion studies of the human placenta. V. Metabolism of ^{3}H-estrone-^{35}S-sulfate and ^{14}C-estradiol-17β at mid-pregnancy. *Biochemistry*, **5**, 337.

ARINSTEIN B. (1926) On proteolytic enzymes of the placenta. *Biochem. Zeitschr.* **171**, 15.

ARION W.J. & NORDLIE R.C. (1964) Liver microsomal glucose 6-phosphatase, inorganic pyrophosphatase, and pyrophosphate-glucose phosphotransferase. *J. Biol. Chem.* **239**, 2753.

AXELROD L.R., MATTHIJSSEN C., RAO P.N. & GOLDZIEHER J.W. (1965) The fate of carbon-19 in the course of estrogen biosynthesis from testosterone-19-^{14}C. *Acta endocrinol.* **48**, 383.

AYAVOU T., BAYLET J.C., CHAPON J.P., FLANDRE O. & ERISTOL P. (1966) On some enzyme activities of early placenta cultures. *Compt. Rend. Soc. Biol.* **160**, 148.

BAILLIE A.H., CAMERON E.H.D., GRIFFITHS K. & HART D.M. (1965) 3β-Hydroxysteroid dehydrogenase in the adrenal gland and placenta. *J. Endocrinol.* **31**, 227.

BASTIDE P., DASTUGUE G., BAUDON J. & MEUNIER S. (1962) Activity of creatine phosphokinase in the human placenta and the blood of the mother and the newborn. *Compt. Rend. Soc. Biol.* **156**, 1296.

BASTIDE P., MEUNIER S. & DASTUGUE G. (1963) Benzoylarginine ethyl esterase and carbamoyltransferase activities in the placenta, maternal blood, and blood of the newborn. *Ann. Biol. Clin. (Paris)*, **21**, 265.

BATTAGLIA F.C., MESCHIA G., BLECHER J. & BARRON D.H. (1961) Effect of insulin and poisons on glucose uptake of sheep and goat placenta. *Am. J. Physiol.* **200**, 64.

BAULIEU E.E. & DRAY F. (1963) Conversion of ^{3}H-dehydroepiandrosterone sulfate to ^{3}H-estrogens in normal pregnant women. *J. Clin. Endocrinol. Metab.* **23**, 1298.

BAULIEU E.E., WALLACE E. & LIEBERMAN S. (1963) The conversion *invitro* of Δ^{5}-androstene-3β,17βdiol-17α-H^{3} to testosterone-17α-H^{3} by human adrenal and placental tissue. *J. Biol. Chem.* **238**, 1316.

BEACONSFIELD P., GINSBURG J. & JEACOCK M.K. (1964) Glucose metabolism via the pentose phosphate pathway relative to nucleic acid and protein synthesis in the human placenta. *Developmental Med. Child. Neurol.* **6**, 469.

BENAGIANO G., KINCL F.A., ZIELSKE F., WIQVIST N. & DICZFALUSY E. (1967) Studies on the metabolism of C-19 steroids in the human foeto-placental unit. 2. Metabolism of androstenedione and testosterone in the intact foeto-placental unit. *Acta endocrinol.* **56**, 203.

BERLINER D.L. & SALHANICK H.A. (1956) The presence of 6β-hydroxylase in human placenta. *J. clin. Endocrinol.* **16**, 903.

BETZ G. & WARREN J.C. (1963) Hydrolysis of norethindrone acetate by fetal and placental tissue. *New Eng. J. Med.* **268**, 1171.

BETZ G. & WARREN J.C. (1965) Studies with glucose-6-phosphate dehydrogenase from human placenta. *Acta endocrinol.* **49**, 47.

BLOCH E. & NEWMAN E. (1966) Comparative placental steroid synthesis. I. Conversion of 7-^{3}H-dehydroepiandrosterone to ^{3}H-androst-4-ene-3,17-dione. *Endocrinology*, **79**, 524.

BOLTÉ E., MANCUSO S., ERIKSSON G., WIQVIST N. & DICZFALUSY E. (1964a) Studies on the aromatization of neutral steroids in pregnant women. 1. Aromatization of C-19 steroids by placentas perfused *in situ*. *Acta endocrinol.* **45**, 535.

BOLTÉ E., MANCUSO S., ERIKSSON G., WIQVIST N. & DICZFALUSY E. (1964b) Studies on the aromatization of neutral steroids in pregnant women. 2. Aromatization of dehydroepiandrosterone and of its sulfate administered simultaneously into a uterine artery. *Acta endocrinol.* **45**, 560.

BOLTÉ E., MANCUSO S., ERIKSSON G., WIQVIST N. & DICZFALUSY E. (1964c) Studies on the aromatization of neutral steroids in pregnant women. 3. Overall aromatization of dehydroepiandrosterone circulating in the fetal and maternal compartments. *Acta endocrinol.* **45**, 576.

BOLTÉ E., MANCUSO S., ERIKSSON G., WIQVIST N. & DICZFALUSY E. (1964d) Conversion of testosterone-17α-^{3}H into 17β-estradiol-17α-^{3}H by human placentas perfused *in situ*. *Steroids*, **4**, 613.

BOSS J.H. & CRAIG J.M. (1962) Histochemical distribution patterns of oxidative enzymes in the human placenta. *Obst. Gynecol.* **20**, 572.

BOYER S.H. (1961) Alkaline phosphatase in human sera and placentae. *Science*, **134**, 1002.

BREUER H. & GRILL P. (1961) Formation of formaldehyde in the aromatization of neutral steroids to phenolic steroids. *Zeitschr. f. Physiol. Chem.* **324**, 254.

BRINCK-JOHNSEN T., BENIRSCHKE K. & BRINCK-JOHNSEN K. (1967) Hormonal steroids in the armadillo, *Dasypus novemcinctus*. I. Oestriol in pregnancy and its *in vitro* biosynthesis by the placenta. *Acta endocrinol.* **56**, 675.

BRITTON H.G., HUGGETT A.ST.G. & NIXON D.A. (1967) Carbohydrate metabolism in the sheep placenta. *Biochim. Biophys. Acta*, **136**, 426.

BRODY S. (1953) Studies on ribonuclease and deoxyribonuclease activities in homogenates from human placenta. *Acta Chem. Scand.* **7**, 721.

BRODY S. (1957) Ribonuclease activity and cellular growth. *Biochim. Biophys. Acta*, **24**, 503.

BROWN J.J., DAVIES D.L., DOAK P.B., LEVER A.F. & ROBERTSON J.I.S. (1963) Plasma renin in normal pregnancy. *Lancet*, ii, 900.

BROWN J.J., DAVIES D.L., DOAK P.B., LEVER A.F., ROBERTSON J.I.S. & TREE M. (1964) The presence of renin in human amniotic fluid. *Lancet*, ii, 64.

BULL G., HEBB C. & RATKOVIC C. (1961) Choline acetylase in the human placenta at different stages of development. *Nature*, **190**, 1202.

BULL G., FEINSTEIN A. & MORRIS D. (1964) Sedimentation behaviour and molecular weight of choline acetyl transferase. *Nature*, **201**, 1326.

BULMER D. (1962) β-Glucuronidase in the rat placenta. *Nature*, **195**, 805.

BULMER D. (1965) Histochemical studies on glycosidases of the rat ovary and placenta. *J. Histochem. Cytochem.* **13**, 396.

BUSSE O. (1936) Studies of the metabolism of human placenta. *Zeitschr. f. Physiol. Chem.* **242**, 271.

CAGNAZZO G., MISURALE F., ROX A. & MONTESSORI G. (1962) Chromatographic analysis of the pregnene-derived steroids in extracts of human placenta. In *Biological and Clinical Aspects of Placental Steroidogenesis*, p. 50. F.Polvani & A.Bompiani, eds. S.Karger AG, Basel.

CAMPBELL A.G., DAWES G.S., FISHMAN A.P., HYMAN A.I. & JAMES G.B. (1966) The oxygen consumption of the placenta and foetal membranes in the sheep. *J. Physiol.* **182**, 439.

CARTER J.E. & WEBER G. (1966) Glucose-6-phosphatase-like activity in the human placenta, fetal liver, and decidual tissue. *Am. J. Obst. Gynecol.* **95**, 914.

CEDARD L., FILLMANN B., KNUPPEN R., LISBOA B.P. & BREUER H. (1964) Metabolism and aromatization of 7-substituted C-19 steroids in the placenta. *Zeitschr. f. Physiol. Chem.* **338**, 89.

CEDARD L. & KNUPPEN R. (1965) 6α-Hydroxylation in human placenta perfusion. *Steroids*, **6**, 307.

CEDARD L., VARANGOT J. & YANNOTTI S. (1962) Biosynthesis of estriol by the human placenta perfused *in vitro*, etc. *Compt. Rend. Acad. Sci. (Paris)*, **254**, 3896.

CEDARD L., VARANGOT J. & YANNOTTI S. (1963) Biosynthesis of estrogens in human placentas perfused *in vitro*. *Compt. Rend. Soc. Biol.* **257**, 2725.

CEDARD L., VARANGOT J. & YANNOTTI S. (1966) Biosynthesis of estrogens in the human placentas perfused *in vitro*. Influence of age of pregnancy. *Compt. Rend. Acad. Sci. (Paris)*, **262**, 379.

CEDARD L., YANNOTTI S. & VARANGOT J. (1961) Perfusion of the placenta *in vitro* applied to a study of the biosynthesis of the estrogens. *Compt. Rend. Soc. Bio.* **155**, 458.

CERLETTI P. & ZICHELLA L. (1960) Adenylate kinase of human placenta. *Clin. Chim. Acta*, **5**, 748.

CHARGAFF E. (1945) The isolation of preparations of thromboplastic protein from human organs. *J. biol. Chem.* **161**, 389.

CHIEFFI O. & MANGIAROTTI M. (1962) Evaluation of transaldolase and transketolase, and the process of nonoxidative heptose formation in the human placenta at full term and in that of the rat at various periods of pregnancy. *Riv. Obstet. Ginecol.* **17**, 645.

CHIEFFI O. & MANGIAROTTI M.A. (1963a) Fructose phosphorylation in multi-enzymatic preparations of human placenta. *Riv. Ostet. Ginecol.* **18**, 239.

CHIEFFI O. & MANGIAROTTI M.A. (1963b) Metabolism of glucose and fructose in the human placenta. *Riv. Ostet. Ginecol.* **18**, 615.

CHIEFFI O., MANGIAROTTI M.A., VALLERINO V. & GUASTALLA L. (1963a) Activity of glucose 6-phosphate dehydrogenase and 6-phosphogluconic acid dehydrogenase in the human placenta. *Boll. Soc. Ital. Biol. Sper.* **39**, 443.

CHIEFFI O., MANGIAROTTI M.A., VALLERINO V. & MONTIXI S. (1963b) On the presence of the enzymes phosphoketopentose epimerase and phosphopentose isomerase in extracts of human placenta. *Boll. Soc. Ital. Biol. Sper.* **39**, 445.

CHRISTIE G.A. (1968) Distribution of hydroxysteroid dehydrogenases in the placenta of the pig. *J. Endocrinol.* **40**, 285.

COLÁS A. & HEINRICHS W.L. (1965) Petenkofer chromogens in the maternal and fetal circulations: anencephalic pregnancies, cesarean sections, and tentative identification of 3β,17β-dihydroxyandrost-5-ene-16-one in umbilical cord blood. *Steroids*, **5**, 753.

COLÁS A., HEINRICHS W.L. & TATUM H.J. (1964) Petenkofer chromogens in the maternal and fetal circulations: detection of 3β,16α-dihydroxy-androst-5-ene-17-one in umbilical cord blood. *Steroids*, **3**, 417.

COMLINE R.S. & WHATLEY F.R. (1948) Inactivation of FAD by tissue extracts. *Nature*, **161**, 350.

CONTE D. (1965) Preliminary observations on the behavior of β-glucuronidase in the chorionic villus of the placenta in the first and second half of pregnancy. *Boll. Soc. Ital. Biol. Sper.* **41**, 1585.

CRIST R.D. & WARREN J.C. (1966) Transhydrogenation in the human placenta. *Acta endocrinol.* **53**, 205.

CURZEN P. (1964) Variations in the enzyme histochemistry of the placenta. *J. Obstet. Gynaec. Brit. Comm.* **71**, 388.

DA CUNHA D.P. (1937) Research on placenta enzymes, phosphoesterase. *Compt. Rend. Soc. Biol.* **124**, 1023.

DA CUNHA D.P. & AZEVEDO M.D. (1956) On the thiaminase of placenta. *Compt. Rend. Soc. Biol.* **149**, 1833.

DA CUNHA D.P. & AZEVEDO M.D. (1961) On the presence of transaminase in the placenta. *Compt. Rend. Soc. Biol.* **155**, 207.

DA CUNHA D.P. & JACOBSOHN K.P. (1936) Investigations of placenta enzymes: fumarase. *Compt. Rend. Soc. Biol.* **123**, 609.

DAHM K. & BREUER H. (1966) Biogenesis of estriol-16α-monoglucuronide and estriol-17β-monoglucuronide. *Acta endocrinol.* **52**, 43.

DANCIS J., BRAVERMAN N. & LIND J. (1957) Plasma protein synthesis in the human fetus and placenta. *J. clin. Invest.* **36**, 398.

DANESINO V., ADINOLFI G. & BUDILLON G. (1961) Enzymatic activities for the metabolism of carbohydrate in the human placenta. *Arch. Obstet. Gynec. (Naples)*, **68**, 1.

DAWKINS J.J.R. (1963) Glycogen synthesis and breakdown in fetal and newborn rat liver. *Ann. N.Y. Sci.* **111**, 203.

DEANE H.W. & RUBIN B.L. (1965) Identification and control of cells that synthesize steroid hormones in the adrenal glands, gonads, and placentae of various mammalian species. *Arch. Anat. Micr. Morph. Exptl.* **54**, 49.

DEANE H.W., RUBIN B.L., DRICKS E.C., LOBEL B.L. & LEIPSNER G. (1962) Trophoblastic giant cells in placentas of rats and mice and their probable role in steroid hormone production. *Endocrinology*, **70**, 407.

DELLAPIANE G. (1926) The enzyme reactions attributed to the placenta in the metabolism of carbohydrate. *Boll. Soc. Ital. Biol. Sper.* **1**, 431.

DELL'ACQUA S., MANCUSO S., ERIKSSON G., RUSE J.L., SOLOMON S. & DICZFALUSY E. (1967b) Studies on the aromatization of neutral steroids in pregnant women. 6. Aromatization of 16α-hydroxylated C-19 steroids by mid-term placentas perfused *in situ*. *Acta endocrinol.* **55**, 401.

DELL'ACQUA S., MANCUSO S., ERIKSSON E., WIQVIST N. & DICZFALUSY E. (1965) Estrogen formation from 19-*nor*-testosterone and testosterone following *in situ* perfusion of human placenta at mid-term. *Acta endocrinol.* **50** (Suppl. 100), 81.

DELL'ACQUA S., MANCUSO S., WIQVIST N., RUSE J.L., SOLOMON S. & DICZFALUSY E. (1967a) Studies on the aromatization of neutral steroids in pregnant women. 5. Metabolism of androst-5-ene-3β,16α,17β-triol in the intact foeto-placental unit at mid-pregnancy. *Acta endocrinol.* **55**, 389.

DE MARIA F. (1964) Placental monoamine oxidase in normal and toxemic patients *Am. J. Obst. Gynecol.* **88**, 490.

DIBELLA S., REVELLI E., PANAZZOLO A. & SCARPA F. (1966) Anaerobic glycolytic activity of the human placenta. *Boll. Soc. Ital. Biol. Sper.* **42**, 1794.

DICZFALUSY E., BARR M. & LIND J. (1964) Estriol metabolism in an anencephalic monster. *Acta endocrinol.* **46**, 511.

DICZFALUSY E., CASSMER O., ALONSO C. & DE MIQUEL M. (1961) Estrogen metabolism in the human fetus and newborn. *Recent Progress Hormone Research*, **17**, 147.

DICZFALUSY E., PION R. & SCHWERS J. (1965) Steroid biogenesis and metabolism in the human feto-placental unit at mid-pregnancy. *Arch. Anat. Micr. Morph. Exptl.* **54**, 67.

DICZFALUSY E., TILLINGER K.G., WIQVIST N., LEVITZ M., CONDON G.P. & DANCIS J. (1963) Disposition of intra-amniotically administered oestriol-C^{14}-sulphate and oestradiol-C^{14}-sulphate in women. *J. Clin. Endocrinol.* **23**, 503.

DICZFALUSY E. & TROEN P. (1961) Endocrine functions of the human placenta. *Vitamins and Hormones*, **19**, 229.

DIPIETRO D.L., GUTIERREZ-CORREA J. & THAIDIGSMAN J.H. (1967) Glucose metabolism by human placental villi. *Biochem. J.* **103**, 246.

DIPIETRO D.L. & ZENGERLE F.S. (1967) Separation and properties of three acid phosphatases from human placenta. *J. Biol. Chem.* **242**, 3391.

DIXON M. & WEBB E.C. (1964) *Enzymes.* 2nd edition. Academic Press, New York.

DIXON R. & PENNINGTON G.W. (1965) The isolation and biosynthesis of highly polar steroids found in placental tissue. *Experientia*, **21**, 298.

DOLLEFELD E. & BREUER H. (1966) Demonstration of estradiol: NAD-17α,17β-oxidoreductases in the cytoplasm fraction of horse placenta. *Biochim. Biophys. Acta*, **124**, 187.

DORFMAN R.I., GUAL C., MORATO T., HAYANO M. & GUT M. (1962) Estrogen synthesis by the human placenta. In *Biological and Clinical Aspects of Placental Steroidogenesis*, p. 68. F.Polvani & A.Bompiani, eds. S.Karger AG, Basel.

DYMLING J.F. (1966) Separation of serum and placental alkaline phosphatase by agarose gel electrophoresis and sephadex chromatography. *Scand. J. Clin. Lab. Invest.* **18**, 129.

EBERHAGEN D. (1963) On the lipids of the human placenta. *Zeitschr. f. Physiol. Chem.* **333**, 179.

EISENBERG S., STEIN Y. & STEIN O. (1967) The role of placenta in lysolecithin metabolism in rats and mice. *Biochim. Biophys. Acta*, **137**, 115.

EMERMAN S., DANCIS J., LEVITZ M., WIQVIST N. & DICZFALUSY E. (1965) Metabolism of estrone-6,7-^{3}H-sulfate-^{35}S in the perfused human fetus. *J. Clin. Endocrinol. Metab.* **25**, 639.

ENGEL L.L., BAGGETT B. & HALLA M. (1958) The formation of ^{14}C-labelled estriol from 16-^{14}C-labelled-estradiol-17β by human fetal liver slices. *Biochim. Biophys. Acta*, **30**, 435.

ENGEL L.L., BAGGETT B. & HALLA M. (1962) *In vitro* metabolism of estradiol-17β by human fetal liver: formation of estriol, 16-epiestriol, estrone and an estriol glucosiduronic acid. *Endocrinol.* **70**, 907.

EWALD W., WERBIN H. & CHAIKOFF I.L. (1964) Δ^{5}-3-Ketosteroid isomerase. *Steroids*, **3**, 505.

FERGUSON M.M. & CHRISTIE G.A. (1967) Distribution of hydroxysteroid dehydrogenases in the placenta and fetal membranes of various mammals. *J. Endocrinol.* **38**, 291.

FISHMAN J. & DIXON D. (1967) Hydroxylation of estradiol by human placental microsomes. *Biochemistry*, **6**, 1683.

FISHMAN W.H. & ANLYAN A.J. (1947) β-Glucuronidase activity in human tissues. *Cancer Research*, **7**, 808.

FISHMAN W.H., INGLIS N.R. & GHOSH N.K. (1968) Distinctions between intestinal and placental isoenzymes of alkaline phosphatase. *Clin. Chim. Acta*, **19**, 71.

FONDA E. & PEYRE A. (1965) Localization of Δ^{5}-3β-hydroxysteroid dehydrogenase in the placenta of *Chiroptera* during pregnancy. *Compt. Rend. Acad. Sci.* (*Paris*), **261**, 2963.

FREINKEL N. & GOODNER C.J. (1960) The metabolism of insulin by human placental tissue. *Steroids*, **6**, 865.

FRENCH A.P. & WARREN J.C. (1966) Sulfatase activity in the human placenta. *Steroids*, **8**, 79.

FRENCH A.P. & WARREN J.C. (1967) Properties of steroid sulphatase and arylsulphatase activities of human placenta. *Biochem. J.* **105**, 233.

FRIEDMAN E.A., LITTLE W.A. & SACHTLEBEN M.R. (1962) Placental oxygen consumption *in vitro*. *Am. J. Obst. Gynecol.* **84**, 561.

GALIL A.K. & DEANE H.W. (1966) Δ^{5}-3β-hydroxysteroid dehydrogenase activity in the steroid-hormone producing organs of the ferret (*Mustela putorius furo*). *J. Reprod. Fertil.* **11**, 333.

GAULL G., HAGERMAN D.D. & VILLEE C.A. (1960) Preparation and properties of glutamic dehydrogenase from human placenta. *Biochim. Biophys. Acta*, **40**, 552.

GEORGATSOS J.G. (1967) Specificity and phosphotransferase activity of purified placental alkaline phosphatase. *Arch. Biochem.* **121**, 619.

GILES C. & GRIFFITHS K. (1964) Inhibition of the aromatizing activity of human placenta by SU 4885. *J. Endocrinol.* **28**, 343.

GINSBURG J. & JEACOCK M.K. (1964a) The placental barrier. In *Absorption and Distribution of Drugs, Symp.*, p. 86. T.B.Binns, ed. Livingstone, Edinburgh.

GINSBURG J. & JEACOCK M.K. (1964b) Pathways of glucose metabolism in human placental tissue. *Biochim. Biophys. Acta*, **90**, 166.

GINSBURG J. & JEACOCK M.K. (1964c) Effect of adrenaline on human placental lactate production *in vitro*. *Am. J. Obst. Gynecol.* **90**, 794.

GINSBURG J. & JEACOCK M.K. (1966) Some aspects of placental carbohydrate metabolism in human diabetes. *J. Obstet. Gynaec. Brit. Comm.* **73**, 452.

GNIOT-SZULZYCKA J. & DZIALOSZYNSKI L.M. (1964) Aryl sulfatases of human placenta. *Clin. Chim. Acta*, **9**, 334.

GNIOT-SZULZYCKA J. & DZIALOSZYNSKI L.M. (1966) Some properties of human placental soluble arylsulphatases. *Acta Biochim. Pol.* **13**, 171.

GOEBELSMANN U., ERIKSSON G., DICZFALUSY E., LEVITZ M. & CONDON G.P. (1966b) Fate of oestriol-3-sulphate and oestriol-16-glucosiduronate in the intact foeto-placental unit at mid-pregnancy. *Acta endocrinol.* **53**, 391.

GOEBELSMANN U., WIQVIST N., DICZFALUSY E., LEVITZ M., CONDON G.P. & DANCIS J. (1966a) Fate of intra-amniotically administered estriol-15-^{3}H-3-sulphate and estriol-16-^{14}C-16-glucosiduronate in pregnant women at midterm. *Acta endocrinol.* **52**, 550.

GOETZE T., FRANKE H., GOETZE E. & MAAK B. (1964) *In vitro* incorporation of glycine-1-C^{14} in maternal and fetal liver and placenta proteins. *Acta Biol. Med. Germ.* **12**, 259.

GOLDSTEIN H.B., HOCKSTEIN P. & MCKAY D.G. (1964) Tissue metabolism in experimental toxemia of pregnancy. *Am. J. Obstet. Gynecol.* **88**, 791.

GROSS F., SCHAECHTELIN G., ZEIGLER M. & BERGER M. (1964) A renin-like substance in the placenta and uterus of the rabbit. *Lancet*, i, 914.

GUAL C., MORATO T., HAYANO M., GUT M. & DORFMAN R.I. (1962) Biosynthesis of estrogens. *Endocrinol.* **71**, 920.

GUERRITORE A. & DELLAPIANE G. (1955) The acetylphosphatase activity of the human placenta. *Boll. Soc. Ital. Biol. Sper.* **31**, 636.

GUETTNER J. & GOETZE T. (1964) Tyrosine-α-ketoglutaric acid transaminase in placenta, liver and kidney of pregnant rats and in the fetal liver under normal and pathological conditions. *Acta Biol. Med. Ger.* **12**, 297.

HAFEZ E.S.F. (1964) Uterine and placental enzymes. A review. *Acta endocrinol.* **46**, 217.

HAGERMAN D.D. (1964) Enzymatic capabilities of the placenta. Federation Proceedings, **23**, 785.

HAGERMAN D.D. (1966) Monomer-trimer polymerization of human placenta estradiol dehydrogenase. *Federation Proceedings*, **25**, 281.

HAGERMAN D.D., SMITH O.W. & DAY C.F. (1966) Mechanism of the stimulatory effect of clomid on aromatization of steroids *in vitro*. *Acta endocrinol.* **51**, 591.

HAGERMAN D.D. & VILLEE C.A. (1959) Separation of human placental estrogen-sensitive transhydrogenase from estradiol-17β dehydrogenase. *J. Biol. Chem.* **234**, 2031.

HAGERMAN D.D. & VILLEE C.A. (1960) Transport functions of the placenta. *Physiol. Rev.* **40**, 313.

HAGERMAN D.D. & VILLEE C.A. (1961) A mechanism of action for estrogenic steroid hormones. In *Mechanism of Steroid Hormone Actions*, p. 178. C.A.Villee & L.L. Engel, eds. Pergamon, Oxford.

HAGERMAN D.D. & VILLEE C.A. (1965) Kinetics of pyridine nucleotide transhydrogenation by human placenta. *Biochem. J.* **95**, 150.

HAGERMAN D.D. & WELLINGTON F.M. (1959) Serum lactic dehydrogenase activity during pregnancy and in the newborn. *Am. J. Obst. Gynecol.* **77**, 348.

HAGOPIAN M., PINCUS G., CARLO J. & ROMANOFF E.B. (1956) Isolation of an unknown substance and 6-ketoprogesterone from perfusates of human placenta. *Endocrinol.* **58**, 387.

HAWKINS D.F. & WHYLEY G.A. (1966) The nature of the lactate dehydrogenase isoenzymes in human placenta and related tissues. *Clin. Chim. Acta*, **13**, 713.

HAYAKAWA S. (1964) Studies on carbohydrate metabolism in chorionic villi of the human placenta. *Tohoku J. Exptl. Med.* **83**, 81.

HAYANO M., LONGCHAMPT J.E., KELLY W., GUAL C. & DORFMAN R.I. (1960) Studies on the biosynthesis of estrogens by human placental microsomes. *Acta endocrinol.* **33** (Suppl. 50), 699.

HAYASHI T.T. (1965) Studies on placental metabolism. 2. Purine nucleotide catabolism in early placenta. *Am. J. Obst. Gynecol.* **93**, 266.

HAYASHI T.T., BALDRIDGE R.C., OLMSTED P.S. & KIMMEL D.L. (1964) Purine nucleotide catabolism in placenta. *Am. J. Obst. Gynecol.* **88**, 471.

HAYASHI T.T. & OLMSTED P.S. (1965) Studies on placental metabolism. 3. Pyrimidine nucleotide catabolism in human placenta. *Am. J. Obst. Gynecol.* **91**, 711.

HAYNES R.C., MIKHAIL G., ERIKSSON G., WIQVIST N. & DICZFALUSY E. (1964) Oestradiol metabolism in the previable human foetus and in the foeto-placental unit. *Acta endocrinol.* **45**, 297.

HEBB C.O. & RATKOVIC D. (1962) Choline acetylase in the placenta of man and other species. *J. Physiol.* **163**, 307.

HECKER E. & FARTHOFER-BOECKH G. (1963) On the metabolism and mechanism of action of estrogens. *Biochem. Zeitsch.* **338**, 628.

HELLMAN L.M., HARRIS B.A. & ANDREWS M.C. (1950) Oxygen consumption of human placenta *in vitro*. *Bull. Johns Hopkins Hosp.* **87**, 203.

HEMSWORTH B.A. & MORRIS D. (1964) A comparison of the N-alkyl group specificity of choline acetyl transferase from different species. *J. Neurochem.* **11**, 793.

HOLCENBERG J.S. & ROSEN S.W. (1965) Enzymatic sulfation of steroids by bovine tissues. *Arch. Biochem.* **110**, 551.

HOLLANDER N. (1962) The conversion of radioactive testosterone to estrogen by placental microsomes in the presence of other steroids. In *Biological and Clinical Aspects of Placental Steroidogenesis*, p. 78. F.Polvani & A.Bompiani, eds. S.Karger AG, Basel.

HOOPER K.C. (1959) The action of inhibitors on placental oxytocinase and vasopressinase. *J. Physiol.* **148**, 283.

HOOPER K.C. (1960) Preparation of soluble vasopressinase from human placenta. *Biochem. J.* **74**, 297.

HOOPER K.C. & JESSUP D.C. (1959) The distribution of enzymes destroying oxytocin and vasopressin. *J. Physiol.* **148**, 283.

HOPSU V.K., RUPONEN S. & TALANTI S. (1961) Leucine aminopeptidase in the placenta of the rat. *Acta Histochemica*, **12**, 305.

HOSOYA N., HAGERMAN D. & VILLEE C.A. (1960) Stimulation of fatty acid synthesis by oestradiol *in vitro*. *Biochem. J.* **76**, 297.

HOSOYA N. & KAWADA N. (1958) Malonate metabolism in human placenta. *J. Biochem.* (*Tokyo*), **45**, 363.

HOSOYA N., KAWADA N., MORIUCHI S. & YOSSHIOKA M. (1961) Organic acids in human placenta. *Iagku to Seibutsugaku*, **61**, 29.

HOWARD P.D. (1968) Progesterone metabolism in ovary, placenta and uterus and regulation of progesterone function. Thesis. Washington University, Saint Louis, Missouri.

HSÜ C.H. (1958) Pyrophosphatase of placenta. *J. Formosan Med. Assoc.* **57**, 736.

HUMKE W. (1963) Alkaline phosphatase in human placenta. *Gynaecologia*, **155**, 400.

ICHIKAWA S. & YAMADA J. (1964) Polyunsaturated fatty acids in rat placenta. *Bull. Univ. Osaka* (*Series B*), **15**, 181.

JAFFE R.B. & LEDGER W.J. (1966) *In vivo* steroid biogenesis and metabolism in the human term placenta. I. *In situ* placental perfusion with isotopic pregnenolone. *Steroids*, **8**, 61.

JAFFE R., PION R., ERIKSSON G., WIQVIST N. & DICZFALUSY E. (1963) Studies on the aromatization of neutral steroids in pregnant women. 4. Lack of estrogen formation from progesterone. *Acta endocrinol.* **48**, 413.

JAMES H.P., ELLIOTT H.W. & PAGE E.W. (1948) Oxygen uptake of human placental tissue as affected by selected substrates and drugs. *Proc. Soc. Exptl. Biol. Med.* **67**, 130.

JARABAK J., ADAMS J.A., WILLIAMS-ASHMAN H.G. & TALALAY P. (1962) Purification of a 17β-hydroxysteroid dehydrogenase of human placenta and studies on its transhydrogenase function. *J. Biol. Chem.* **237**, 345.

JEACOCK M.K., MORRISS N.F. & PLESTER J.A. (1963) The activity of alkaline and acid phosphatases in the human placenta. *J. Obst. Gynaecol. Brit. Comm.* **70**, 267.

JOEL P.B., HAGERMAN D.D. & VILLEE C.A. (1961) Effects of estradiol added *in vitro* on the metabolism of human placenta. *J. Biol. Chem.* **236**, 3151.

JOZWIK M., GLOWACKA D. & POPOWICZ J. (1967) Hexosamine synthesis in human placenta *in vitro*. *Am. J. Obst. Gynecol.* **99**, 258.

JUCHAU M.R., NISWANDER K.R. & YAFFEE S.J. (1968) Drug metabolizing systems in homogenates of human immature placentas. *Am. J. Obst. Gynecol.* **100**, 348.

JUNGMANN A. & SCHWEPPE J.S. (1967) Biosynthesis and metabolism of neutral steroids by human mid-term placenta and fetal liver. *J. Clin. Endocrinol.* **27**, 1151.

KAPELLER-ADLER R. (1965) Recent attempts at the purification and identification of human placental 'histaminase'. *Clin. Chim. Acta*, **11**, 191.

KARAVOLAS H.J. & ENGEL L.L. (1966) Human placental 17β-estradiol dehydrogenase. 3. The separation of a 17β-estradiol-dependent transhydrogenase. *J. Biol. Chem.* **241**, 3454.

KAWAHARA F.S., WANG S.F. & TALALAY P. (1962) The preparation and properties of crystalline Δ^5-3-ketosteroid isomerase. *J. Biol. Chem.* **237**, 1500.

KELLOGG D.A. & GLENNER G.S. (1960) Histochemical localization of human term placenta 17β-estradiol dehydrogenases. *Nature*, **187**, 763.

KIRSCHNER M.A., WIQVIST N. & DICZFALUSY E. (1966) Studies on oestriol synthesis from dehydroepiandrosterone sulphate in human pregnancy. *Acta endocrinol.* **53**, 584.

KITCHIN J.D., PION R.J. & CONRAD S. (1967) Metabolism of progesterone by the term placenta perfused *in situ. Steroids*, **9**, 263.

KLAUSNER D.A. & RYAN K.J. (1964) Estriol secretion by the human term placenta. *J. Clin. Endocrinol. Metab.* **24**, 101.

KLEINE U. (1967) Studies on the lipid metabolism of villi of mature human placentas. *Clin. Chim. Acta*, **17**, 95.

KLEINER H., WILKIN P. & SNOECK J. (1962) Localization of the steroid dehydrogenases and the leucine aminopeptidase in the human placenta. *Geburtshilfe Frauenheilkunde*, **22**, 986.

KLINGE E., PENTTILÄ O. & TISSORI A. (1964) The content of 5-hydroxytryptamine in human uterus and placental tissue, and their 5-hydroxytryptophan decarboxylase and monoamine oxidase activities in normal and toxemic pregnancies. *Acta Obstet. Gynec. Scand.* **43**, 107.

KNUPPEN R. & BREUER H. (1963) Biogenesis of oestratetraenol by human placenta. *Acta endocrinol.* **42**, 129.

KOIDE S.S. & MITSUDO S.M. (1965) Histochemical study of 3β- and 17β-hydroxysteroid dehydrogenases in human term placenta. *Endocrinology*, **76**, 403.

KOIDE S.S. & TORRES M.T. (1965) Distribution of 3β-hydroxysteroid dehydrogenase and Δ^5-3-oxosteroid isomerase in homogenate fractions of human term placenta. *Biochim. Biophys. Acta*, **105**, 115.

KOIDE S.S. & TORRES M.T. (1966) Isolation of 3-oxosteroid Δ^4-Δ^5-isomerase of human term placenta. *Biochim. Biophys. Acta*, **122**, 151.

KOMINE S. (1960) The biosynthesis of serum proteins in human placenta. *J. Jap. Biochem. Soc.* **32**, 290.

KUCZYNSKI J., PYDZIK T. & WENCLEWSKI A. (1964) Aryl sulfatase activity in fetal liver and brain and in the placenta. *Ginekol. Polska*, **35**, 373.

KYANK H. (1958) The enzymes in the normal and toxemic placenta. *Gynaecologica*, **145**, 222.

LAMB E., MANCUSO S., DELL'ACQUA S., WIQVIST N. & DICZFALUSY E. (1967) Studies on the metabolism of C-19 steroids in the human foeto-placental unit. I. Neutral metabolites formed from dehydroepiandrosterone and dehydroepiandrosterone sulphate by the placenta at mid-pregnancy. *Acta endocrinol.* **55**, 263.

LANGER L.J. & ENGEL L.L. (1958) Human placental estradiol-17β dehydrogenase. I. *J. Biol. Chem.* **233**, 583.

LANGER L.J., ALEXANDER J.A. & ENGEL L.L. (1959) Human placental estradiol-17β dehydrogenase. II. *J. Biol. Chem.* **234**, 2609.

LAPAN B. & FRIEDMAN M.M. (1965) Tissue enzymes in gestation: comparative activities in the placenta and fetal membranes. *Am. J. Obst. Gynecol.* **93**, 1157.

LEONARDI R. & RIGANO A. (1960) On the lipase activity of the placenta. *Arch. Ostet. Ginec.* **65**, 669.

LEVITZ M., CONDON G.P., MONEY W.L. & DANCIS J. (1960) The relative transfer of estrogens and their sulfates across the guinea-pig placenta: sulfurylation of estrogens by the placenta. *J. biol. Chem.* **235**, 973.

LEVITZ M., EMERMAN S. & DANCIS J. (1962) Sterol synthesis in the perfused placenta. In *Biological and Clinical Aspects of Placental Steroidogenesis*, p. 4. F.Polvani & A.Bompiani, eds. S.Karger AG, Basel.

LEWIS J., Jnr. (1962) Serum leucine aminopeptidase values in patients with trophoblastic tumours and in normal pregnancy. *Am. J. Obst. Gynecol.* **84**, 1407.

LINDAHL K.M. (1960) *In vitro* studies on histamine metabolism in placenta. *Archiv. Kemi*, **16**, 1.

LINDBERG S. (1963) ^{14}C-Histamine inactivation *in vitro* by human myometrial and placental tissues. *Acta Obstet. Gynec. Scand.* **43** (Suppl. 1), 26.

LINDBERG S. & WESTLING H. (1962) Placental monoamine oxidase and toxaemia of pregnancy. *Lancet*, ii, 46.

LISTER U.M. (1966) Ultrastructure of the placenta in hypertensive states. The localization of enzymes hydrolyzing adenosine triphosphate in placentae from normal and toxaemic pregnancies. *J. Obstet. Gynaec. Brit. Comm.* **73**, 439.

LITTLE B., DIMARTINIS J. & NYHOLM B. (1959) Conversion of progesterone to Δ^4-pregnene-20α-ol-3-one by human placenta *in vitro*. *Acta endocrinol.* **30**, 530.

LITTLE B. & SHAW A. (1961) Conversion of progesterone to 17α-hydroxyprogesterone by human placenta *in vitro*. *Acta endocrinol.* **36**, 455.

LITTLE B., SHAW A. & PURDY R. (1963) Conversion of progesterone to 16α-hydroxyprogesterone and Δ^4-androstenedione by human placenta *in vitro*. *Acta endocrinol.* **43**, 510.

LÖB W. & HIGUCHI S. (1909) On the knowledge of placental enzymes. *Biochem Zeitschr.* **22**, 316.

LOBEL B.L., DEANE H.W. & ROMNEY S.L. (1962) Enzymic histochemistry of the villous portion of the human placenta from six weeks of gestation to term. *Am. J. Obst. Gynecol.* **83**, 295.

LOKE K.H. (1964) Metabolism of testosterone by human placenta. *Abst. 6th Intl. Congr. Biochem., I.U.B.* **32**, 584.

LONGCHAMPT J.E., GUAL C., EHRENSTEIN M. & DORFMAN R.I. (1960) 19-Hydroxyandrostenedione, an intermediate in estrogen biosynthesis. *Endocrinol.* **66**, 416.

LOUROS N., MIRAS C. & VRETTOS A. (1964) Deiodination *in vitro* of thyroxine by human placenta. *Ann. Endocrinol. (Paris)*, **25**, 417.

LUCIS O.J. (1965) Biological methylation of estrogens by tissues from human genital tract. *Steroids*, **5**, 163.

LUSCHINSKY H.L. (1951) The activity of glutaminase in the human placenta. *Arch. Biochem.* **31**, 132.

LUSCHINSKY H.L. & SINGHER H.O. (1948) Identification and assay of monamine oxidase in the human placenta. *Arch. Biochem.* **19**, 95.

LUST J., HAGERMAN D.D. & VILLEE C.A. (1954) The transport of riboflavin by human placenta. *J. Clin. Invest.* **33**, 38.

MA L. & CHEN M.C.C. (1965) Phosphatases in tissues of hydatidiform mole and normal placenta. *Clin. Chim. Acta*, **12**, 153.

MACDONALD P.C. & SIITERI P.K. (1965) Origin of estrogen in women pregnant with an anencephalic fetus. *J. Clin. Invest.* **44**, 465.

MAEDA K. (1923) On the enzymes in the placenta. *Biochem. Zeitschr.* **143**, 347.

MAGENDANTZ H.G. & RYAN K.J. (1964) Isolation of an estriol precursor, 16α-hydroxydehydroepiandrosterone from human umbilical cord sera. *J. Clin. Endocrinol.* **24**, 1155.

MALLOW S. & ALOUSI A.A. (1965) Lipoprotein lipase activity of rat and human placenta. *Proc. Soc. Exper. Biol. Med.* **119**, 301.

MANCUSO S., DELL'ACQUA S., ERIKSSON G., WIQVIST N. & DICZFALUSY E. (1965) Aromatization of androstenedione and testosterone by the human fetus. *Steroids*, **5**, 183.

MANGIAROTTI M.A. & CHIEFFI O. (1963) Activity of phosphoglucomutase in the human placenta at term. *Boll. Soc. Ital. Biol. Sper.* **39**, 1652.

MANGONI C., MAGRI E., PALMIERI A., MANZI A. & SCARANO E. (1964) Deoxycytidylic aminohydrolase activity in human placenta tissue. *Boll. Soc. Ital. Biol. Sper.* **40**, 1596.

MARUYAMA K. (1955) Dephosphorylation of adenylic acid by rat placenta homogenate. *J. Fac. Sci. Tokyo (Sect. IV)*, **7**, 411.

MATTHAEI J.H. & SCHOECK G.K. (1967) Human gene expression. I. An aminoacyl-RNA binding system from human placenta. *Biochem. Biophys. Res. Commun.* **27**, 638.

MEADE B.W. & ROSALKI S.B. (1963) The origin of increased maternal serum enzyme activity in pregnancy and labour. *J. Obst. Gynaecol. Brit. Comm.* **70**, 862.

MEIGS R.A. & ENGEL L.L. (1961) The metabolism of adrenocortical steroids by human tissues. *Endocrinology*, **69**, 152.

MESSER R.H. (1967) Heat-stable alkaline phosphatase as an index of placental function. *Am. J. Obst. Gynecol.* **98**, 459.

MEYER A.S. (1955) Conversion of 19-hydroxy-Δ^4-androstene-3,17-dione to estrone by endocrine tissue. *Biochim. Biophys. Acta*, **17**, 441.

MIKHAIL G., WIQVIST N. & DICZFALUSY E. (1963) Oestriol metabolism in the human foeto-placental unit. *Acta endocrinol.* **43**, 213.

MITSUDO S.M. & KOIDE S.S. (1966) Histochemical demonstration of the hydroxysteroid oxidoreductases in the umbilical cord and membranes of human term and immature placenta. *Endocrinology*, **78**, 333.

MORATO T., HAYANO M., DORFMAN R.I. & AXELROD L.R. (1961) The intermediate steps in the biosynthesis of estrogens from androgens. *Biochem. Biophys. Res. Commun.* **6**, 334.

MORATO T., LEMUS A.E. & GUAL C. (1965) Efficiency of dehydroepiandrosterone sulfate as an estrogen precursor. *Steroids* (Suppl. I), 59.

MORATO T., RAAB K., BRODIE H.J., HAYANO M. & DORFMAN R.I. (1962) The mechanism of estrogen biosynthesis. *J. Am. Chem. Soc.* **84**, 3764.

MORI M. (1965) Study of protein biosynthesis in fetus and placenta. 1. Incorporation of ^{14}C-amino acids into the human placenta. *Am. J. Obst. Gynecol.* **93**, 1164.

MORI M. & ISO H. (1965) Study of protein biosynthesis in fetus and placenta. 2. Transfer of ^{35}S-methionine across the placenta and mechanism of protein biosynthesis in the fetus. *Am. J. Obst. Gynecol.* **93**, 1172.

MORRIS D. (1966) The choline acetyltransferase of human placenta. *Biochem. J.* **98**, 754.

MORRISON G., MEIGS R.A. & RYAN K.J. (1965) Biosynthesis of progesterone by the human placenta. *Steroids* (Suppl. 2), 177.

NAVRATIL E. (1939) Does the human placenta contain cholinesterase? *Klin. Wochenschr.* **18**, 963.

NEALE F.C., CLUBB J.S., HOTCHKISS D. & POSEN S. (1965) Heat stability of human placental alkaline phosphatase. *J. Clin. Path.* **18**, 359.

NEIL M.W., WALKER D.G. & WARREN F.L. (1961) The occurrence of phosphorylcholine and phosphorylethanolamine in goat placenta. *Biochem. J.* **80**, 187.

NELSON G.H., KENIMER B.K. & JONES A.E. (1967) Thin-layer chromatography of placental phospholipids. *Am. J. Obst. Gynecol.* **99**, 262.

NISSELBAUM J.S. & BODANSKY O. (1961a) Purification and properties of human heart lactic dehydrogenase. *J. Biol. Chem.* **236**, 323.

NISSELBAUM J.S. & BODANSKY O. (1961b) Reactions of human tissue lactic dehydrogenases with antisera to human heart and liver lactic dehydrogenases. *J. Biol. Chem.* **236**, 401.

NISSELBAUM J.S. & BODANSKY O. (1963) Purification, kinetic and immunochemical studies of the major variants of lactic dehydrogenase from human liver, hepatoma, and erythrocytes; comparison with the major variant of human heart lactic dehydrogenase. *J. Biol. Chem.* **238**, 969.

NISSELBAUM J.S., PACKER D.E. & BODANSKY O. (1964) Comparison of the actions of human brain, liver and heart lactic dehydrogenase variants on nucleotide analogues and on substrate analogues in the absence and in the presence of oxalate and oxamate. *J. Biol. Chem.* **239**, 2830.

NISSIM J.A. & ROBSON J.M. (1952) The conversion of pregnenolone to a more active progestational substance by incubation with endocrine tissue *in vitro*. *J. Endocrinol.* **8**, 329.

NORDLIE R.C. & ARION W.J. (1964) Evidence for the common identity of glucose-6-phosphatase, inorganic pyrophosphatase, and pyrophosphate-glucose phosphotransferase. *J. Biol. Chem.* **239**, 1680.

NORUM K.R. (1966) The organ and the subcellular distribution of palmityl-CoA: carnitine palmityltransferase in man. *Acta Physiol. Scand.* **66**, 172.

OGINO W. (1956) Studies on the fermentative action of the villous tissue of human placenta. *Naika Hôkan*, **3**, 863 (cf. *Chem. Abst.* **53**, 9411 f., 1959).

O'KELLY D.A. & GRANT J.K. (1967) Formation of 3β,19-dihydroxyandrost-5-en-17-one and its sulphate by human placenta *in vitro*. *Europ. J. Steroids*, **2**, 209

ORD M.G. & THOMPSON R.H.S. (1950) Nature of placental cholinesterase. *Nature*, **165**, 927.

OSINSKI P.A. (1960) Steroid 11β-ol-dehydrogenase in human placenta. *Nature*, **187**, 777.

PADYKULA H.A. (1958) A histochemical and quantitative summary of enzymes of the rat's placenta. *J. Anat.* **92**, 118.

PAGE E.W. (1945) DOPA decarboxylase activity of human and animal tissues. *Arch. Biochem. Biophys.* **8**, 145.

PAGE E.W. (1946) The value of plasma pitocinase determinations in obstetrics. *Am. J. Obst. Gynecol.* **52**, 1014.

PAGE E.W. & GLENDENNING M.B. (1955) Enzymes of the human placenta. In *Gestation*, p. 225. L.B. Flexner, ed. Josiah Macy, Jnr., Foundation, New York.

PALMER R., BLAIR J.A., ERIKSSON G. & DICZFALUSY E. (1966) Studies on the metabolism of C-21 steroids in the human foeto-placental unit. 3. Metabolism of progesterone and 20α- and 20β-dihydroprogesterone by mid-term placentas perfused *in situ*. *Acta endocrinol.* **53**, 407.

PALMER R., ERIKSSON G., WIQVIST N. & DICZFALUSY E. (1966) Studies on the metabolism of C-21 steroids in the human foeto-placental unit. 2. Metabolism of pregnenolone sulphate by mid-term placentas perfused *in situ*. *Acta endocrinol.* **52**, 598.

PASQUALINI J.R., CEDARD L., NGUYEN B.L. & ALSATT E. (1967) Differences in the activity of human term placenta sulphatases for steroid ester sulphates. *Biochim. Biophys. Acta*, **139**, 177.

PEARLMAN W.H., CERCEO E. & THOMAS M. (1954) Conversion of Δ^5-pregnenolone into progesterone by homogenates of human placental tissue. *J. Biol. Chem.* **208**, 231.

PERROTTA A. & LEWIS P.R. (1958) A histochemical study of placental esterases in the guinea-pig and in the human. *J. Anat.* **92**, 110.

PETERSON D.M. & WARREN J.C. (1966) Effect of steroids and cofactors on the activity and stability of human placental glutamate dehydrogenase. *Acta endocrinol.* **51**, 599.

PETIT J.F., PANIGEL M. & JOLLES P. (1963) Purification and analysis of lysozyme extracted from human placenta. *Bull. Soc. Chim. Biol.* **45**, 211.

PION R.J., CONRAD S.H. & WOLF B.J. (1966) Pregnenolone sulfate–an efficient precursor for the placental production of progesterone. *J. Clin. Endocrinol.* **26**, 225.

PION R.J., JAFFE R., ERIKSSON G., WIQVIST N. & DICZFALUSY E. (1965) Studies on the metabolism of C-21 steroids in the human feto-placental unit. I. Perfusion with pregnenolone and 17α-hydroxypregnenolone. *Acta endocrinol.* **48**, 234.

PORCELLATE G., CURTI B. & LUCIANI S. (1959) Presence of phosphorous precursors of the phospholipids in human placenta. *Rev. Espanola Fisiol.* **15**, 139.

PRUDDEN J.F., LANE N. & LEVISON J. (1949) Lysozyme titres. *Proc. Soc. Exptl. Biol. Med.* **72**, 220.

PULKKINEN M.O. (1961) Arylsulfatase and hydrolysis of some steroid sulphates in the developing organism and placenta. *Acta Physiol. Scand.* **52**, Suppl. 180.

PULKKINEN M.O. & PAUNIO I. (1963) Hydrolysis of aromatic steroid sulfates during pregnancy. *Ann. Med. Exptl. Biol. Fenn.* **41**, 283.

PULKKINEN M.O. & WILLMAN K. (1966) *In vitro* regulation of human placental aspartate aminotransferase by sulfate esters of estrogens. *Steroids*, **8**, 51.

PULKKINEN M.O. & WILLMAN K. (1967) Human placental steroid-dependent pyridine nucleotide transhydrogenase. *Acta Obstet. Gynec. Scand.* **46**, 494.

PURDY R.H., HALLA M. & LITTLE B. (1964) 20α-Hydroxysteroid dehydrogenase activity a function of human placental 17β-hydroxysteroid dehydrogenase. *Biochim. Biophys. Acta*, **89**, 557.

QUINTO P., ORLANDI C. & SEGATA L. (1964) Effect of hormones on the incorporation of radioactive amino acids in homogenates of term human placenta. *Boll. Soc. Ital. Biol. Sper.* **40**, 1903.

RECOMMENDATIONS 1964 OF THE INTERNATIONAL UNION OF BIOCHEMISTRY. *Enzyme Nomenclature*. Elsevier, New York.

REIS J. (1937) Activity of 5-nucleotidase in animal and human tissues. *Enzymologia*, **2**, 183.

Report of the Commission on Enzymes of the International Union of Biochemistry (1961). Pergamon Press, Oxford.

RICCIARDI I., SALLUSTO A. & MALATO M. (1963) Adenosine tri-phosphatase, phosphoglucomutase and glucose 6-phosphatase activities in the human placenta. *Arch. Obstet. Ginecol.* **68**, 35.

RITTER P. & LEUTHARDT F. (1963) Formation of fructose and sorbitol from glucose in the human placenta. *Helv. Physiol. Pharmacol. Acta*, **21**, 212.

ROBERTSON A. & SPRECHER H. (1966) Human placental lipid metabolism. I. Synthesis of phosphatidylcholine from lysophosphatidylcholine. *Pediatrics*, **38**, 1028.

ROBSON E.B. & HARRIS H. (1965) Genetics of the alkaline phosphatase polymorphism in the human placenta. *Nature*, **207**, 1257.

ROBSON J.M. & SENIOR J.B. (1964) The 5-hydroxytryptamine content of the placenta and foetus during pregnancy in mice. *Brit. J. Pharmacol.* **22**, 380.

ROUX J.F., HAGERMAN D.D. & VILLEE C.A. (1959) Studies of the mechanism of fructose production by human placenta. *J. Physiol.* **146**, 98.

ROUX J.F. & VILLEE C.A. (1960) Effects of anoxia on metabolism of placenta. *Am. J. Obst. Gynecol.* **80**, 224.

ROVERSI G.D. & POLVANI F. (1963) Corticosteroid biosynthesis in the placenta. *Ann. Ostet. Ginecol.* **85**, 1048.

RYAN K.J. (1959a) Biological aromatization of steroids. *J. Biol. Chem.* **234**, 268.

RYAN K.J. (1959b) Metabolism of C-16 oxygenated steroids by human placenta: the formation of estriol. *J. Biol. Chem.* **234**, 2006.

RYAN K.J. (1960) Metabolism of 16-ketoestrone by human placenta. *Endocrinology*, **66**, 491.

RYAN K.J. & ENGEL L.L. (1953) The interconversion of estrone and estradiol by human tissue slices. *Endocrinology*, **52**, 287.

RYAN K.J., MEIGS R. & PETRO Z. (1966) The formation of progesterone by the human placenta. *Am. J. Obst. Gynecol.* **96**, 676.

SAMUELS L.T., HELMREICH M.L., LASATER M.B. & REICH H. (1950) An enzyme in endocrine tissues which oxidizes Δ^5-3-hydroxysteroids to α,β-unsaturated ketones. *Science*, **113**, 490.

SANDLER M. & COVENY J. (1962) Placental monoamine oxidase activity in toxemia of pregnancy. *Lancet*, ii, 1096.

SCHREINER W. & VILLEE C.A. (1965) Oxidative phosphorylation in mitochondria from human placenta. *Am. J. Obst. Gynecol.* **91**, 961.

SCHUBERTH J. (1966) Choline acetyltransferase. Purification and effect of salts on the mechanism of the enzyme-catalysed reaction. *Biochem. Biophys. Acta*, **122**, 470.

SCHWERS J., ERIKSSON G. & DICZFALUSY E. (1965) Metabolism of estrone and estradiol in the human feto-placental unit at mid-pregnancy. *Acta endocrinol.* **49**, 65.

SCHWERS J. & GOVAERTS-VIDETZKY M. (1964) Metabolism of estrogens by human placenta. *Ann. Endocrinol.* (*Paris*), **24**, 920.

SCHWERS J. & RODESCH F. (1964) Metabolism of estrogens by human placenta. *Ann. Endocrinol.* (*Paris*), **24**, 931.

SHAROV I.I. (1963) Phosphatases in human placenta. *Byull. Eksp. Biol. Med.* **56**, 64.

SHIRASU H. (1964) Effect of synthetic estrogens on NAD(P) transhydrogenase of rat placenta. *J. Biochem.* (*Tokyo*), **55**, 462.

SIITERI P.K. & MACDONALD P.C. (1963) The utilization of circulating dehydroepiandrosterone sulfate for estrogen synthesis during human pregnancy. *Steroids*, **2**, 713.

SILVERSTEIN J. & BONDY P.K. (1966) An RNA fraction in human placenta with template activity. *Biochim. Biophys. Acta*, **119**, 407.

SIMMER H.H., EASTERDAY W.E., Jnr., PION R.J. & DINGMAN W.J. (1964) Neutral C-19 steroids and steroid sulfates in human pregnancy. I. Dehydroepiandrosterone sulfate in fetal blood, etc. *Steroids*, **4**, 125.

SLAUNWHITE W.R., KARSAY M.A., HOLLMER A., SANDBERG A.A. & NISWANDER K. (1965) Fetal liver as an endocrine tissue. *Steroids* (Suppl. 2), 211.

SMITH J.K. (1967) The purification and properties of placental histaminase. *Biochem. J.* **103**, 110.

SMITH O.W. & DAY C.F. (1963) Effect of clomiphene on aromatization of steroids by the human placenta *in vitro*. *Acta endocrinol.* **44**, 519.

SOBREVILLA L., HAGERMAN D.D. & VILLEE C.A. (1964) The metabolism of pregnenolone and 17α-hydroxyprogesterone by homogenates of human term placentas. *Biochim. Biophys. Acta*, **93**, 665.

SOLOMON S. (1960) In *The Placenta and Fetal Membranes*, pp. 200–203. C.A.Villee, ed. Williams & Wilkins, Baltimore.

SOMA H., EHRMANN R.L. & HERTIG A.T. (1961) Human trophoblast in tissue culture. *Obst. Gynecol.* **18**, 704.

SOUTHREN A.L., KOBAYASHI Y., JUNG W., CARMODY N.C. & WEINGOLD A.B. (1966) *In vitro* production of diamine oxidase by the perfused human placenta. *J. Clin. Endocrinol.* **26**, 1005.

STARK G. & JUNG W. (1955) Phosphatase content of placenta and its different cell fractions. *Arch. Gynaec.* **187**, 398.

STARK G. & OWEIS E. (1963) Transaminases and dehydrogenases in normal and pathological placentas. *Arch. Gynaekol.* **199**, 124.

STARKA L. & BREUER H. (1966) Biosynthesis of non-phenolic aromatic C-18 steroids in perfused human placenta. *Biochim. Biophys. Acta*, **115**, 306.

STARKA L., BREUER H. & CEDARD L. (1966a) Biosynthesis of equilin and related ring B unsaturated oestrogens in perfused human placenta. *J. Endocrinol.* **34**, 447.

STARKA L., BREUER J. & BREUER H. (1965) Biogenesis of estrogen in the placenta of the horse. *Naturwissenschaften*, **52**, 540.

STARKA L., JANATA J. & NOVAK J. (1966b) Aromatization of 7α-hydroxydehydroepiandrosterone and of its 3-sulphate by ovarian and placental tissue cultures. *J. Endocrinol.* **34**, 57.

STETTEN M.R. (1964) Metabolism of inorganic pyrophosphate. *J. Biol. Chem.* **239**, 3576.

STETTEN M.R. & TAFT H.L. (1964) Metabolism of inorganic pyrophosphate. *J. Biol. Chem.* **239**, 4041.

SWANBERG H. (1950) Histaminase in pregnancy. *Acta Physiol. Scand.* **23** (Suppl. 79), 1.

SYBULSKI S. & TREMBLAY P.C. (1967) Uptake and incorporation into protein of radioactive glycine by human placentas *in vitro*. *Am. J. Obst. Gynecol.* **97**, 1111.

TALALAY P. & WILLIAMS-ASHMAN H.G. (1958) Activation of hydrogen transfer between pyridine nucleotides by steroid hormones. *Proc. Natl. Acad. Sci. (U.S.)*, **44**, 15.

TARANTINO C. & PASQUINELLI F. (1947) Metabolism of arginine in the human placenta. *Sperimentale*, **98**, 578.

TESAURO G. (1935) On the presence of some fatty acid dehydrogenases in human placenta. *Boll. Soc. Ital. Biol. Sper.* **10**, 325.

THEIL S. (1966) The activity of glycerokinase in the placenta and in maternal and fetal liver in rats. *Naturwissenschaften*, **53**, 436.

TORDA C. (1942) Choline esterase content of tissue without innervation (the placenta). *Proc. Soc. Exptl. Biol. Med.* **51**, 398.

TOWNSLEY J.D. & BRODIE H.J. (1966) A new placental metabolite of oestr-4-ene-3,17-dione: A possible source of error in oestrogen estimation. *Biochem. J.* **101**, 25c.

TOWNSLEY J.D., POSSANZA G.J. & BRODIE H.J. (1966) Stereochemical studies on estrogen biosynthesis. *Federation Proceedings*, **25**, 282.

TROEN P. (1961) Perfusion studies of the human placenta. II. Metabolism of ^{14}C-17β-estradiol with and without added human chorionic gonadotropin. *J. Clin. Endocrinol.* **21**, 895.

TROEN P., DEMIGUEL M. & ALONSO C. (1962) Sulfurylation of estriol by perfused human placenta: a preliminary report. In *Biological and Clinical Aspects of Placental Steroidogenesis*, p. 63. F.Polvani & A.Bompiani, eds. S.Karger AG, Basel.

TROEN P., DEMIGUEL M. & ALONSO C. (1966) Perfusion studies of the human placenta. IV. Conjugation of estriol-16-^{14}C. *Biochemistry*, **5**, 332.

VAN BOGAERT E.C., DI PERETTI E. & VILLEE C.A. (1967) Electrophoretic studies of human placental dehydrogenases. *Am. J. Obst. Gynecol.* **98**, 919.

VAN LEUSDEN H. & VILLEE C.A. (1965) The *de novo* synthesis of sterols and steroids from acetate by preparations of human term placenta. *Steroids*, **6**, 31.

VARANGOT J., CEDARD L. & YANNOTTI S. (1965) Perfusion of the human placenta *in vitro*: study of the biosynthesis of estrogens. *Am. J. Obst. Gynecol.* **92**, 534.

VELARDO J.T. & ROSA C.G. (1963) Histochemistry of enzymes in the female genital system. In *Handbuch der Histochemie*. W.Grauman & K.Neumann, eds. Fischer Verlag, Stuttgart.

VELLE W. & ENGEL L.L. (1964) Enzymes from bovine placenta and seminal vesicle that oxidize D(-)-1,2-propanediol and other polyols. *Endocrinology*, **74**, 429.

VENNING E. & SYLBULSKI S. (1962) *In vitro* biosynthesis of steroids in placental tissue. In *Biological and Clinical Aspects of Placental Steroidogenesis*, p. 13. F.Polvani & A.Bompiani, eds. S.Karger AG, Basel.

VESCIA A. & FIDANZA A. (1948) The peptidases of human placenta. *Boll. Soc. Ital. Biol. Sper.* **24**, 832.

VILLEE C.A. (1953a) The *in vitro* metabolism of placental and fetal tissues. In *Pregnancy Wastage*, p. 71. E.T.Engle, ed. C.C.Thomas, Springfield.

VILLEE C.A. (1953b) The metabolism of human placenta *in vitro*. *J. Biol. Chem.* **205**, 113.

VILLEE C.A. (1953c) Regulation of fetal blood glucose. *J. Appl. Physiol.* **5**, 437.

VILLEE C.A. (1962) Metabolism of the placenta. *Am. J. Obst. Gynecol.* **84**, 1684.

VILLEE C.A. & GORDON E.E. (1955) Further studies on the action of estradiol *in vitro*. *J. Biol. Chem.* **216**, 203.

VILLEE C.A. & HAGERMAN D.D. (1961) Hormonal effects on pyridine nucleotide metabolism in human placenta. *Gen. Comp. Endocrinol.* **1**, 317.

VILLEE C.A., VAN LEUSDEN H. & ZELEWSKI L. (1966) *Advances Enzyme Regulat.* **4**, 161.

VINSON G.P. & JONES I.C. (1964) Capacity of mouse fetus and placenta to synthesize steroids from progesterone *in vitro*. *Gen. Comp. Endocrinol.* **4**, 415.

VON WARTBURG J.P., BETHUNE J.L. & VALLEE B.L. (1964) Human liver-alcohol dehydrogenase. Kinetic and physiochemical properties. *Biochemistry*, **3**, 1175.

WACHSTEIN M., MEAGHER J.G. & ORTIZ J. (1963) Enzymatic histochemistry of the term human placenta. *Am. J. Obst. Gynecol.* **87**, 13.

WALKER D.G., LEA M.A., ROSSITER G. & ADDISON M.E.B. (1967) Glucose metabolism in the placenta. *Arch. Biochem.* **120**, 646.

WARREN J.C. & CHEATUM S.G. (1964) Demonstration of a 17,20-desmolase in the human placenta. *Canad. J. Biochem.* **42**, 143.

WARREN J.C. & CRIST R.D. (1967) Site specificity and mechanism of human placental 17β-hydroxysteroid dehydrogenase. *Arch. Biochem.* **118**, 577.

WARREN J.C. & FRENCH A.P. (1965) Distribution of steroid sulfatase in human tissues. *J. Clin. Endocrinol. Metab.* **25**, 278.

WARREN J.C. & TIMBERLAKE C.E. (1962) Steroid sulfatase in the human placenta. *J. Clin. Endocrinol. Metab.* **22**, 1148.

WARREN J.C. & TIMBERLAKE C.E. (1964) Biosynthesis of estrogens in pregnancy: precursor role of plasma dehydroepiandrosterone. *Obst. Gynecol.* **23**, 689.

WEHEFRITZ B. & GIERHAKE E. (1928) Enzyme studies in the placenta. *Arch. Gynaek.* **135**, 212.

WELCH R.M., HARRISON Y.E. & CONNEY A.H. (1968) Cigarette smoking: stimulatory effect on metabolism of 3,4-benzpyrene by enzymes in human placenta. *Science*, **160**, 541.

WHIPPLE H.E. & STERLING J.A. (1963) Fetal and infant liver function and structure. *Ann. N.Y. Acad. Sci.* **111**, 1–558.

WIENER M. & ALLEN S.H.G. (1967) Inhibition of placental steroid synthesis by steroid metabolites: possible feedback control. *Steroids*, **9**, 567.

WIENER M., LUPU C.I. & PLOTZ E.J. (1961) Metabolism of 17α-hydroxyprogesterone-4-C^{14}-17α-caproate by homogenates of rat liver and human placenta. *Acta endocrinol.* **36**, 511.

WIGGERT B.O. & VILLEE C.A. (1964) Multiple molecular forms of malic and lactic dehydrogenases during development. *J. Biol. Chem.* **239**, 444.

WILCOX R.B. & ENGEL L.L. (1965a) Kinetic studies on the role of 19-hydroxy-androst-4-ene-3,17-dione in estrogen biosynthesis. *Steroids* (Suppl. 1), 49.

WILCOX R.B. & ENGEL L.L. (1965b) The aromatization of 10-methyl and 10-hydroxymethyl steroids by human placental microsomes. *Steroids* (Suppl. 2), 249.

WINICK M., COSCIA A. & NOBLE A. (1967) Cellular growth in human placenta. I. Normal placental growth. *Pediatrics*, **39**, 248.

WINKLER L. (1963) On the lipids of the rat placenta. *Zeitschr. f. Physiol. Chem.* **333**, 199.

WINKLER L. (1964) Activity of phosphatidase A and lysophosphatidase in placenta, maternal liver and fetal liver of pregnant rats. *Naturwissenschaften*, **51**, 340.

WU C.H., FLICKINGER G.L. & TOUCHSTONE J.C. (1967) Conversion of dehydroepi-androsterone-7α-3H to oestrogens by corpus luteum, placenta, and placenta plus foetal viscera in early human pregnancy. *Acta endocrinol.* **54**, 181.

WYNN R.M. (1965) Electron microscopic contributions to placental physiology. *J. Obst. Gynaec. Brit. Comm.* **72**, 955.

YAMAZAKI E., NOGUCHI A. & SLINGERLAND D.W. (1960) The *in vitro* metabolism of iodide, diiodotyrosine and thyroxine by human placenta. *J. Clin. Endocrinol. Metab.* **20**, 794.

ZANDER J. (1963) Hormone synthesis in the placenta and its significance for the fetus. *Arch. Gynaek.* **198**, 113.

ZELEWSKI L. & VILLEE C.A. (1966) The biosynthesis of squalene, lanosterol and cholesterol by minced human placenta. *Biochemistry*, **5**, 1805.

ZOCH E. (1965) Peptidase activity in human placenta. *Enzymologia*, **28**, 325.

ZSOLNAI B., SOMOGYI J., SZARVAS Z. & PUSKAS E. (1964) On the role of proteolytic enzymes in pregnancy. I. Leucine aminopeptidase. *Acta Chir. Acad. Sci. Hung.* **5**, 207.

9

The Assessment of Placental Function in Clinical Practice

ARNOLD KLOPPER

'These arteries, together with the umbilical vein, are supposed to do the same office in the placenta, which is afterward performed in the lungs, by the pulmonary artery and vein, until the child is delivered and begins to breathe.'

WILLIAM SMELLIE, *A Treatise on the Theory and Practice of Midwifery*, Second edition, 1752.

The functions of the placenta have long excited interest and, as the quotation from Smellie shows, by the 18th century the respiratory function was recognized. Since then a great many other functions have been ascribed to this organ and the list will doubtless be still further extended in the future. The clinician who is required to examine placental function, has a number of dissimilar activities to consider. For the most part these can be defined only in the most general terms, and little is known about the mechanisms involved. There can be no single test which embraces all aspects of placental function. It is the purpose of this section to select some placental functions which have been measured; to consider how these measurements can best be made and what their significance is. No attempt will be made to review all the functions of the placenta, nor indeed to examine all the functional tests which have been devised. Only a selection of techniques presently used in clinical practice will be considered.

In recent years the concept of the foetus and placenta as a single functional entity has gained ground. Often a functional effect is the result of inter-related activity between the foetus and placenta. In this sense tests of placental function are properly tests of foeto-placental function. Some tests, such as measurements of the rate of transfer of materials from the maternal to the foetal circulation, are more relevant to the placenta alone, but more often a combined function is being measured and any abnormalities revealed by the test could arise from the foetus as well as the placenta. The group in Stockholm associated with Egon Diczfalusy has done much to establish the view of foetus and placenta as a unit so far as oestrogen production is concerned, and it is likely that the same concept applies to other steroid hormones originating within the uterus. It is of interest that the foetus appears to play little part in the production of chorionic gonadotrophin which finds its way into the maternal circulation (cf. Chapter 6). Measurements of this protein hormone have relevance only to the placenta, as attested by its persistence in the urine after foetal death, provided placental tissue survives.

It is seldom possible to make observations directly on the foetus and placenta until after delivery and this detracts from their usefulness. The practice of amniocentesis is increasing and in the case of some constituents of the liquor amnii, e.g. bilirubin metabolites in erythroblastosis, –it is evident that this sample of the uterine contents gives valid information concerning the state of the foetus. It is likely that measurement of other substances in the liquor will give useful information about the function of the foeto-placental unit but generally observations have to be made on the blood or urine of the mother. This introduces a third variable–maternal effects. Any abnormalities in functional tests may result, not from the foeto-placental unit, but may be reflections of alterations in maternal cardiac, liver or renal function. In this context uterine blood flow may be an important factor in determining the amount of any foetal or placental product available for measurement. Indeed there is reason to believe that alterations of uterine blood flow may be the basis of many pathological changes in foetus and placenta. If this is so, measurements which are dependent on uterine blood flow may have particular clinical significance as they are relevant not only to the functional defect in the foeto-placental unit but to the underlying cause of that defect.

In assessments of placental function these three factors should be kept in mind. Firstly, the placenta has many functions and any single test may not be relevant. Secondly, the placenta and foetus are functionally inter-dependent and functional tests are as likely to measure processes in the foetus as in the placenta. Thirdly, most tests have, of necessity, to be made on the mother and may detect changes in her rather than in the placenta or foetus.

METHODS OF ASSESSMENT

A ASSESSMENT OF NON-ENDOCRINE FUNCTIONS OF THE PLACENTA

A.1 MORPHOLOGICAL CHANGES WHICH MAY ACCOMPANY FUNCTIONAL ALTERATIONS

Examination of the gross or microscopic anatomy of the placenta is widely used in retrospective assessments of its function. It is usual to find some statements concerning placental morphology in descriptions of stillbirths and few maternity units fail to record the weight of the placenta even in normal deliveries. The growth of the placenta is illustrated in Fig. 9.1. This graph shows the weight of the placenta week by week from its formation in the 10th week after the last menstrual period. It is very similar to the figure published by Hendricks (1964) who

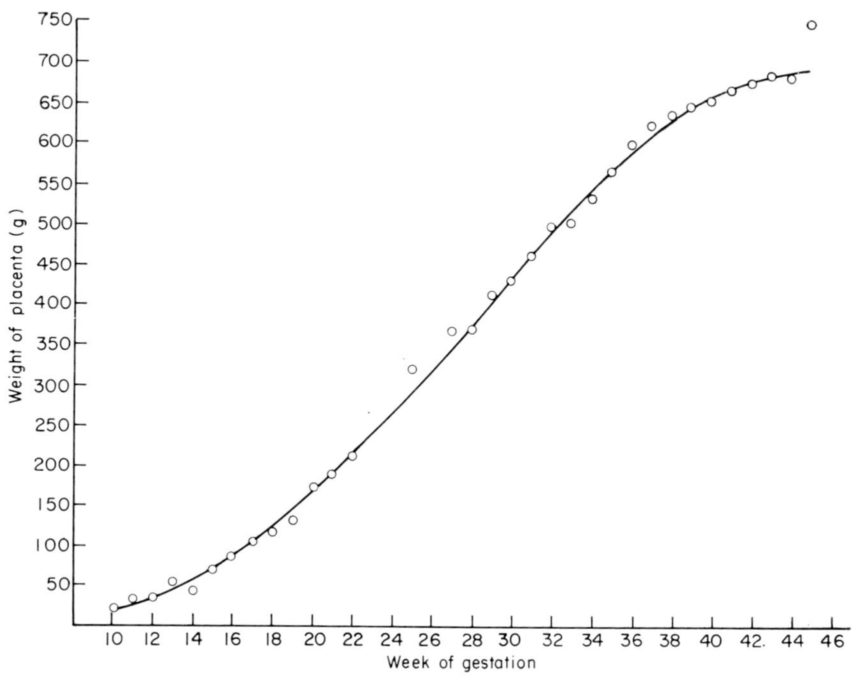

FIG. 9.1. Weight increase of the placenta during gestation.

studied placental weight during the latter half of pregnancy in a different population.

The data on which Fig. 9.1 is based were supplied by Mr W. Billewicz and were derived from 8,006 placentae examined in the Aberdeen Maternity Hospital in 1948 to 1952.

When the placental weight at term was compared with that of the foetus it was found that they were to some extent related, the index of correlation being 0·538 for females and 0·558 for males. Parous women had heavier placentae on average than primigravidae. Taller women also had heavier placentae but there was no significant difference in the placental weight associated with the sex of the foetus. Because of the relationship between foetal and placental weights, the weight of the placenta may be regarded as a very rough indication of its efficiency.

Aherne & Dunnill (1964) have pointed out that the relationship between foetal and placental weights at various stages of gestation can be expressed by the equation:

$$y = ax^b$$

where y is the weight of the placenta, a is a proportionality constant, x is the weight of the foetus and b is the relative growth ratio. Empirically, b is roughly 0·7. Zeuthen (1953) showed that the total oxygen consumption of the foetus is also related to foetal weight by a similar equation. It is reasonable therefore to suppose that placental weight and total foetal metabolism are directly related. The weight of the placenta and the extent of the chorionic villous surface are also proportional. In postnatal life total metabolism is directly related to pulmonary alveolar surface area (Tenney & Remmers 1963). As Smellie observed the placenta serves the foetus in the office of a lung.

Little has been done about expressing the correlation between placental structure and function in quantitative terms other than crude measurements of placental weight. Both the chorionic villous surface area and the volume of the intervillous space probably have a more direct bearing on placental function. Measurements of the villous surface area using planimetry are too laborious and skilled for any but the research situation. Aherne & Dunnill record an area of $11{\cdot}0 \pm 1{\cdot}3\ \text{m}^2$ in a study of ten normal placentae at term. When maternal hypertension was present the figure dropped to $7{\cdot}7 \pm 1{\cdot}6\ \text{m}^2$ and when the baby was abnormally small for the stage of gestation, the average villous surface was only $6{\cdot}4 \pm 1{\cdot}4\ \text{m}^2$. Other forms of placental dysfunction may be associated with an increase in the villous surface area. In haemolytic disease the size of the placenta is greatly increased (Hellman & Hertig 1938) and in two such cases Aherne & Dunnill found the villous surface area to be 15·0 m^2 and 17·0 m^2. The placenta of a diabetic woman was also found to have an increased villous area totalling 13·7 m^2.

Estimations of the volume of the intervillous space are more subject to error. It is possible to arrive at a fair approximation of the volume of this space in the delivered placenta but it is open to question how far this figure is related to the functioning space in a living pregnancy. Aherne & Dunnill found the intervillous volume to have a mean value of 144 ml in ten placentae with an average total placental volume of 488 ± 99 ml. The placental volume was reduced to 363 ± 77 ml when there was maternal hypertension with a proportionate reduction in the intervillous space. Placentae associated with an abnormally small baby also had a reduced volume (350 ± 65 ml) with a proportionate reduction of the intervillous space. The measurement of total placental volume is, of course, not nearly as difficult as measuring the intervillous space. As the intervillous space appears to constitute a fairly fixed proportion of the total placental volume in a variety of conditions associated with placental dysfunction there is much to be said for routine measurements of placental volume in obstetric hospitals.

Presumably, the essential feature concerned in all measurements of this kind is the total placental diffusing area. A further drastic reduction of this occurs with infarction of the placenta. In five cases associated with stillbirths Aherne & Dunnill found that the villous surface was reduced to 4·5 m^2 or less. Placental infarction is a puzzling lesion which has been recorded in documents concerned with obstetrics for centuries and it seems appropriate here briefly to review some of the modern views on the functional significance of this lesion.

Although these lesions are true infarcts in so far as they involve a circumscribed area of tissue necrosis; they are not, as infarcts usually are, the consequence of a sudden occlusion of a blood vessel. The description of the origin of placental infarcts which best fits the evidence is that of Hellman (1952). He thought that the first stage in the process was the deposition of fibrin round the villus whereby it was cut off from the intervillous circulation and became fibrosed. The evaluation of the functional significance of placental infarcts is dependent on how they are caused; it is thus worth while to consider the development of our ideas on this subject. The tissues of the chorionic villus have contact with two circulations–the maternal circulation in the intervillous space, and the foetal blood in the central vessels of the villus–and it could be supposed that obstructions in either or both these circulations could give rise to infarction. The belief that placental infarcts arose from lesions of the foetal circulation was widely held at the turn of the century. Eden (1897) described the process as originating from an obliterating endarteritis and periarteritis of the foetal vessels. This view gradually fell into disrepute but was revived in a modified form by Bartholomew (1947) who suggested that placental infarcts arose as a result of retrograde thrombosis arising from a spasm of a placental vein. The suggestion that placental infarcts arose from defects in the foetal circulation was severely criticized by Thomsen (1954) who summarized the evidence that the syncytiotrophoblast, at least, derived its nourishment from the maternal blood in the intervillous space, and Bartholomew *et al.* (1957) have now withdrawn the original hypothesis. The role of the foetal circulation cannot, however, be entirely discounted. Its importance has been revived by Ten Berge (1955) who lays great stress on the role played by capillary pulsation in the vessels of the villus as a determinent of the intervillous circulation.

Although the emphasis is now firmly placed on the maternal circulation, it is by no means clear whether the primary defect is to be sought within the intervillous space or in the maternal decidual vessels leading to this space. Zeek & Assali (1952) have put forward the view that the prime cause lies in abnormalities of the spiral arteries of the endometrium. The role of the maternal decidual vessels is more fully discussed by Dixon & Robertson in Chapter 1.

Although there is little doubt that in their most severe form, placental infarcts are a pathological entity indicative of functional derangement, the degree of infarction is not necessarily indicative of the amount of functional impairment. Indeed, attempts to measure the degree of infarction have not been conspicuously successful, and their evaluation has been further hindered by the lack of any clear-cut functional criteria by which infarcts might be judged. From a study of 1,000 placentae, Torpin & Swain (1966) concluded that there was no close correlation between placental infarcts and toxaemia.

In essence infarction is only one of several related degenerative processes in the placenta. Another such process is calcification. Chemical analysis has shown the deposits to consist of the carbonates or phosphates of calcium and magnesium. Little is known about the processes which cause these deposits and it is therefore difficult to assess their significance. On somewhat empirical grounds they have come to be associated with deterioration of placental function and various attempts have been made to quantitate the calcium deposition. Burnstein *et al.* (1957) have associated calcification in the placenta particularly with the dysfunction induced by pre-eclamptic toxaemia and have elaborated a scoring system to measure the degree of calcification. Tindall & Scott (1965) came to the opposite conclusion on the basis of measuring the degree of calcification by x-ray examination. The connection between calcification and deterioration of placental function is a good deal less certain than it is with infarction and it is generally agreed that the degree of calcification is valueless as a measure of placental function.

The macroscopic features which have so far been discussed are only a few of the degenerative changes in the placenta, some of which lend themselves admirably to microscopic examination. The placenta is an organ in which growth and age changes are greatly speeded up as compared with other organs in the body. Microscopic changes suggesting tissue degeneration and accompanied by evidence of functional deterioration are part of the normal life cycle of the placenta. It is very difficult in such a dynamic organ to define the limits of normality in morphology. Very often pathological processes in the placenta are either extreme degrees of normal physiological degeneration or the premature occurrence of degenerative changes.

The ageing changes of the placenta first evidence themselves by a retraction and autolysis of the nuclei of the syncytiotrophoblast. According to Wislocki & Dempsey (1946), by the end of pregnancy, the cells contain much less fat and there is no glycogen in the syncytium. The number of mitochondria (phospholipids) and the degree of basophilism declines while the quantity of phosphatase increases. It is probable that the basophilism is caused by ribonucleoprotein in the cytoplasm and by desoxyribonucleoprotein in the nuclei, and that the staining change is due to the disappearance of these nucleoproteins and their gradual replacement by acid phosphates (Dempsey & Wislocki 1945).

Recent work by Tominaga & Page (1966) has cast a new light on the so-called degenerative changes in the placenta. They cultured terminal villi for 48 hours at various oxygen tensions. At the end of this time the tissues kept at 26 per cent oxygen were normal but histological examination of cultures kept at lower oxygen tensions showed lesions exactly the same as the degenerative changes described by Tenney (1936) and by

Wislocki & Dempsey (1946) in toxaemia. When the low oxygen tension was maintained for only six hours similar thinning of the syncytiotrophoblast with retraction and heaping up of the nuclei occurred but if the oxygen tension was then raised these changes regressed. Tominaga & Page interpret these histological changes as representing a physiological adaptation to hypoxia. They presume that the thinning of the trophoblast reduces the thickness of tissue which the oxygen must traverse before reaching the foetal circulation and so increases oxygen transport. This is a slower temporary adaptation which is reversible as long as the hypoxia is not prolonged.

These findings emphasize the fact that, by and large, histological changes are more related to oxygen transport than any other placental function. In this histology is particularly valuable since oxygen transport is a prime placental function on which many other functions are dependent. Histological changes do not lend themselves easily to quantitative description and even when such quantitative histological measurements are made, it is difficult to find other functional criteria by which they might be evaluated. The most successful attempt at this was made by Lenters (1958) who elaborated separate scoring systems for the microscopic anatomy of the intervillous space, the villous epithelium and the stroma and compared these histological findings with the urinary oestriol excretion by the mother and the outcome of the pregnancy. He was able to show that there was a fairly close relationship between the histological findings, the oestriol output and the clinical picture, but it is evident from his data that different functional lesions will affect these parameters in different degrees. There is a great deal of overlap between the normal and the abnormal and occasional discrepancies between the measurements.

A.2 HISTOCHEMICAL CHANGES IN THE PLACENTA

Advances in histochemical techniques have led to attempts to examine specialized placental functions by more refined methods. These have mainly been applied to the localization and measurement of placental enzymes and the functional aspect of this is dealt with by Hagerman in Chapter 7. A few observations on the assessment of placental function by histochemical examination of the tissue are, however, germane here.

The placental constituents for which more or less specific methods of histochemical analysis exist consist of (a) nucleoproteins and acid mucopolysaccharides, (b) carbohydrates, (c) lipids, (d) enzymes, (e) miscellaneous compounds such as iron or the sulphydryl and amino groups of proteins.

a *Nucleoproteins and acid mucopolysaccharides*

These substances are conspicuously basophilic. Basophilia is intense in the early part of gestation and diminishes in the second half of pregnancy. It is associated with rapidly growing cells and with the synthesis of specific proteins by the placenta. The amount of basophilia is therefore in rough measure an indication of placental age. It was suggested by Wislocki *et al.* (1948) that one of the functions of the ribonucleoprotein of the syncytium is to make the proteins of the foetal blood plasma before the foetal liver becomes sufficiently differentiated to take on this function.

b *Carbohydrates*

These substances are shown by the periodic acid-Schiff stain. The periodic acid oxidases the 1,2-glycol linkages in sugars to aldehydes which are then coloured by the Schiff's reagent. Most of the placental investigations have centred around the distribution of glycogen which can be distinguished from other PAS-positive material such as glycoproteins by the use of saliva or malt diastase. Up to six weeks gestation, before the glycogenic function of the foetal liver becomes active, the chorionic villi are rich in glycogen but later stainable glycogen disappears completely.

c *Lipids*

From the point of view of assessing placental function most interest has centered on the amount of lipid material which reacts positively in tests for carbonyl groups and which also gives rise to coloured products in the Liebermann-Burchardt reaction for cholesterol. Seligman & Ashbel (1951) directed attention to the possibility that such stains could be demonstrating ketonic steroids in the placenta. Karnovsky & Deane (1955) have now shown that the positive carbonyl reaction is due to aldehydes formed by the oxidation of unsaturated fatty acids but the belief is still widely held that the intensity of the staining reaction correlates with secretory activity.

d *Enzymes*

A whole host of enzymes have been demonstrated in the placenta by histochemical means. As possible indicators of placental function, alkaline and acid phosphatases, Δ^5-3β-hydroxysteroid dehydrogenase, lactic hydrogenase, succinic hydrogenase, glucose-6-phosphate dehydrogenase, adenosine triphosphatase and adenosine mono-phosphatase have attracted most attention. Dempsey & Wislocki (1945) pointed out that many substances depend on phosphatases for transfer across cell boundaries and they suggested that a layer of different phosphatases in the placental barrier may participate in the transfer of metabolites. The concentration of alkaline phosphatase increased as cytoplasmic basophilia decreased during the course of pregnancy. Curzen (1964) noted that alkaline phosphatase activity increased in late pregnancy and that pre-eclamptic toxaemia was associated with a more rapid rise in activity reaching a peak at 37 weeks gestation. There was no obvious difference in alkaline phosphatase between hypertensive and normal pregnancy. Curzen (1964) was not able to confirm the observation of Thomsen (1955) who reported a reduction in alkaline phosphatase activity after 40 weeks. It is of interest that Lobel *et al.* (1962) found Δ^5-3β-hydroxysteroid dehydrogenase both in the syncytium and in the cytotrophoblast, suggesting that the latter might also be involved in steroid hormone production. No reports have been published of changes in Δ^5-3β-hydroxysteroid activity associated with placental dysfunction although Lobel *et al.* (1962) did note that there was a decline in activity as the placenta aged. This is a somewhat puzzling finding as urinary steroid hormone output continues to increase until term although Zander (1959) noted that placental progesterone concentration was higher at ten weeks than at term.

It was claimed by Curzen (1964) that glucose-6-phosphatase showed a similar earlier rise in pre-eclamptic toxaemia to that which he had noted with alkaline phosphatase. In addition to those authors already quoted Wielenga & Willighagen (1962), Wachstein *et al.* (1963) and Hafez (1964) have published work on the histochemistry of the placenta.

As ways in which to measure placental function, all examinations of the gross or microscopic anatomy of the placenta have serious disadvantages. At best they come after the event. Such retrospective assessments may enhance understanding of placental function but they do little to help clinical control of the dangers which beset the foetus. The object of good placental function is foetal well-being; a state which does not readily lend itself to quantitation in the newborn. Many placental functions combine to create the endpoint–a healthy baby. Even where morphological changes can be measured by a generally agreed scale, one often does not know to which placental function these changes pertain, how far the function is affected, or how much that function ultimately contributes to foetal wellbeing.

e *Miscellaneous compounds*

Although occasional attempts have been made to measure by histochemical means placental constituents such as iron or sulphydryl groups these studies have not been systematically pursued and do not appear very promising.

A.3 EXTRACTION AND ESTIMATION OF VARIOUS PLACENTAL CONSTITUENTS

These methods share the disadvantage of assessment of function by placental morphology by also being retrospective; in many instances they are only a more sophisticated means of quantitating the elements observed in morphology.

For the most part, the work done on various constituents of the placenta has been identifications of particular substances with measurements of their concentration in the organ. In a few instances, attempts have been made to correlate the tissue concentration with other parameters of placental function or to compare tissue concentrations in placentae from normal and abnormal pregnancies. It must be admitted that in such studies, one constantly encounters the problem that tissue concentration may bear no relevance to the production of a particular substance if it is not stored in the placenta but secreted and rapidly carried away.

Among other substances, the placental concentration of hormones, lipids, nitrogen, amino acids, glycogen and a host of enzymes have been studied. The tissue concentrations of the placental hormones, chorionic gonadotrophin, oestrogen and progesterone at various stages of gestation have all been determined. Much of the work in this area rests on the normal pregnancy values determined by Diczfalusy (1953) for chorionic gonadotrophin and oestrogens. Sporadic attempts have been made to relate the placental concentration of chorionic gonadotrophin to diseases in which placental function may be affected such as pre-eclampsia or postmaturity. Drescher (1956), using the glucoprotein content of the placenta as a measure of chorionic gonadotrophin, found a considerable decrease in such malfunctioning placentae, but the test has not proved useful in clinical practice. Progesterone has been isolated from human placentae (Salhanick *et al.* 1952), but the very short biological life of this compound, even in the tissue from which it is supposed to originate, results in a very low concentration, which does not bear any relevance to placental function.

In recent times the emphasis has shifted from examination of the hormonal content of the placenta to the enzymes concerned with steroid metabolism. Many enzymes concerned with steroid biogenesis have been isolated from the placenta, notably those concerned with the insertion of a particular substituent, e.g. 6-β-hydroxylase (Berliner & Salhanick 1956). Presumably, the tissue concentration of these enzymes is an indication of the capacity of the placenta to perform a particular endocrine function but there is as yet no data connecting tissue concentration and hormone production *in vivo*. In this context, the oestrogen dependent transhydrogenase described by Villee & Hagerman (1953) is of particular interest as it may be connected with the energy supply mechanism of the placenta.

A variety of other enzymes in the placenta have attracted attention. The glycogen content of the placenta is high in early pregnancy and then declines, so that glycogen concentration may be some indication of age changes in the placenta. Thus the increased glycogen content in the placenta of the diabetic mother has been interpreted as evidence of placental immaturity (Heijkenskjöld & Gemzell 1957). The enzymes connected with carbohydrate metabolism have been studied, notably glucose-6-phosphatase, hexokinase and isomerase. Enzymes connected with carbohydrate metabolism which warrant particular study are the alkaline and acid phosphatases. As suggested by Dempsey & Wislocki (1945) they may be essential to active transport across the placenta. The blood levels of these enzymes during pregnancy can also be measured. These findings will be discussed later. Jeacock *et al.* (1963) have examined the activity of alkaline and acid phosphatase in placentae from normal and abnormal pregnancies. They conclude that the alkaline phosphatase rises and the activity of the acid phosphatase declines from the second month of gestation onward. The only significant deviation they could find in pathological pregnancies was a rise in alkaline phosphatase in toxaemic patients delivered between 33 and 36 weeks gestation, and an alkaline and acid phosphatase concentration at 33–36 weeks in macerated stillbirths which corresponded to the normal term values.

Attention has also been directed to the placental content of enzymes possibly concerned in the regulation of blood pressure. Luschinsky &

Singher (1948) identified and assayed monoamine oxidase in the placenta. They surmised that the function of this enzyme was to detoxify amines, such as noradrenaline, which have a vasomotor effect, and that in the placenta the enzyme might serve to protect the foetus from maternal vasoactive substances. Sandler & Coveney (1962) found that the placental content of monamine oxidase was reduced in patients with toxaemia of pregnancy and thought that this fall might be concerned in the genesis of toxaemia. They suggested that a failure to deaminate 5-hydroxytryptamine could result in placental vasospasm and further anoxic damage. This hypothesis was refuted by Klinge *et al.* (1964) who examined the monamine oxidase activity in normal and toxaemic placentae and also the 5-hydroxytryptamine content and the activity of the enzyme, 5-hydroxytryptophan decarboxylase, which sets 5-hydroxytryptamine free from its precursor. They found that there was very little 5-hydroxytryptamine or 5-hydroxytryptophan decarboxylase in the placenta and that there was no difference between normal and toxaemic placentae. There was a high concentration of monamine oxidase but this did not fall in the toxaemic placenta. Speculation about the role of monamine oxidase in placental function has now been revived by the work of De Maria & See (1966). They found that there was indeed less monamine oxidase activity in the toxaemic placenta and a corresponding rise in the concentration in noradrenaline. They surmised that these changes were the result of poor placental oxygenation following reduced blood flow.

Choline acetylase activity in the placenta declines during gestation (Bull *et al.* 1961), as does the glutaminase activity (Luschinsky 1951). Histaminase has also been found in the placenta (Kapeller-Adler 1965).

Among the non-enzymic constituents of the placenta, the lipids have occasionally been studied (Cole *et al.* 1953, Helmy & Hack 1964). There is no evidence as to whether lipid concentration reflects placental function, nor is there data on the significance of the vitamins in the placenta (Pratt *et al.* 1946).

Many theories concerning the aetiology of toxaemia have involved altered placental function due to the accumulation of toxic material in the organ. One group of substances which has been investigated is the components of the nucleic acids. Hoover & Bartholomew (1959) examined the acid-soluble nucleotides in placentae from normal and toxaemic patients. There was a tendency for the triphosphate nucleotides to be reduced and the xanthine to be raised in toxaemia. The technical problems of separating and estimating these materials make it impossible to assess the significance of any particular component in terms of placental function.

Mischel (1956) summarized a series of scholarly studies on the functional significance of placental composition. He paid particular attention to trace elements such as nickel, aluminium and zinc and also studied biological amines such as choline, nicotinamide and creatinine. He found significant changes in mineral content of pathological placentae and particularly noted a 50 per cent drop in choline content in eclampsia which he thought might be of aetiological significance.

A.4 FUNCTIONAL TESTS ON THE PLACENTA AFTER DELIVERY

For more than two decades, the oxygen consumption of placental tissue has engaged the attention of workers interested in the measurement of placental function. The pioneer studies were done by Wang & Hellman (1943) who found that there was a progressive decline in oxygen uptake as the placenta grew older. In view of the general belief that toxaemia hastens senescent changes in the placenta, they examined placentae from patients suffering from this disease but were unable to show a significant decrease in the oxygen consumption of the toxaemic placenta. The effect of toxaemia on the oxygen consumption of the placenta was studied by several groups of workers but no definite conclusion was arrived at, although Hellman *et al.* (1950) were again unable to find any significant difference between toxaemic and normal placentae of the same gestational age. MacKay (1958) studied a large number of placentae and confirmed the now generally agreed view that the oxygen consumption of fresh placental tissue falls as pregnancy advances to term and is even lower in the postmature placenta. She also claimed to show a definite reduction of oxygen uptake by the toxaemic placenta. In her study essential hypertension did not cause a fall in oxygen consumption and the findings on the diabetic placenta were inconclusive. MacKay's work was criticized by Friedman & Sachtleben (1960) on methodological grounds and it became apparent that the oxygen consumption could be influenced by factors such as the storage of the placenta, the incubation media, the gas phase or the placental area sampled, all of which are not relevant to placental function. Neither Friedman & Sachtleben nor

Kyank (1955) were able to confirm MacKay's finding of a significantly reduced oxygen consumption in the toxaemic placenta and she herself pointed out that her findings did not give a true indication of placental functional capacity but merely demonstrated some evidence of accelerated ageing in the healthier areas of the toxaemic placenta. These contrary findings are to some extent reconciled in another study by Friedman *et al.* (1962) who now examined the total oxygen consumption of the whole placenta. They found that the total oxygen consumption was unrelated to gestational age and after 28 weeks also not related to placental or foetal weight, remaining essentially constant during the last trimester of pregnancy. The total consumption was reduced in toxaemia or when foetal distress was present. Later studies by Tremblay *et al.* (1965) again showed no reduction in oxygen uptake by the toxaemic placenta but emphasized the relationship between retarded foetal growth and reduced oxygen consumption by the placenta.

In vitro studies on the placenta have shown it to have metabolic patterns of much the same kind as the liver. Its capacity to use carbohydrates for energy production through the tricarboxylic acid cycle has been particularly studied. The findings have not provided a means to measure placental function but have cast some light on the changes in placental function as gestation advances. Villee (1962) made some interesting comparisons between the capacity of the liver and of slices of term placenta to metabolise pyruvate, glucose and fructose to lactate, lipids and carbon dioxide. He was particularly interested in examining the metabolic patterns found under anaerobic *in vitro* conditions as these might reflect the sort of functional changes which occur in placental hypoxia *in vivo*. He found that the term placenta was as active as the young or adult liver, or as the placenta at an earlier stage of gestation, and felt that this weakened the concept of a general decline in metabolic function as the placenta ages.

Attempts have been made to study the function of the placenta by perfusion of the organ after delivery. Such a technique should make it possible to measure various aspects of placental metabolism, also the release of hormones into the perfusate and the permeability of the placenta to metabolites, respiratory gases, drugs and other substances. The perfusion experiments of Panigel (1962) have been helpful in this respect but so far most of the work has been concerned with normal placentae and very little is known about the changes which may take place in these parameters with placental malfunction.

A.5 FUNCTIONAL TESTS ON THE PLACENTA IN UTERO

a *Measurement of uterine or placental blood flow*

There is good evidence that many functions of the placenta, such as oxygen transfer, are dependent upon the amount of maternal blood which passes through the intervillous space per unit time. On the assumption that placental blood flow is a fairly fixed proportion of the total uterine blood flow it seemed possible that measurements of uterine blood flow would provide an index of placental function.

The history of attempts to measure uterine blood flow is not a happy one. The rate of transfer of an inert gas such as nitrous oxide has been used to measure blood flow through other organs and this technique was applied to the uterus by Assali *et al.* (1953). This technique can only be applied to patients undergoing laparotomy as it involves catheterization of the uterine vein. Assali and his colleagues were able to do this successfully only in four out of 14 attempts. It is doubtful how representative of the total venous flow their samples were and Huckabee (1962) pointed out that nitrous oxide equilibrium could not be obtained between the blood and uterine tissue. Assali *et al.* did not themselves regard their results as anything but an approximation. It is noteworthy that the figure for normal term pregnancy–750 ml per minute–still accords well with the later results achieved by more sophisticated means. Metcalfe *et al.* (1955) using the same technique came to the somewhat lower figure of 500 ml per minute. The 4-aminoantipyrine method of estimating blood flow avoids some of the pitfalls of the nitrous oxide technique and was successfully applied to uterine blood flow by Huckabee *et al.* (1961). They arrived at a figure of 700–800 ml per minute.

Studies on the measurement of uterine blood flow received great impetus from the work of Browne & Veall (1953). They injected radioactive sodium chloride directly into the retroplacental space in normal and in toxaemic women and measured the rate at which the radioactivity disappeared. They calculated that in normal pregnancy, the blood flow at term was in the order of 600 ml per minute whereas in hypertensive pregnancy, it was reduced to about 200 ml per minute. Although this work made a considerable contribution to our understanding of the mechanism of placental malfunction in toxaemia, the test was not of a kind which could be applied to routine clinical measurements. With a view to clinical measurement, it was adapted by Morris *et al.* (1955) who injected ^{24}Na, not into the placental circulation, but directly into the uterine wall, and measured the rate at which radioactivity was dispersed. Of course this did not give them any direct measure of uterine blood flow, but they were able to make comparisons of the time taken for the activity to fall by half in normal and toxaemic pregnancy. Somewhat surprisingly, they found a marked difference between the normal values and even mild pre-eclampsia while in severe pre-eclampsia the time to half value was nearly four times longer than the normal. These findings gave rise to great expectations which have not, however, come to fruition. Other workers have been unable to get results as consistent as those of Morris and his colleagues and the test has now fallen into disuse. Its epitaph was written by Cox *et al.* (1963a) who were able to do the test successfully only in 54 patients out of 79 and wrote a good exposition of the mechanical reasons for their failures. They found that the clearance time was not prolonged in pre-eclampsia and that the test could not be used for the prediction of placental insufficiency.

b *Tests of placental permeability*

The study of what substances are transmitted across the placenta and of how they are conveyed across the layers of cells between the maternal and the foetal circulations has been the subject of many laboratory investigations. The transmission of material between mother and foetus is a fundamental function of the placenta and it is surprising that efforts to use this activity as a clinical test of placental function have met with so little success. In part this has arisen from the difficulty of defining the accumulation of material in the foetal compartment. In many instances one can estimate the concentrations of a test material in foetal and maternal circulations at birth, but as a test of placental function it is largely academic if the foetus has to be delivered to make the test possible. Sampling the foetal circulation *in utero* is now possible and its application to tests of placental function will be discussed later, but for the moment such tests on the foetus are possible only at the end of pregnancy when the decision to induce labour has already been taken. It is now feasible to sample another part of the foetal environment without being committed to the induction of labour; *viz.*, the aspiration of liquor amnii by transabdominal puncture. In many instances the liquor concentration of a particular substance is liable to be influenced by many factors other than placental transmission, but there may be circumstances in which the time taken for a substance to appear in the liquor after injection into the mother, has a direct relation to placental permeability. Placental transmission is such a critical function of this organ, and there are so many inert substances which can easily be detected in low concentration that this is a line of research which would be well worth pursuing.

It may not be necessary to sample the foetal environment directly in order to detect the appearance of a substance. The transmission of a radio-opaque contrast medium can be detected by radiography, and a test of this nature was devised by Lampé *et al.* (1960). Attitudes at the present time about irradiation of the foetus make it unlikely that this line can be pursued very far.

An ingenious test of placental transmission was devised by Hellman *et al.* (1963). They gave the mother an intravenous injection of atropine. When this substance was transmitted to the foetus its appearance in the foetal circulation was signalled by an increase in foetal heart rate. Unfortunately, the change in foetal heart rate is a subtle and complex one and Hellman and his colleagues found it necessary to study separately several elements in this change. They measured when a significant change in the mean rate began, when the new rate was established, how long it lasted, when it started to fall again and when the decline stopped. In order to do these complex calculations on running means it was necessary to feed the data into a computer. Hellman & Fillisti (1965) tested patients with toxaemia, with chronic hypertension and with diabetes in this fashion and found that a significant proportion of the pre-eclamptics did not transfer atropine while patients with chronic hypertension did not differ from normal controls. The diabetic patients also were not significantly different from the normals. In spite of the elaborate instrumental refinements they were obliged to conclude that the test was not of use in clinical circumstances.

A.6 FUNCTIONAL TESTS ON THE FOETUS IN UTERO

a *Phonocardiography and electrocardiography of the foetus*

Foetal cardiac function is very sensitive to deleterious changes in the foetal environment and monitoring the foetal heart rate is a standard test for foetal distress the world over. Simple changes in foetal heart rate are, however, usually reflections of relatively sudden changes such as acute hypoxia, whereas many forms of placental malfunction are only slowly established. Complex electronic systems have been devised for the continuous monitoring of foetal heart rate but they are intended for use in labour rather than the diagnosis and control of placental insufficiency in earlier pregnancy.

Foetal electrocardiography has found some application in the assessment of placental function. The electrical activity of the foetal heart can be detected as early as 12 weeks but throughout gestation the signal from the foetal heart is very weak compared with the electric impulses arising from the maternal myocardium and voluntary muscles. It is very difficult to screen off these unwanted signals but even in early pregnancy the foetal electrocardiogram has been used to distinguish between a viable conceptus and a hydatidiform mole or a dead baby. Southern (1957) studied the changes in the foetal electrocardiogram with changes in placental function. When intra-uterine anoxia occurred during labour he found constant changes in the electrocardiogram but did not find the tracings of value in diagnosing placental malfunction in toxaemia or in postmaturity. A more optimistic view was taken by Scholl (1963) who felt that the size of the QRS complex gave some indication of foetal heart size and hence its maturity. It is not likely that the many electronic refinements which are being introduced in this field will add much to the rather dubious value of observations on foetal cardiac function as a means of assessing placental function.

b *Ultrasonic studies of foetus and placenta*

High frequency sound waves travelling in a liquid are reflected at the surface of any body of different density immersed in the liquid. This technique has been used for many years to locate underwater obstructions or submarines and has now been applied to outlining the placenta or the foetal head *in utero*. MacVicar & Donald (1963) applied this method successfully to the diagnosis of hydatidiform mole and missed abortion in early pregnancy. Further studies from the same centre (Donald 1965), have been concerned with measuring the growth of the foetal head by weekly ultrasound recordings in order to detect growth failure resulting from placental insufficiency. Although the apparatus is now in commercial production, it is a temperamental instrument and its operation requires skill, patience and experience. It is, of course, quite harmless to mother and foetus. In later pregnancy, its main use is limited to those forms of placental malfunction associated with poor foetal growth. Its applicability is too restricted for widespread clinical use but in specialized circumstances it has proved valuable.

A.7 TESTS ON LIQUOR AMNII

The view put forward by Walker (1957) that amniocentesis is not a particularly dangerous procedure and might well be used when an assessment of placental function is urgently necessary, has gained ground steadily in the intervening time. It seems likely that transabdominal aspiration of liquor amnii will become a procedure that is widely used in the near future. It is therefore a matter of some importance to consider what substances there are whose concentration in liquor bears any relevance to placental function, and which particular function of the placenta is thereby reflected.

a *The appearance and volume of the liquor*

The appearance of green staining in liquor by meconium has long been a valuable qualitative indication of foetal distress but there is little evidence to support the assertion, which is frequently made, that a thick inspissated liquor is necessarily associated with declining function in the foeto-placental unit. This assumption arises from the belief that a low liquor volume is indicative of malfunction. Although a low liquor volume often accompanies other evidence of inadequate function, the association is by no means constant. The findings on liquor volume have recently been reviewed by Fuchs (1966). In the last trimester of pregnancy the values show a great variation but the average remains fairly constant around 850 ml. Although the mean value declines after term, individual values are so variable that they cannot be used as a measure of postmaturity or any other form of placental malfunction.

b *Metabolites of foetal haemoglobin in amniotic fluid*

In Rh-sensitized pregnancies, the products of foetal haemolysis find their way into the amniotic fluid where their presence and concentration may be valuable indicators of the state of the foetus. Much of the subsequent work in this field is owed to the findings of Bevis (1953). He examined 205 specimens of liquor amnii from 98 patients and did analyses for chloride, glucose, protein, cholesterol, urea, bile pigment, icteric index, urobininogen, laevulose, iron and copper. He found that the increase in the concentration of non-haematin iron was of value in predicting the prognosis of foetuses affected by haemolytic disease. Walker (1957) found that, in Rh-sensitized pregnancies, he could distinguish the affected foetuses from non-affected ones, by examining the adsorption spectrum of the liquor. Liley (1961) did spectrometric analyses of the liquor in 101 Rh-sensitized pregnancies. He found that amniotic fluid from a normal pregnancy showed a more or less straight line adsorption curve from 365 mμ to 550 mμ. When the degradation products of blood were present in the liquor, as in antepartum haemorrhage or when the foetus is affected by haemolytic disease, an adsorption peak was found at 450 mμ. He showed that in Rh-sensitized pregnancies the size and the progress of the 450 mμ peak with advancing gestation, gives a reliable indication of the severity of the anaemia and of the prognosis for the foetus. This peak appears to be caused by bilirubin but somewhat surprisingly is poorly correlated with the cord bilirubin at birth. Liley also concluded that attempts to assess the liquor bilirubin concentration by more refined means than crude direct spectrophotometry did not improve the results. In addition to non-haemin iron and bilirubin the concentration of coproporphyrin in the liquor from Rh-sensitized pregnancies has been examined (Goodlin & Schwartz 1962). It was found that the concentration of coproporphyrin was elevated if the foetus had erythroblastosis. Of the three tests, spectrophotometry of the liquor, being both simple and directly related to the state of the foetus, has proved most acceptable in clinical practice.

c *Examinations of other liquor constituents*

The tension of CO_2 and particularly of O_2 in the amniotic fluid has attracted attention as possible indicators of the capacity of the placenta to perform its respiratory function. The tension of these gases in the amniotic fluid is influenced by many factors and the results are also very subject to variation according to the technique of assay. Not surprisingly, even normal mean values have varied very much with different authors. For Po_2 Vasicka & Hutchinson (1964) quote a range of 1·3 to 16·2 mmHg while Romney *et al.* (1962) found the mean value of their group was 25·5 mmHg. Quilligan (1962) found a normal Po_2 and Pco_2 in the liquor in cases where the foetus was dead and could not correlate the foetal arterial gas tensions with those in the liquor amnii. It is likely that Po_2 is related to many factors such as maternal arterial blood Po_2, foetal heart rate, medication of the mother and the rate of diffusion through the foetal skin and the amnion as well as through the placenta. Such measurements of gas tension are unlikely therefore to be an adequate measure of the respiratory function of the placenta.

d *Amnioscopy*

A new technique for examination of the liquor amnii does not involve puncturing the membranes at all. An endoscope is passed through the cervix and the membranes viewed by reflected light. In this way, some impression of the appearance of the liquor can be gained, especially the amount of vernix caseosa and it can be determined whether any meconium staining is present. Although a useful improvement in foetal salvage by the use of this technique has been claimed by its originator (Saling 1962), it is, in view of the variability of normal liquor, inherently unlikely that simple inspection–'seen through a glass, darkly'–will be of much value in the assessment of placental function.

A.8 TESTS ON THE FOETUS AFTER RUPTURE OF MEMBRANES

When the evidence for placental malfunction is so strong that labour has to be induced, it is possible to obtain foetal blood after rupture of the membranes and therefore to make a more accurate assessment of the situation. The technique for these measurements has been evolved largely by Saling (1963). The presenting part, either scalp or buttock, is sprayed with ethyl chloride and a small skin nick made in the resulting area of reactive hyperaemia. From this a capillary tube of heparinized blood can be drawn which is largely arterial in nature. A large range of micro-analyses can be done on this specimen,–blood sugar, haemoglobin, haematocrit, Coombes test, pH, P_{O_2} and P_{CO_2}. The pH appears to be most helpful in the control of treatment. This technique has roused a great deal of interest and it may be of value in helping to monitor the foetal state during labour. It is, however, applicable only to studies done immediately before or during labour and commits the obstetrician to proceeding with delivery. It is therefore not applicable in the large area where chronic placental insufficiency may require repeated assessment in late pregnancy.

A.9 TESTS ON MATERNAL BLOOD

During gestation some of the constituents of the mother's blood are either derived from the foeto-placental unit or else elaborated partly in response to the stimulus of the pregnancy. It may be supposed that measurement of such substances will give some insight into placental function. Many such materials have been proposed for study. Among the non-endocrine substances which have appeared most promising there is:

a *Serum alkaline phosphatase*

Numerous studies have shown that the concentration of this enzyme in the maternal serum increases during pregnancy and there is evidence which suggests that part of the complex which is measured as alkaline phosphatase is a specific isoenzyme derived from the chorionic villi. It might be expected therefore that the production of this enzyme would be depressed in conditions affecting the function of the chorionic villi. Lee & Lewis (1963) examined the serum levels of alkaline phosphatase in toxaemic pregnancy and somewhat surprisingly found them to be significantly higher than in normal pregnancy and in non-pregnant women. This conclusion was disputed by Curzen & Morris (1965) who found no significant rise in alkaline phosphatase in toxaemia or in hypertensive pregnancy. Nor was there any marked change when intra-uterine death of the foetus occurred. Levine & Wood (1965) showed that there were several constituents in the serum alkaline phosphatase complex, only some of which, the enzymes from the chorionic villi, increased in pregnancy. They also found no significant change in toxaemia and even patients with an intra-uterine foetal death had values within the normal pregnancy range. It is difficult to agree with their conclusion that serum alkaline phosphatase assay is a useful test of placental function in view of the fact that there was a considerable overlap between the values at term and in the non-pregnant women, and that there was no consistent change accompanying conditions of major placental dysfunction.

b *Diamine oxidase*

This is another enzyme complex present in maternal serum, at least part of which is derived from the foeto-placental unit, with a consequent rise in the concentration in maternal serum during the course of gestation. The main substrate for diamine oxidase is histamine and this somewhat remote connection with blood pressure and uterine contractility has served to maintain interest in the assay of the enzyme during pregnancy. There is, however, no sound evidence to support the view that it is of any value in the assessment of placental function.

c *Serum proteins*

During pregnancy the total serum protein concentration and the level of serum albumin fall, owing presumably to the haemodilution of pregnancy. At the same time there is an increase in certain globulin fractions notably α_1-, α_2-, and β-globulins. There are also data suggesting that specific new protein fractions appear in the maternal serum during pregnancy. MacGillivray & Tovey (1957) examined the changes which take placein certain protein fractions during gestation and concluded that in toxaemia there was a more marked fall in albumin and in γ globulin than in normal pregnancy. The test does not appear to be sufficiently closely correlated with the severity of placental malfunction to be of use in the measure- ment of placental function.

d *Plasma renin*

Recent work (Brown *et al.* 1966) has shown that in hypertensive disease the plasma concentration of this substance falls within the range found in normal pregnancy but that the more severe forms of pre-eclampsia tended to have plasma renin values below the normal mean and in pregnant Negro women with hypertension it was significantly lower (Bonar *et al.* 1966). Although it is not suggested that this substance derives from the foeto-placental unit it may be possible that its concentration in the maternal blood bears some relation to the state of affairs within the uterus.

e *Plasma volume*

The development of dye dilution techniques has made it possible to measure plasma volume accurately in pregnant women. Although changes are of great interest to the study of fluid changes during pregnancy their connection with placental function is somewhat tenuous. The plasma volume may be connected with placental size and a recent publication (Thomson *et al.* 1967), demonstrated a clear association between maternal oedema and foetal size.

B ASSESSMENT OF THE ENDOCRINE FUNCTIONS OF THE PLACENTA

The foeto-placental unit is concerned in the production of a number of hormones and in essence this mode of assessing placental function consists of measuring by indirect means the production of one or other of these hormones. Although a great variety of substances may be concerned, these measurements have in practice resolved themselves to the metabolites of three hormones, chorionic gonadotrophin, oestrogen and progesterone. As far as the last two are concerned, they are not unique to the foeto-placental unit, and at least in early pregnancy, it is difficult to decide how far any measurement represents ovarian function and how far foeto-placental function. Some techniques also do not discriminate between the two steroid hormones. They will be considered briefly before passing on to measurements of the metabolites of particular hormones.

B.I VAGINAL CYTOLOGY

The cells of the vaginal mucosa are constantly being shed. If a smear of such cells is fixed and stained the microscopic appearance will depend, *inter alia*, on the admixture of steroid hormones acting on the vagina. Once standard procedures for taking and preparing the smears had been evolved it became possible to produce more or less agreed descriptions of the appearance of smears in various endocrine states, during the normal menstrual cycle, in pregnancy and after the menopause. It was found that vaginal, rather than cervical, cells gave the most characteristic picture and today smears are usually taken by spatula from the lateral vaginal wall.

It is necessary to quantitate the various features of the vaginal smear, and, in order to do so, several indices have been evolved, notably those concerned with the demonstration of eosinophilic cells (eosinophilic index), and with the degree of pyknosis of cell nuclei (karyopyknotic index). The changes in vaginal cytology which take place during pregnancy were described in detail by Pundel & Van Meensel (1951). The eosinophilic and karyopyknotic indices are low and in a fully established normal pregnancy are characteristically below 5 per cent. The proportion of superficial cells diminishes and there is an increasing tendency for the cells to adhere together in clusters. The cells of the intermediate layer are shed in increasing numbers and often present a characteristic 'boat-like' appearance – the so-called navicular cell. There is some controversy about further changes which may take place at the very end of pregnancy, although there is some evidence for claiming that the full term smear can be distinguished from that of normal pregnancy before term. After delivery and possibly in severe *antepartum* depression of placental function regressive changes can be detected in the pattern of vaginal cytology.

The pattern of vaginal cytology is subject to many influences, notably infection, oestrogens and progesterone. Administration of oestrogens to a castrated woman causes the appearance of many superficial squamous cells and a rise in eosinophilic and karyopyknotic indices. On the other hand progesterone causes the shedding of more intermediate cell types and a fall in these indices. Normal pregnancy, therefore, shows a picture more closely related to progesterone than to oestrogen. It is usually claimed that the smear pattern depends on the relative amounts of each hormone, but this can be true only up to a point. There is some evidence to suggest that the absolute amounts of either hormone present also exert an influence. In the most general terms the normal pregnancy picture is the result of intense oestrogen stimulation acting on a high progesterone background. This view is supported by the work of Stamm *et al.* (1959) and to some extent also by MacRae and his colleagues (1965). Both groups studied vaginal cytology and the urinary excretion of pregnanediol and of oestriol in women with a jeopardized pregnancy. Neither could find any correlation between vaginal cytology and the pregnanediol output although Stamm *et al.* did find that when the eosinophilic and karyopyknotic indices rose the oestriol output tended to fall.

Studies of vaginal cytology have been directed mainly toward two situations in which placental function could be failing. The first is in patients with signs of threatened abortion or a history of recurrent abortion and the second is in the diagnosis of term pregnancy or of a decline in placental function at or after term. Cox *et al.* (1964) found vaginal smears to be as reliable as urinary pregnanediol assay in the prognosis of threatened abortion. Gaudefroy (1959), Soule (1964) and Hassan (1965) all found vaginal cytology to be of value in predicting the outcome of pregnancy in patients likely to abort.

Opinions concerning the value of vaginal cytology at term have not been unanimous. Lichtfus (1959) described three types of smear in late pregnancy. The first he considered to be representative of pregnancy prior to term, the second of full term pregnancy and the third of the post-partum period or of severe placental malfunction. Lichtfus took smears from 715 women who were by dates at the end of their pregnancy. He found that of those who had a smear 'prior to term' only 3 per cent delivered spontaneously within five days of taking the smear. On the other hand, 92 per cent of those who had an 'at term' smear delivered within five days. Eight of the 713 patients had a 'post-partum' type of smear. Labour was induced immediately but four of the eight babies died of postmaturity soon after birth. Lichtfus therefore concluded that vaginal cytology was a reliable guide to the changes in hormone production which initiate labour and could be used as an indication of declining placental function. This conclusion is somewhat surprising in that no convincing demonstration has yet been made of changes in hormone production associated with the onset of labour. His conclusion was not supported by Abrams & Abrams (1962) who found that the change from the normal pregnancy to the 'at term' smear pattern was a gradual one which occurred 12–42 days before the onset of labour and did not occur at all in 66 per cent of the patients examined. Soule (1964) could not support the finding that a regressive 'postpartum' type of smear indicated declining placental function and Frampton (1966) who studied a group of normal pregnant women by weekly serial smears in late pregnancy also found that about half went into labour without changing from the normal pregnancy pattern to the 'at term' type of smear. It seems likely from the work of most of these authors that a change to the 'at term' type of smear, when it does occur, is indicative of the close approach of the onset of labour in a large proportion of patients.

Vaginal cytology is a quick and easy way to assess placental function but a number of shortcomings have been overlooked by the more enthusiastic advocates of this technique. At first the interpretation of the smear was largely a subjective matter. Even with the present day methods for quantitation of some aspects of the usual impression, there is no indication that these indices bear a close proportionate relationship to hormone production. Nor is there any evidence of the time relationship between the decline in hormone production and the change in vaginal cytology. Time is often of the essence in the assessment of placental function. If the change in vaginal cytology is a consequence of a fall in the production of a particular hormone, it would be more logical to study that hormone directly. If, as seems likely, the vaginal smear picture is the outcome of a certain ratio of oestrogen to progesterone, this ratio could be maintained over a great range of absolute values of the hormones. The fact that the smear is not representative of any single hormone is a grave disadvantage.

In clinical practice some practical difficulties appear. Factors other than hormone levels may influence the vaginal cytology. Infection may have marked effects. Occasionally extensive cytolysis occurs during pregnancy and a fair proportion of smears cannot be read on this account.

In summary, vaginal cytology has severe limitations as a technique for the assay of placental function. As long as it is not presumed to bear too close a relationship to the circulating level of any particular hormone it has some application in the clinical evaluation of abortion.

B.2 CERVICAL MUCUS

The appearance, viscosity, volume and electrolyte content of the mucus secreted by the cervix are all to some extent under hormonal influence. The effect of oestrogen is to make the fluid watery and more copious, and to increase greatly the content of sodium chloride. When mucus, which is secreted under oestrogen stimulation, is smeared on a glass slide and allowed to dry the salt crystallizes out in characteristic aborescent patterns, a phenomenon which has been called ferning. The effect of progesterone is opposite in kind; the mucus becomes scanty and tacky, contains much less salt and does not exhibit ferning. These changes have been made the basis of a test of placental function in early pregnancy. It is supposed that as long as ovarian and placental hormone production are normal, the progesterone effect is dominant, but if the function declines the oestrogen effect predominates and ferning begins to appear. Thus MacDonald (1963) found that eight out of 16 patients who showed ferning eventually aborted while only four pregnancies were lost in 41 patients who did not show ferning.

The ferning test is so simple to perform that it has struck the clinical imagination and a voluminous literature has grown up about it. Among the more sophisticated projects have been attempts to quantitate the chloride concentration of the mucus. Thus McSweeney & Sbarra (1964) have designed a test whereby the mucus is spotted on filter paper impregnated with silver nitrate and potassium chromate. The amount of chloride is estimated from the size of the resulting clear spot. According to their findings, in normal pregnancy the mucus has a chloride concentration of 0·1–0·2 per cent. Concentrations above 0·3 per cent indicate an unstable pregnancy in danger of abortion.

The ferning test is a non-specific procedure which gives no measure of the hormone production. It is hard to define what process, if any, in the placenta it indicates. The data on its prognostic value in abortion are not convincing. Taken in conjunction with the clinical picture it may be of some use in deciding therapy but wherever possible measurements of specific hormones or their urinary metabolites are to be preferred as means of assessing placental function.

B.3 CHORIONIC GONADOTROPHIN

Recent work on this protein hormone are reviewed in detail in Chapter 6 and only a few considerations relevant to the measurement of placental function will be examined here. The hormone can be assayed in either blood or urine. Serum estimations have the advantage of eliminating the delay and error of urine collections. Most of the definitive work has been done on serum and for the estimation of placental function this source is to be preferred.

Interest in the use of HCG assay as a means of assessing placental function dates back to the early 1940's. An early publication by White & Hunt (1943) compared the urinary pregnanediol and HCG excretion in pregnant women with diabetes. They used a crude rat corpus luteum method for the HCG assay and the techniques for pregnanediol assay were also at that time in the early stages of their development. It is somewhat surprising that they were able to sort their patients into two clear groups; one of which had normal hormone levels and a very low incidence of prematurity, toxaemia and perinatal mortality. The other had abnormal levels (either low pregnanediol or high HCG or both), and if left untreated had a very high incidence of prematurity, toxaemia and perinatal mortality. If the patients were treated with progesterone or stilboestrol, White & Hunt claimed that the incidence of such complications was much reduced. This paper was one of the starting points of a false lead which was to be pursued vigorously for the next twenty years. It is only in recent years that, by using properly designed double blind therapeutic trials, and much more accurate hormone assay techniques, it has become apparent that, although hormone assays give useful information about the existing state of placental function, they do not forecast what the state of affairs will be in weeks or months, nor does substitution therapy affect the outcome.

The problem of whether hormone changes preceded the onset of toxaemia in diabetic patients continued to intrigue obstetricians. Rubin *et al.* (1946) did serial studies of oestrogen, pregnanediol and HCG in pregnant diabetics. They found that both toxaemia and foetal death may or may not be associated with increased serum HCG. There was no reciprocal relationship between the steroids and HCG and they could find no support for the theory that increased HCG output occurs in an attempt to compensate for lowered steroid production.

In order to assess the value of HCG assay as a measure of placental function in obstetric disease, it was necessary to have reliable data on HCG levels in normal pregnancy. The first definitive study of normal pregnancy was done by Wilson *et al.* (1949). This publication became the yardstick for HCG estimation for many years and their graphs and figures are still reproduced in many textbooks today. Although at the present time one would have reservations about their experimental design (they did only single assays in 112 women at various stages of pregnancy), and their method is now superseded, there is little doubt that the picture they produced is substantially correct. They found that in serum the HCG concentration rose rapidly in early pregnancy to a mean peak of 70 i.u./ml at 55 days gestation; then fell away to a mean mid-pregnancy low of 20 i.u./ml. Although they do not comment upon it their graph shows a small rise in HCG at the end of pregnancy. Haskins & Sherman (1952) used an inferior assay technique but were able substantially to confirm the work of Wilson *et al.* (1949). Again a small secondary rise in HCG in late pregnancy was noted. The same finding can be seen in the publication by Behrman & Niemann (1955). It seems very likely that on the average there is a small rise in HCG level in the last weeks of pregnancy. No acceptable explanation of the significance of this phenomenon has yet been offered.

Haskins & Sherman (1952) noted an increased output of HCG in pre-eclamptic toxaemia, an observation which had cropped up repeatedly in the literature since it was first recorded by Smith & Smith (1934). These investigations were carried a stage further by Watts & Adair (1943) who found that HCG excretion was increased, not only in pre-eclamptic toxaemia, but also in pregnancy complicated by essential hypertension and concluded that the raised HCG level was a consequence rather than the cause of the pathology. The matter rests at present on the work of Loraine & Matthew (1950) who found that a significant rise in mean HCG levels occurred only in severe toxaemia. The change in HCG excretion was inconsistent and they concluded that routine HCG assays were not of much value in the clinical management of pre-eclamptic toxaemia.

In addition to the interest in diabetic pregnancy and toxaemia already mentioned much of the early work on HCG assays as a measure of placental function centred on abortion, hydatidiform mole, and Rh incompatible pregnancies. The impressions derived from this work will have to be revised now that much improved HCG assay techniques are available but some of the earlier publications are worthy of note in passing. It is evident from the work of Delfs & Jones (1948), Hon & Morris (1956) and Vermelin, Ribon & Ribon (1957) that falls in HCG levels often occur in association with the process of abortion. The clinical material in these surveys is poorly categorized and it is seldom clear at what stage of the abortion process the assays were done. Not surprisingly, many aberrant findings are recorded. It is reasonable to conclude that extensive placental damage incompatible with foetal life is often reflected in a fall of HCG level but there is no evidence that such a fall is causative of the abortion or indeed precedes the placental damage. When intra-uterine foetal death takes place without placental damage, HCG levels may remain within the normal range for some time. Clearly a large category of abortion is not associated with a fall in HCG soon enough for such assays to be of any clinical value.

HCG assays in hydatidiform mole and chorionepithelioma do not fall strictly within the context of placental function and the literature on this field is reviewed in Chapter 6.

The large, immature placenta which is found in Rh incompatible pregnancies has led to the suggestion that HCG output may be increased in this condition. Bradbury & Goplerud (1963) noted a correlation between serum HCG and hydrops foetalis although three non-hydropic affected babies and two Rh-negative infants with raised HCG levels also occurred in their series. McCarthy & Pennington (1964a) using an improved assay technique were able to demonstrate a closer correlation between raised serum HCG and hydrops foetalis, but a companion study (McCarthy & Pennington 1964b) showed that the HCG concentration in the liquor amnii of severely affected foetuses did not differ significantly from normal.

The field of HCG assay has been transformed by the development of immunological assay techniques, and it is likely that impressions derived from the earlier biological assays will have to be revised as fresh data becomes available. The immunological techniques are analysed in detail in Chapter 6 and will not be considered here except to note how the general state of knowledge in a particular field will lead to the evaluation of very similar methods in different places at the same time. Thus in one year three independent methods were published. The first, by Brody & Carlstrom (1960) depends upon complement fixation, the second by Wide & Gemzell (1960) on haemaglutination inhibition and the third, by McKean (1960) is a precipitin test.

It is not possible at this stage to give a final assessment of the relative merits of each method. Various modifications of the Wide & Gemzell technique have been widely used and the publications in many languages on the application of this method to the study of placental function are probably now at their peak. Brody & Carlstrom's method has been less widely applied but has the advantage of having been used by its originators in a number of very well designed and strictly controlled clinical studies (Brody & Carlstrom 1962, Brody & Carlstrom 1965). It is becoming clear that the two methods give slightly different results and that immunoassay techniques altogether give rather different results from earlier biological methods. Many workers (e.g. Danielsson 1965) have found that immunological methods give higher values than the biological assays. This, especially in urine, is supposed to be due to the existence of an immunologically active fraction which is biologically inactive. Some workers (Toaff *et al.* 1965), have gone so far as to state that there is no statistical correlation between values obtained by biological or by immunological methods.

Brody & Carlstrom (1962) published a carefully designed survey of the changes in serum HCG during pregnancy which is likely to replace the old data of Wilson *et al.* (1949). They were able to show clearly that the normal mean curve was biphasic in nature with a secondary smaller rise at 35 weeks. For a while it looked as if this might be a real point of difference with the Wide & Gemzell method as Wide & Gemzell (1962) found no late pregnancy rise in morning urines, but Connon (1964) using a modification of this method did note a rise in urinary HCG between 32 and 36 weeks gestation.

The new immunological methods indicate that HCG assay may be much more useful in the assessment of placental function than could be concluded from the biological assay data. Immuno-assay of HCG appears to be particularly applicable to studies in early pregnancy. Brody & Carlstrom (1965) studied a group of patients admitted to hospital with threatened abortion in whom it was not possible to tell on clinical grounds whether the abortion process had proceeded to an inevitable stage. Fifty patients had low serum values and all aborted, while 23 with normal values all went to term. In their earlier work, (Brody & Carlstrom 1962), some of the findings suggested that a fall in HCG may precede signs of extensive placental damage. Carlsson (1964) using the Wide technique was able to confirm Brody & Carlstrom's optimistic view of the value of HCG assay in threatened abortion but found that later in pregnancy normal values occurred in patients with pre-eclamptic toxaemia. Danielsson (1965) found that no change of HCG values took place in prolonged pregnancy, further strengthening the view that these assays are of less value as a measure of placental function in late pregnancy.

The failure of HCG assays in late pregnancy to provide a reliable index of placental function may be related to the wide fluctuation of values from time to time in the same subject; even larger than those of urinary steroids. So far we have no reasonable evidence of what factors determine the normal levels of HCG in blood and urine and have little prospect of elucidating the day to day fluctuations. Present data show that the levels do not appear to be related to the size of the placenta, the presence of placental infarcts, the size or the sex of the infant or the maternal parity. Further studies on the fundamental physiology of HCG, –its serum life, the renal handling of HCG, indeed its very function in late pregnancy, are necessary to bring us to the point where assays in late pregnancy can be most usefully performed in conditions of placental malfunction. In this context, the concept elaborated by Lauritzen (1965) provides an important new perspective and may well supply an explanation of the control of endocrine function in the foeto-placental unit. He has adduced evidence to show that HCG levels determine the production of dehydroepiandrosterone by the foetal adrenal. The supply of this steroid in turn determines the production of oestriol by the foeto-placental unit. He has further suggested that a feedback control mechanism may exist between oestriol and HCG. Thus a fall in oestriol will stimulate HCG secretion and vice versa.

B.4 PROGESTERONE AND ITS METABOLITES

Progesterone is elaborated by the foeto-placental unit. Its concentration in body fluids may then reflect the capacity of the foetus or placenta to perform this endocrine function. The idea that a single specific hormone is secreted has now been replaced by the realization that molecules like progesterone or oestradiol are links in a metabolic chain and have an evanescent existence. Measurements of single, short-lived, molecular entities may bear little relationship to the physiological processes with which the whole series of compounds is concerned. In the foeto-placental unit, progesterone is partly reduced to its C-20 hydroxyl derivatives which are then oxidized back to progesterone (Solomon 1966). These derivatives are also progestationally active and it is therefore impossible to say which particular molecular species is the active hormone. Indeed we know so little about the physiological function of progesterone in pregnancy that the argument for progesterone measurement on the ground that this represents the concentration of a physiologically active substance is a very insecure one. Progesterone concentration in the retroplacental blood may bear some relevance to endocrine conditions obtaining in the foeto-placental unit, but, in practice, it is peripheral maternal venous, and not retro-placental, blood which is available for assay. Progesterone disappears very rapidly from the circulation, (Zander 1954), and its concentration in peripheral venous blood is as likely to be representative of the rate of removal as it is to reflect its production in the foeto-placental unit. Reliable methods for the estimation of progesterone in blood have been in use for some time (Short 1958, Zander 1962) and the range of concentration at various stages of gestation determined, (Zander 1957, 1959, Short & Eton 1959), but progesterone assay has not proved of much value in the assessment of placental function. This view was formulated by Coyle *et al.* (1962) who examined blood progesterone levels in women with severe pre-eclampsia and found that the results bore no relation to the imminence of intra-uterine foetal death. In some cases no fall in progesterone concentration took place for several days after foetal death.

Pregnanediol is an end product of progesterone metabolism. It may be therefore that its concentration in peripheral maternal venous blood will reflect progesterone production in the foeto-placental unit more accurately than does progesterone itself. Methods for the estimation of pregnanediol in blood were first introduced some years ago (Sommerville & Deshpande 1958, Oertel *et al.* 1960). They have not proved to be reliable in clinical practice, and adequate data on normal pregnancy levels are still lacking. No extensive findings on blood pregnanediol as a measure of placental function have been published, but the recent introduction of gas chromatographic techniques for the assay of pregnanediol can be expected to lead to a revival of interest in this possibility.

The approach which has been most adequately explored is the measurement of pregnanediol in urine. The value of urinary pregnanediol assays will depend *inter alia*, on the urinary pregnanediol being a more or less constant proportion of the progesterone produced in the body. Klopper & Michie (1956) examined the quantitative relationship between progesterone and urinary pregnanediol by measuring the urinary recovery of pregnanediol after administration of the active hormone. The average conversion of progesterone to urinary pregnanediol was 12·9 per cent with a range of 5·1 per cent to 16·8 per cent. The conversion did not alter in pregnant women. Plotz *et al.* (1963) using progesterone-4-C^{14} obtained a similar conversion figure in pregnant women. Although such conversion studies support the view that there is a reasonably constant relationship between progesterone production and urinary pregnanediol there are some serious reservations to be made about this thesis. In the first instance, the curve of urinary pregnanediol during gestation and of blood progesterone do not coincide. Secondly pregnanediol has been isolated from the faeces of a pregnant woman (Klopper & Macnaughton 1959), and one never knows whether a change in pregnanediol output represents an alteration of progesterone production or a shift in the relative amounts of pregnanediol excreted in urine and faeces. Whatever its relationship to progesterone production, the level of urinary pregnanediol has frequently been used as a measure of placental function and this index requires to be examined in some detail.

The value of urinary pregnanediol estimations as a measure of placental function is dependent upon the reliability of the method used for the assay. In the first two decades after the isolation of this progesterone metabolite from pregnancy urine a good many methods for its quantative estimation were devised. Basically they all depended upon a crude purification of urinary extracts by precipitation of the steroid from mixtures of various organic solvents and water. By its very nature such a step cannot be either quantitative or specific and, in spite of the optimism of many authors, the results published before 1950 are little more than rough indications of the nature of the changes to be expected with advancing gestation and in foeto-placental pathology. In the early 1950's chromatographic methods were first applied in this field and by 1955 a method devised by Klopper, and his colleagues made it possible to obtain reliable estimates of the changes in pregnancy.

The interpersonal variation and change in pregnanediol excretion with gestation have been adequately defined in the studies of normal pregnancy published by Coyle *et al.* (1956), Shearman (1959), Kankaanrinta (1963), and by Klopper & Billewicz (1963), but so far little is known about what makes one normal pregnant woman excrete more pregnanediol than another. The findings on day to day variation in the same subject are discouraging. Klopper (1964) found the average co-efficient of variation between successive 24 hour urines from the same subject to be 24 per cent!

Because of the supposed causal relationship between progesterone production and maintenance of pregnancy most of the first studies on the clinical applications of urinary pregnanediol assay were done on patients liable to abortion. This involved studies in early pregnancy when it was impossible to determine what proportion of the steroid came from the ovary and what from the foeto-placental unit. In spite of many manifest difficulties the initial reports were enthusiastic. The extensive investigation of Guterman (1953) was done before sound methods were available, but it called the tune in abortion studies for the next decade. He found that pregnancy was maintained when pregnanediol output was normal and that abortion tended to occur when the trend of excretion was low. Many workers strongly supported this contention (de Watteville 1951, Furuhjelm 1953, Alder & Krieger 1957, Rawlings 1965), although from the beginning some investigators were severely critical of this conclusion (Robson & Gornall 1955, Baker *et al.* 1955, Langmade *et al.* 1961). A more critical evaluation of the results of serial assays has shown that they have little prognostic value in recurrent abortion, (Macnaughton & Michie 1960) and there seems no doubt that pregnanediol output shows little change until the foeto-placental unit is irretrievably damaged (Klopper & Macnaughton 1965). This narrows the field in which pregnanediol assays might usefully be applied, but still leaves an area where they are of value. They are helpful in determining the presence and functional state of the corpus luteum or trophoblast in such conditions as incomplete abortion, missed abortion, hydatidiform mole or pseudocyesis. The finding that pregnanediol assays have little prognostic value in abortion has an important therapeutic implication. The therapy of recurrent abortion by progesterone is based on the presumption that a substantial proportion of abortions is caused by progesterone deficiency. The presumption of progesterone deficiency was derived from the finding of low urinary pregnanediol, which now turns out to be a consequence, not a cause of abortion. The progesterone deficiency–low pregnanediol belief was discredited in a critical review by Goldzieher & Benigno as early as 1958. The introduction of synthetic oral progestogens lead to further experimental examination by double blind therapeutic trials, (Shearman & Garrett 1963 and Klopper & Macnaughton 1965) and there can be little doubt that progesterone deficiency is not a major cause of recurrent abortion.

Pregnanediol assays have been extensively applied as a measure of placental function in later pregnancy. Sufficient data have now accumulated from laboratories all over the world to make it possible to assess the value of this technique in a variety of placental malfunction states. As it is likely that pregnanediol excretion will vary with the cause of the placental malfunction, the findings in various common obstetric complications will be separately examined.

Pre-eclamptic toxaemia of pregnancy

The early crude techniques for urinary pregnanediol assay were soon brought into use to examine the state of placental function in this disease. Unfortunately, the technical problems were compounded by clinical naïvety. The early investigators seldom had adequate information about the normal values obtaining under their circumstances, and took little account of day to day variation. Most of the investigations were based on casual urine collections from poorly categorized material, and the results did not lend themselves to any critical statistical evaluation. At first the view of Smith & Smith (1948), that pregnanediol output was greatly reduced in toxaemia was more or less uncritically supported by other investigators. It was elaborated by de Watteville (1951) who claimed that the pregnanediol level was a good guide to foetal prognosis and by Borth (1954) who found a correlation between the urinary pregnanediol and the condition of the toxaemic infant at birth.

These conclusions have been modified by subsequent experience. Although it is still generally agreed that pregnanediol output tends to be low in toxaemia, this is not invariably the case. Strand (1966) found that the percentage of low values was much larger in toxaemic patients than in normal women but, even so, large numbers of toxaemic women had a pregnanediol output within the normal range; only 68 per cent of toxaemic patients having values below the lower limit of the normal range. As a guide to prognosis pregnanediol has proved much less reliable than was at first presumed. As early as 1955 Trolle pointed out that pregnanediol values could not be correlated with the severity of the toxaemia or with the outcome as regards foetal survival. Albeit often based on few cases the volume of criticism has swollen. Van der Molen & Hart (1961) could find no clear correlation with foetal prognosis and Coyle *et al.* (1962) found that in two patients with severe toxaemia the urinary pregnanediol levels gave no indication of impending foetal death.

A systematic investigation of pregnanediol excretion in toxaemia was published by Kankaanrinta in 1963. His survey presents the most reliable and critical evaluation to date in this field. It is based on adequate examination of the normal universe and systematic enquiry in a carefully categorized group of toxaemic women. He found that in mild pre-eclamptic toxaemia the pregnanediol fell to 60 per cent of the normal average. In view of the large range in the normal values this fall was not statistically significant. In mild pre-eclamptic toxaemia, even when a series of observations on each individual was taken into account, there was a notable variation between patients. Thus some patients had more than twice the mean toxaemic output while the lowest was 23 per cent of the toxaemic mean. In mild toxaemia there was still a tendency for pregnanediol excretion to rise with advancing gestation, but patients with severe toxaemia remained at a low level which, on the whole, was 51 per cent of the normal value. Even in severe pre-eclampsia the pregnanediol output was not consistently depressed. In severe pre-eclampsia, the values were also very variable. The co-efficient of variation was 32 per cent; more than twice as variable as the normal series. When severe and mild pre-eclampsia are considered together, the average values are just below the 95 per cent confidence limits of the normal range. There is a good deal of overlap between the normal and toxaemic values so that prediction in the individual case is hazardous. Serial observations are, of course, more helpful, but even here a falling output may be obscured by the high day to day variability. Although the effect of the disease on pregnanediol output can be more clearly discerned in the severer forms of toxaemia, there is no correlation between pregnanediol values and individual features of toxaemia. Thus there is no correlation with age, parity, body weight, blood pressure, proteinuria, oedema or urine volume.

Retarded intra-uterine foetal growth

Retardation of foetal growth is often associated with toxaemia and few authors make any effort to distinguish between underweight babies born to women with toxaemia and those from non-toxaemic mothers. Not surprisingly, therefore, the pattern of results in foetal retardation has been much the same as in toxaemia. An early enthusiastic advocate of the value of pregnanediol assay in foetal retardation was Rawlings, but his views have now become somewhat more tempered (Rawlings 1965), and he now believes that a rising or falling curve is of more prognostic value than the actual level.

In all measurements of placental function by hormone assay, the information gained by serial observations is a good deal more secure than the results of a single assay. This applies particularly to poor foetal growth where a failure of pregnanediol excretion to rise as gestation progresses correlates closely with the failure of the foetus to grow. This view is supported by the findings with a variety of assay techniques, including the most recent gas chromatographic methods (Brush *et al.*

1966). Whether, in fact, the excretion of urinary pregnanediol and the weight of the newborn baby are related, is open to question. In normal pregnancy many investigators have found a correlation between foetal weight and pregnanediol excretion, (Shearman 1959, Van der Molen & Hart 1961), while others are equally emphatic that the two are not related (Klopper & Billewicz 1963, Kankaanrinta 1963). The explanation may be that the very process which causes retardation of foetal growth will also depress pregnanediol output. Any series which contains a proportion of such retarded babies will produce a spurious correlation between foetal weight and pregnanediol by virtue of the fact that both are adversely affected by the unknown pathological cause of retardation.

Premature labour

The supposed causal relationship between progesterone production and the onset of premature labour has stimulated many investigators to look at pregnanediol excretion by these patients. Premature labour is probably due to a variety of causes, and it is unlikely that all would affect placental function and thereby pregnanediol output equally. The difficulties of etiological classification and of predicting who would go into premature labour have raised formidable problems which have not been satisfactorily solved. At most it can be said that some patients show dramatic falls in pregnanediol output shortly before going into premature labour.

Postmaturity

It has long been a subject of controversy whether a dangerous decline in placental function takes place in pregnancies which go past term. Pregnanediol assays would appear to be an admirable means to examine this question, but surprisingly few systematic studies have been published. All authors are agreed that the curve of pregnanediol output flattens off in the last few weeks of pregnancy, and most believe that it actually declines at term. The available data indicate that this decline continues after term, e.g. Strand (1966). A persistent fall in pregnanediol output constitutes a reasonable indication for termination of pregnancy in a woman past term.

Diabetes

At first high hopes were entertained of pregnanediol assays as a measure of placental function in diabetes. This view has had to be modified as better assay techniques and experimental designs were employed. In a patient who is desperately ill with severe or uncontrolled diabetes, or in one with superimposed toxaemia, pregnanediol output is often depressed, but on such occasions, the clinician hardly needs pregnanediol assays to read the signs of placental malfunction. A reliable measure of placental function is most needed in the well controlled diabetic liable to unheralded intra-uterine foetal death near term, and it is precisely in such cases that pregnanediol measurements may, upon occasion, give no warning of impending foetal death. Such patients often have bulky, immature placentae, and it is possible that this placental state compensates, as far as progesterone production is concerned, for the pathological process which leads to foetal death.

Rhesus incompatibility

The Rh incompatible pregnancy in an immunized woman is another obstetric situation where the clinician is much in need of a secure means of assessing the foeto-placental state. Klopper & Stephenson (1966) did serial pregnanediol assays in a group of immunised women. They found that there was no significant difference between the pregnanediol output in women bearing foetuses so severely affected as to require exchange transfusion after birth, and those whose babies were only mildly affected. The pregnanediol output in affected pregnancies ranged about the normal mean but showed a greater scatter, both above and below the average, than the range of normal. In Rh incompatible pregnancy, the steroidogenic process may be deranged but the effect is not consistent enough to be of use in assessing placental function. The placenta in such pregnancies is also notably bulky and immature, and it is possible that a similar process to that obtaining in diabetic pregnancy operated here.

Factors determining urinary pregnanediol output

Pregnanediol assays have proved less useful as a means of assessing placental function than at first hoped. In part this is due to the great variability in the excretion of the steroid, and in part this is due also to the fact that the processes which urinary pregnanediol represents are the consequences, not the cause of placental malfunction. Thus changes in pregnanediol output occur after the onset of placental malfunction and may coincide with, rather than precede, other consequences of placental malfunction, such as irretrievable placental damage or foetal death. As much as anything else, the failure of pregnanediol assay is due to the fact that we have little knowledge of what determines the amount of pregnanediol normally excreted. Pigeaud & Burthiault (1951) have adduced some evidence to show that pregnanediol excretion is lowered in renal disease, but the main weight of the evidence supports the view that the primary determinant of urinary pregnanediol is the amount of precursor produced by the foeto-placental unit. Pregnanediol output tends to be lower in conditions where it can be presumed that uterine blood flow is less, and it may be that utero-placental haemodynamics have a bearing on pregnanediol levels. But even here it is at least as likely that a reduced blood flow causes reduced precursor production as it is that the reduced flow impedes transport of formed material.

A critical problem in the control of pregnanediol output is the relative role of the foetus and the placenta. Until recently it was thought that progesterone production and metabolism proceeded in the placenta and mother only, and that the foetus played no part in the process. The urinary pregnanediol output therefore reflected only placental or maternal events, and foetal activity as such did not affect pregnanediol. This view was in part supported by the experiments of Cassmer (1959) who showed that when the foetus was killed by ligation of the cord, little change in pregnanediol output occurred as long as the placenta remained *in situ*. There was, however, a small drop, (20 per cent) in pregnanediol excretion; a finding later substantiated by Klopper *et al.* (1966) in studies done following the death of the foetus after intra-amniotic injection of hypertonic saline as a means of therapeutic abortion. It is possible, therefore, that at least 20 per cent of the pregnanediol in the mother's urine is of foetal origin. It will be evident from Chapter 5 that progesterone metabolism in the foeto-placental unit is the result of a complex interplay between foetus and placenta. Urinary pregnanediol reflects mainly, but not entirely, placental activity. The foetus plays some part, albeit quantitatively a lesser role, in determining how much pregnanediol is present in the mother's urine.

B.5 OESTROGEN ESTIMATION AS A MEASURE OF PLACENTAL FUNCTION

Although some 20 different oestrogens have been found in the urine of pregnant women, interest in the clinical applications of urinary assays has centred on one particular compound–oestriol. It is excreted in very large quantities during pregnancy as compared with the other oestrogens and is relatively easy to assay reliably. As far as non-pregnant women are concerned, oestriol is looked upon as a weakly active metabolite of more potent oestrogens, but in pregnancy new biosynthetic pathways peculiar to oestriol are opened so that the rise in oestriol production is disproportionately large. Nearly all the data on clinical applications of oestriol assay pertain to urinary studies but blood methods are now being evolved and more information is becoming available concerning the plasma levels of oestriol which occur during normal pregnancy. Although these techniques are yet in their infancy and we know little about the changes which may take place when foeto-placental function is affected, assays on blood have some advantages and are likely to be used more in the future. It is proposed therefore also briefly to mention blood assay techniques and results in considering the application of urinary determinations.

Methods of assay

Much of the value of an oestriol assay is dependent on the technique employed. The value of the best assay is vitiated by the high variability of the oestriol excretion from day to day in the same subject and from subject to subject. If to this disadvantage still has to be added an element of variability due to an unreliable method, a single estimation becomes almost useless.

The best methods are expensive in laboratory time, skill and equipment. Biochemists are constantly under pressure to evolve shorter, simpler methods. Many such short methods have been produced in the last decade, all sacrificing specificity for speed, and some notably unreliable in other respects. They are to be eschewed.

The biological oestrogen assay methods gave way to chemical techniques in the 1940's. One of the earliest methods to be widely applied was that of Jayle *et al.* (1943). This was followed in short order by the techniques of Stimmel (1946), Cohen & Bates (1947) and Jailer (1948). Compared to the sophisticated techniques of to-day, these methods are crude. They have all been superseded by the method of Brown (1955), later modified by Brown, Bulbrook & Greenwood (1957). This work has dominated the field for the last decade. It is still the standard technique today and most subsequent methods are based on it. Three other independent methods were evolved at roughly the same time as the Brown technique. They were published by Finkelstein (1952), Aitken & Preedy (1956) and Bauld (1956). They were all a good deal better than previous methods but have not gained the wide acceptance of the Brown method. Each has been applied to a number of investigations by their originators, but only one, (Finkelstein), was used to any extent in studies of placental function notably by workers in Europe and Israel.

The need for shorter, simpler methods of oestriol assay has led many investigators to attempt modifications of the Brown procedure. Those who set their reliability criteria reasonably high found themselves with methods not much different from the original procedure. This criticism may be applied to the techniques published by Eberlein *et al.* (1958) and later modified by Dale *et al.* (1965) and also to the methods of Taylor *et al.* (1961), of Klopper & Wilson (1962) and of Brown & Coyle (1963). The reliability criteria for these methods when applied to pregnancy urine are adequate. They give closely comparable results and the clinical application studies which have been done with them are acceptable. In the method devised by Frandsen (1963) the simplification is achieved by omitting all chromatography of the steroids. This probably involves an unacceptable sacrifice of specificity. This tendency is carried still further in the method of Ittrich (1958) in which all chemical purification is omitted; the Kober colour being directly developed from urine and subsequently extracted. This method has had a considerable vogue. It has a limited usefulness in following the day to day trend in a patient but designating these measurements as 'oestriol' as though they were comparable with the results of more laborious techniques is not warranted. A further short method pioneered by Wotiz & Martin (1962) involves the use of gas-liquid chromatography and seems very promising. Insufficient clinical application studies using such techniques have been published on which to form a judgment at the present time.

It seems unlikely that substantial improvements on the time taken to do a reliable urinary oestriol assay can be achieved. Each new technique, whatever its advantages, will still require a number of manipulations to sort the oestriol from the large spectrum of related substances in urine. The best that can be looked for is that when a urine specimen reaches the laboratory in the morning, the assay results are reported by the end of that working day. For certain kinds of clinical application a speedy answer is an essential requirement. For this purpose it seems more hopeful to set about a reduction of the time taken to collect the specimen rather than a shortening of the time spent in the laboratory. The coefficient of variability of repeated 24 hour urinary oestriol assays on the same subject is 27 per cent; for 48 hour urine collections it is 20 per cent

(Klopper 1964). A reduction in urine collection time is unpromising, the only other resort is fluids like blood or liquor amnii which can be sampled immediately.

The possible advantages which accrue from blood assays have engendered much pressure for the development of suitable methods. The initial stumbling block has been sensitivity. At best the concentration of oestriol in plasma is very much less than in urine and it is not practicable to take much more than 10 ml of blood for routine assays. Initial attempts to solve the problem of sensitivity involved the use of spectrophotometry on very small volumes of reagents (Roy & Brown 1960, Ittrich 1960), or of fluorimetry (Finkelstein 1952, Preedy & Aitken 1957, Ittrich 1960). Radio-isotope techniques have greatly advanced the possibilities of blood assays, and in one form or another are likely to be a *sine qua non* in future techniques. Radio-isotope methods have been used in two ways; either as double isotope dilution methods which, as designed by Svendson (1960), use fully the tremendous increase of sensitivity inherent in the technique but are laborious, inconvenient and demand high skill; or simple radio-isotope internal standards which use non-radio-active endpoints and are either applicable only to free oestrogens (Ichii *et al.* 1963) or else involve the use of labelled conjugates not available to the ordinary investigator (Nachtigall *et al.* 1966). The most promising development in blood assay techniques appears to be a combination of a radio-active internal standard and a gas chromatographic endpoint. The work of Wotiz & Martin (1962) might well form a starting point in this respect. Other gas chromatographic methods have been published by Touchstone & Murawec (1965) and by Kroman *et al.* (1966). It has not been sufficiently realized that blood is not a fluid to which urinary methods can be applied without change. More exacting purification techniques are necessary to achieve adequate specificity and the virtue of a gas chromatographic endpoint lies in its sensitivity, not in any presumed capacity to spare the investigator the labour of extensive purification. Elaborate purification involves large variable losses of steroid which can only be compensated for by the use of a radioactive internal standard and by gas chromatography to read the minute quantities of final residue.

Oestriol levels in normal pregnancy

Accurate information about the values obtaining in normal pregnancy is a *sine qua non* for the use of oestriol assays as a measure of placental

TABLE 9.1

Normal urinary oestriol excretion in the second half of pregnancy (mg per 24 hours)

	Authors									
Weeks pregnant	Taylor *et al.* 1961	Frandsen *et al.* 1966	Klopper *et al.* 1963	Hobkirk *et al.* 1962	Ittrich *et al.* 1959	Brown 1956	Würtele 1963	Coyle *et al.* 1963	Zondek *et al.* 1959	Average
20	—	6·1	5·6	5·0	5·2	—	—	—	—	—
21	—	6·2	6·7	4·6	—	—	—	—	—	—
22	4·0	7·9	7·6	9·5	—	—	—	—	4·2	—
23	—	7·7	9·4	—	—	—	—	—	—	—
24	4·2	8·7	10·0	8·2	8·5	—	—	—	5·0	—
25	—	10·2	10·6	5·9	—	—	—	—	—	—
26	7·3	10·4	13·0	10·5	—	—	—	—	—	—
27	—	11·6	13·8	—	—	—	—	10·5	—	—
28	5·6	11·9	13·0	9·8	12·5	—	—	10·8	6·8	10·1
29	—	12·0	14·7	—	—	—	—	12·4	—	—
30	8·8	14·0	15·2	9·6	—	—	—	12·5	—	—
31	—	13·5	15·2	13·5	—	—	—	12·7	—	—
32	10·6	13·6	17·5	13·0	24·4	—	12·4	13·3	8·4	14·2
33	—	16·8	18·1	—	—	—	—	14·3	—	—
34	11·3	18·6	18·8	12·6	—	—	—	16·3	—	—
35	—	21·6	22·6	14·7	—	—	—	16·2	—	—
36	16·8	22·1	23·4	19·5	20·6	28·0	17·1	19·7	11·0	19·8
37	—	25·9	28·6	22·1	—	26·0	—	19·8	—	—
38	18·1	23·4	31·3	15·0	—	32·0	—	20·0	—	—
39	—	29·7	33·3	31·2	—	—	—	21·6	—	—
40	15·7	29·8	34·5	19·4	37·2	29·0	19·3	23·1	—	26·0
41	—	24·7	33·2	—	—	—	—	25·0	—	—

function. It is not enough to know the normal range recorded by other investigators using the same method; there should be a small test series on normal subjects done by every laboratory for comparison with published results before embarking on studies of abnormal pregnancy.

As might be expected the normal values in the early studies varied according to the method used. In recent years the values in different publications have been very similar, whatever the assay technique used. Although a great many normal oestriol studies have now been published, it is not possible to prepare an accurate comprehensive list of normal values because few authors have published tabulated data as well as mean curves. Table 9.1 has been constructed from a few recent publications in which figures were given.

Any method giving mean normal values much different from the averages listed in Table 9.1 should be critically examined.

The mean excretion figures give no impression of the large individual scatter of normal values. In the few publications where statistical data such as standard deviations are given the coefficient of variation works out at around 30 per cent in all the series. There is no consistent change in variability during the course of gestation, so that a value has to be at least 60 per cent below the normal means listed in Table 9.1 before it can be said to be lower than the 95 per cent probability range. This emphasizes the value of serial assays as compared with a single observation, but even here the means of repeated assays in different individuals still show considerable scatter.

When blood oestriol levels are considered there is less unanimity concerning mean normal values. Some mean figures culled from recent publications are shown in Table 9.2. It is generally agreed that oestriol concentrations are a good deal higher in the foetal than in the maternal circulation. The spread of *mean* values in peripheral maternal blood is discouraging. There is a 7-fold difference between the highest and lowest recorded mean concentrations. To some extent the differences are methodological and are an indication that assay techniques are being applied before they are adequate for their purpose, but the results do not augur well for the usefulness of blood assays in clinical applications. No final verdict is possible until a reliable assay method is developed and applied to a thorough study of day-to-day and patient-to-patient variation in normal subjects to provide a basis for the evaluation of results in obstetric disease. It is to be hoped that such a programme will be applied to the promising new gas chromatographic and radioisotope techniques

TABLE 9.2

Blood oestriol levels at term pregnancy (All figures are in μg per 100 ml plasma)

Source of blood	Authors									
	Schild *et al.* 1963	Kubli *et al.* 1963	Keller *et al.* 1963	Wodrig *et al.* 1964	Aitken *et al.* 1958	Klausner *et al.* 1964	Roy 1962	Troen *et al.* 1961	Slaunwhite *et al.* 1959	Oertel *et al.* 1959
Cord vein	51·2	—	—	—	—	89·0	55·0	—	—	—
Cord artery	45·1	—	—	—	—	94·8	54·0	—	—	—
Mixed cord blood	24·9	—	49·2	16·5	134·3	—	49·0	49·9	—	—
Retro-placental	18·5	—	28·8	—	—	18·0	—	—	—	—
Maternal venous	13·0	9·3	8·8	9·6	21·0	11·2	9·2	—	6·1	2·9

now being evolved. If maternal blood levels are reasonably stable under normal circumstances and do not change significantly until foeto-placental function deteriorates, a great advance in assessment of placental function will have been achieved. It is, however, imperative that methods should be accurate and specific, and that present doubts concerning the degree of protein binding, the efficacy of extraction and hydrolysis procedures, the uptake of oestriol by red cells and whether to measure free, conjugated or total oestriol should be resolved before assays are applied to an extensive study of the normal universe, and to strictly defined categories of patients with abnormalities of foeto-placental function.

A further possibility remains to be explored. One of the attractions of blood oestriol assays is that they carry the investigation one stage nearer the foetus than the mother's urine. It is tempting to try to sample the foetal environment more directly. Foetal blood cannot be tested until delivery, but amniocentesis is now approaching the status of a routine procedure and repeated sampling of the liquor amnii is now feasible. The amniotic fluid contains a high concentration of oestriol but there is no evidence on whether liquor concentrations reflect foetal blood levels. If the two are at all rapidly equilibrated, tests on liquor may become of prime importance in the assessment of foeto-placental function.

Oestrogen production in the foeto-placental unit

The biosynthetic pathways for oestrogen synthesis are discussed in full by Diczfalusy & Mancuso in Chapter 4 and will not be considered here. The oestriol in the mother's urine gets there as a result of metabolic processes in the foeto-placental unit. Alterations in foetal metabolism are a very likely cause of changes in maternal urinary oestriol output. It is therefore necessary briefly to consider some of the normal metabolic processes which may have a bearing on urinary levels.

The concept that neither the foetus nor the placenta are of themselves complete endocrine organs but that their combined activity is required for oestriol synthesis has been clearly established by the Diczfalusy school in Stockholm. Here and elsewhere the steps by which oestriol is made from neutral steroid precursors have been worked out one by one. Some of these steps, e.g. hydroxylation at C16 or sulphurylation, can only be done in the foetus. Others, like aromatization of C5–6 unsaturated steroids happen only in the placenta, while other steps are carried out at both sites. Maternal urinary oestriol therefore reflects metabolic processes in both foetus and placenta and is apt to be affected by pathological changes in either.

A further metabolic factor which is likely to have some bearing on maternal urinary levels is the supply of raw material for oestriol synthesis. The investigations of Frandsen & Stakemann (1963a) and (1964) have pointed to the possibility that oestriol is synthesized from precursors produced by the foetal adrenal. It is therefore possible that a fall in maternal urinary oestriol may be due to a decline in precursor production by the foetal adrenal. Alternatively, pathological processes may affect any of the subsequent steps. There is very little information about what factors control these biosynthetic steps or by what mechanisms pathological processes exert their effects, but some speculations on clinical grounds might be permissible. It is possible that the rate of maternal blood flow through the uterus has an important bearing on the amount of oestriol being delivered to the maternal circulation. A number of observations can be marshalled in support of this view. Uterine blood flow is known to be reduced in pre-eclamptic toxaemia, (Browne & Veall 1953) a condition also accompanied by lowered oestriol output. The oestriol level rises when a normal pregnant woman is put to bed (Roy 1962), possibly as a result of improved uterine blood flow. The effect of uterine blood flow need not be a purely mechanical consequence of reduced outflow from the oestriol pool in the foeto-placental unit. This is likely to be corrected by a raised oestriol concentration in the blood draining from the uterus. If uterine blood flow has an effect on oestriol production it is more likely to exert this by way of a reduced input of factors concerned in oestriol synthesis, such as oxygen. It must be acknowledged that in the last resort we do not know what foetal factors affect oestriol production, but many parallels can be drawn between foetal oxygenation and oestriol production. Cassmer (1959), suggested reduced oxygenation as the cause of the rapid fall in oestriol when the cord is ligated. Many authors are agreed that oestriol output is reduced when intra-uterine foetal growth is retarded; a state supposed often to be associated with reduced foetal oxygenation. Some authors have gone further and claimed that the weight of a normal foetus at birth and the preceding maternal oestriol output is related (Frandsen & Stakemann 1960, Beling 1967), but others have failed to find such a correlation (Klopper & Billewicz 1963, Turnbull *et al.* 1967). Normal foetal growth is the outcome of many factors and it is inherently unlikely that there is a single dominant one simultaneously operative on growth and oestriol production.

The concentration of oestriol is very much higher in the foetal than in the maternal circulation. It clearly does not cross the placenta by simple diffusion, and placental transmission may have an important bearing on maternal urinary output. It is tacitly assumed that maternal urinary excretion reflects production in the foeto-placental unit and clinical experience bears this out, but it is still possible that in particular situations, placental transmission may play a definitive role. Oestriol in the foetus is very largely in the form of oestriol sulphate (Troen *et al.* 1961). Klausner & Ryan (1964) found that, on the other hand, oestriol in the placenta is present mainly as the free compound. The sequence of events as traced by successive investigations of the Stockholm school is that foetal oestriol sulphate is conveyed to the placenta which is rich in sulphatase. It is hydrolysed in the placenta and part of the free compound transmitted to the maternal circulation. In the maternal organism it is reconjugated and excreted as the glucosiduronate. The possibility therefore arises that measurements of maternal oestriol output may be little more than indirect measurements of placental sulphatase. It is unlikely that placental sulphatase will be the only, or indeed a dominating, factor in determining oestriol output in conditions of impaired placental function, but it is an interesting speculation that this may be the mechanism by which the supply of free oestriol to the myometrium is controlled. If retroplacental oestriol concentration has any role in the onset of labour, this may be the key by which the foeto-placental unit eventually unlocks the door of its shelter.

Oestriol conjugation may be of some significance in placental function in another respect. The oestriol in the mother's urine is conjugated either at C_3 or C16 or in both positions. The substitution may be either with glucosiduronate or with sulphate. A number of these conjugates have been isolated in urine and there is evidence that the pattern of urinary oestriol conjugates changes during the course of gestation (Beling 1960). It is not known what such a change in pattern signifies, nor whether any specific alterations take place when placental function is affected. It may be that studies of particular fractions of urinary oestriol will give a much more definitive assessment of placental function in certain obstetric diseases. In blood, where oestriol may be free, protein bound, or conjugated, one is still more at a loss to know which is the physiologically significant fraction.

The process which eventually leads to oestriol in the maternal urine is a complex one, and there are many points at which it may be affected.

It is unlikely that all obstetric diseases will act in the same manner at the same points. It is necessary to consider oestriol assays as a test of placental function, not in the overall view, but in terms of individual obstetric diseases. In many instances, e.g. retarded intra-uterine foetal growth, obstetric disease is poorly categorized, and a single classification may embrace several entities. If we are to come to a critical evaluation of oestriol assays it is essential that the diseases under study be as rigorously defined as possible.

Oestriol excretion in prolonged pregnancy

An acceptable definition of prolonged pregnancy would be a pregnancy which extends more than 14 days beyond 280 days from the last menstrual period in a woman who previously had a regular 28 day cycle. It is a matter of controversy whether prolongation of pregnancy without any pathological features is dangerous to the foetus, and therefore worthy of special measures. The simple time definition surely includes a number of diverse entities. Sometimes the dating may be in error. At any stage in pregnancy oestriol assays are only of use if the gestation is accurately known, as the oestriol value for the subject has to be set against the normal range for that stage. The spread of values in the last eight weeks of pregnancy is so large that oestriol assays are useless as a means of assessing maturity. One woman may excrete as much oestriol at 32 weeks as another does at term. Several investigators have studied the changes in blood and urinary oestriol in the last few days of pregnancy and after the onset of labour (Kubli & Keller 1963, Ittrich *et al.* 1962, Zondek & Pfeifer 1959). Although Lundwall & Stakemann (1966) have suggested that oestriol output falls once contractions begin, all authors are agreed that there is no consistent change preceding labour, and changes of oestriol output in prolonged pregnancy should not be ascribed to imminent labour.

There is sound evidence that one of the entities associated with prolonged pregnancy is post-maturity. Its clinical features such as reduced liquor amnii, meconium staining and desquamation of superficial skin in a large infant, have often been described. It is a condition associated with a high perinatal mortality, and it is therefore important that means be devised to distinguish it from simple prolonged pregnancy. It is here that oestriol assays can play a vital part.

Two groups of investigators have done serial oestriol assays in prolonged pregnancy. Smith *et al.* (1966) examined 67 such patients and

Lundwall & Stakemann (1966) studied 171 patients. The latter had sufficient data to consider separately such factors as parity and degree of prolongation of pregnancy. Both groups found some patients with low or falling oestriol output, and some with a normal excretion. Their conclusions were similar. As long as oestriol output remained normal, the babies were well, while there was a high concentration of perinatal morbidity and mortality in the babies of patients with a low oestriol output. If labour is induced on account of low oestriol output alone, a fair proportion of the babies born will be normal and healthy and might well have been left longer *in utero*.

There can be little doubt that prolonged pregnancy is a clinical situation where oestriol assay can be of great value. It is less easy to decide what constitutes lowering of oestriol output in this situation. In part, the answer depends on what view is taken of normal oestriol output after term. There is little doubt that it continues to rise sharply until term. Does it continue to rise thereafter, or does it flatten out, or even fall? Lundwall & Stakemann found a continuing rise in the absence of the postmaturity syndrome, and therefore set their lower normal limit in prolonged pregnancy high, – 16 mg per 24 hours. Smith *et al.* made it lower, – 12 mg. Zondek & Pfeifer made their criterion a dynamic one and suggested a drop of 60 per cent from the previous value was a strong indication to proceed to delivery. To some extent all these absolute values derived from other circumstances are misleading, and the obstetrician is well advised to evolve his own criterion in the light of local findings. As good a rule of thumb as any other would be two successive falls, whatever the absolute values. Of course complications, such as toxaemia, with prolonged pregnancy constitute a strong indication for induction of labour, irrespective of the oestriol output. When induction is undertaken on grounds of oestriol output, it is wise to do so by rupture of the membranes, and if the liquor is meconium stained to proceed directly to Caesarean section. Used with discrimination, and set against the whole clinical picture, there is no doubt that oestriol assays are of great value in the management of prolonged pregnancy.

Oestriol excretion with retarded foetal growth

Retardation of foetal growth *in utero* is an entity which is attracting more and more attention from obstetricians. It is associated with a high perinatal mortality which, as other more easily dealt with causes of foetal death are disposed of, has resulted in retarded foetal growth becoming a more prominent component of perinatal mortality. For purposes of definition it is generally accepted that a birth weight more than two standard deviations below the mean weight for the stage of gestation constitutes growth retardation. In practice this means a birth weight of less than 2,500 g ($5\frac{1}{2}$ lb) at term. Of course, a good many babies are born weighing less than 2,500 g. According to Gruenwald (1964), two thirds such cases are normally grown babies prematurely expelled from the uterus. Premature birth and growth retardation are probably separate entities and it is a matter of importance to distinguish between them in considering their effect on oestriol output. Even when prematurity is excluded, retarded foetal growth probably comprises several discrete conditions and it would be well to try and distinguish between them. One author to have done so is Michie (1968), who considered separately oestriol excretion in retarded foetal growth in pregnancies complicated by hypertension and those without raised blood pressure. She studied 38 pregnant women whose babies were thought to be growth retarded on clinical grounds. Twenty-two of these were found at birth to have weights within the normal range, although less than average. Three of these had a depressed oestriol output, while of the remaining 16 women with proven retarded foetal growth, nine had a low oestriol output.

Many authors writing on this subject have not sought to define specific factors in growth retardation or to pursue generalizations of the pattern of oestriol excretion which might be encountered but have contented themselves with 'typical examples' from their experience, frequently under the vague diagnosis of 'placental insufficiency'. Notable among such studies are the publications of Zondek & Pfeifer (1959), Banerjea (1962), Bentele (1963) and Bell *et al.* (1964). Publication of 'typical cases' implies a selection of material and leaves the reader to wonder how many cases were disregarded on what grounds. Frequently, the data consist of varying numbers of serial assays on patients at different stages of pregnancy which are difficult to render into a uniform format with means and standard deviations. If, however, oestriol assays are to be fully exploited in the assessment of placental function, it is essential to have a clearly defined picture of how the spread of values in a particular disease differs from the normal universe.

Nearly all authors are agreed that there is a tendency for oestriol output to be reduced when foetal growth is retarded. There is less unanimity about how frequently normal oestriol values may occur when retardation of foetal growth is present, or low values when growth is normal. As for the latter, it may reasonably be supposed that when serial assays are done very few consistently low values will be found when the stage of gestation can be accurately fixed. As regards the former, Frandsen & Stakemann (1963b) found that four out of 32 women with normal oestriol output gave birth to babies weighing less than 2,500 g. Klopper (1966) found a very similar result, three out of 37 women with retarded babies having an oestriol output in the normal range. Yousem *et al.* (1966) record one out of 12 patients with retarded foetal growth having a normal oestriol value. It can therefore be accepted that roughly 10 per cent of patients with retarded foetal growth have an oestriol output within the normal range. It should be realized that one is here dealing with a continuous spectrum of values from normal to abnormal in two respects. Firstly, normal foetal growth shades into retardation; the lower limits of normal birthweight are reasonable criteria but will certainly not discriminate between normal and abnormal in every case. Secondly, the normal range of oestriol excretion is similarly a statistical limitation which cannot cover every contingency. Almost all normal oestriol values in retarded growth are less than average and fall in the grey border between normal and abnormal. It may be of some interest to examine the characteristics of this twilight zone. Klopper (1965) tried to do so by examining the oestriol output of a group of women who gave birth to babies of less than average birthweight and within 10 per cent of the lower limit of the normal range. This corresponds to the group of patients having babies less than 6½ lb examined by Coyle & Brown (1963). Both conclude that, although many more oestriol values fell in the normal range than with frankly retarded foetal growth, there was still a significant tendency for oestriol output to be reduced in these intermediate cases. The interpretation of results in these cases is a matter for controversy. Many authors, notably Coyle & Brown (1963), Frandsen (1963) and Beling (1967), contend that there is a close correlation between foetal weight and oestriol excretion in normal pregnancy, while Klopper & Billewicz (1963) found that no such relationship existed and believe that retarded foetal growth and low oestriol output are both secondary effects of a pathological state in the foeto-placental unit which is not present in normal pregnancy.

Several authors have defined the limits of oestriol excretion at various stages of gestation, below which retardation of foetal growth might confidently be anticipated. Most content themselves with a value more than two standard deviations below the mean. Jayle *et al.* (1965) regard a value less than 25 per cent of the mean as being in the zone of severe oestrogen deficiency. Others offer absolute values. Yousem *et al.* (1966) put the lower limit of normal in late pregnancy as 7 mg, while MacLeod *et al.* (1967) give the limits as below 8 mg at 28–32 weeks and below 12 mg at 38–41 weeks.

Although it is generally agreed that oestriol output is almost always reduced when growth of the foetus is retarded, clinicians differ about how useful these assays are in diagnosis and treatment. Booth *et al.* (1965) found that when oestriol was low, the growth retardation was clinically obvious, and oestriol assays were not of value. Others are less confident of the clinical diagnosis and find oestriol assay useful in distinguishing an 'at risk' group. Klopper (1965), for instance, had 125 patients in his series who were diagnosed on clinical grounds as having retarded foetal growth, but only 34 gave birth to babies more than two standard deviations below the mean birthweight. Martin & Hahnel (1964) found no difference between the oestriol output of mothers with retarded babies who succumbed and those who survived, but they are alone in considering oestriol assays to be of no value in the treatment of the condition. Most clinicians have found the assay to be of great value in deciding when delivery should be effected and there seems little doubt that if used with discretion serial assays can be a potent factor in reducing foetal wastage in this condition. The use of *serial* assays is of crucial importance in this context. For instance, both premature and retarded babies may cause a low oestriol output by the mother. Prematures are very likely to die if delivered, while retarded babies will survive (North 1966). Premature babies show a rising oestriol output, indicating that they may safely be left *in utero*, while retarded babies show a flat or falling curve as their uterine environment becomes dangerous.

The present dearth of information concerning the process which leads to a lowering of oestriol output in retarded growth, detracts from the value of the assay. In some way the oestriol output appears to be bound up with foetal growth but we do not know whether it reflects events in the placenta or in the foetus or both. Klopper & Billewicz (1963) speculated that the late pregnancy rise in oestriol output was essentially a foetal process superimposed on a relatively static placental production and both Klopper (1965) and Coyle & Brown (1963) noted that the essential feature of oestriol output in retarded growth was the absence of this late pregnancy, presumably foetal, rise. These suggestions do not, however, dispose of the attractive hypothesis that the primary fault is one of placental transmission, or due to inadequate maternal uterine circulation. It seems likely that all three factors–foetal, placental, and maternal –may be concerned to a greater or lesser extent in different subjects. In terms of the biosynthesis of oestriol in the foeto-placental unit, a number of points at which the defect may be operative, can be suggested. Among likely mechanisms are: (1) A lack of precursor steroid, (dehydroepiandrosterone sulphate, or pregnenolone sulphate), from the foetal adrenal. (2) A failure of C16 hydroxylating enzyme system in the foetal liver. (3) A failure of placental sulphatase which is essential to speedy placental transmission of oestriol. Such mechanisms are, at present, entirely hypothetical; but the hypotheses have the attraction of being capable of experimental verification. If, for instance, the mechanism is a sulphatase defect, the low urinary oestriol glucosiduronate will be associated with high oestriol sulphate levels in liquor and in the foetal circulation. The possibility of dynamic tests of oestrogen biosynthesis or of placental transmission by injecting dehydroepiandrosterone sulphate or oestriol sulphate into the liquor amnii is an intriguing one and is being explored in several centres.

In summary there is good evidence that oestriol output is almost invariably reduced when foetal growth is retarded; that oestriol assays are helpful in arriving at a diagnosis which may be difficult on clinical grounds alone; that serial assays provide a good basis for assessing the results of treatment and deciding when delivery should take place.

Oestriol excretion in pre-eclamptic toxaemia

Retardation of foetal growth is often associated with toxaemia, particularly when it is of long duration. It is generally agreed that in such cases, oestriol output is reduced. It is less easy to determine whether toxaemia of itself can result in a reduced oestriol output. In order to resolve this, some categorization of toxaemia is necessary. Many classifications according to the degree of hypertension and the presence or amount of albuminuria have been put forward. For the present purpose, it matters little precisely where the lines are drawn. The different grades of severity shade into one another and so do the changes in oestriol output. Any system which separates toxaemia into mild or severe categories will also delimit roughly two universes of oestriol excretion. In addition, the effect of pre-existing essential hypertension needs to be separately considered.

The picture of oestriol excretion in mild toxaemia is not a clear one. Most authors, like Würtele (1962) find no very great change from normal.

Kellar *et al.* (1959) noted a wider scatter than normal. Some findings, published by Klopper (1965), are shown in Fig. 9.2.

Although there is a downward trend, most values fall within the normal range and the reduction is most marked and occurs most frequently when there is also retardation of foetal growth.

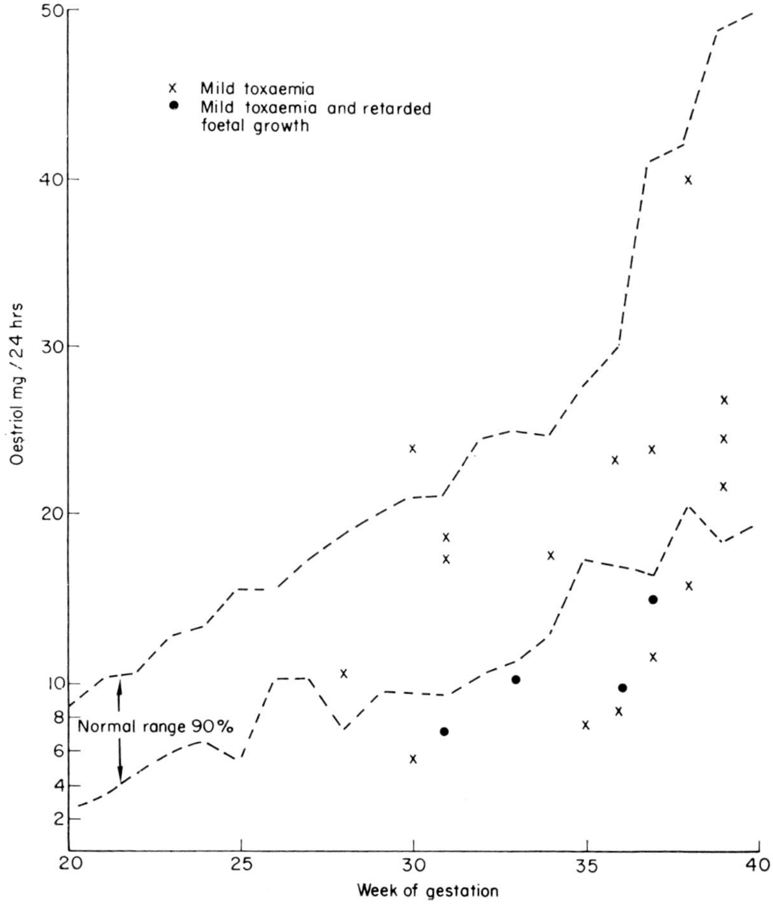

FIG. 9.2. Oestriol excretion in mild pre-eclampsia.

Taylor and his colleagues in 1958 pointed out that, in toxaemia, the oestriol output is reduced according to the severity of the disease, and many authors have since confirmed this claim. There is less agreement about what proportion of patients with severe toxaemia show a reduced output or what levels indicate a dangerous impairment of function in toxaemia. Lenters (1958) found that with blood pressures between 130/80 and 160/100, 42 per cent of subjects have an oestriol excretion in the normal range. Strand (1966) found that all subjects with toxaemia had an oestriol output below average and 74·5 per cent were below the normal limit, while Würtele (1962) found only 50 per cent of subjects with severe toxaemia had an oestriol excretion below the normal limit.

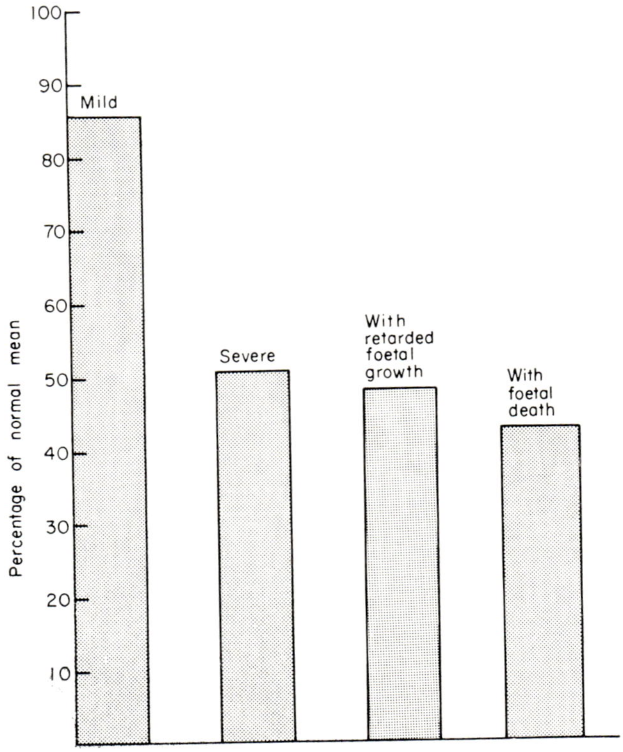

FIG. 9.3. Oestriol excretion in various categories of toxaemia.

It is of interest to know not only what proportion of patients have a reduction in oestriol output but also what the average excretion in toxaemia is. The average excretion in various categories of toxaemia was calculated by Klopper (1965) and his findings are shown in Fig. 9.3.

For the purposes of this figure the oestriol excretion of each patient was calculated as a percentage of the mean normal excretion for the stage of gestation and the percentages in each category then averaged. The reduction in mild toxaemia is slight, averaging 85 per cent of normal while in severe toxaemia, the average is 51 per cent of normal. This is in contrast with the findings of Timonen & Hirvonen (1964) who found no oestriol reduction in severe toxaemia at term. When toxaemia is complicated by retarded foetal growth, or in those patients who eventually lose their baby from retarded growth or other effects of toxaemia, the average output is slightly less than in severe toxaemia. In the group which ended in foetal death, all the values were taken seven to ten days before the intra-uterine death. If the readings had been taken closer to the death, a more dramatic reduction in mean oestriol might have been expected.

TABLE 9.3

Danger levels of oestriol output in toxaemia

Reference	Level of oestriol indicating impending foetal death (mg per 24 hour urine)
Lenters (1958)	12 mg
Zondek & Pfieffer (1959)	1–3 mg
Ten Berge (1961)	10 mg
Furuhjelm (1962)	7·5 mg
Würtele (1962)	2–5 mg
McLeod *et al.* (1967)	12 mg

When using oestriol output to monitor foeto-placental function in toxaemia, some criterion of danger level is a *sine qua non*. Various authors differ in what they regard as levels indicating impending foetal death. To some extent this is a methodological difference but the best modern techniques give very similar results and the nub of the question is the limits which are assigned to the grey zone between the lower end of the normal range and the results when the foetus has died. This will depend on the data which an author has on his normal range and the care and sophistication with which toxaemic patients have been categorised and the results analysed. A few of the figures which have been suggested are recorded in Table 9.3.

Personal experience suggests that few babies die while the oestriol output is above 5 mg per 24 hours, but that such low levels may be close to foetal death and that in toxaemia after 37 weeks, a value below 8 mg is a signal for rapid delivery. As in other types of obstetric disease, serial oestriol estimations are of much more value in toxaemia as they reflect changes in the foeto-placental state.

While the findings in mild toxaemia may be equivocal nearly all authors are agreed that in severe toxaemia, oestriol output is usually reduced. Both Würtele (1962) and Beling (1967) point out that a normal excretion may, on occasion be found when the toxaemia is of short duration. Indeed, in toxaemia, almost any kind of result may be recorded, depending on what type of patient is selected and when in the course of the disease the readings are taken. Toxaemia is a dynamic condition and often responds to treatment. If the question being investigated is whether oestriol output is reduced in toxaemia then only values from patients immediately after admission to hospital, before the picture is blurred by the effects of treatment, should be considered. On the other hand, if the point at issue is whether oestriol output can be used as a measure of foetal vitality in toxaemia, then serial studies would seem to be best suited to the purpose.

The crux of the matter is how useful oestriol assays are for the control of treatment in clinical practice. Booth *et al.* (1965) were not enthusiastic. They felt that any fall in oestriol output was usually accompanied by obvious clinical signs which would warn the obstetrician of increasing danger to the foetus. They also found a poor correlation between oestriol levels and the outcome of the pregnancy; the oestriol might be low on occasions when the foetus survived and normal or rising when the foetal state was deteriorating. MacLeod *et al.* (1967) came to the opposite conclusion. They found a close correlation between oestriol levels and the foetal state and decided that oestriol assays were a most useful means of monitoring the foetal state. Most other workers agree more or less with this favourable assessment of the value of oestriol assays. A personal finding is that they are valuable in proportion to the degree of supervision of the patients, the closeness of the link between ward and laboratory, the number and duration of urine collections and the degree to which oestriol values are taken in conjunction with the day-to-day clinical findings.

Since the use of oestriol assays was first introduced by Zondek, a slow change of attitude concerning these tests has come about. The first workers thought they were measuring an entirely placental activity and concentrated their attention on comparisons between oestriol excretion and the placental state. Indeed, Lenters' thesis in 1958 was devoted completely to this aspect and by detailed examinations of placentae from toxaemic mothers he was able to demonstrate that there was a correlation between the findings on microscopic examination of the placenta and urinary oestriol. The point was pursued by Taylor *et al.* (1958) who, although they assumed that the basic pathology lay in the placenta, also studied the clearance of radio-active sodium from the uterus and wondered whether the reduction of uterine blood flow did not play a part in the lowered oestriol output. It is widely believed that reduced uterine blood flow is a feature of toxaemia. It is difficult to see how this could be a direct cause of reduced oestriol output. Unless there was a concomitant fall in oestriol production, there would presumably be a formidable build-up of oestriol on the foetal side. A reduced uterine blood flow could act by lowering oestriol production by impairment of the supply of oxygen or other essentials for the biogenesis of the steroid. It is an attractive hypothesis to assume that reduced uterine blood flow may be the common factor linking retarded growth and low oestriol excretion.

Würtele (1963) also directed his attention to placental damage as the cause of the fall in oestriol output in toxaemia and is, indeed, one of the few workers to have found a correlation between placental weight and oestriol output. He was, however, aware of the work of Cassmer (1959) and considered the role of the foetal circulation but mistakenly assumed that this effect was exerted via the oxygenation of the placenta without considering the possibility that essential foetal steps in oestriol biogenesis might be affected. Further attempts to seek a correlation between the state of the placenta and the oestriol output were undertaken by Breborowicz, Krzywinska & Pisarski (1965). They found a low correlation between oestriol excretion and placental weight but were unable to demonstrate any correlation between oestriol levels and the amount of degenerative change in the placenta nor with the amount of syncytium present in it. Their histological analysis was not nearly as detailed as that of Lenters and the oestriol assays were done by a crude method which could only have given a very rough approximation of the amount of the steroid in the urine. It is fair to say that there is no clear evidence linking placental state and oestriol level in toxaemia and the tentative conclusion may be drawn that the cause of the decreased oestriol production must be sought in the foetus rather than the placenta.

A few workers have addresssed themselves to the question of the role played by hypertension in the lowered oestriol output of toxaemia. Klopper (1966) studied 11 patients with essential hypertension, seven of whom later developed a superimposed toxaemia. He found that a fall in oestriol output did not occur until toxaemic signs appeared and concluded that high blood pressure *per se*, was not the cause of the depressed oestriol level.

A further possibility concerning oestriol excretion in toxaemia which needs to be considered is that the lowered output may not be a reflection, so much of lowered production in the foeto-placental unit as a failure of maternal renal function. Brown *et al.* (1964) have shown that oestriol is excreted by tubular secretion as well as by glomerular filtration. It is therefore possible that in part, the lowered urinary oestriol is due to impaired renal function. This possibility is also raised by the work of Taylor *et al.* (1963) who found oestriol excretion to be lowered in six patients with pyelonephritis. There is, however, no evidence of an accumulation of oestriol in the maternal circulation as might be expected if the lowered urinary content were due to impaired excretion, and many toxaemic subjects with low oestriol show no evidence of a renal lesion, while others with overt renal malfunction have a normal oestriol excretion.

A further central question concerning oestriol excretion in toxaemia remains unresolved. This is whether the oestriol decline plays a part in the causation of the toxaemia or any of its manifestations. If this were so, it might be expected that the drop in oestriol output would precede the onset of the toxaemia. A number of workers have recorded more or less casual examples of a fall in oestriol preceding the onset of toxaemia. This was noted by Brown (1960) and by Jayle *et al.* (1965). A systematic investigation of this point was undertaken by Klopper (1966). He assayed the oestriol output of 19 subjects who later developed toxaemia. His findings are recorded in Table 9.4.

TABLE 9.4

Oestriol excretion prior to onset of toxaemia

Stage of gestation (weeks)	No. of subjects	Normal value mean and S.D. (mg per 24 hour)	Pre-toxaemic value (mg per 24 hour)	Percentage of normal
13	3	0·58 ± 0·25	0·41	71
20	7	5·59 ± 1·93	3·70	66
30	5	15·21 ± 3·49	14·14	93
34	4	18·82 ± 3·57	12·25	65

Although the average values are below the normal mean for the corresponding stage of pregnancy, there is not a significant depression of oestriol output. The point is more convincingly demonstrated in Table 9.5 which shows the oestriol excretion in a further four subjects for whom values both before and after the onset of toxaemic signs are available.

TABLE 9.5

Oestriol excretion before and after onset of toxaemia

Subject	Value before onset of toxaemia (percentage of normal)	Value after onset of toxaemia (percentage of normal)
NW	101	75
MT	93	81
IS	129	115
CM	65	50
Average	97	80

There is no clear evidence that the reduction of oestriol output has any aetiological significance in toxaemia. It is a more reasonable assumption that both the toxaemic signs and the fall in oestriol output are reflections of an underlying disease process affecting the foeto-placental unit.

Oestriol excretion in association with intra-uterine foetal death

Two problems in particular have interested investigators in relation to oestriol assays in intra-uterine foetal death. The first concerns the possibility of being able to predict by means of oestriol assay when foetal death is imminent and the second is the use of the assays to determine whether foetal death has taken place.

Although much care has been devoted to ascertaining what level of oestriol excretion indicates impending death and how long before foetal death such levels may occur, the necessity to consider such values in the light of the underlying disease leading to the foetal death has not been realized. A foetus may die from a great variety of causes and it is unlikely that they will all affect oestriol production equally or for the same length of time beforehand, yet few authors have categorized their intra-uterine deaths by cause. There is little doubt that in the common causes of intra-uterine death such as toxaemia, retarded intra-uterine growth or foetal abnormality, the impending disaster is foreshadowed by the oestriol excretion. Many authors have reported series of this kind, notably Zondek (1954), Zondek & Goldberg (1957), Frandsen & Stakemann (1960), Banerjea (1962), Coyle *et al.* (1962), Wray & Russel (1964) and Jayle *et al.* (1965). All are agreed that low levels of oestriol generally precede foetal death in these diseases, although estimates of what constitutes a dangerous level in late pregnancy vary from 1 to 12 mg per 24 hours. When the cause is placental rather than foetal in origin as in antepartum haemorrhage, the findings may be equivocal although Beisher *et al.* (1967) have reported that in bleeding from placenta praevia or in bleeding of unknown origin when placental function is not affected the oestriol output is normal whereas when placental function is deleteriously affected the oestriol output falls. They conclude that oestriol assay has a useful place in the management of antepartum haemorrhage.

The significance of the underlying pathology in determining oestriol levels before foetal death becomes more obvious when a wider range of causes is considered. The changes which might be expected before the silent intra-uterine death of the postmature foetus which most frequently occurs in elderly primigravidae have never been fully documented. The oestriol levels which may occur with intra-uterine death caused by diabetes are very variable and will be more fully analysed in the section on diabetes. Klopper & Stephenson (1966) found that oestriol excretion remained within the normal range in erythroblastotic pregnancies until foetal death.

Many investigations of oestriol after foetal death has occurred have been published. There is no doubt that once the foetus is dead, the oestriol output drops rapidly to very low levels, whatever the state of the placenta. In late pregnancy values of less than 1 mg per 24 hours urine are a secure indication of foetal death and below 3 mg there is a strong possibility of intra-uterine death. The value found after intra-uterine death will depend on how soon after foetal death the urine collection was done and on the cause from which the foetus died. Unfortunately, few publications have specified how soon after foetal death the assays were done and almost none have considered the results in terms of the cause of death. Although oestriol assay will invariably give the correct answer when the foetus has been dead for a week or more, by this time the diagnosis is usually obvious on clinical grounds. When oestriol excretion is examined in relation to the manner of foetal death, the impression is gained that when the foetal death takes place by slow degrees with widespread deterioration of foeto-placental function as in retarded intrauterine growth or chronic toxaemia, the oestriol output falls to very low levels *pari passu* with the decline in foetal vitality so that very low levels

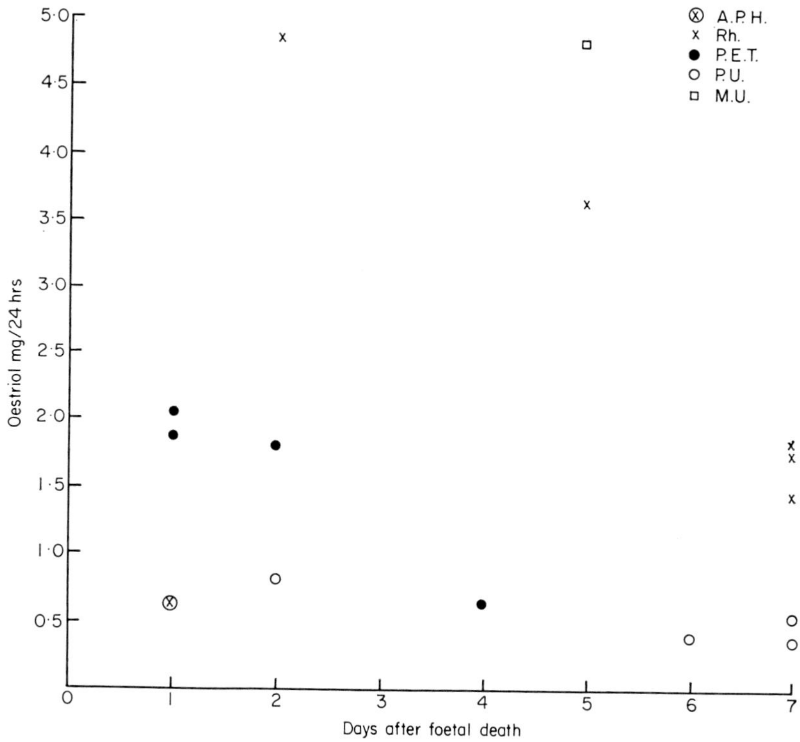

FIG. 9.4. Oestriol excretion after foetal death: A.P.H., Antepartum Haemorrhage; Rh., Rhesus Incompatibility; P.E.T., Pre-Eclamptic Toxaemia; P.U., Premature, Unknown cause; M.U., Mature, Unknown cause. From *Research on Steroids*, Vol. 2, with kind permission of the publishers, Il Pensiero Scientifico, Rome.

are recorded soon after foetal death. On the other hand, if foetal death takes place very suddenly as in acute toxaemia or as a result of a selective pathology involving only certain vital functions as with Rh incompatibility, much higher levels may obtain for a few days after foetal death. The findings in a group of intra-uterine deaths are considered in terms of cause of death and length of time after death in Fig. 9.4.

There is another sense in which prognosis about foetal death is useful in clinical practice. Patients sometimes present themselves for antenatal examination with a history of recurrent foetal loss or near loss, often with an ill-defined obstetric cause. In such circumstances, it is of value to have

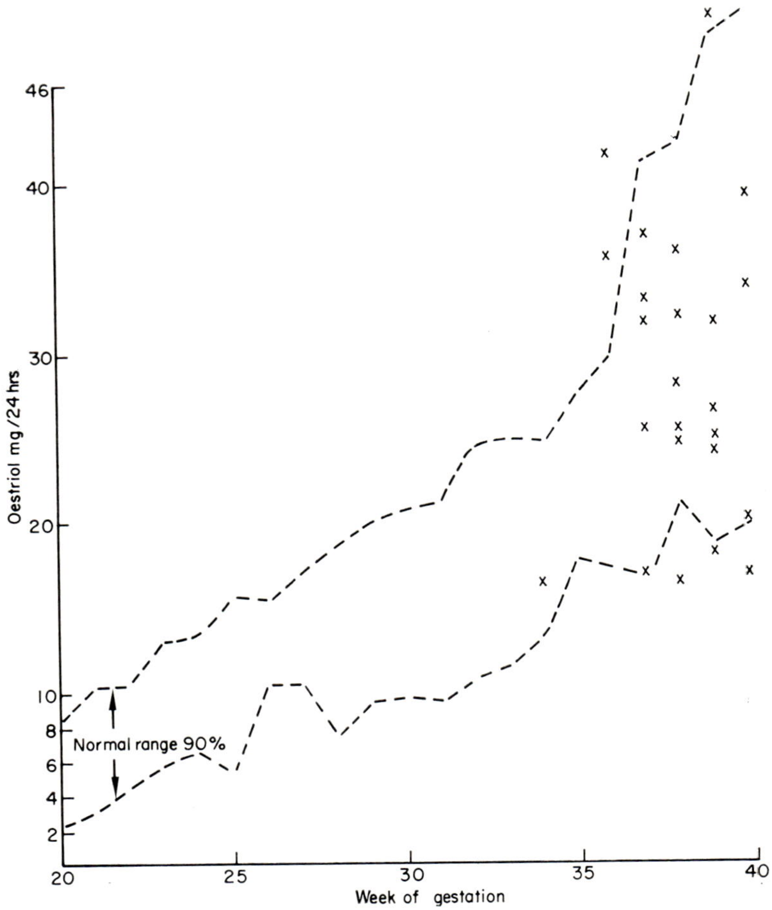

FIG. 9.5. Oestriol excretion in patients with a poor obstetric history–favourable outcome.

information about the likely outcome of the present pregnancy. It would appear that such patients can be roughly sorted into two groups on the grounds of their oestriol excretion in late pregnancy. Figure 9.5 shows that those with a favourable outcome have a normal oestriol output while

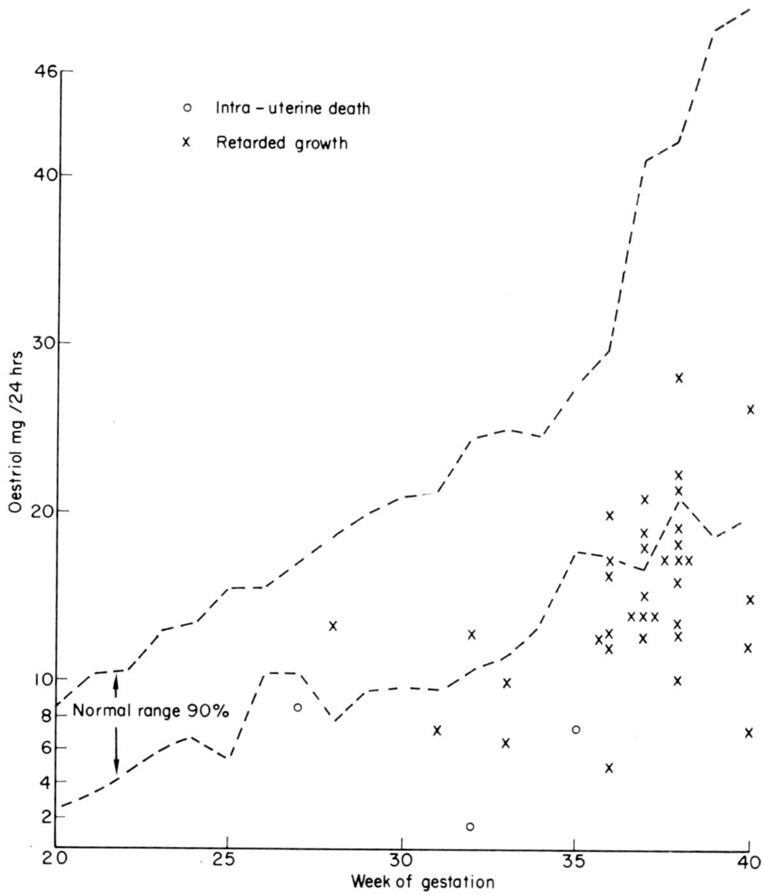

FIG. 9.6. Oestriol excretion in patients with a poor obstetric history–unfavourable outcome.

those who will ultimately lose the baby or give birth to a growth retarded child have a lowered excretion, as shown in Fig. 9.6.

Oestriol excretion in diabetic pregnancy

Because of the high perinatal mortality in diabetic pregnancy a good deal of attention has been paid to means of assessing placental function in this condition. One of the earliest surveys of oestrogen levels was done in diabetic pregnancy (Smith & Smith 1937). The assays were actually carried out on blood and would today be considered to have no quantitative significance. Nevertheless, the general conclusion was little modified by the flood of investigation which followed the development of reliable chemical methods of investigation.

It appears to be securely established that in diabetic pregnancies the oestriol output is generally less than average but only rarely falls below the lower limit of the normal range. This conclusion was supported by the studies of Rubin *et al.* (1946), Hobkirk *et al.* (1960), Hobkirk & Nilsen (1962), Coyle & Brown (1963), Greene *et al.* (1965), Taylor *et al.* (1965) and also Beling (1967). Ten Berge *et al.* (1957) appear to be alone in the belief that oestriol output may be higher than normal in diabetes, although several authors remark on the fact that the scatter of values tends to be larger than normal.

The blanket statement that oestriol output tends to be below average but not outwith the normal range in diabetes does not answer two important questions–whether the oestriol output is related to the severity of the diabetes and whether serial assays provide a means of deciding when to effect delivery. Beling (1967) is one of the few authors to have considered oestriol output in relation to the severity of the diabetes and he showed that the lower values were concentrated among the most severe grades of diabetes. Even this does not explore the point adequately for he did not consider the foetal state in this respect. Beling believes that oestriol output is closely related to foetal size and one would expect on these grounds that diabetics with large babies would tend toward high oestriol outputs while the occasional patient with a small baby would have a low output.

Some workers, notably Beling, have viewed oestriol assays with enthusiasm as a means of deciding when delivery should be effected. A caveat should be entered here. Diabetes is a very variable disease and the foeto-placental unit may be affected in different ways. A diabetic baby may die *in utero* from toxaemia, from maternal ketosis, from retarded growth or it may be an unheralded silent death of an unusually large infant. It is unlikely that all such foetuses would be equally affected in their oestriol production. A large foetus or the bulky, immature placenta often found in diabetics may counterbalance the deleterious effect upon oestriol production of the lowered vitality of the diabetic foetus. The results pertaining in any particular case may be the fortuitous outcome of diverse, occasionally contending, influences. Hence the wide scatter frequently commented upon.

One way to judge the value of oestriol assays in diabetes is to consider the effect of such assays on foetal salvage. Of course oestriol assays are of little use before 34 weeks gestation as it is not feasible to effect delivery before then whatever the oestriol level. A proportion of pregnancies are therefore lost before oestriol assays can be effectively used. Barnes, in the discussion on the paper of Greene *et al.* (1965), stated that oestriol assay had not, in his experience, improved foetal salvage in diabetic pregnancy. The improvement, if any, is likely to be small. How small, will not be known, except in the unlikely event that a proper control study is set up in which two groups of diabetic pregnancies differ in their treatment only by whether or not the clinicians have access to oestriol assays in making their decisions.

Because the urinary levels of oestriol in diabetics are so variable, several groups have turned to blood oestriol measurements. There is little reason to expect that these would be more stable than the urinary levels; particularly as the technical problems of assay would add an element of laboratory variation to the physiological variability. In the event, the results recorded by Roy & Kerr (1964) give the same picture as the urinary values,–within the normal range but less than average. Wodrig & Göretzlehner (1964) looked at the oestriol concentration of the liquor amnii as well as maternal and foetal blood but were unable to show any significant difference in the liquor although they concluded that the oestriol concentration in both maternal and foetal blood was significantly lowered.

Oestriol excretion in Rhesus incompatibility

The problem of placental hypertrophy counteracting the effect of declining foetal vitality on oestriol output as mentioned in connection with diabetic pregnancy is more to the fore here. The mechanism by which a foetus dies *in utero* from Rh incompatibility is clearly different from that operative in retarded growth, postmaturity or toxaemia. Very possibly different physiological functions are impaired beforehand and those involved in erythroblastosis may not have a bearing on oestriol production. On the other hand, if Cassmer's (1959) speculation that oestriol biosynthesis is an oxygen sensitive process is correct, erythroblastosis is *par excellence* a condition which might impede oestriol production. In addition erythroblastosis impairs foetal liver function and the foetal liver is an important site of oestrogen metabolism in the foetus. These reasonable expectations led Klopper & Stephenson (1966) to undertake a large scale survey of oestriol excretion in Rh incompatible pregnancies. They found that the oestriol output a few days before delivery of mothers giving birth to severely affected babies was no different from those delivering mildly affected babies and was, on average, 113 per cent of the normal mean for the stage of gestation. Although the oestriol output fell rapidly once an intro-uterine death had taken place, there was not sufficient change in advance of the event to give adequate warning. A few patients showed a consistently high output and they considered that oestriol production might be raised in some forms of Rh incompatible pregnancy. This possibility had earlier been raised by Taylor *et al.* (1963) who also found a raised oestriol output in Rh incompatible pregnancy.

Oestriol excretion in abnormalities of early gestation

The use of oestriol assays before 20 weeks gestation is vitiated by the fact that one does not know whether one is measuring the activity of the ovary, the placenta or the foetoplacental unit. Diczfalusy & Borell (1961) examined the oestriol output in a pregnant woman who had all ovarian tissue removed 78 days after her last menstrual period. They found no decline in oestriol output after operation and concluded that by this stage in pregnancy the ovarian contribution to oestriol production was negligible. The same conclusion need not, of course, apply to the hyperstimulated ovaries found in pathological pregnancy like hydatidiform mole. The relative preponderance of oestriol over oestrone and oestradiol becomes evident in the urinary oestrogen soon after the first missed period. Presuming that this oestriol excess, which is characteristic of pregnancy, is produced by the conceptus rather than the ovary, it is likely that the foetoplacental contribution is a significant proportion of the urinary output from very early in pregnancy. It is no more than a reasonable guess to suppose that a foetal contribution by way of precursor steroid from the foetal adrenal for later placental oestrogen synthesis also starts very early in pregnancy, but that if this foetal contribution is deficient it can be wholly substituted by the maternal adrenal supply of precursor steroid, so that no fall in urinary oestriol occurs unless placental biosynthesis also becomes deficient.

There are two situations in early pregnancy where oestriol assays may be helpful. The first is in relation to abortion and the second concerns hydatidiform mole and chorionepithelioma. Many cases present with the symptoms of threatened abortion, and it may be very difficult to forecast what the outcome may be. Borth (1960) found oestriol assays to be more helpful than measurement of pregnanediol and went so far as to suggest that oestrogen deficiency may play the more important role. Booth *et al.*

(1965) also considered the causative role of oestrogen deficiency in threatened abortion and found only one patient in 19 where oestriol assays indicated that hormone therapy would have helped. Frandsen & Stakemann (1966) concentrated on the more important question of whether oestriol assay gave a reliable indication of the likely outcome of threatened abortion. They found in 106 cases of threatened abortion that abortion almost invariably occurred if the oestriol output was low but that 75 per cent of cases with a normal output went to term. Of course, many cases which present the appearance of threatened abortion are already so far advanced as really to be inevitable or indeed incomplete abortions. In such instances, the oestriol excretion can be expected to be low and the results are not a true reflection of the capacity of oestriol assays to forecast the outcome of cases which are really in doubt.

Even when there is presumptive evidence of a missed abortion, it may be very difficult to decide on clinical grounds whether the foetus is dead. Bengtsson & Forsgren (1966) considered the use of oestriol assays in this situation and found them most helpful, not only in the diagnosis of missed abortion, but in deciding how long the foetus had been dead.

Women with a history of recurrent abortion present a challenge to the endocrinologist. Here oestriol assays may have an application, not only in prognosis, but in assessing the value of therapy. It is in particular, a situation where it may be possible to initiate assays well before the abortion process starts and thus to study step by step the genesis of abortion. Klopper & Macnaughton (1965) did serial assays in such a group of women with a history of recurrent abortion and came to the conclusion that oestriol assays were more reliable than assays of pregnanediol and that the former assays frequently gave warning of an impending abortion long before it was clinically evident. The cause of the recurrent abortion may have some bearing on the likelihood of a preceding drop in oestriol output. Booth *et al.* (1965) have pointed out that recurrent abortions due to an incompetent cervix do not have an antecedent fall in oestriol output while other types of abortion may show this change.

Hydatidiform moles and chorionepithelioma have roused some interest in respect of oestriol assay both in terms of how useful the assays can be in establishing the diagnosis and for the light which this pathology may shed on the mechanism of oestriol production in early pregnancy. Frandsen & Stakemann (1964), who have studied the largest series, concluded that there was a tendency for oestriol excretion to be low, upon occasion in the non-pregnant range. A few patients however, excreted amounts in the normal range, which much detracts from the diagnostic possibilities of the technique. They found the ratio of oestriol to oestrone plus oestradiol to be similar to that of non-pregnant women and presumed that the source of the oestriol was the hyperstimulated ovaries rather than the placenta. Macnaughton (1965) studied five patients with hydatidiform moles and found two in whom the oestriol output was normal. He concluded that in this condition placental biogenesis of oestriol does upon occasion proceed at normal levels from precursors supplied by the maternal adrenal.

CONCLUSION

The placenta has a great variety of functions. No one test measures all. The concern of placental function tests in clinical practice is not with placental function as such but with its effect on the foetus. In respect of oestrogen biogenesis, the foetus and placenta act as a single integrated unit. For clinical purposes, oestriol assays have much to recommend them over the other tests which have been discussed. They must be used with discrimination knowing that their usefulness varies with the basic pathology and that the day-to-day value is subject to much variability. There is still room for technical improvement in the application of oestriol assay–by measurements in blood and liquor, by measurement of specific oestriol conjugates or by dynamic measurements of oestriol biogenesis following supply of oestriol precursors. But in the end, the main possibilities of advance lie in the elucidation of the function of oestriol in pregnancy and of the control of its rate of manufacture. Until we know what processes in foetus and placenta we are measuring by oestriol assay, we are groping in the dark. For the future Goethe's dying words apply–'Mehr licht!'

REFERENCES

Abrams R. & Abrams J. (1962) Vaginal cytology in the final weeks of pregnancy *Acta cytol.* **6**, 359.

Aherne W. & Dunnill M.S. (1966) Morphometry of the human placenta. *Br. med. Bull.* **22**, 5.

AITKEN E.H. & PREEDY J.R.K. (1956) The estimation of oestrone, oestradiol-17β and oestriol in human urine by gradient elution partition chromatography. *Biochem. J.* **62**, 15P.

AITKEN E.H., PREEDY J.R., ETON B. & SHORT R.V. (1958) Oestrogen and progesterone levels in foetal and maternal plasma at parturition. *Lancet*, ii, 1096.

ALDER R.M. & KRIEGER V.I. (1957) Hormonal therapy and the significance of the pregnanediol excretion test in recurrent abortion. *Med. J. Aust.* **2**, 122.

ASSALI N.S., DOUGLASS R.A., BAIRD W.W., NICHOLSON D.B. & SUYEMOTO R. (1953) The measurement of uterine blood flow and uterine metabolism. *Am. J. Obstet. Gynec.* **66**, 248.

BACHMAN C. (1941) Excretion of oestrogen and pregnanediol preceding normal parturition. *Am. J. Obstet. Gynec.* **42**, 599.

BAKER W.S., BANCROFT C.E., LYDA E.W. & LEHMAN J.J. (1955) The value of urinary pregnanediol determinations as an indication for the use of progesterone in the treatment of threatened abortion. *Am. J. Obstet. Gynec.* **69**, 405.

BANERJEA S.K. (1962) Index of placental function by endocrine assay and its clinical application in obstetrical practice. *J. Obstet. Gynaec. Br. Cwlth.* **69**, 963.

BARTHOLOMEW R.A. (1947) The possible etiologic significance of thrombosis of a placental vein on the mechanism of placental infarction and associated toxaemia of pregnancy. *Am. J. Obstet. Gynec.* **53**, 650.

BARTHOLOMEW R.A., COLVIN E.D. & GRIMES W.H. (1957) Facts pertinent to the etiology of eclamptic toxaemia. *Am. J. Obstet. Gynec.* **74**, 64.

BAULD W.S. (1956) A method for the determination of oestriol, oestrone and oestradiol-17β in human urine by partition chromatography and colorimetric estimation. *Biochem. J.* **65**, 488.

BEHRMAN S.J. & NIEMANN P. (1955) Serum gonadotrophins in normal and abnormal pregnancy. *Fert. Steril.* **6**, 236.

BEISHER N.A., BROWN J.B., MACLEOD S.C. & SMITH M.A. (1967) The value of urinary oestriol estimation in patients with antepartum vaginal bleeding. *J. Obstet. Gynaec. Br. Cwlth.* **74**, 51.

BELING C.G. (1960) Gel filtration of conjugated urinary oestrogens and its application in clinical assays. *Acta endocr.* Suppl. **79**.

BELING C.G. (1967) Estriol excretion in pregnancy and its application to clinical problems. In *Advances in Obstetrics and Gynecology*, p. 88. S.C.Marcus & C.C. Marcus, eds. Williams & Wilkins Co., Baltimore.

BELL E.T., LORAINE J.A., MCEWAN H.P. & CHARLES D. (1964) Serial hormone assays in patients with uteroplacental insufficiency. *Am. J. Obstet. Gynec.* **97**, 562.

BENGTSSON L.P. & FORSGREN B. (1966) The diagnosis of intra-uterine foetal death and elucidation of the aetiology of 'missed abortion' by means of semi-quantitative gas chromatographic determination of urinary oestriol and pregnanediol. *Acta Obst. et Gynec. Scandinav.* **45**, 155.

BENTELE W. (1963) Harnoestrogenbestimmung und Indikation zur Schmittentbindung beim Fetus Dysmaturus. *Arch. für Gynak.* **198**, 313.

BERLINER D.L. & SALHANICK H.A. (1956) The presence of 6-β-hydroxylase in human placenta. *J. clin. Endocr.* **16**, 903.

BEVIS D.C. (1953) The composition of the liquor amnii in haemolytic disease of the newborn. *J. Obstet. Gynaec. Br. Emp.* **60**, 1953.

BONAR J., DAVIES D.L. & LANGFORD H.G. (1966) Plasma renin concentration in American Negro women with hypertensive disease of pregnancy. *J. Obstet. Gynaec. Br. Cwlth.* **73**, 418.

BOOTH R.T., STERN M.I., WOOD C., SHARPLES M.J. & PINKERTON J.H. (1965) Urinary hormone excretion in abnormal pregnancy. *J. Obstet. Gynaec. Br. Cwlth.* **72**, 229.

BORTH R. (1954) Elimination du pregnandiol au cours de la grossesse. *Gynec. Obstet.* **53**, 27.

BORTH R. (1960) *Prenatal Care*, p. 57. Noordof, Groningen.

BRADBURY J.T. & GOPLERUD C.P. (1963) Serum chorionic gonadotrophin studied in sensitized Rh-negative patients. *Obstet. Gynec.* **21**, 330.

BREBOROWICZ H., KRZYWINSKA F. & PISARKI T. (1965) The relationship between placental structure and urinary oestrogen levels. *Am. J. Obstet. Gynec.* **91**, 1107.

BRODY S. & CARLSTROM G. (1960) Estimation of human chorionic gonadotrophin in biological fluids by complement fixation. *Lancet*, ii, 99.

BRODY S. & CARLSTROM G. (1962) Immuno-assay of human chorionic gonadotrophin in normal and pathological pregnancy. *J. clin. Endocr.* **22**, 564.

BRODY S. & CARLSTROM G. (1965) Human chorionic gonadotrophin in abnormal pregnancy. Serum and urinary findings using immunoassay techniques. *Acta Obst. et Gynec. Scandinav.* **44**, 32.

BROWN C.H., SAFFAN B.D., HOWARD C. & PREEDY J.R. (1964) The renal clearance of endogenous oestrogens in late pregnancy. *J. Clin. Invest.* **43**, 295.

BROWN J.B. (1955) A chemical method for the determination of oestriol, oestrone and oestradiol in human urine. *Biochem. J.* **60**, 185.

BROWN J.B. (1956) Urinary excretion of oestrogens during pregnancy, lactation and the re-establishment of menstruation. *Lancet*, i, 704.

BROWN J.B. (1960) In *Advances in Clinical Chemistry*, p. 157. C.P.Stewart, ed. Academic Press, New York, Vol. 3.

BROWN J.B. & COYLE M. (1963) Urinary excretion of oestriol during pregnancy. A shortened procedure. *J. Obstet. Gynaec. Br. Cwlth.* **70**, 219.

BROWN J.B., BULBROOK R.D. & GREENWOOD F.C. (1957) An additional step for a method for estimating oestriol oestrone and oestradiol-17β in human urine. *J. Endocr.* **16**, 49.

BROWN J.J., DAVIES D.L. & DOAK P.B. (1966) Plasma-renin concentration in hypertensive disease of pregnancy. *Lancet*, ii, 1219.

BROWNE J.C. & VEALL N. (1953) The maternal placental blood flow in normotensive and hypertensive women. *J. Obstet. Gynaec. Br. Emp.* **60**, 142.

BRUSH M.G., TAYLOR R.W. & MAXWELL R. (1966) Gas chromatographic determination or urinary pregnanediol in toxaemia of pregnancy and suspected dysmaturity. *J. Obstet. Gynaec. Br. Cwlth.* **73**, 954.

BULL G., HEBB C. & RUTKOVIC O. (1961) Choline acetylase in the human placenta at different stages of development. *Nature*, **190**, 1202.

BURNSTEIN R., BLUMENTHAL H.J. & SOULE S.D. (1957) Placental lesions in toxaemia and hypertension. *Am. J. Obstet. Gynec.* **74**, 85.

CARLSSON MATS G. (1964) The use of haemagglutination-inhibition reaction for qualitative and quantitative determinations of HCG in normal and pathological pregnancies. *Acta endocr. (Copenh.)*, **46**, 142.

CASSMER O. (1959) Hormone production of the isolated human placenta. *Acta endocr. (Kbh.)*, Suppl. 45.

COHEN H. & BATES R.W. (1947) A single quantitative colorimetric method for oestrogenic steroids. *J. clin. Endocr.* **7**, 701.

COLE P.G., LATHE G.H. & RUTHVEN C.R. (1953) The application of countercurrent methods to the fractionation of lipid material from the human placenta. *Biochem. J.* **55**, 17.

CONNON A.F. (1964) The excretion of human chorionic gonadotrophin in normal pregnancy. An immunological investigation. *J. Endocr.* **30**, 79.

COX L.W., MUNDAY R.M. & SAUER H.H. (1963) The use of radioactive isotopes in determining placental function. *Aust. N.Z. J. Obstet. Gynaec.* **3**, 119.

COX L.W., COX R.I. & SKIPPER J.S. (1964) The management of threatened abortion by pregnanediol estimation and vaginal cytology. *Aust. N.Z. J. Obstet. Gynaec.* **4**, 160.

COYLE M.G. & BROWN J.B. (1963) Urinary excretion of oestriol during pregnancy. *J. Obstet. Gynaec. Br. Cwlth.* **70**, 225.

COYLE M.G., MITCHELL F.L. & RUSSELL C.S. (1956) A report on the chromatographic assay of urinary pregnanediol in pregnancy. *J. Obstet. Gynaec. Br. Emp.* **63**, 560.

COYLE M.G., GREIG M. & WALKER J. (1962) Blood-progesterone and urinary pregnanediol and oestrogens in foetal death from severe pre-eclampsia. *Lancet*, ii, 275.

CURZEN P. (1964) Variations in the histochemistry of the placenta. *J. Obstet. Gynaec. Br. Cwlth.* **71**, 388.

CURZEN P. & MORRIS I. (1965) Serum alkaline phosphatase in the hypertensive disorders of pregnancy. *J. Obstet. Gynaec. Br. Cwlth.* **72**, 397.

DALE E., GREENE J.W. & DUHRING J.L. (1965) Comparison of three methods for determination of urinary estriol during late pregnancy. *Am. J. Obstet. Gynec.* **92**, 112.

DANIELSSON M. (1965) Urinary excretion of human chorionic gonadotrophin during prolonged pregnancy and labor. *Am. J. Obstet. Gynec.* **91**, 895.

DELFS E. & JONES G.E.S. (1948) Endocrine patterns in abortion. *Obstet. Gynaec. Surv.* **3**, 360.

DE MARIA F.J. & SEE H.Y. (1966) Role of the placenta in pre-eclampsia. *Am. J. Obstet. Gynec.* **94**, 471.

DEMPSEY E.W. & WISLOCKI G.B. (1945) Histochemistry of the placenta. *Am. J. Anat.* **76**, 277.

DE WATTEVILLE H. (1951) Pregnanediol determinations in the clinic and in research. *J. clin. Endocr.* **11**, 251.

DICZFALUSY E. (1953) Chorionic gonadotrophin and oestrogens in the human placenta. *Acta endocr. (Copenh.)*, **12**, 78.

DICZFALUSY E. & BORELL U. (1961) Influence of oophorectomy on steroid excretion in early pregnancy. *J. clin. Endocr.* **21**, 1119.

Donald I. (1965) Diagnostic uses of sonar in obstetrics and gynaecology. *J. Obstet. Gynaec. Br. Cwlth.* **72**, 907.

Drescher J. (1956) Die glukoproteinanalyse des plazentargewebes und ihre bedeutung für eine beurteilung der choriongonadotrophin-konzentration. *Z. Geburtsh. Gynak.* **146**, 233.

Eberlein W.R., Bongiovanni A.M. & Francis C.M. (1958) A simplified method for the routine measurement of oestriol. *J. clin. Endocr.* **18**, 1274.

Eden T.W. (1897) A study of the human placenta, physiological and pathological. *J. Path. Bact.* **4**, 265.

Finkelstein M. (1952) Fluorimetric determination of micro amounts of oestrone, oestradiol-17β and oestriol in urine. *Acta endocr.* **10**, 149.

Frampton J. (1966) Fluorescence microscopy applied to vaginal cytology at the end of pregnancy. *J. Obstet. Gynaec. Br. Cwlth.* **73**, 249.

Frandsen V.A. (1963) *The Excretion of Oestriol in Normal Human Pregnancy.* Munksgaard, Copenhagen.

Frandsen V.A. & Lundwall F. (1966) The excretion of oestrone-oestradiol and oestriol in normal human pregnancy. *Acta endocr.* **53**, 93.

Frandsen V.A. & Stakemann G. (1960) Urinary excretion of estriol during normal pregnancy. *Danish Medical Bulletin,* **7**, 95.

Frandsen V.A. & Stakemann G. (1963a) The site of production of oestrogenic hormones in human pregnancy II. *Acta endocr.* **43**, 184.

Frandsen V.A. & Stakemann G. (1963b) The clinical significance of oestriol estimations in late pregnancy. *Acta endocr. (Kbh.),* **44**, 183.

Frandsen V.A. & Stakemann G. (1963c) The urinary excretion of oestriol during the early months of pregnancy. *Acta endocr.* **44**, 196.

Frandsen V.A. & Stakemann G. (1964a) The site of production of oestrogenic hormones in human pregnancy III. *Acta endocr.* **47**, 265.

Frandsen V.A. & Stakemann G. (1964b) The excretion of hormones in cases of hydatidiform mole and chorionepithelioma. *Acta endocr.* Suppl. **90**, 81.

Frandsen V.A. & Stakemann G. (1966) The excretion of oestrone-oestradiol and oestriol in normal human pregnancy. *Acta endocr. (Kbh.),* **53**, 93.

Friedman E.A. & Sachtleben M.R. (1960) Placental oxygen consumption *in vitro*. I. Baseline studies. *Am. J. Obstet. Gynec.* **79**, 1058.

Friedman E.A., Little W.A. & Sachtleben M.R. (1962) Placental oxygen consumption *in vitro*. II. Total uptake as an index of placental function. *Am. J. Obstet. Gynec.* **84**, 561.

Fuchs F. (1966) Volume of amniotic fluid at various stages of pregnancy. *Clin. Obstet. Gynec.* **9**, 449.

Furuhjelm M. (1953) Pregnanediol excretion in women. *Acta endocr. (Kbh.),* **14**, 353.

Furuhjelm M. (1962) The excretion of oestriol and of pregnanediol in toxaemia of pregnancy and postmaturity. *Acta Obst. et Gynec. Scandinav.* **41**, 370.

Gaudefroy M. (1959) Vaginal cytology as a prognostic method in pregnancy disorders. *Acta cytol.* **3**, 228.

Goldzieher J.W. & Benigno B.B. (1958) The treatment of threatened and recurrent abortion: a critical review. *Am. J. Obstet. Gynec.* **75**, 1202.

GOODLIN R.C. & SCHWARTZ S.P. (1962) Coproporphyrin content of the amniotic fluid in normal and diseased infants. *Am. J. Obstet. Gynec.* **84**, 808.

GREENE J.W., SMITH K., KYLE G.C., TOUCHSTONE J.C. & DUHRING J.L. (1965) The use of urinary estriol excretion in the management of pregnancies complicated by diabetes mellitus. *Am. J. Obstet. Gynec.* **91**, 684.

GRUENWALD P. (1964) Chronic fetal distress. *Clin. Pediat.* **3**, 141.

GUTERMAN H.S. (1953) Progesterone metabolism in the human female: its significance in relation to reproduction. *Rec. Prog. Horm. Res.* **8**, 293.

HAFEZ E.S. (1964) Uterine and placental enzymes. A review. *Acta endocr.* **46**, 217.

HASKINS A.L. & SHERMAN A.I. (1952) The quantitative assay of serum chorionic gonadotrophin in pregnancy using the modified male frog technique. *J. clin. Endocr.* **12**, 385.

HASSAN S. (1965) A vaginal smear study in cases of threatened abortion. *J. Obstet. Gynaec. Br. Cwlth.* **72**, 416.

HEIJKENSKJOLD F. & GEMZELL C.A. (1957) Glycogen content in the placenta of diabetic mothers. *Acta paediat.* **46**, 74.

HELLMAN L.M. (1952) Placental infarction. In *Gynaecological and Obstetrical Pathology*, p. 161. E.Novak, ed. 3rd edition. W.B.Saunders Co., Philadelphia and London.

HELLMAN L.M. & FILLISTI L.P. (1965) Analysis of the atropine test for placental transfer in gravidas with toxaemia and diabetes. *Am. J. Obstet. Gynec.* **91**, 797.

HELLMAN L.M. & HERTIG A.T. (1938) Pathologic changes in the placenta associated with erythroblastosis fetalis of the fetus. *Am. J. Path.* **14**, 111.

HELLMAN L.M., HARRIS B.A. & ANDREWS M.C. (1950) Studies of the metabolism of the human placenta. Oxygen consumption and anaerobic glycolysis in relation to ageing and severe toxaemia. *Bull. Johns Hopkins Hosp.* **87**, 203.

HELLMAN L.M., MORTON G.W., TOLLES W.E. & FILLISTI L.P. (1963) A computer analysis of the atropine test for placental function. *Am. J. Obstet. Gynec.* **85**, 610.

HELMY F.M. & HACK M.H. (1964) Histochemical and lipid studies on human and rat placentas. *Am. J. Obstet. Gynec.* **88**, 578.

HENDRICKS C.H. (1964) Patterns of fetal and placental growth: the second half of normal pregnancy. *Obstet. Gynec.* **24**, 357.

HOBKIRK R. & NILSEN M. (1962) Observations on the occurrence of six estrogen fractions in human pregnancy urine. *J. clin. Endocr.* **22**, 142.

HOBKIRK R., BLAHEY P.R., ALFHEIM A., RAESIDE J. & JORON G.E. (1960) Urinary oestrogen excretion in normal and diabetic pregnancy. *J. clin. Endocr.* **20**, 805.

HON E.H. & MORRIS J. (1956) Further experience with the toad method of testing for chorionic gonadotrophin in normal and disturbed pregnancy. *J. clin. Endocr.* **16**, 1355.

HOOVER C.R. & BARTHOLOMEW R.H. (1959) Acid-soluble nucleotides in placentae from normal and toxic patients. *Obstet. Gynec.* **14**, 309.

HUCKABEE W.E. (1962) Uterine blood flow. *Am. J. Obstet. Gynec.* **84**, 1623.

HUCKABEE W.E., METCALFE J., PRYSTOWKY H. & BARRON D.H. (1961) Measurement of uterine blood flow. *Am. J. Physiol.* **200**, 274.

ICHII S., FORCHIELLI E., PERLOFF W.H. & DORFMAN R.I. (1963) Determination of plasma estrone and estradiol-17β. *Analyt. Biochem.* **5**, 422.

ITTRICH G. (1958) Eine neue methode zur chemischen Bestimmung der oestrogen Hormone im Harn. *Z. physiol. Chem.* **312**, 1.

ITTRICH G. (1960) Eine methode zur chemischen Bestimmung von öestrogenen Hormonen in Blut, Milch und Colostrum. *Hoppe-Seylers Zeitschrift fur physiologische Chemie*, **320**, 103.

ITTRICH G. & IGEL H. (1959) Bestimmung der Harnöstrogene in der Schwangerschaft. *Zentralb für Gynak.* **81**, 255.

ITTRICH G., IGEL H., BERGMANN K.H. & KLIETZ H. (1962) Oestrogenausscheidung unter der Geburt. *Zentralb für Gynak.* **84**, 1928.

JAILER J.W. (1948) A fluorometric method for the determination of oestrogens. *J. clin. Endocr.* **8**, 564.

JAYLE M., CREPY O. & JUDAS O. (1943) Dosage colorimetrique de la folliculine urinaire. *Bull. soc. chim. biol.* **25**, 301.

JAYLE M.F., SCHOLLER R., VEYRIN-FORRER F. & MEGE F. (1965) Clinical importance of oestrogen and pregnanediol estimations in pathological pregnancies. *Europ. Rev. Endocrinol.* Suppl. **1**, 77.

JEACOCK M.K., MORRIS N.F. & PLESTER J.H. (1963) The activity of alkaline and acid phosphatase in the human placenta. *J. Obstet. Gynaec. Br. Cwlth.* **70**, 267.

KANKAANRINTA T. (1963) On the pregnanediol excretion in the urine during the last trimester of normal and toxaemic pregnancy. *Scand. J. Clin. Lab. Invest.* **5**, Suppl. 7.

KAPELLER-ADLER R. (1965) Recent attempts at purification and identification of human placental histaminase. *Clinica chim. Acta*, **11**, 191.

KARNOVSKY M.L. & DEANE H.W. (1955) Aldehyde formation in the lipide droplets of the adrenal cortex during fixation, as demonstrated chemically and histochemically. *J. Histochem. Cytochem.* **3**, 85.

KELLAR R., MATTHEW G.D., MACKAY R., BROWN J.B. & ROY E.J. (1959). Some applications of oestrogen assay. *J. Obstet. Gynaec. Br. Cwlth.* **66**, 804.

KELLER M. & KUBLI F. (1963) Plasmaoestrogenbestimmungen im normalen cyclus, während der normalen Gravidität im Retroplacentarblut, im Nabelschurblut und beim Neugeboren. *Archiv. für Gynak.* **197**, 605.

KLAUSNER D.A. & RYAN K.J. (1964) Estriol secretion by the human term placenta. *J. clin. Endocr.* **24**, 101.

KLINGE E., PENTTILÄ O. & TISSARI A. (1964) The content of 5-hydroxytryptamine in human uterine and placental tissue and their 5-hydroxytryptophan decarboxylase and mono-amine oxidase activities in normal and toxaemic pregnancies. *Acta obstet. gynec. Scand.* **43**, 107.

KLOPPER A. (1959) The effect of oestriol on plasma water content. *J. Obstet. Gynaec. Br. Cwlth.* **66**, 822.

KLOPPER A. (1964) Variability of urinary sex steroid hormone output in pregnancy. *Research on Steroids*, Vol. 1, p. 119. C.Cassano, ed. Il Pensiero Scientifico, Rome.

KLOPPER A. (1965) Assays of urinary oestriol as a measure of placental function. In *Research on Steroids*, Vol. 2, p. 63. C.Cassano, ed. Il Pensiero Scientifico, Rome.

KLOPPER A. (1966) A critical review of urinary oestriol excretion in the assessment of placental function. Abhandlungen der deutschen Akademie der Wissenshaften Zu Berlin. *Akademie-Verlag, Berlin*, p. 247.

Klopper A. & Billewicz W. (1963) Urinary excretion of oestriol and pregnanediol during normal pregnancy. *J. Obstet. Gynaec. Br. Cwlth.* **70**, 1024.

Klopper A. & Macnaughton M.C. (1965) Hormones in recurrent abortion. *J. Obstet. Gynaec. Br. Cwlth.* **72**, 1072.

Klopper A. & Macnaughton M. (1959) The identification of pregnanediol in liquor amnii, bile and faeces. *J. Endocr.* **18**, 319.

Klopper A. & Michie Eileen M. (1956) The excretion of urinary pregnanediol after the administration of progesterone. *J. Endocr.* **13**, 360.

Klopper A. & Stephenson R. (1966) The excretion of oestriol and of pregnanediol in pregnancy complicated by Rh immunisation. *J. Obstet. Gynaec. Br. Cwlth.* **73**, 282.

Klopper A. & Wilson G. (1962) A method for the assay of oestriol in pregnancy urine. *J. Obstet. Gynaec. Br. Cwlth.* **69**, 28.

Klopper A., Michie E.A. & Brown J.B. (1955) A method for the determination of urinary pregnanediol. *J. Endocr.* **12**, 209.

Klopper A., Turnbull A.C. & Anderson A.B. (1966) Changes in steroid hormone excretion during abortion in mid-pregnancy by the intra-amniotic injection of hypertonic saline. *J. Obstet. Gynaec. Br. Cwlth.* **73**, 390.

Kroman H.S., Bender S.R., Brest A.N., Moskovitz M.C. & King M.O. (1966) Estrogens in human plasma. *Clin. Chem.* **12**, 670.

Kubli F. & Keller M. (1963) Plasmaoestrogene in der pathologischen Swangerschaft und unter der Geburt. *Arch. für Gynak.* **198**, 139.

Kyank H. (1955) Der stoffwechsel der toxikoseplacenta *in vitro. Arch. Gynaek.* **186**, 1955.

Lampe L., Kapu L. & Peter F. (1960) Untersuchung der plazentapermeabilität mit intravenös verabreichbarem kontrastmittel. *Z. Geburtsh. Gynäk.* **155**, 294.

Langmade C.G., Notrica S., Demetriou J. & Ware A. (1961) Pregnanediol excretion in threatened abortion. *Am. J. Obstet. Gynec.* **81**, 1149.

Lauritzen C. (1965) Action of HCG and steroids on physiological processes in the neonatal period. In *Research on Steroids*, Vol. 2, p. 109. C.Cassano, ed. Il Pensiero Scientifico, Rome.

Lee A.B. & Lewis P.L. (1963) Alkaline phosphatase in normal and toxaemic pregnancies. *Am. J. Obstet. Gynec.* **87**, 1071.

Lenters G.J. (1958) Oestrioluitscheiding in de urine en de anatomische toestand van de placenta. M.D. thesis at the University of Groningen, J.B.Wolters, Groningen.

Levine B. & Wood W. (1965) Maternal serum alkaline phosphatase and placental function. *Am. J. Obstet. Gynec.* **91**, 967.

Lichtfus C.J. (1959) Vaginal cytology at the end of pregnancy. *Acta cytol.* **3**, 247.

Liley A.W. (1961) Liquor amnii analysis in the management of the pregnancy complicated by rhesus sensitization. *Am. J. Obstet. Gynec.* **82**, 1359.

Lobel B.L., Deane H.W. & Romney S.L. (1962) Enzyme histochemistry of the villous portion of the human placenta from six weeks of gestation to term. *Am. J. Obstet. Gynec.* **83**, 295.

Loraine J.A. & Matthew G.D. (1950) Chorionic gonadotrophin in toxaemias of pregnancy. *J. Obstet. Gynaec. Br. Emp.* **57**, 542.

LUNDWALL F. & STAKEMANN G. (1966) The urinary excretion of oestriol in postmaturity. *Acta Obst. et Gynec. Scandinav.* **45**, 301.

LUSCHINSKY H.L. (1951) The activity of glutaminase in the human placenta. *Arch. Biochem. Biophys.* **31**, 132.

LUSCHINSKY H.L. & SINGHER H.O. (1948) Identification and assay of monoamine oxidase in the human placenta. *Arch. Biochem.* **19**, 95.

MCCARTHY C. & PENNINGTON G.W. (1964a) Maternal chorionic gonadotrophin concentration as an aid to the antenatal prediction of haemolytic disease of the newborn. *Am. J. Obstet. Gynec.* **89**, 1069.

MCCARTHY C. & PENNINGTON G.W. (1964b) Immunological determination of chorionic gonadotrophin in liquor amnii and its application in Rh incompatability. *Am. J. Obstet. Gynec.* **89**, 1074.

MACDONALD R.R. (1963) Cervical mucus and the management of abortion. *J. Obstet. Gynaec. Br. Cwlth.* **70**, 580.

MACGILLIVRAY I. & TOVEY J.E. (1957) A study of serum protein changes in pregnancy and toxaemia using paper strip electrophoresis. *J. Obstet. Gynaec. Br. Cwlth.* **64**, 361.

MACKAY R.B. (1958) Studies of the oxygen consumption of fresh placental tissue from normal and abnormal pregnancies. *J. Obstet. Gynaec. Br. Emp.* **65**, 791.

MCKEAN C.M. (1960) Preparation and use of antisera to human chorionic gonadotrophin. *Am. J. Obstet. Gynec.* **80**, 596.

MACLEOD S.C., BROWN J.B., BEISCHER N.A. & SMITH M.A. (1967) The value of urinary oestriol measurements during pregnancy. *Aust. N.Z. J. Obstet. Gynaec.* **7**, 25.

MACNAUGHTON M.C. (1965) Urinary excretion of oestrogen and pregnanediol in hydatidiform mole. *J. Obstet. Gynaec. Br. Cwlth.* **72**, 249.

MACNAUGHTON M.C. & MICHIE E.M. (1960) Some observations on the excretion of pregnanediol in the urine of women with a bad obstetric history. *Advance Abstracts of Short Communications, First International Congress of Endocrinology*, p. 669. F.Fuchs, ed. Periodica, Copenhagen.

MACRAE D.J., IRANI J.B., BOWLER R.G. & LONGHURST P.L. (1965) A comparison between the vaginal cytology and urinary hormone excretion during pregnancy. *J. Obstet. Gynaec. Br. Cwlth.* **71**, 586.

MCSWEENEY D.J. & SBARRA A.J. (1964) A new cervical mucus test for hormone appraisal. *Am. J. Obstet. Gynec.* **88**, 705.

MACVICAR J. & DONALD I. (1963) Sonar in the diagnosis of early pregnancy and its complications. *J. Obstet. Gynaec. Br. Cwlth.* **70**, 387.

MARTIN J.D. & HAHNEL R. (1964) Urinary oestrogen excretion and retarded intrauterine growth of the foetus. *J. Obstet. Gynaec. Br. Cwlth.* **71**, 260.

METCALFE J., ROMNEY S.C., RAMSEY L.H., REID D.E. & BURWELL C.S. (1955) Estimation of uterine blood flow in normal human pregnancy at term. *J. Clin. Invest.* **34**, 1632.

MICHIE E.M. (1967) Urinary oestriol excretion in pregnancies complicated by suspected retarded intrauterine growth, toxaemia or essential hypertension. *J. Obstet. Gynaec. Br. Cwlth.* **74**, 896.

MISCHEL W. (1956) Übner die chemische zusammensetzung der menschlichen plazenta mit besonderer berücksichtigung des biogenen amin cholin. *Zentbl. Gynak.* **78**, 1089.

MORRIS M., OSBORN S.B. & WRIGHT H.P. (1955) Effective circulation of the uterine wall in late pregnancy measured with ^{24}MaCl. *Lancet*, i, 323.

NACHTIGALL C., BASSETT M., HOGSANDER U., SLAGLE S. & LEVITZ M. (1966) A rapid method for the assay of plasma estriol in pregnancy. *J. clin. Endocr.* **26**, 941.

NORTH A.F. (1966) Small-for-dates neonates. *Pediat.* **38**, 1013.

OERTEL G.W., WEST C.D. & EIK-NES K.B. (1959) Isolation and identification of estrone, estradiol-17β and estriol in human pregnancy plasma. *J. clin. Endocr.* **19**, 1619.

OERTEL G.W., BECKMANN INGE N. & EIK-NES K.B. (1960) The measurement of pregnane-3α,20α-diol and its isomers in human plasma. *Arch. Biochem. Biophys.* **86**, 148.

PANIGEL M. (1962) Placental perfusion experiments. *Am. J. Obstet. Gynec.* **84**, 1664.

PIGEAUD H. & BURTHIAULT R. (1951) Etude de elimination du pregnandiol urinaire dans 21 cas de nephropathies gravidiques. *Gynec. Obstet.* **50**, 23.

PLOTZ E.J., WIENER M. & DAVIS M.E. (1963) Effect of administered progesterone on urinary excretion of endogenous pregnanediol in pregnancy. *Am. J. Obstet. Gynec.* **87**, 1.

PRATT J.P., RODERICK C., CORYELL M. & MACY I.G. (1946) Composition of the human placenta. Vitamin content. *Am. J. Obstet. Gynec.* **52**, 783.

PREEDY J.R.K. & AITKEN E.H. (1957) Plasma oestrogen levels in late pregnancy, in the normal menstruating female, and in the male. *Lancet*, i, 191.

PUNDEL J.P. & VAN MEENSEL F. (1951) *Gestation et Cytologie Vaginale.* Masson et cie, Paris.

QUILLIGAN E.J. (1962) Amniotic fluid gas tensions. *Am. J. Obstet. Gynec.* **84**, 20.

RAWLINGS W.J. (1965) Pregnanediol excretion and placental insufficiency. *Fert. Steril.* **16**, 323.

ROBSON T.B. & GORNALL A.G. (1955) Pregnanediol assays and the abortion problem. *Can. med. Ass. J.* **72**, 830.

ROMNEY S.C., KANEOKA T. & GABEL A. (1962) Polographic determinations of oxygen tension in umbilical cord blood and amniotic fluid of normal term newborn infants. *Am. J. Obstet. Gynec.* **84**, 25.

ROY E. (1962) The concentration of oestrogens in maternal and foetal blood obtained at Caesarean Section and the effect of hospitalisation on maternal blood oestrogen levels. *J. Obstet. Gynaec. Br. Cwlth.* **69**, 196.

ROY E.J. & BROWN J.B. (1960) A method for the estimation of oestriol, oestrone and oestradiol-17β in the blood of the pregnant woman, and of the foetus. *J. Endocr.* **21**, 9.

ROY E.J. & KERR M.G. (1964) The concentration of oestrogens in the peripheral blood of the diabetic women. *J. Obstet. Gynaec. Br. Cwlth.* **71**, 106.

RUBIN BETTY, DORFMAN R.I. & MILLER M. (1946) Hormone metabolites in blood and urine of diabetic pregnant patients with and without toxaemia. *J. Clin. Endocr.* **6**, 347.

SALHANICK H.A., NOALL M.W., ZARROW M.X. & SAMUELS L.T. (1952) The isolation of progesterone from human placentae. *Science*, **115**, 708.

SALING E. (1962) Amnioscopy, a new method for the diagnosis of conditions hazardous to the fetus when membranes are intact. *Geburtsh. Frauenheilk*, **22**, 830.

SALING E. (1963) Erstmalige Blutanalysen und PH Messungen am Feten unter Geburt und die klinische Bedeutung dieses neuen Verfahrens. *Arch. für Gynak.* **198**, 82.

SANDLER M. & COVENEY J. (1962) Placental mono-amine oxidase activity in toxaemia of pregnancy. *Lancet*, i, 1096.

SCHILD W. (1961) Qualitative and quantative Bestimmung von freien und konjugiertem Oestron, 17β-Oestradiol un Oestriol in biologischem material. *Zeitschrift für die gesamte experimentelle Medizin*, **135**, 13.

SCHILD W., SCHURHOLZ K. & SEUKEN A. (1963a) Untersuchungen über den Gehalt an Oestron, 17β-Oestradiol und Oestriol in Nabelschurvene und Nabelschurarterien. *Zeitschrift für die gesamte experimentelle Medizin.* **136**, 552.

SCHILD W., SCHURHOLTZ K. & SEUKEN A. (1963b) Untersuchungen über den Oestrogengehalt in den Nabelschurgefassen und im Retroplacentenblut. *Archiv. für Gynak.* **198**, 136.

SCHOLL O. (1963) Die Klinische bedeutung pränatuler elektrokardiographischer und phonokardiographischer vorsogeutersuchungen. *Arch. Gynaek.* **198**, 103.

SELIGMAN A.M. & ASHBEL R. (1951) Histochemical demonstration of ketosteroids in virilizing tumours of the adrenal cortex. *Endocrinology*, **49**, 110.

SHEARMAN R.P. (1959) Some aspects of the urinary excretion of pregnanediol in pregnancy. *J. Obstet. Gynaec. Br. Emp.* **66**, 1.

SHEARMAN R.P. & GARRETT W.J. (1963) Double-blind study of the effect of 17-hydroxyprogesterone caproate on abortion rate. *Br. med. J.* i, 292.

SHORT R.V. (1958) The chemical determination of progesterone in peripheral blood. *J. Endocr.* **16**, 415.

SHORT R.V. & ETON B. (1959) Progesterone in the peripheral blood of pregnant women. *J. Endocr.* **18**, 418.

SLAUNWHITE W.R. & SANDBERG A.A. (1959) Phenolic steroids in human subjects. III Estrogens in plasma of pregnant women. *Proc. Soc. exp. Biol.* **101**, 544.

SMITH G.V. & SMITH O.W. (1934) Excessive gonad-stimulating hormone and subnormal amounts of estrin in the toxemias of late pregnancy. *Am. J. Physiol.* **107**, 128.

SMITH G.V. & SMITH O.W. (1948) Internal secretions and toxaemia of late pregnancy. *Physiol. Rev.* **28**, 1.

SMITH O. & SMITH G.V. (1937) Prolan and estrin in the serum of diabetic and non-diabetic women during pregnancy. *Am. J. Obstet. Gynec.* **33**, 365.

SMITH K., GREENE J.W. & TOUCHSTONE J.C. (1966) Urinary estriol determination in the management of prolonged pregnancy. *Am. J. Obstet. Gynec.* **96**, 901.

SOLOMON S. (1966) Formation and metabolism of neutral steroids in the human placenta and fetus. *J. clin. Endocr.* **26**, 762.

SOMMERVILLE I.F. & DESPHANDE G.N. (1958) The quantitative determination of progesterone and pregnanediol in human plasma. *J. clin. Endocr.* **18**, 1223.

SOULE S.D. (1964) The practical value of vaginal cytology in pregnancy. *Acta cytol. (Balt.)*, **8**, 364.

SOULE S.D. (1964) The practical value of vaginal cytology in pregnancy. II. Vaginal smears during labour. *Acta cytol.* **8**, 368.

SOUTHERN E.M. (1957) Fetal anoxia and its possible relation to changes in the prenatal fetal electrocardiogram. *Am. J. Obstet. Gynec.* **73**, 233.

STAMM O., RAWYLER V. & RIOTTON G. (1959) Hormonal basis of the cytological changes during pathological pregnancies. *Acta cytol.* **3**, 201.

STIMMEL B.F. (1946) The fractionation and photometric estimation of the estrogens in human pregnancy urine. *J. Biol. Chem.* **162**, 99.

STRAND A. (1966) The function of the placenta and placental insufficiency with especial reference to the development of prolonged foetal distress. *Acta Obstet. Gynec. Scandinav.* **45**, Suppl. 1.

SVENDSON R. (1960) A double isotope derivative method for the quantitative determination of oestrone and 17β-oestradiol in plasma. *Acta endocr.* **35**, 161.

TAYLOR E.S., BRUNS P.D., HEPNER H.J. & DROSE V.E. (1958) Measurements of placental function. *Am. J. Obstet. Gynec.* **76**, 983.

TAYLOR E.S., BRUNS P.D., DUNCAN I.W. & DROSE V.E. (1961) Urinary estriol determinations in normal pregnancy. *Am. J. Obstet. Gynec.* **81**, 625.

TAYLOR E.S., HASSNER H., BRUNS P.D. & DROSE V.E. (1963) Urinary estriol excretion of pregnant patients with pyelonephritis and Rh immunisation. *Am. J. Obstet. Gynec.* **85**, 10.

TAYLOR E.S., BRUNS P.D. & DROSE V.E. (1965) Estriol excretion in normal and complicated pregnancies. *Clin. Obstet. Gynec.* **8**, 550.

TEN BERGE B.S. (1955) De bloodstroom in de placentavlokken. *Ned. Tijdschr. Geneesk*, **99**, 2371.

TEN BERGE B.S. (1961) The influence of the placenta on cerebral injuries. *Cereb. Palsy. Bull.* **3**, 323.

TEN BERGE B.S., WEEKE A. & GROEN A. (1957) Oestriolbestimmung während der swangerschaft. *Arch. für Gynak.* **189**, 140.

TENNEY B. (1936) Syncytial degeneration in normal and pathologic placentas. *Am. J. Obstet. Gynec.* **31**, 1024.

TENNEY S.M. & REMMERS J.E. (1963) Comparative quantitative morphology of the mammalian lung. *Nature, Lond.* **197**, 54.

THOMSEN K. (1954) Zur morphologie und genese der sog. Placentarinfarkte. *Arch. Gynäk.* **185**, 221.

THOMSEN K. (1955) Über die aktivität der alkalischen phosphates in der menschlichen placenta. *Arch. Gynaek.* **187**, 1.

THOMSON A.M., HYTTEN F.E. & BILLEWICZ W.Z. (1967) The epidemiology of oedema during pregnancy. *J. Obstet. Gynaec. Br. Cwlth.* **74**, 1.

TIMONEN S. & HIRVONEN E. (1964) Urinary excretion of oestrogens in pre-eclamptic toxaemia of pregnancy. *Annls Chir. Gynaec. Fenn.* **53**, 96.

TINDALL V.R. & SCOTT J.S. (1965) Placental calcification; a study of 3025 singleton and multiple pregnancies. *J. Obstet. Gynaec. Br. Cwlth.* **71**, 379.

TOAFF R., AYALON D., LUNENFIELD B. & ESHKOL A. (1965) Immuno-titrations and quantitative bioassays of pregnancy urine. *J. Obstet. Gynaec. Br. Wwlth.* **72**, 236.

TOMINAGA T. & PAGE E.W. (1966) Accommodation of the human placenta to hypoxia. *Am. J. Obstet. Gynec.* **94**, 679.

TORPIN R. & SWAIN B. (1966) Placental infarction in 1000 cases correlated with clinical findings. *Am. J. Obstet. Gynec.* **94**, 284.

TOUCHSTONE J.C. & MURAWEC T. (1965) In *Gas Chromatography of Steroids in Biological Fluids*, p. 243. M.B.Lipsett, ed. Plenum Press, New York.

TREMBLAY P.C., SYBULKI S. & MAUGHAN G.B. (1965) Role of the placenta in fetal malnutrition. *Am. J. Obstet. Gynec.* **91**, 597.

TROEN P., NILSSON B., WIQUIST N. & DICZFALUSY E. (1961) Pattern of oestriol conjugates in human cord blood, amniotic fluid and urine of newborns. *Acta endocr.* **38**, 361.

TROLLE D. (1955) Experimental and clinical investigation on the pregnanediol excretion in human urine. *Acta endocr.* **19**, 217.

TURNBULL A.C., ANDERSON A. & WILSON G. (1967) Maternal urinary oestrogen as evidence of a foetal role in determining gestation at labour. *Lancet*, ii, 627.

VAN DER MOLEN H.J. & HART P.G. (1961) Die uitscheiding van 5β-pregnaan-3α,20α-diol in urine tijdens de zwangerschap. *Ned. T. v Verlosk en Gyn.* **61**, 391.

VASICKA A. & HUTCHINSON H.T. (1964) Oxygen tension in amniotic fluid and fetal distress. *Am. J. Obstet. Gynec.* **88**, 530.

VERMELIN H., RIBON M. & RIBON C. (1957) Interet et limites d'interpretation du dosage de prolan dans les avortements. *Bull. Fed. Socs. Gynec. Obstet. Lang. fr.* **9**, 210.

VILLEE C.A. (1962) Metabolism of the placenta. *Am. J. Obstet. Gynec.* **84**, 1684.

VILLEE C.A. & HAGERMAN D.D. (1953) Effects of estradiol on the metabolism of the human placenta *in vitro*. *J. biol. Chem.* **205**, 873.

WACHSTEIN M., MEAGHER J.G. & ORTIZ J. (1963) Enzyme histochemistry of the human placenta. *Am. J. Obstet. Gynec.* **87**, 13.

WALKER A.H. (1957) Liquor amnii studies in the prediction of haemolytic disease of the newborn. *Br. med. J.* ii, 376.

WANG H.W. & HELLMAN L.M. (1943) Studies in the metabolism of human placenta. Oxygen consumption in relation to ageing. *Bull. Johns Hopkins Hosp.* **73**, 31.

WATTS R.M. & ADAIR F.L. (1943) Excretion of estrogen and gonadotrophin in late pregnancy. *Am. J. Obstet. Gynec.* **46**, 183.

WHITE PRISCILLA & HUNT HAZEL (1943) Pregnancy complicating diabetes. *J. clin. Endocr.* **3**, 500.

WIDE L. & GEMZELL C.A. (1960) An immunological pregnancy test. *Acta endocr.* **35**, 261.

WIDE L. & GEMZELL C.A. (1962) Determinations of gonadotrophins in urine by a haemagglutination-inhibition technique. *Ciba Fdn. Colloq. Endocr.* **14**, 296. Churchill, London.

WIELENGA G. & WILLIGHAGEN R.G. (1962) The histochemistry of the syncytiotrophoblast and the stroma in the normal full-term placenta. *Am. J. Obstet. Gynec.* **84**, 1059.

WILSON R.B., ALBERT A. & RANDALL L.M. (1949) Quantitative study on the production, destruction and elimination of chorionic gonadotrophin in normal pregnancy. *Am. J. Obstet. Gynec.* **58**, 960.

WISLOCKI G.B. & DEMPSEY E.W. (1946) Ageing of placental villi. *Endocrinology*, **38**, 90.

WISLOCKI G.B., DEMPSEY E.W. & FAWCETT D.W. (1948) Some functional activities of the placental trophoblast. *Obstet. Gynec. Surv.* **3**, 604.

WODRIG W. & GORETZLEHNER W. (1964) Untersuchungen über den Östrogenspeigel im Blutserum und Fruchtwasser bei Diabetes mellitus und Schwangerschaft. *Z. Geburtsh. Gynak.* **162**, 89.

WOTIZ H.H. & MARTIN H.F. (1962) Gas chromatographic determination of estrogens in human pregnancy urine. *Analyt. Biochem.* **3**, 97.

WRAY P.M. & RUSSEL C.S. (1964) Maternal urinary oestriol levels before and after death of the foetus. *J. Obstet. Gynaec. Br. Cwlth.* **71**, 97.

WÜRTELE A. (1962) Ostrogenausscheidung bei Spätgestosen. *Z. Geburtsh. Gynak.* **159**, 287.

WÜRTELE A. (1963) Das Verhalten der Harnausscheidung von oestron 17β-oestradiol und oestriol bei Spätgestosen. *Arch. für Gynak.* **198**, 131.

YOUSEM H., SEITCHIK J. & SOLOMON D. (1966) Maternal estriol excretion and fetal dysmaturity. *Obstet. and Gynec.* **28**, 491.

ZANDER J. (1954) Progesterone in human blood and tissues. *Nature, Lond.* **174**, 406.

ZANDER J. (1957) Die gestagen wirksamen hormone in organismus. *Geburtsh. Frauenheilk.* **17**, 876.

ZANDER J. (1959) Gestagens in human pregnancy. In *Recent Progress in the Endocrinology of Reproduction*, p. 255. C.W.Lloyd, ed. Academic Press, London.

ZANDER J. (1962) Progesterone. In *Methods in Hormone Research*, Vol. 1, p. 91. R.I. Dorfman, ed. Academic Press, London.

ZEEK P.M. & ASSALI N.S. (1952) The formation, regression and differential diagnosis of true infarcts of the placenta. *Am. J. Obstet. Gynec.* **64**, 1191.

ZEUTHEN E. (1953) Oxygen uptake as related to body size in organisms. *Q. Rev. Biol.* **28**, 1.

ZONDEK B. (1954) Some problems related to ovarian function and to pregnancy. *Recent Prog. Horm. Res.* **10**, 395.

ZONDEK B. & GOLDBERG S. (1957) Placental function and foetal death. *J. Obstet. Gynaec. Br. Emp.* **64**, 1.

ZONDEK B. & PFEIFER V. (1959) Urinary oestriol during pregnancy and its significance for the estimation of placental function. *Acta Obst. et Gynec. Scandinav.* **38**, 742.

10
Endocrinology of the Foetus

M.C.MACNAUGHTON

'What a piece of work is a man.' *Hamlet*

INTRODUCTION

The development of the normal foetus involves the normal physiological specialization of tissues and organs, and the development of the foetal endocrine glands is an integral part of this evolution. Interactions of foetal glands, and their effects during intrauterine life, were suggested as early as 1836 by Hilaire and much of the experimental work since then has supported his view. It is also now clear that there may be great differences between species and that it is unwise to draw conclusions about one mammal from data derived from another.

The work of Jost and his colleagues has pointed the way in experimental foetal endocrinology, and techniques such as decapitation have been particularly useful in delineating the extent of foetal endocrine gland activity, and its effect on growth and development.

Diczfalusy and his colleagues have shown how intimately the foetus and placenta are related in the process of hormone production and metabolism. It is often therefore, well-nigh impossible, in a given set of circumstances, to say whether a hormone level in the foetus is due to foetal or placental production.

This chapter is primarily concerned with the physiology of development of the foetal endocrine glands, and emphasis is placed on the human foetus when information is available. However, much of the information has been obtained from animal experiments and frequently little is known of conditions in man owing to technical difficulties; in these areas reference is made to the relevant animal work.

The endocrine glands at birth seem to be as well developed, and as ready for extrauterine activity as are any of the other physiological systems of the neonate. There may be some temporary imbalance of homeostatic mechanisms of the adrenal cortex, pancreas, parathyroid and posterior pituitary glands, but these could be explained by failure of target organ response as well as by failures of hormone production.

In the adult most of the endocrine glands are in a homeostatic state, but it is not known whether or not this is so in the foetus. The environment of the foetus is to a great extent regulated by the mother through the placenta. For instance, maternal hyperglycaemia is accompanied by foetal hyperglycaemia. It is, however, possible that foetal hormones may regulate biochemical processes in the foetus and Jost & Picon (1958) found an influence of the thyroid on the lipid content of the body in thyroidectomized rabbit foetuses.

It is also possible (Jost 1961a), that the foetal hormones exert effects on target organs at definite stages of development, and it is therefore important to discover the effect of foetal hormones on target organs. It should be remembered, however, that no foetal endocrine gland has so far been found to be indispensible to the survival of the foetus. Animal foetuses have survived in spite of the removal of the pituitary, thyroid, parathyroid and adrenal glands.

Histological and histochemical evidence is becoming available about the possible function of foetal endocrine glands, but the finding of a hormone in a particular situation only proves its presence, and not its synthesis or storage. The use of autoradiography, and perfusion with radioactive precursors, has increased our knowledge, and where large accumulations of activity have been found, it seems reasonable to conclude that storage in that area is likely.

In vitro techniques of incubation of foetal glands show that the glands under the conditions of the experiment have certain properties, but it is again unwise to extrapolate from the *in vitro* to the *in vivo* situation.

Certain endocrine disorders of the mother, such as diabetes and adrenal disease have effects on the foetus during intrauterine life, making specialized management necessary in the neonatal period to restore normal conditions in the foetus. A full knowledge of the foetal endocrine system and the interrelationship of foetal and maternal endocrine secretions is necessary for this purpose.

In the present chapter the development of the endocrine system, and its function in intrauterine life will be discussed under the headings of the various glands.

PITUITARY GLAND

The endocrine role of the foetal pituitary and the effect of its trophic secretions on other foetal endocrine glands has been studied in certain animals, and it seems likely that at least some of the foetal endocrine glands are under the control of the foetal pituitary. The foetal pituitary seems to be active from very early in pregnancy, and its trophic factors probably play an important part in stimulating the secretion of some of its dependant glands.

I ACTH

There has been much discussion of the effect of the foetal pituitary on the size of the foetal adrenal cortex. Foetal pituitary ACTH has been detected in the gland by the 10th week of gestation, (Taylor, Loraine & Robertson 1953), and is thought by Lanman (1961) to be the trophic hormone responsible for foetal adrenal hypertrophy. Lanman (1962) considered that foetal adrenal enlargment reflected an intense stimulus to the gland, and that there was apparently the same type of feedback control mechanism as in the adult. Jost *et al.* (1962) have shown that decapitation of the foetus produces atrophy of the adrenal glands, with altered histology of the cortex and changes in lipid distribution and ascorbic acid content. These alterations can be prevented by giving ACTH to decapitated animals.

More recently Jost & Cohen (1966) have suggested that this 'atrophy' which occurs in decapitated rat foetuses results from a special mode of development which takes place in the absence of the pituitary.

Margolis *et al.* (1966) found in the foetal rat, that the activity of phenyl ethanolamine-N-methyl transferase, the enzyme that methylates noradrenaline to form adrenaline increases in the foetal rat during the day preceding adrenaline accumulation. These developments could be prevented by foetal hypophysectomy but administration of ACTH or cortisol acetate reversed the effects of foetal decapitation showing that the activity of adrenal cortex and medulla are closely related and that the medulla also is influenced by ACTH secretion from the pituitary gland.

The maximum relative weight of the human foetal adrenal gland is greatest about the 4th month of pregnancy (Eckholme & Niemineva 1950).

The human foetal adrenal cortex is characterized by the greatly enlarged foetal zone which regresses after birth. This zone is very atrophic in fullgrown anencephalic foetuses.

Some anterior pituitary tissue is present in almost all human anencephalics (Angevine 1938, Lanman 1953), and ACTH has been found in the pituitary of an anencephalic monster at term, although the adrenal cortex was hypoplastic. In anencephalics the neurohypophysis is most markedly deficient. Lanman (1962) treated an anencephalic monster, which survived for 18 days with ACTH and found that normal hypertrophic adrenals with a foetal zone were present after this time. He believes that the growth of the foetal zone is dependant on ACTH produced by the foetal pituitary. This view has been supported by recent work by Bearn (1967). He found that when foetal rats were hypophysectomized by decapitation *in utero* that, although the headless foetuses continued to grow at the same rate as controls, the adrenals were significantly reduced in size and the thymus was hypertrophied. In a second series when depot ACTH was injected into each foetus at the time of decapitation the changes in the adrenal and thymus did not occur. This again confirms that the development and functional activity of the foetal adrenals is controlled by the foetal pituitary.

It seems likely that the hypoplasia of the anencephalic adrenal cortex results from insufficient release of ACTH from the foetal pituitary.

ACTH appears to cross the placenta readily but the amount crossing to the foetus is insufficient to stimulate adequately the foetal adrenal cortex, and no adrenocorticotrophic activity has so far been demonstrated in cord blood (Gemzell *et al.* 1955).

2 GONADOTROPHINS

There is good histological and histochemical evidence that foetal or neonatal ovaries are able to respond to gonadotrophin stimulation (Spivak 1934, Ober & Bernstein 1955, Pinkerton 1959). Whether this gonadotrophin is produced by the foetal or maternal pituitary or by the placenta is not clear. A possible foetal origin is suggested by Rosa (1954), who found a correlation between the histological appearance of the foetal ovaries and the number of chromophil cells in the foetal pituitary. There is, however, some evidence that gonadal development in anencephalic monsters, who lack a pituitary gland, is normal.

It seems, certainly in animals, that gonadotrophic stimulation is required by the foetus for the proper development of certain target organs. For instance, Jost (1948, 1951b) found definite abnormalities in the genital tract, if male rabbit embryos were decapitated on day 18–19, before differentiation of the genital tract was initiated. He interpreted this as resulting from a diminution of testicular activity, which could be prevented by giving gonadotrophic hormone to the decapitated foetuses.

He concluded that, in the rabbit, there is a hypophyseal stimulation of the gonads about day 22–24, when the male structures are being established. Jost (1953b), and Bettendorf *et al.* (1962) estimated the total gonadotrophic activity in the human foetal hypophysis and found very low values. In children they could detect no gonadotrophic activity at all. It is just possible that the activity found in the foetus might therefore have been maternal or placental in origin.

It therefore seems probable that a time factor is involved, and Jost (1961a) has suggested that there may be a period of high secretory activity of the foetal pituitary followed by a period of lesser activity. The finding by Rosa (1954) of a gonadotrophic effect on the ovaries of intact immature mice, which had been implanted with pituitary tissue from human embryos, does suggest the formation of some gonadotrophin by the human foetal pituitary.

It is obvious that further work is required on this subject. It seems, however, that conditions are quite different in the human where genital development, for instance, is apparently normal in the anencephalic foetus, whereas in the rabbit, effects on the accessary reproductive organs are evident. These effects are less pronounced in other species e.g. hamster (Foote 1955), and are absent in the mouse and rat foetus (Jost 1953b).

3 GROWTH HORMONE

While it has been stated by Smith & Dortzbach (1929) that growth hormone has been detected in foetal pig pituitaries, this must be viewed with caution. It is the development of radioimmuno assay methods for growth hormone which have permitted the accurate assessment of growth hormone secretion at delivery and in the early weeks of life.

High levels of growth hormone in umbilical vein blood at delivery have been reported by Greenwood *et al.* (1964), and this was confirmed by Daughaday *et al.* (1964), who also found that these high levels persisted during the first 48 hours of neonatal life. The latter workers found in addition that the mean half-life of growth hormone in infants was 13 minutes compared with a rate of between 20 and 30 minutes in adults (Parker *et al.* 1962). From these observations it seems evident that the disappearance rate of growth hormone from the plasma is accelerated in infancy and the high concentration of hormone reported probably represents true hypersecretion.

It seems likely, therefore, that the human foetal pituitary does produce growth hormone at least in the later stages of pregnancy although, in the human, somatic development is normal in anencephalic monsters (Nanangas 1925). There is also a growth hormone-like factor in the human placenta which has immunologic properties which differ from growth hormone itself. This was first suggested by the work of Josimovich & MacLaren (1962) and later followed by Daughaday *et al.* (1964). Further work by Josimovich & Atwood (1964) has done much to elucidate the function of this placental lactogen. It is possible that the placental factor may be operative in early pregnancy, while later in gestation the foetal pituitary takes over the function by the production of growth hormone.

Laron *et al.* (1966) have shown that there is no transfer of growth hormone through the placenta in rabbits during gestation so that any effect that maternal growth hormone may have on the foetus can only be indirect. There is also an exaggerated response of growth hormone to hypoglycaemia in early infancy, although it is possible that the secretion of growth hormone only begins at delivery. Whether the growth hormone secreted by the foetal pituitary is related to baby size is not known, but Greenwood (1964) did not find that the higher levels in children were related to differences in growth rate, so it seems improbable that there is a relation between secretion and foetal growth. Attempts have been made to incriminate growth hormone as the cause of the large babies in diabetic mothers but the evidence for this is inconclusive.

The findings in general suggest that foetal growth hormone derives from the foetal pituitary and not from the placenta and lends further support to the view that the foetal pituitary is an actively functioning organ.

4 THYROID STIMULATING HORMONE (TSH)

There is much confusing evidence about the presence and role of thyrotrophin in the foetus. Embryonic growth and differentiation are intrinsic properties of embryonic thyroid epithelium which can be carried out in the absence of thyrotrophin (Purvis 1964). Differentiation of the basophil cells in the anterior pituitary lobe in rats (Jost & Tavernier 1956) and rabbits (Jost & Danysz 1952) begins only about three days before birth. TSH has been demonstrated in the anterior pituitary of a human foetus from the 8th week of foetal life (Mizusawa 1966). In the guinea-pig secretion of the thyrotrophin from the pituitary gland may be demonstrated during the latter half of pregnancy. Furthermore after ablation of the hypophysis by decapitation, or its destruction by irradiation, a retardation of the histological differentiation of the foetal thyroid gland occurs in the mouse (Raynaud & Frilley 1948), in the hamster (Foote & Foote 1949), in the rabbit (Jost 1953a), and in the rat (Noumura 1959). Decreases in iodine trapping, hormonal synthesis and secretion have also been reported in animals (Jost, Morel & Marois 1952, Jost 1961b, Geloso 1958).

These disorders can be corrected when thyrotrophin is given (Geloso 1964). These investigations suggest that, in the foetus, the hypophysis is necessary for normal thyroid development and function. It is however, apparent from the work of Jost & Tavernier (1956), that some degree of differentiation and development of the foetal thyroid may occur without stimulus from the foetal pituitary. These workers found that when rat foetuses are decapitated on day 16 of gestation, no thyroidal trapping of iodine occurs at this stage, and there are no histological signs of thyrotrophic activity in the foetal hypophysis. However, the thyroid glands of these foetuses show slight trapping of radioiodide on day 18, and the extent of this becomes greater at the end of pregnancy. When the thyroid extracts were subjected to analysis, thyroxine was found. In a human anencephalic infant, lacking a hypophysis, thyroxine has been found in the gland (Yamazaki *et al.* 1959). These workers also showed that in the human foetal thyroid, iodine can be accumulated at 14 weeks, and at about 19 weeks thyroxine can be synthesized. Lampé, Kertesz & Dzvonyar (1964) also suggested that iodine storage occurred in the thyroid after the 12th week of pregnancy. The TSH activity of cord blood, however, differs little from that of the maternal peripheral venous blood (Yamazaki *et al.* 1961), but it has been reported that in rabbits the maternal thyrotrophin does not pass the placental barrier (Osorio & Myant 1960a). If it is true that there is no passage of TSH through the placenta then the foetal pituitary must be producing the circulating thyrotrophin. This view, however, is in conflict with the evidence that anencephalics or an infant with a congenitally absent pituitary gland may have a morphologically normal thyroid gland (Blizzard & Albert 1956).

The evidence, therefore as to whether thyrotrophin does pass the placenta, is confusing and it is possible that species differences may account for the varying reports.

It seems most probable that normal development of the foetal thyroid requires the presence of foetal thyrotrophin from the anterior pituitary, but that if this gland is absent, some degree of development of the thyroid with some iodine trapping and synthesis of thyroxine can occur, but not to a normal extent. This view is suggested, in animals at least, by Jost *et al.* (1949), who found that decapitation of rabbit embryos greatly reduced the radioiodine uptake of the foetal thyroid. In the reverse direction, Geloso (1964) has shown that when thyroxine is administered to rat foetuses, results similar to those of decapitation are obtained and hormonal secretion is markedly inhibited. An excess of thyroid hormone in the foetal blood diminishes adenohypophyseal hormone production and thereby reduces thyroid secretion. It is probable that there is considerable species difference in respect of the production and effect of TSH during foetal life.

5 ANTIDIURETIC HORMONE (ADH) AND OXYTOCIN

The hormones of the posterior pituitary are probably elaborated in the hypothalamus but stored in and released from the posterior pituitary. Niemineva (1950) found that the hypophyseal-portal system is fully developed in human foetuses at term and it seems that the neurohypophysis is capable of function by this time.

Dicker & Tyler (1953) estimated the vasopressor and oxytocic activities of the pituitary gland of 25 human foetuses varying in gestational age from 55–195 days. Neither activity was present earlier than 70 days but from 70–110 days both activities could be demonstrated. Quantitative assays were possible from 110 days onwards. In all the foetuses the amount of vasopressor activity greatly exceeded the oxytocic activity but the ratio of vasopressor to oxytocic activity at full term is about 1:1 (Heller & Zaimis 1949).

It has been suggested (Heller & Zaimis 1949) that lack of vasopressin might be responsible for the apparent inability of the newborn infant to concentrate urine to the same extent as the adult. This seems unlikely as the relative amount of vasopressor activity in newborn animals is not very different from that found in adults. A more likely explanation is that the kidneys of the newborn may not have the same ability to respond as in the adult, and Heller (1952) has demonstrated that the kidneys of newborn rats are less responsive to exogenous posterior pituitary ADH than adults. However, the premature infant does show a substantial response to I.V. Pitressin and it cannot, therefore, be assumed that a diminished response to ADH is the cause of the apparently decreased ability to concentrate urine (Barnett & Vesterdal 1953). McCance & Widdowson (1953) conclude that the foetal kidney is not under ADH control.

In newborn animals the antidiuretic-vasopressor activity of the neurohypophyseal tissue of newborn animals is mature, but the oxytocic function is immature. The main function of oxytocin is concerned with parturition and milk ejection, so it is somewhat surprising to find relatively large amounts present in the full term foetus. It is possible that some of this oxytocin might have come from the mother, but there is no information about the trans-placental passage of this hormone. Injection of vasopressin into the foetus has been reported to cause a rise in arterial tension in the mother in animals, suggesting some passage of vasopressin from foetus to mother (Snoeck 1958) but further work is necessary to confirm this observation.

Congenital amputations have been induced by ADH (Jost 1950, 1951a), so it is possible that this hormone may play some part in the pathogenesis of malformations.

THE THYROID GLAND

DEVELOPMENT OF THE THYROID GLAND

In mammals including man it is almost certain that normal growth and development does not occur when thyroid hormone is absent. This results in the human, in congenital hypothyroidism leading to mental deficiency and retarded ossification. Knowledge of foetal thyroid development and function is therefore of considerable interest and importance.

Early studies in mammals (Fenger 1912) indicated that the foetal thyroid gland has biological activity early in pregnancy. Rumph & Smith (1926) induced metamorphosis of hypophysectomized tadpoles with thyroid or pituitary gland implants from foetal pigs.

In the human, there is every appearance of thyroid activity in many foetuses by the end of the third month of development. Experiments using I_{131} indicate that there is an uptake of iodine by the human foetal gland at the time when the colloid is first seen (Chapman *et al.* 1948, Hodges *et al.* 1955). Anderson and co-workers (quoted by Kaijser 1959) administered I_{131} to women at different times before legal abortion and found that the thyroid gland of the foetus first concentrated the isotope at the 12th to 14th week of pregnancy. The uptake increased progressively up to 25 weeks of gestation. The initial stage of uptake found by these workers corresponds well with the histological changes found in the gland (Shepherd *et al.* 1964). These workers, examining human foetal thyroid glands, observed scallop-like vacuolization of the outer parts of the colloid cavity, indicative of utilization of thyroid hormone in embryos of 70–80 mm crown-rump length and this became more prominent in foetuses of 89 mm and over. The 70–80 mm length corresponds to 75–80 days of gestation. Shepherd *et al.* also reported that the human thyroid does not develop synchronously throughout. There is much variation in the state of maturity seen in the same section and in different foetuses of the same length. Aboul-Khair *et al.* (1966) have confirmed that the growth and iodine trapping function of the human foetal thyroid is age dependent at least until the 23rd week of gestation.

More recent work on the human foetus confirms that storage of iodine starts in the 12th week of pregnancy and increases throughout pregnancy (Lampé *et al.* 1964), and these workers also point out that the thyroid accumulates ^{131}I to a concentration 10–100 times greater than in other foetal organs. The hazards of treatment with ^{131}I during pregnancy are obvious from this observation.

PASSAGE OF THYROID HORMONE FROM MOTHER TO FOETUS

Since normal foetal development requires thyroid hormone, this could reach the foetus from the foetal thyroid, or from the mother via the placenta. The experiments of Peterson & Young (1952) indicated that thyroid hormone does cross from mother to foetus in the guinea-pig. Knobil *et al.* (1959) have shown that tri-iodo thyronine and thyroxine cross the placenta in rats. Hirvonen & Lybeck (1956) injected thyroxine and tri-iodo thyronine into guinea pigs in late pregnancy and found that the concentration in the foetal serum was much lower than that in the maternal two to four and a half hours later, suggesting that the passage of the hormone across the guinea-pig placenta is very slow. The permeability of the rat placenta to tri-iodo thyronine seems much greater than that of guinea-pig, rabbit or man (Osorio & Myant 1960b). The effectiveness with which the thyroid passes from maternal to foetal circulation is probably influenced in some way by the foetal pituitary, Hamburgh *et al.* (1962). Hall & Myant (1956) and Myant (1958) found that radioactive thyroxine in the rabbit was transferred across the placenta more rapidly in late than in early pregnancy, and they consider that conditions for the transfer of the hormone across the placenta become more favourable as pregnancy advances. These workers have also shown that neither deiodination or storage occurs to any extent in the foetus.

In human beings the transfer of hormone from mother to foetus resembles that found in the rabbit. Grumbach & Werner (1956) injected radioactive thyroxine into the mother in late pregnancy and demonstrated a relatively high concentration in the foetal serum at birth. Myant (1958), found, on the other hand, that relatively little activity reached the foetus if the injection was made early in pregnancy. Tri-iodo thyronine appears to pass from mother to foetus more readily than thyroxine at all stages of pregnancy. Carr *et al.* (1959), gave large doses of dessicated thyroid during their third pregnancy to two women who had previously given birth to two cretins. Each gave birth to a living infant whose clinical appearance, cord blood PBI and BEI concentrations, and I_{131} uptake suggested that an adequate amount of thyroid hormone had been transferred across the placenta. Huge doses of thyroid were given by these workers; amounts up to 20 g daily.

It would appear, therefore, that although some maternal thyroid hormone does reach the foetus the amount is inadequate to ensure completely normal development if the foetal thyroid production is inadequate. Newborns with cretinism do not have myxoedema but they frequently show pathological changes of skeletal and brain growth (Grumbach & Werner 1956). It has also been shown that totally athyroid women can conceive and bear normal children while myxoedematous

(Hodges *et al.* 1952), although in some, while the newborn did not show signs of hypothyroidism, there was some physical and mental retardation

ROLE OF BINDING SUBSTANCES IN THE DISTRIBUTION OF THYROID HORMONE BETWEEN MOTHER AND FOETUS

Thyroid hormone in the blood is reversibly adsorbed to thyroxine-binding protein (TBP). This fact influences the passage of hormone from mother to foetus. If the placenta is impermeable to TBP only a small amount of circulating hormone will be available for exchange across the placenta at any one time. The concentrations of total hormone in the maternal and foetal circulations at equilibrium will be in the ratio of their thyroxine binding power. The binding power of foetal rabbit TBP for thyroxine is greater than that of adult TBP (Myant & Osorio 1959). The proportion bound by foetal TBP is greater at the lowest concentrations of thyroxine; if this relationship is also true *in vivo* it would ensure that the foetus has an adequate supply where a deficiency is present.

These findings in rabbits are not directly transferable to man because TBP in the human foetus cannot be distinguished from that found in adults. However, Osorio & Myant (1960b) have shown that the thyroxine binding capacity of TBP in the serum from the human foetus at the 15th week of gestation is much lower than in the maternal serum.

PASSAGE OF THYROID HORMONE FROM FOETUS TO MOTHER

There is little reliable evidence on the passage of thyroid hormone from foetus to mother. The measurement of butanol-extractable iodine and PBI in maternal and cord blood suggests some exchange (Mann *et al.* 1952, Dowling *et al.* 1956). It has also been found, that in some women untreated myxoedema is temporarily relieved during pregnancy, (Zondek 1940) and this has been put forward as showing that the hormone secreted by the foetus is available to the mother. However, Hall & Myant (1956) found very little radio-activity in the maternal serum four hours after injection of radioactive thyroxine into rabbit foetuses.

The question as to whether thyroid hormone passes from foetus to mother is still open although it seems likely that some passage does occur.

FUNCTION OF THE FOETAL THYROID

There is good evidence suggesting that synthesis of thyroid hormones does occur in the foetal gland. This has been demonstrated in man, Yamazaki *et al.* (1959), the monkey, Pickering *et al.* (1961) and several other mammals, and it is probable that these hormones are secreted into the blood. Thus, Geloso (1958), and Nataf & Sfez (1961) have shown that at the end of gestation the plasma of the foetuses of thyroidectomized rats injected with I_{131} contains labelled thyroxine. Geloso (1964) has also demonstrated that, in the rat, radio-active thyroxine is absent from the plasma of thyroidectomized foetuses where the mother has also had her thyroid removed. This seems to show that the foetal blood thyroxine is secreted by the thyroid gland of the foetus.

Hormonal synthesis begins before differentiation of the gland is complete (Waterman & Gorbman 1956). It therefore seems that follicular structure may not be necessary for hormone synthesis (Geloso 1961, Nataf & Sfez 1961). The stage of gestation at which the various iodinated compounds appear varies greatly with the species. This difference is probably due more to differences in the degree of maturity of the young at birth than to differences in the maturity of the thyroid at a given stage of the development of the foetus as a whole. There does not seem to be any reason to think that the foetal thyroid could supply the foetus with hormone at a particular stage of development in one species and not in another. For example, the thyroid begins to function both in rats and in man shortly after the appearance of the first centres of ossification (Osorio & Myant 1960b). In man at 14 weeks gestation iodide alone is found, and at 19 weeks all iodinated compounds are present (Yamazaki *et al.* 1959).

PHYSIOLOGICAL ROLE OF THYROID HORMONE IN THE MAMMALIAN FOETUS

The effects of thyroid deficiency on postnatal development have been studied in relation to skeletal growth (Scow *et al.* 1948), muscle development Scow (1964), and the central nervous system (Eayrs & Taylor 1951, Legrand *et al.* 1961). There are however, scanty data on the foetal period.

The effect on foetal growth

There is considerable variation in information about the effect of foetal or maternal thyroidectomy or suppression of the thyroid with drugs on foetal growth. It does seem to be established that the presence of the foetal thyroid is not necessary for gains in body weight by the rabbit foetus (Jost 1961b). It has also been reported (Andersen 1960) that the weight of an athyrotic infant is normal.

When considering the results of maternal thyroidectomy or suppression with antithyroid drugs Jost (1961b) observed that any type of maternal thyroid suppression can reduce foetal weight. The maternal diet may also influence foetal growth and Picon (1957) observed no weight change in the foetuses of hypophysectomized rats when operated mothers were pair-fed with controls.

The effect on ossification

Weiss & Noback (1949) reported that in rats thiouracil treatment of the mother produced delayed ossification in the foetus, the defect being almost certainly due to a deficiency of thyroid hormone within the foetus. Jost *et al.* (1960) have disputed these interpretations and consider that the apparent delay in ossification is the consequence of a generalized delay in total development and not a specific effect on ossification. Jost *et al.* (1963) studied the effect of the administration of antithyroid drugs to pregnant rats and observed an increased foetal calcium without any change in maternal levels. They further observed histological modifications in the foetal parathyroid gland and considered that in the rat foetus hypothyroidism leads to hyperparathyroidism. This latter observation is of particular interest in view of the observations of Mégevand, Mathieu & Royer (1961) of the occurrence of hypercalcaemia in some hypothyroid infants. In view of a report by Dorff (1934) of congenital aplasia of the thyroid in a neonate whose bones indicated thyroid deficiency, detailed studies of the effects of thyroidectomy *in utero* are required.

The effect on lipids

An influence of the foetal thyroid on the lipid content of the body as a whole and the liver in particular has been demonstrated by Jost & Picon (1958), and Bearn *et al.* (1961) who demonstrated an increase in foetal plasma cholesterol.

There seems, however, to be no information on the effect of thyroidectomy *in utero* on the development of the nervous system and skeleton although these systems are known to be influenced by thyroid hormone in postnatal life.

It appears, therefore, that normal activity of both foetal and maternal thyroid glands is essential for normal development of the human foetus.

PARATHYROID GLANDS

There is remarkably little information about the foetal parathyroid glands. Scothorne (1964) explanted parathyroid glands from a pair of twin human foetuses of 12–13 weeks gestational age, to the chorio-allantoic membrane of nine or ten day chick embryos in close contact with pieces of neonatal rat parietal bone. Resorption of bone, with perforation occurred close to the parathyroid. The experiments were repeated with sheep parathyroid glands. The results suggest that the parathyroid glands in the human foetus are functional at this gestational age. In the sheep function begins earlier, at the end of the first fifth of its gestational age.

Technical difficulties make experiments in foetuses under 12 weeks unsatisfactory but it seems possible, from evidence in the sheep, that the human glands may function at an even earlier stage than 12 weeks gestational age.

TRANSPLACENTAL PASSAGE OF PARATHYROID HORMONE

Injections of parathyroid hormone into dog foetuses caused foetal hypercalcaemia but no elevation in maternal serum calcium. This suggests that the hormone does not cross the placenta at least in the dog (Hoskins & Snyder 1928).

The amount of maternal parathyroid hormone which crosses the placenta in the human is probably small. Even in severe cases of maternal hyperparathyroidism with marked bone disease, histological and x-ray signs of bone disease are not usually found in the babies. This implies that large amounts of maternal hormone do not cross the placental barrier. However, high plasma alkaline phosphatase levels found in a few infants probably indicate that small amounts may cross (Wagner *et al.* 1964).

FUNCTION OF FOETAL PARATHYROID HORMONE

Jost *et al.* (1963) gave propyl-thiouracil to pregnant rats just before term and found an increase in foetal calcium without any similar change in the maternal level. These workers noticed a diminution in the calcium level in decapitated foetal rats deprived of the thyroid and parathyroid glands. Administration of an antithyroid drug to the mother five days before term produced hypercalcaemia of the foetus, suggesting that some stimulation of the foetal parathyroid had occurred. The parathyroid glands of the foetuses of treated mothers were smaller than those of the controls.

When the thyroid function of the rat foetus was depressed by partial decapitation, the hypophysis being destroyed but the thyroid and parathyroids being left intact, hypercalcaemia resulted in the foetus. This suggests that the thyroid of the foetus participated in control of the parathyroids. Jost *et al.* (1963) conclude that the rat foetus has its own calcium regulatory mechanism which is independent of that of the mother.

The degree of parathyroid activity in foetal life and its relationship to maternal hormone production is uncertain (Smith 1959). Parathyroidectomized animals are not protected from hypocalcaemia by the presence of a foetus. Human mothers with hyperparathyroidism and elevated blood calcium may have hypoparathyroid infants who may develop neonatal tetany. In these babies it is possible that the depression of their parathyroid function is a result of foetal environment. However, hyperparathyroid mothers do not always have hypoparathyroid infants (Walton 1954), so the effect of maternal hyperparathyroidism is not constant. In these subjects it is possible that the effect of excessive maternal parathyroid hormone could be indirect. Some of the excess maternal calcium could pass into the foetal circulation and exert an inhibiting effect on foetal parathyroid function and development.

It seems, therefore, that the parathyroid gland of the foetus is active from an early stage in intrauterine life and that the actions of the foetal thyroid and parathyroid glands are in some way connected during this time.

GONADS

I TESTES

DEVELOPMENT

The process of sexual differentiation of the gonads begins in the human foetus of 14–16 mm in length. The suggestion that the embryonic testes might influence the later differentiation of the genital tract which begins in the human foetus of 30 mm length is supported by the observation of freemartins in certain bovine species.

This condition is also seen in twin pregnancy; the secretions of the foetal testes cause male differentiation of the genital tract in the female twin, due to early connection of the circulation in twins of opposite sex.

In the rabbit, gonadal sex may be recognized on the 15th day of pregnancy (Allen 1904) but other parts of the future sex apparatus remain identical in males and females until day 20. During the next few days differentiation of the genital tract takes place. The female retains the undifferentiated condition until day 23; thereafter the Müllerian duct develops and the Wolffian duct disappears (Jost 1953b, 1961a). In the male, however, rapid change occurs between day 20 and 22. The Müllerian ducts regress and a large seminal vesicle develops.

In the human foetus a similar series of events occurs. The Wolffian duct is well differentiated by the 5th week of intrauterine life and the Müllerian duct appears one week later; both sets of ducts are well developed by the 8th week. About the third month the upper part of the vagina, the uterus and Fallopian tubes develop from the Müllerian ducts in the female while the Wolffian ducts regress leaving vestigial elements such as the epöophoron, and Gaertner's duct. In the male foetus the epididymis, vas deferens and seminal vesicles form from the Wolffian ducts while the Müllerian ducts regress (Grumbach *et al.* 1955).

When male foetuses were castrated before day 23 or the early gonads were destroyed by X-rays in mice (Raynaud & Frilley 1947, Raynaud 1950) no masculine features appeared and sex organogenesis became female in character (Jost 1961a). Genital abnormalities in castrated foetal rats could be prevented by testosterone propionate (Wells *et al.* 1954).

In organ culture experiments with explanted genital tracts Price (1957) and Price & Pannabecker (1959) confirmed these observations. When their castrated explants were cultured on standard medium for four days no seminal vesicles developed and the Wolffian ducts began to regress. When the same type of explant, without testes, was cultured on a medium containing testosterone the seminal vesicles developed and Wolffian ducts were retained. In other words testosterone achieved the same results as the hormone of the foetal testis. However, it has not yet been shown whether foetal testis hormone and testosterone are one and the same. Furthermore, the experiments of Price (1957) and

Price & Pannabecker (1959) took place where no circulation was present, suggesting a local effect of the foetal testis hormone on the genital tract. When an explanted tract was cultured for four days on a standard clot differentiation continued, seminal vesicles developed from dilations in the Wolffian ducts and prostatic buds grew out from the urogenital sinus. When the tracts were cultured with both testes removed the Wolffian ducts regressed; no seminal vesicles formed but there were a few prostatic buds. If, in a similar experiment, one or both testes were removed and one replaced, development went on as if both testes were present only when the two sides of the tract were close together; if the two sides were further apart the seminal vesicle was smaller or absent on that side without the testis and the Wolffian duct was not so well retained. Price (1957) considered that the testes hormone might have been coming down the Wolffian duct itself.

In the guinea-pig foetus of 30–36 days of age, Zaaijer *et al.* (1966) have also shown that the testes can secrete an androgenic hormone which maintains normal histological structure in prostate explants, and conclude (Ortiz *et al.* 1966) that the foetal testes is capable of secretory activity at very early stages of differentiation.

This 'local' effect of the testes hormone gains support from the existence of gynandromorphic mice (Hollander *et al.* 1956). These animals have a normal ovary, tube and uterus on the ovarian side and a normal testis and male duct system on the testicular side.

These experimentally induced abnormalities have their clinical counterpart and cases of gonadal dysgenesis represent the equivalent of the castrated male rabbit embryos (Grumbach *et al.* 1955). In these subjects the bodily characteristics do not reveal their genetic sex which may be XO or XY. Cases of true hermaphroditism or gonadal intersex have been described e.g. Harnden & Armstrong (1959). These subjects have a vas deferens and testis on one side, and a fallopian tube and ovary or an ovotestis on the other. In some of these subjects both gonads may contain only testicular tissue (Shah *et al.* 1961). The nuclear sex of these individuals may be chromatin positive or chromatin negative.

In the human true hermaphrodite there is a suggestion that the foetal testis hormone has a similar local action to that in the rat. The development of the homolateral genital duct and gonad correspond although the appearance of the external genitalia is variable. Furthermore Wilkins (1957) observed in female pseudohermaphroditism resulting from congenital adrenal hyperplasia, that female development of the genital ducts is not altered, although there are masculine changes in the urogenital sinus and external genitalia.

Similar cases of female pseudohermaphroditism were noted in babies born to women who had taken synthetic progestational agents in early pregnancy (Wilkins 1960). Norethindrone and various forms of ethisterone have been responsible for most cases. Severe virilization may be caused by methyl testosterone in doses as small as 3 mg daily even though androgenic effects are not noticable in the mother.

Testosterone has been shown to cross the placental barrier as early as in the 12th week of pregnancy (Salhanick 1959).

It is interesting to note how well some of the human abnormalities correspond to the experimental work designed to elucidate the development of the gonads. The extrapolation of some of this work from animal to human is not unreasonable.

FUNCTION OF THE FOETAL TESTIS

Differentiation and development of the accessory reproductive tract in the normal male mammalian foetus is controlled by functional testes secreting androgenic hormones. It is not known whether these hormones are the same as those made in the adult testes; but they may, at least in part, consist of C_{19} steroids similar to those found in the adult.

Acevedo *et al.* (1961a,b), reported that human foetal testicles from the second trimester of pregnancy can convert progesterone to several steroids including testosterone and androstenedione, and Bloch *et al.* (1962a) also demonstrated the ability of human foetal testes of 15 weeks gestational age to convert progesterone to 17α-hydroxy progesterone, testosterone and androstenedione. It is therefore evident that in the human testes at this early stage the 17α hydroxylating, 20α and 20β reducing, side-chain splitting, and 21-hydroxylating enzyme systems are active. Acevedo *et al.* (1963) have confirmed the presence of these metabolites in incubation of progesterone 4-^{14}C and pregnenolone–7α-H^3 with human foetal testis. In addition, they demonstrated the pathway from Δ^5 pregnenolone to Δ^4-androstenedione by isolation of 17α hydroxy Δ^5 pregnenolone and dehydroepiandrosterone. These workers also found that in pregnenolone substrate incubations with two foetuses 23·0 cm and 20·0 cm C.R. length, the larger foetus formed a smaller percentage of $\alpha\beta$unsaturated 3-ketones. This evidence of lack of 3β-hydroxydehydrogenase might explain the inability of the newborn to synthesize male hormone until puberty.

More recently Bloch (1964), using reverse isotope dilution methods, isolated 17α and 16α hydroxylated progesterone from human foetal testes of nine to 11 weeks gestational age and testosterone and 17α hydroxyprogesterone from those of 12 to 15 weeks gestational age. This would indicate that 16α hydroxylase is also present in the human foetal testes of this age. Ling *et al.* (1969) have now isolated testosterone and androstenedione from the human foetal testes at 22 weeks gestation after perfusion of the intact foeto-placental unit with 17α -hydroxyprogesterone.

Although these reports do not prove that the foetal testes secrete testosterone in early pregnancy, they demonstrate that they have the ability to perform the essential steps leading to formation of the main androgenic hormones, testosterone and androstenedione. Furthermore these *in vitro* observations agree, in general, with the *in vivo* endocrine activities of the foetal gonads.

The majority of studies of steroid conversion by foetal gonads have been confined to man but Bloch and Benirschke (1965) have demonstrated that the testis of the foetal 9-banded armadillo near term possessed the capacity to convert progesterone to 17α hydroxyprogesterone, testosterone and androstenedione. Bloch (1967) suggested that the capacity of the adult mammalian testes to synthesize C_{19} steroids, particularly testosterone is established during foetal development.

It would appear from the published evidence that mammalian foetal testicular tissue is remarkably similar in different species both in its development and hormone production.

2 OVARY

THE FOETAL OVARY AND SEX DIFFERENTIATION

The development of the ovary has been outlined in the previous section together with the testis and minimal mention will be made of it here.

When the rabbit foetus is castrated at an early stage of gestation (day 19) the appearance of masculine structures does not occur (Jost 1953b). In experiments with the genital tract explants of female foetal rats (Price 1957) the Wolffian ducts underwent regression. When the Mullerian ducts were well established at the time of explantation, they were retained whether ovaries were present or not and were not inhibited by testosterone. Furthermore, when foetal testes, which had apparently been secreting hormones, were placed directly against the Mullerian ducts, the growth of the latter was not at all inhibited.

Bronski (1950) showed that Mullerian duct tissue of either male or female guinea-pig foetuses developed into uteri when grafted into the anterior chamber of the eye of normal or castrated adult female guinea-pigs. The differentiation of the uterus seemed to be independant of the influence of host hormones. Bronski concluded that, in the guinea-pig, ovarian hormones are not necessary for the development and differentiation of the uterus and that testicular hormone does not inhibit it. Hence, it appears that, in the female rodent foetus, the absence of foetal testis hormone results in regression of the Wolffian ducts, and the further development of the female Mullerian system does not depend on foetal ovarian secretion. The secretion of the foetal ovary does not therefore seem to be necessary for sex organogenesis.

It does not follow that the development of the genital tract is uninfluenced by ovarian hormones and it has been shown (Greene *et al.* 1940) that prenatal treatment of the mother with oestradiol causes inhibition and degeneration of the Wolffian derivatives in the male rat embryo, with only a moderate degree of persistence and stimulation of the Mullerian derivatives.

It appears that the Wolffian duct in both the male and female opossum can be stimulated with oestrogen (Moore 1939).

PRODUCTION OF HORMONES BY THE FOETAL OVARY

There is no direct evidence, as yet, that the foetal ovary, *in vivo*, synthesizes oestrogen or progesterone. Even the possible presence of oestrogen in foetal ovaries does not mean that the hormone is secreted, although an oestrogenic effect was demonstrated in a castrated female rat after an embryonic human ovary from the 8th month of pregnancy had been implanted (Rosa 1954). There is also some histological evidence suggesting possible oestrogen production by the ovaries in the newborn, and Tillinger *et al.* (1957) found measurable quantities of oestriol, but no oestradiol-17β or oestrone, in the urine of newborn boys. At present no endocrine function has been demonstrated for the ovary during foetal life.

In the human nearly all full term babies show genital signs due to oestrogens derived from the mother, the supply of which suddenly stops at birth. This is frequently referred to as 'the genital crisis of the newborn'. Female babies at birth have prominent labia and clitoris, small tags on the labia and hymen and a vaginal discharge. The breasts are engorged and slightly swollen in many full term infants, male and female, and the secretion of milk (witch's milk), may occur. It seems unlikely that these effects are in any way due to foetal ovarian secretion, considering the huge amounts of oestrogen circulating in the foeto-placental unit, and derived from the placenta (see Diczfalusy & Troen 1961).

METABOLISM OF HORMONES BY THE FOETAL OVARY

The ability of the human foetal ovary to metabolize progesterone *in vitro* has been demonstrated by Bloch (1964). Homogenates of ovaries from human foetuses aged nine to 11, 12 to 15 and 19 weeks of age were incubated with $4^{14}C$ progesterone. The ovarian tissue from the two older foetal age groups reduced progesterone to 20α hydroxy-4-pregnene-3-one and some evidence for the formation of 16α and 17α hydroxyprogesterone was also found. No synthesis of C_{19} or C_{18} steroids could be demonstrated. Thus the human foetal ovary seems to be relatively inactive in the metabolism of progesterone, except for reduction to 20α hydroxy-4-pregnene-3-one. This finding instances the ability of most human foetal tissues to reduce progesterone to 20α hydroxy progesterone (Zander 1961), Greig & Macnaughton (1966).

Roberts & Warren (1964) incubated bovine foetal ovarian tissue with $4^{14}C$ androstenedione and $4^{14}C$ progesterone. Incubation with progesterone yielded 17α, 20α-dihydroxy-4-pregnene-3-one, 17α-hydroxy-4-pregnene-3-one, 16α-hydroxy-4-pregnene-3-one, testosterone and androstenedione. After incubation with androstenedione, testosterone was recovered. This demonstrates that the bovine foetal ovary has most of the capabilities of the adult bovine ovary (Sweat *et al.* 1960), and that it is capable of effecting 17α-hydroxylation, 16α-hydroxylation, 20α-reduction, 17β-reduction, side chain cleavage and aromatization. It may be that in fact, the foetal ovary, like the foetal testis does have some degree of activity *in utero* in some species.

It is probable that the foetal ovary is capable of performing steroid biosynthesis but this is only minimally used. The two principal hormones which the ovary produces in adult life, namely oestrogen and progesterone, are already being supplied in large quantities to the foetus by the placenta. The problem for the foetus is how to deal with these compounds and not how to manufacture more. It is possible that foetal ovarian activity is inhibited during pregnancy by the very large amounts of oestrogen and progesterone which are present in the foetal circulation.

On the present evidence the ovary seems to be a rather inactive organ during foetal life.

THE ENDOCRINE PANCREAS

DEVELOPMENT

The pancreas can first be seen in the 3 mm human embryo, and by the time it is 15 mm in length the pancreas is a single mass composed of branching ducts embedded in a small amount of loose connective tissue. The acini which are the secretary portions of the pancreas appear during the third month, and shortly before this time a few islands of Langerhans can be found. These are primary islands and they continue to enlarge during the 3rd month, when the β cells occupy only about one third to one quarter of the total volume of each island. Most primary islands begin to degenerate during the 6th month. Islands of the second generation appear first during the 4th month. The islands of Langerhans in the pancreas of most mammals contain A, β and D cells. β cells are known to produce insulin. A cells probably produce glucagon and D cells are of unknown significance. It appears therefore, that insulin and glucagon are produced early in foetal life by the pancreas. The primary islands are relatively few in number. As they grow the three types of cells increase in number; they reach full development in the 5th month of gestation and then begin to degenerate. Degeneration appears temporarily to involve all A cells, and suggests the occurrance of physiological changes which lessen the requirement of A cells. Ferner & Stoechenius (1950) found a predominance of A cells over β cells in the foetus, equal numbers of both cells in newborn infants and a marked increase of β cells in the adult; A cells constituted only 20 per cent of all islet cells. Ferner & Stoechenius suggested that the decrease in the number of A cells might be explained by the slowing rate of body growth with diminished glucogen requirement. The same explanation was postulated in other observations on the human foetus (Hsiang Mei Liu & Potter 1962), since there is a diminished rate of growth during the latter part of foetal life in the human foetus.

FUNCTION

In the rat Fryre (1957) and Kim *et al.* (1960) found that the foetal islets begin functioning at the 17th or 18th day of gestation, β granules being seen by the 18th day. Munger (1958), using the electron microscope identified β granules in the mouse islets by the 15th or 14th day of development. Both insulin and glucagon have been demonstrated in foetal pancreatic tissue in animals, and in the earliest stages of work on insulin Banting & Best (1922) extracted insulin from the pancreas of foetal calves of under five months development. This insulin was present in higher concentrations than in the adult glands. Dixit *et al.* (1964) demonstrated a progressive increase in the insulin content of the islets from the 18th day to birth.

It is probable, therefore, that foetal insulin production begins early in pregnancy. The gestation period at which insulin had been found corresponds well with development of the β cells; it thus seems likely that the β cells produce some insulin during prenatal life. Insulin has been demonstrated both by the fluorescent antibody technique and by immunoassay in the pancreatic extracts of human foetuses of over 80 mm CR length (Grillo & Shima 1966). These workers did not find insulin in the extract of the pancreas of a 35 mm foetus. They suggest that since β-granulation occurred in foetuses of 90–110 mm CR length insulin formation starts before β-granulation.

It has also been shown that when neonatal or foetal pancreatic tissue from hamsters or rats is grafted into alloxan diabetic or pancreatectomized hosts the carbohydrate metabolism of the diabetic host is completely controlled (House *et al.* 1958, Gonet 1961).

In alloxan diabetic rats Dixit *et al.* (1964) found that the pancreas of the foetuses from diabetic mothers had a lower insulin content than the normal controls. Fryre (1957) and Kim *et al.* (1960) had previously found diminished numbers of β granules in the pancreatic islets of foetuses of diabetic mothers. The diminished insulin content of the islets in foetuses of the diabetic mothers correlates with the cytological studies, which indicates a decreased insulin content. It is possible that the decrease in the insulin content may result from a release of insulin from the foetal islets in response to hyperglycaemia, maternal or foetal.

PLACENTAL TRANSFER OF INSULIN

There seems to be considerable species difference concerning the transport of insulin across the placenta. Transplacental transport has been noted in the rat and rhesus monkey (Knobil & Josimovich 1959,

Josimovich & Knobil 1961), but not in the rabbit (Davis & Lacy 1957). Some workers have failed to find evidence that insulin crosses the placental barrier in the rat (Goodner & Freinkel 1961). The effect of foetal insulin secretion on foetal carbohydrate metabolism must vary greatly, in part because the maternal insulin contribution is so variable and also because the foetuses of certain species are extremely resistant to the effects of insulin even in very large doses (Schlossman 1938, Passmore & Schlossman 1938). Schlossman (1933) administered insulin to a foetus *in utero* and found that the maternal blood sugar always remains higher than that of the foetus. There was some fall in the maternal level but this Schlossman attributed to the transfer of glucose from mother to foetus to compensate for the lowering of the blood sugar of the foetus. Seller (1964) found that, in rats, a rise in maternal blood sugar level follows injection of insulin into the foetus and she accounted for this by the prolonged ether anaesthesia. The findings of Seller (1964), in fact, differed from those of Knobil & Josomovich (1959) in that she did not find that insulin passed the placenta. This was considered to be due to differences in experimental technique, so that the question in the rat is not yet decided.

There is no evidence in the human that insulin can cross the placenta (Buse *et al.* 1962). The results obtained by Milner & Hales (1965) supported this view. They found that after a rise in maternal blood sugar concentration there was also a rise in the foetal blood sugar and plasma insulin concentration. They considered that the rise in foetal plasma insulin was more likely the result of stimulation of the foetal pancreas by the rise of foetal blood sugar concentration than due to transfer of maternal insulin.

There seems to be little grounds for the belief first expressed by Carlson & Drennan (1911) that insulin passed from foetus to mother during pregnancy. They observed that, in pancreatectomized dogs, the diabetes was less severe during late pregnancy than in non-pregnant animals, and attributed this to insulin produced by the foetus crossing the placenta to the mother. This observation was apparently confirmed by Cuthbert *et al.* (1936) who found however that the pancreatectomized dog was more improved during lactation than during pregnancy. Increased utilization of carbohydrate by the foetuses and nursing puppies, rather than passage of foetal insulin through the placenta seems to be a better interpretation of these experiments: Hartman (1957) stated that, in the light of further studies, Carlson had, in fact, given up his original interpretation. It seems therefore, unlikely that significant amounts of foetal insulin are transferred to the mother.

RELEASE OF FOETAL INSULIN

In the human pancreas the β cells exhibiting signs of secretory activity are found to be present in the 5th month but there is, so far, no direct evidence that the foetal pancreas does release insulin into the circulation, although some release seems likely. The plasma insulin-activity in cord blood at delivery is very much less than in the peripheral circulation of the mother (Santos *et al.* 1955, Baird & Farquhar 1962).

DIABETES AND PREGNANCY

There has been much discussion on the relationship of diabetes and pregnancy. In diabetic pregnancy there is a high perinatal mortality rate and increased size and weight of the newborn who also have hypertrophy of the islets of Langerhans (Smith 1959). In the years which precede the onset of their diabetes such women tend to have unusually large babies, of which an increased number are stillborn or die soon after birth. The baby born to the pre-diabetic mother also has hypertrophy of the islets of Langerhans, and several mothers with a normal glucose tolerance curve at the time of birth of their infant with islet cell hypertrophy developed diabetes three years later (Woolf & Jackson 1957). Burwell (1957) has reported that women may give birth to prediabetic babies as much as ten years before they develop diabetes.

It has been suggested that the foetus of a diabetic mother is subjected to intermittant hyperglycaemia and that this results in pancreatic islet hyperplasia, increased insulin secretion and greater deposition of fat (Osler 1960).

The infants of diabetic mothers are sometimes described as 'Cushingoid' in appearance. Although Osler & Pedersen (1960) did not consider that hyperadrenocorticism was a major cause of foetal overgrowth in infants of diabetic mothers, it does seem likely (Farquhar 1962) that changes in the adrenal gland occur in these babies. This is suggested by Cathro & Forsyth (1965) who measured corticosteroid excretion in the newborn of diabetic and pre-diabetic mothers. These workers found that infants of mothers with diabetes show greater adrenocortical activity than control infants. This is shown by increased excretion of blue tetrazolium-reducing corticosteroids of all ranges of polarity. These infants also show an excretion of sodium, chloride and potassium above average during the early neonatal period; indicating an alteration in body composition (Zetterstrom & Alberg 1955, Cathro & Forsyth 1965).

Osler (1960) has shown that these babies have less extra-cellular water and less total water than normal. This finding was considered to be consistent with an increased amount of body fat, and was substantiated by Cheek *et al.* (1961) and Clapp *et al.* (1962). It is probable therefore, that there are changes in adrenocortical function in the foetus of diabetic mothers. Other hormone abnormalities have been reported; for example, the amniotic fluid in diabetic pregnancy contains less oestriol than in normal pregnancy.

It seems therefore, that there are multiple hormonal changes in the foetus in diabetic pregnancy, but the relationship between these remains to be worked out.

ADRENAL GLANDS

I ADRENAL CORTEX

The growth and differentiation of the adrenal cortex in foetal life has been the subject of much investigation in a variety of species. The secretion of hormones of the adrenal cortex, and the activity of the hypophyseal-adrenal axis in foetal life, has been reviewed by Jost, Jacquot & Cohen (1962). Cohen (1963) found that in the rat early adrenal growth was independent of pituitary control, and that this period was followed by one in which an intact hypophysis was required to sustain growth. Prior to the 18th day of foetal age, little or no secretory activity was present in the developing adrenal gland but evidence was obtained for secretory activity from day 18–19 onwards.

Adrenalectomy or decapitation of 18 day old rat foetuses was found to retard the accumulation of liver glycogen, and the activity of enzymes regulating glycogen metabolism (Jacquot 1959, Jacquot & Kretchner 1964). Maternal adrenalectomy combined with foetal decapitation resulted in the complete arrest of glycogen deposition. Furthermore, the administration of ACTH or cortisone effected glycogen deposition in decapitated foetal rats. It appears therefore, that liver glycogenolysis in the foetal rat is dependent upon glucocorticoid action, with the glucocorticoids being derived from foetal adrenal secretion, and a maternal contribution.

It seems likely that the foetal adrenal glands may pass through a period of maximum activity before birth, and that their activity does not steadily increase throughout intrauterine life.

FEED-BACK MECHANISMS

In the foetus, as in the adult, there is an equilibrium between the release of ACTH by the pituitary gland and the level of circulating adrenal steroids. Changes at the level of foetal pituitary gland were observed as a consequence of changes in the level of circulating corticosteroids. Foetal adrenalectomy induced a decrease in the number of acidophil cells in the pituitary gland (Tobin 1939), and an increase in the size of the hypophysis (Jacquot 1959), while an excess of cortisteroids injected into rat foetuses produced a reduction in size of the pituitary gland (Noumura 1959); and also an atrophy of the cortex which resembles that produced by decapitation. If ACTH was given at the same time this was prevented (Jost 1957).

Unilateral adrenalectomy of rat foetuses on day 19 is followed by enlargement of the remaining gland (Kitchell & Wells 1952a, Noumura 1959). The hypertrophy can be prevented either by giving cortisone to the foetus (Kitchell & Wells 1952b) or by decapitation (Noumura 1959).

It is evident from these data that an endocrine interrelationship between pituitary gland and adrenal cortex is present in the rat foetus before birth.

GLYCOGEN STORAGE IN FOETAL LIVER AS CONTROLLED BY ADRENOCORTICAL HORMONES

It is thought that the glycogen content of the foetal liver increases at a definite stage of gestation. Endocrine factors are considered to be important in this respect, particularly as Jost & Jacquot (1955) observed, in rabbit foetuses, that this increase could be prevented by decapitation. In a number of experiments they showed that the secretion of the adrenal gland controlled the glycogen deposition in the foetal liver. The impaired glycogen deposition can be restored to normal by administration of cortisone to the mother or to the foetus (Jacquot 1959). In decapitated rabbit foetuses cortisol also induced glycogen deposition under particular experimental circumstances (Jost & Jacquot 1955, Jost 1961a). Similarly, in the rat foetus, the heart contains a large quantity of glycogen which decreases if the foetus is deprived of corticoids (Picon & Bouhnik 1966).

STEROID SYNTHESIS

Some observations on corticosteroid synthesis or secretion by mammals during intra-uterine life have been made. Jones *et al.* (1964) found cortisol and corticosterone in adrenal vein blood from foetal lambs at a late stage of gestation. Bloch & Benirschke (1965) found cortisol and corticosterone during *in vitro* incubations of the adrenal tissues of foetal armadillos. In this species, like the human, a foetal zone is present during intra-uterine life. In these experiments, which were conducted on adrenal glands from late gestation, 3β-hydroxy Δ^5 steroid formation could not be demonstrated.

There is now good evidence from various sources that the human foetal adrenal is functional during intra-uterine life. The maximum concentration of cholesterol occurs about the 18th to 19th week of gestation. This is of particular interest as far as steroid biosynthesis is concerned. Studies of the biosynthesis of steroids in the foetal adrenal have been made both *in vivo* and *in vitro*.

The human foetal gland is relatively, 10 to 20 times, larger than the adult gland and the bulk of this hypertrophied organ is composed of a histologically distinct central reticular zone known as the foetal zone. Within a few days after birth this zone involutes and the gland does not regain its birth weight until well after puberty. In addition much interest has centred around the anencephalic foetus in which the pituitary is almost always absent. This has the effect of producing a physiological decapitation in the human. Here the adrenal hypertrophy and the foetal zone are lacking.

All the evidence available at present supports the view that the human foetal adrenal is capable of forming a number of steroids. Two methods of investigation have been employed: (1) Incubation of adrenal glands or slices with various steroids and their precursors (e.g. Villee & Villee 1964); and (2) Isolation of metabolites from human foetuses following perfusion with steroids or their precursors, e.g. Zander (1961), Solomon *et al.* (1964), Greig & Macnaughton (1967).

Results from incubation studies

Bloch & Benirschke (1959) demonstrated the ability of human foetal tissue to synthesize steroids from acetate during *in vitro* incubations, and showed that the human foetal adrenal contains the necessary enzyme systems to convert acetate to steroids as does the adult gland. Dehydroepiandrosterone, pregnenolone, androstenedione, 11β hydroxy androst-4-ene-3,17-dione and cortisol were found. They could not demonstrate progesterone, 17α hydroxy progesterone, corticosterone, testosterone or adrenosterone. They further showed that pure foetal zone tissue could

TABLE 10.1

Products of progesterone and pregnenolone in incubations with homogenized foetal adrenals (from Villee & Villee 1964)

Progesterone	Pregnenolone
Androstenedione	16α OH Pregnenolone
11β OH Androstenedione	17 OH Pregnenolone
17 OH Progesterone	Dehydroepiandrosterone
16α OH Progesterone	16α OH DHA
16α 17di OH Progesterone	Progesterone
Deoxycorticosterone	Androstenedione
Corticosterone (+TPNH)	
Cortisol (+TPNH)	

synthesize dehydroepiandrostene, pregnanolone and androstenedione and suggested that there was some restriction of the activity of the 3β ol-dehydrogenase enzyme system in the foetal adrenal compared with that in the adult gland. Solomon *et al.* (1958) showed that the foetal zone tissue could convert progesterone to 17α hydroxy progesterone and androstenedione.

Observations by Bloch *et al.* (1962b) and Dawson *et al.* (1961), which include determination of dehydrogenases, showed the presence of dehydroepiandrosterone dehydrogenase in adrenal tissue including the definitive cortex from foetuses 12 weeks or older.

Villee *et al.* (1959, 1961) examined the activity of certain steroid hydroxylases and dehydrogenases at various times in the development of the foetal adrenal and considered that the metabolism of progesterone in the foetal gland differed with the stage of gestation. They found that homogenized adrenals from foetuses of less than 10 cm crown-rump length produce the steroids shown in Table 10.1. They found that the relative amounts of steroids formed from progesterone depended on the amounts of the incubation medium. Androstenedione however, under all conditions is a major metabolite of progesterone at this gestational stage.

The adrenal from foetuses of more than 10 cm crown-rump length produced only small amounts of androstenedione or 11β-hydroxy-androstenedione from progesterone. These older foetuses formed more cortisol and corticosterone from progesterone than did the earlier foetuses.

Pregnenolone is largely converted to dehydroepiandrosterone by homogenized human foetal adrenals, but small amounts of 17α-hydroxypregnenolone, 16α-hydroxypregnenolone and androstenedione also are found. Villee & Villee (1964) consider from this evidence that the 3β-hydroxydehydrogenases of the foetal adrenal are far less active than those present in the adrenal of the newborn. In this they agree with the findings of Bloch & Benirschke (1959).

It is of interest also that the adrenals of the hydrocephalic foetus make mainly androstenedione *in vitro* while only small amounts are made by the adrenal of the anencephalic foetus. These results might seem to suggest androstenedione is formed primarily in the foetal zone as anencephaly is associated with lack of the foetal zone. However, Bloch & Benirschke (1959) and Solomon *et al.* (1958) could not detect any difference in the amount of steroids formed from radioactive sulphate in the foetal zone and definitive cortex. 16α-Hydroxyprogesterone and 16α-17-dihydroxyprogesterone have been shown to be products of progesterone metabolism in the foetal adrenal, and the 16α-hydroxylases of the human foetal adrenal are very active *in vitro* at all stages of gestation. The conversion of progesterone to 16α-hydroxyprogesterone has recently been demonstrated in the human placenta (Little *et al.* 1963) and it is therefore possible that some of the 16α-hydroxylated steroids found in the urine, and in the cord blood (Zander *et al.* 1962), may originate in the foeto-placental unit. The activity of 16α-hydroxylase, seems, however, to be much greater in the foetal adrenal than in the placenta.

Bernstein (1958) has shown that the 16α-hydroxysteroids have a regulatory effect on the sodium retaining properties of corticoids. This may produce significant electrolyte changes in the foetus, by 16-hydroxylation of deoxycorticosterone or aldosterone.

In short incubations, Villee & Villee (1964) found pregnenolone was converted to very polar material, some of which was dehydroepiandrosterone. About 4 per cent of the initial radioactivity was converted to dehydroepiandrosterone sulphate. In longer incubations steroid sulphates did not accumulate. These findings suggest that the foetal adrenal may sulphate 21 carbon steroids, as it has been shown to do in the case of C19 steroids (Diczfalusy *et al.* 1961a).

It seems likely that the concentration of progesterone in the medium may influence the activity of the 3β-hydroxydehydrogenase and Villee & Villee (1964) found that the adrenal maintained with progesterone was, after two days in culture, still capable of converting progesterone to androstenedione. When culture took place in the absence of progesterone, deoxycorticosterone and 17-hydroxyprogesterone were found but no androstenedione.

It has been shown that the level of progesterone in the umbilical arteries is higher than that in the umbilical vein (Runnebaum & Zander 1962, Greig *et al.* 1962), suggesting that the foetus metabolizes progesterone. The level of this progesterone, presumably produced by the placenta, may determine the activity of the 3β-hydroxydehydrogenase and thus which steroids are formed in the foetal adrenal. In this instance therefore, the activity of the placenta with regard to progesterone production, could control steroidogenesis in the foetal adrenal.

Perfusion studies

Several studies have been performed where the human foetus has been perfused with progesterone [Bengtsson *et al.* (1964), Solomon *et al.* (1964), Zander (1961), Greig & Macnaughton (1966)]. In each of these studies considerable accumulation of radioactivity has been found in the adrenal glands. This suggests that the foetal adrenal is a site of metabolism of progesterone. Solomon *et al.* (1964) isolated 16α-hydroxyprogesterone, 17α-hydroxyprogesterone, corticosterone sulphate and hydrocortisone from the adrenals, the 16α-hydroxyprogesterone and corticosterone sulphate being the most abundant steroids isolated. Formation of corticosterone sulphate supports the view of Villee & Villee (1964) that the foetal adrenal can sulphurylate steroids. Greig & Macnaughton (1966) perfused two previable human foetuses for 14 and 45 minutes respectively, with C_{14} progesterone. The principal compounds found were polar steroids, but 20α- and 20β-hydroxyprogesterone were also isolated from the adrenals following short perfusion for 14 minutes. It was also noted that a considerable amount of conjugation activity took place in the adrenal, and the evidence suggested that the conjugated material in the adrenal was mainly sulphates.

There is evidence that the foetal adrenal is an active centre of steroidogenesis in the human. Oestrogen production in the foetal adrenal has not been unequivocibly demonstrated to date, but it has been shown (Diczfalusy *et al.* 1961b) that the adrenals are capable of sulphurylating oestriol. It seems likely therefore, that in the foetus the adrenal is one of the main users of progesterone secreted from the placenta, that it uses this progesterone to manufacture a number of steroids, and that the outcome depends on the stage of gestation and the level of progesterone in the foetal circulation.

There is good evidence that with advancing gestation there may be a qualitative and quantitative change in the steroids produced by the foetal adrenal, probably reflecting the gradual development of various enzyme systems.

2 ADRENAL MEDULLA AND EXTRA MEDULLARY STRUCTURES

DEVELOPMENT

The precursor of the adrenal medulla can be discerned at a very early stage of intrauterine development in human and rabbit embryos (Coupland 1952). The rudiments of the epithelial adrenal glands may be observed at the 8 mm stage and the chromaffin reaction is seen at the 55 mm stage.

Extra-medullary chromaffin tissue is precocious in development and relatively large amounts are found in the human foetus. The largest amounts of extra-medullary chromaffin tissue are closely related to the origin of the inferior mesenteric artery, and are called the para-aortic bodies or organs of Zuckerkandl (Zuckerkandl 1901).

FUNCTION

Extra-adrenal chromaffin cells were first shown to produce an adrenaline-like substance by Biedl & Wiesel (1902). The cells of the foetal medulla synthesize and store little or no adrenaline, and *nor*-adrenaline is the main product of the foetal chromaffin system. Greenberg & Lind (1961) demonstrated that, whereas the para-aortic tissue contained *nor*-adrenaline in relatively large amounts, almost no adrenaline was present. In the adrenal gland itself, however, both substances were found in almost equal amounts. This might indicate that the adrenal cortex plays a role in the methylation of *nor*-adrenaline, due to its proximity to the medullary region. However, adrenaline has also been demonstrated in the adrenal glands in species, e.g. elasmobranchs, where the medulla and cortex are anatomically separate (West 1955).

Catecholamines are present in the medulla at a very early stage in foetal life and there is little change in total amount during the first trimester of gestation. In the rat adrenal the amount of *nor*-adrenaline has been quantitatively determined from the 16th day of gestation and adrenaline after 17·5 days. After 19·5 days the glands contain more adrenaline than *nor*-adrenaline (Cheoux & Roffi 1965).

The organs of Zuckerkandl in the human foetus contain only *nor*-adrenaline and since this amine is more potent than adrenaline in man, the constant supply may help to maintain vascular tone (West *et al.* 1953). These organs may, therefore, be necessary for the maintenance of foetal blood pressure always presuming, of course, that secretion of the amine does occur in the foetus.

The finding of *nor*-adrenaline and adrenaline in the urine of the neonate (Stern *et al.* 1961) suggests that secretion does occur at any rate in late pregnancy.

Greenberg & Lind (1961) also showed that the catecholamine content of human foetal heart, kidney and lung is roughly similar to values found in the adult, although the percentage of adrenaline was somewhat higher in foetal tissues. The level of both adrenaline and *nor*-adrenaline in the human foetal brain is much lower than in the adult.

It is probable that, during foetal life the emergency demand for adrenaline is lessened, not only by environmental factors but also by a different response of the tissues to *nor*-adrenaline and adrenaline. Comline & Silver (1966) found that a low arterial Po_2 in foetal lambs was the only factor which, under normal circumstance, excited the adrenal medulla *in utero*. Since the organs of Zuckerkandl are probably not innervated (Muscholl & Vogt 1964), they may have properties similar to the adrenal medulla of the foetal calf, and release *nor*-adrenaline as a direct response to asphyxia.

Finally it seems probable that *nor*-adrenaline is the important product of foetal medullary and extra-medullary chromaffin tissue and that its main function may be the maintenance of vascular tone and foetal blood pressure.

CONCLUSIONS

There seems to be good evidence, that the foetal endocrine glands do function during intra-uterine life, and that the function depends to some extent on species and developmental age. During intra-uterine life glandular activity probably undergoes important changes; the more advanced the development, the more the gland approximates to adult function.

Some foetal glands appear to pass through periods of varying activity; maximal activity may be followed by minimal or absent function. Furthermore the sensitivity of the target organs to the effects of hormones may alter during pregnancy resulting in variable effects.

Some of the endocrine glands which are active in foetal life may be suppressed without preventing foetal growth, and others, such as the testis, exercise a morphogenetic effect; a deficiency at certain stages of development leading to abnormalities such as pseudohermaphroditism.

Although the foetal glands are probably able to synthesize hormones which appear to be the same as those found in the adult, there may be no requirement for these during intra-uterine life. In many cases the foetal requirement would, in the event, be tiny and, as it seems likely that small amounts of various maternal endocrine secretions pass to the foetus via the placenta, the foetal requirements of these substances may be adequately provided for by the mother during intra-uterine life. This may result in some suppression of activity of the foetal glands.

Certain other glandular functions, although they occur in the foetus, are unimportant from the point of view of intra-uterine life. For instance although the foetal kidneys produce urine in the first trimester of pregnancy the placenta performs the main secretory function of the foetus and total renal agenesis does not retard foetal development.

It will not therefore, be surprising if further work shows that the foetal endocrine glands are capable of performing biosynthetic procedures such as those found in the adult. This does not mean, however, that these procedures do in fact, take place during intra-uterine life.

There is, for example, little point in the foetus using cholesterol to manufacture progesterone during intra-uterine life, when it already receives large amounts from the placenta. Hence, some of the early steps in the biosynthetic pathways from cholesterol may not occur during intra-uterine life, although experiment may demonstrate that the foetus is capable of metabolizing cholesterol to progesterone.

The endocrinology of the foetus, and particularly the human foetus, is poorly understood but recently more interest has been taken in this subject, and it is to be hoped that this will throw more light on the physiology and pathology of development.

REFERENCES

ABOUL-KHAIR S.A., BUCHANAN T.J., CROOKS J. & TURNBULL A.C. (1966) Structural and functional development of the human foetal thyroid. *Clin. Sci.* **31**, 415.

ACEVEDO H.F., AXELROD L.R., ISHIKAWA E. & TAKARI F. (1961a) Steroidogenesis in the human fetal testis. Abst. No. 39. 43rd Meeting of the Endocrine Society 1961, Abstracts, p. 22. N.Y. 22–24 June 1961.

ACEVEDO H.F., AXELROD L.R., ISHIKAWA E. & TAKARI F. (1961b) Steroidogenesis in the human fetal testis: The conversion of pregnenolone-17α-H^3 to dehydroepiandrosterone, testosterone and 4-androstene-3,17-dione. *J. Clin. Endocr. Metab.* **21**, 1611.

ACEVEDO H.F., AXELROD L.R., ISHIKAWA E. & TAKARI F. (1963) Studies in fetal metabolism II. Metabolism of progesterone-(4-^{14}C) and pregnenolone-7αH^3 in human fetal testes. *J. Clin. Endocr. Metab.* **23**, 885.

ALLEN B.M. (1904) The embryonic development of the ovary and testis of the mammals. *Am. J. Anat.* **3**, 89.

ANDERSEN H.J. (1960) Studies of hypothyroidism in children. *Acta Paediat. Stockh.* Suppl. 125.

ANGEVINE P. (1938) Pathologicanatomy of hypophysis and adrenals in anencephaly. *Archs. Path.* **26**, 507.

BAIRD J.D. & FARQUHAR J.W. (1962) Insulin secreting capacity in newborn infants of normal and diabetic women. *Lancet*, i, 71.

BANTING F.G. & BEST C.H. (1922) Pancreatic extracts. *J. Lab. Clin. Med.* **7**, 464.

BARNETT H.L. & VESTERDAL J. (1953) The physiologic and clinical significance of immaturity of kidney function in young infants. *J. Pediat.* **42**, 99.

BEARN J.G. (1967) Role of the fetal pituitary and adrenal glands in the development of the fetal thymus of the rabbit. *Endocrinology*, **80**, 979.

BEARN J.G., KOERSELMAN H.B. & PILKINGTON R.E. (1961) Function of the foetal thyroid of the rabbit with regard to cholesterol metabolism studied by foetal thyroidectomy. *Nature, Lond.* **190**, 822.

BENGTSSON G., ULLBERG S., WIQVIST N. & DICZFALUSY E. (1964) Auto-radiographic studies on previable human foetuses perfused with radioactive steroids. (1) Distribution of radioactive material following perfusion with 4-^{14}C progesterone. *Acta Endocr.* (*Kbh*), **46**, 544.

BERNSTEIN S. (1958) The chemistry and biological activities of 16 hydroxylated steroids. *Recent Prog. Horm. Res.* **14**, 1.

BETTENDORF G., APOSTOLAKIS M. & VOIGT K.D. (1962) Darstellung von Gonadotropin aus menschlichen Hypophysen. *Acta Endocr. (Kbh)*, **41**, 1.

BIEDL A. & WIESEL J. (1902) Ueber die functionelle Bedeutung der Nebenorgane des Sympathicus (Zuckerkandl) und der Chromaffinen Zellgruppen. *Pflügers. Arch. ges. Physiol.* **91**, 434.

BLIZZARD R.M. & ALBERT S.M. (1956) Hypopituitarism, hypoadrenalism and hypogonadism in the newborn infant. *J. Pediat.* **48**, 782.

BLOCH E. (1964) Metabolism of (4-^{14}C) progesterone by human fetal testis and ovaries. *Endocrinology*, **74**, 833.

BLOCH E. (1967) The conversion of 7-^{3}H-pregnenolone and 4-^{14}C-progesterone to testosterone and androstenedione by mammalian foetal testes *in vitro*. *Steroids*, **9**, 415.

BLOCH E. & BENIRSCHKE K. (1959) Synthesis *in vitro* of steroids by human fetal adrenal gland slices. *J. Biol. Chem.* **234**, 1085.

BLOCH E. & BENIRSCHKE K. (1965) *In vitro* steroid synthesis by fetal newborn and adult armadillo adrenals and by fetal armadillo testes. *Endocrinology*, **76**, 43.

BLOCH E., TISSENBAUM B. & BENIRSCHKE K. (1962a) The conversion of (4-^{14}C) progesterone to 17α-hydroxyprogesterone, testosterone and androstenedione by human fetal testes *in vitro*. *Biochem. Biophys. Acta*, **60**, 182.

BLOCH E., TISSENBAUM B., RUBIN B.L. & DEAN H.W. (1962b) 5-3β-hydroxysteroid dehydrogenase activity in human fetal adrenals. *Endocrinology*, **71**, 629.

BRONSKI M. (1950) Development of embryonic guinea-pig Mullerian ducts in anterior eye chamber grafts. *Proc. Soc. Exp. Biol. Med.* **75**, 426.

BURWELL C.S. (1957) In *Gestation*. Transactions of the 3rd Conference, p. 139. C.A. Villee, ed. Josiah Macy Jnr. Foundation.

BUSE G.B., ROBERTS W.J. & BUSE J. (1962) The role of the human placenta in the transfer and metabolism of insulin. *J. Clin. Invest.* **41**, 29.

CARLSON A.J. & DRENNAN F.M. (1911) The control of pancreatic diabetes in pregnancy by the passage of the internal secretion of the pancreas of the fetus to the blood of the mother. *Am. J. Physiol.* **28**, 39.

CARR E.A., BEIERWALTES W.H., RAMAN G., DODSON V.M., TANTON J. & BETTS J.S. (1959) The effect of maternal thyroid function on foetal thyroid function and development. *J. Clin. Endocr. Metab.* **19**, 1.

CATHRO D.M. & FORSYTH C.C. (1965) Excretion of corticosteroids by infants of diabetic and pre-diabetic mothers. *Archs. Dis. Childh.* **40**, 583.

CHAPMAN E.M., CORNER G.W., ROBINSON D. & EVANS R.D. (1948) The collection of radioactive iodine by the human foetal thyroid. *J. Clin. Endocr. Metab.* **8**, 717.

CHEEK D.B., MADDISON T.G., MALINEK M. & COLDBECK J.H. (1961) Further observations on the corrected bromide space of the neonate and investigation of water and electrolyte status in infants born of diabetic mothers. *Pediatrics, Springfield*, **28**, 861.

CHEOUX G. & ROFFI J. (1965) Dosage de l'adrénaline et de la noradrénaline dans les surrénales du foetus et du nouveau-né de rat. *C.R. Acad. Sci. (Paris)*, **260**, 6702.

CLAPP W.M., BUTTERFIELD J. & O'BRIEN D. (1962) Body water compartments in the premature infant, with special reference to the effects of the respiratory distress syndrome and of maternal diabetes and toxaemia. *Pediatrics, Springfield*, **29**, 883.

COHEN A. (1963) Corrélation entre l'hypophyse et le cortex surrénal chex le foetus de rat. Le cortex surrénal du nouveau-né. *Archs. Anat. microsc. Morph. exp.* **52**, 277.

COMLINE R.S. & SILVER M. (1966) Development of activity in the adrenal medulla of the foetus and newborn animal. *Br. med. Bull.* **22**, 16.

COUPLAND R.E. (1952) The prenatal development of the abdominal para aortic bodies in man. *J. Anat.* **86**, 357.

CUTHBERT F.P., IVY A.C., ISAACS B.L. & GRAY J. (1936) Relation of pregnancy and lactation to extirpation diabetes in dog. *Am. J. Physiol.* **115**, 480.

DAUGHADAY W.H., CORNBLATH M. & PARKER M.L. (1964) Secretion and metabolism of growth hormone in normal and premature infants, p. 985. *Proceeding of the Second International Congress of Endocrinology.*

DAVIS J. & LACY P.E. (1957) Observations on the failure of insulin to pass from the foetus to the mother in the rabbit. *Am. J. Obstet. & Gynec.* **74**, 514.

DAWSON I.M.P., PRYSE-DAVIES J. & SNAPE I.M. (1961) The distribution of six enzyme systems and of lipid in the human and rat adrenal cortex before and after administration of steroid and ACTH with comments on the distribution in human foetuses and in some maternal disease conditions. *J. Path. Bact.* **81**, 181.

DICKER S.E. & TYLER C. (1953) Vasopressor and oxytocic activity of the pituitary glands of rats, guinea-pigs and cats and of human foetuses. *J. Physiol. (Lond.)*, **121**, 206.

DICZFALUSY E. & TROEN P. (1961) Endocrine function of the human placenta. *Vitamins and Hormones*, **19**, 230.

DICZFALUSY E., CASSMER O., ALONSO C. & DE MIQUEL M. (1961a) Oestrogen metabolism in the human foetus and newborn. *Recent Prog. Horm. Res.* **17**, 147.

DICZFALUSY E., CASSMER O., ALONSO C., DE MIQUEL M. & WESTIN B. (1961b) Oestrogen metabolism in the human foetus. II. Oestrogen conjugation by foetal organs *in vitro* and *in vivo*. *Acta Endocr. (Kbh)*, **37**, 516.

DIXIT P.K., LOWE I.P., HEGGESTAD C.B. & LAZAROW A. (1964) Insulin content of micro dissected foetal islets obtained from diabetic and normal rats. *Diabetes*, **13**, 71.

DORFF G.B. (1934) Sporadic cretinism in one of twins. Roentgen demonstration of osseus changes that occurred *in utero*. *Am. J. Dis. Child.* **48**, 1316.

DOWLING J.T., FREINKEL M. & INGBAR S.H. (1956) Thyroxine-binding by sera of pregnant women, newborn infants, and women with spontaneous abortion. *J. Clin. Invest.* **35**, 1263.

EAYRS J.T. & TAYLOR S.H. (1951) The effect of thyroid deficiency induced by methylthiouracil on the maturation of the central nervous system. *J. Anat.* **85**, 350.

ECKHOLME E. & NIEMINEVA K. (1950) On prenatal changes in the relative weights of the human adrenals, the thymus and the thyroid gland. *Acta Pediat. Stockh.* **39**, 67.

FARQUHAR J.W. (1962) Maternal hyperglycaemia and foetal hyperinsulinism in diabetic pregnancy. *Postgrad. Med. J.* **38**, 612.

FENGER F. (1912) On the presence of active principles in the thyroid and suprarenal glands before and after birth. *J. Biol. Chem.* **12**, 55.

FERNER H. & STOECHENIUS W., Jnr. (1950) Die Cytogeneses des Inselsystems beim Menschen. *Z. Zellforsch, mikrosk. Anat.* **35**, 147.

FOOTE C.L. (1955) *Trans. Illinois State Acad. Sci.* **47**, 173. Quoted Jost 1961 Harvey lectures.

FOOTE C.L. & FOOTE F.M. (1949) Changes in the thyroid gland of hamster embryos hypophysectomised by decapitation. *Anat. Rec.* **105**, 559.

FRYRE B.E. (1957) The differentiation of the endocrine pancreas in foetuses of alloxan diabetic and insulin-treated rats. *J. Morph.* **101**, 325.

GELOSO J.P. (1958) Recherches préliminaires sur la sécrétion de thyroxine par la thyroide du foetus de rat en fin de gestation. *C.r. Hebd. Séanc. Acad. Sci. Paris*, **264**, 168.

GELOSO J.P. (1961) Date de l'entrée en function de la thyroide chez le foetus de rat. *C.r. Séanc. Soc. Biol.* **155**, 1239.

GELOSO J.P. (1964) Correlations thyreo-hypophysaires chez le foetus de rat en fin de gestation. 32eme Réunion de l'Association de Physiologistes de Langue Française. *J. Physiol. (Paris)*, **56**, 358.

GEMZELL C.A., HEIJKENSKJÖLD F. & STRÖM L. (1955) A method for demonstrating growth hormone activity in human plasma. *J. Clin. Endocr. Metab.* **15**, 537.

GONET A. (1961) Correction de diabète expérimental du rat par le greffe pancréatique foetale. *Acta Endocr. (Kbh)*, Suppl. 62.

GOODNER C.J. & FREINKEL N. (1961) Carbohydrate metabolism in pregnancy IV. Studies on the permeability of the rat placenta to I^{131} insulin. *Diabetes*, **10**, 383.

GREENBERG R.A. & LIND J. (1961) Catecholamines in tissues of the human foetus. *Pediatrics, Springfield*, **27**, 904.

GREENE R.R., BURRELL M.W. & IVY A.C. (1940) Experimental intersexuality, the effects of oestrogens on the antenatal sexual development of the rat. *Am. J. Anat.* **67**, 305.

GREENWOOD F.C. (1964) Influence of age on growth hormone secretion and plasma levels. *Proceedings of the Second International Congress of Endocrinology*, p. 981.

GREENWOOD F.C., HUNTER W.M. & KLOPPER A. (1964) Assay of human growth hormone in pregnancy, at parturition and in lactation. Detection of a growth-hormone like substance from the placenta. *Br. Med. J.* i, 22.

GREIG M., & MACNAUGHTON M.C. (1967) Radioactive metabolites in the liver and adrenals of the human foetus after administration of [4 ^{14}C] progesterone. *J. Endocr.* **39**, 153.

GREIG M. & COYLE M.G., COOPER W. & WALKER J. (1962) Plasma progesterone in mother and foetus in the second half of human pregnancy. *J. Obstet. Gynaec. Br. Commonw.* **69**, 772.

GRILLO T.A.I. & SHIMA K. (1966) Insulin content and enzyme histochemistry of the human foetal pancreatic islet. *J. Endocr.* **36**, 151.

GRUMBACH M.M. & WERNER S.C. (1956) Transfer of thyroid hormone across the human placenta, at term. *J. Clin. Endocr. Metab.* **16**, 1392.

GRUMBACH M.M., VAN WYK J.J. & WILKINS L. (1955) Chromosomal sex in gonadal dysgenesis (ovarian agenesis): Relationships to male pseudohermaphrodism and theories of human sex differentiation. *J. Clin. Endocr. Metab.* **15**, 1161.

HALL P.F. & MYANT N.B. (1956) Passage of exogenous thyroxine and of iodide between mother and foetus in pregnant rabbits. *J. Physiol.* **133**, 181.

HAMBURGH M., SOBEL E.H., KOBLIN R. & RINESTONE A. (1962) Passage of thyroid hormone across the placenta in intact and hypophysectomized rats. *Anat. Rec.* **144**, 219.

HARNDEN D.G. & ARMSTRONG C.N. (1959) The chromosomes of a true hermaphrodite. *Br. Med. J.* ii, 1287.

HARTMAN C.G. (1957) In *Gestation*. Transaction of the Third Conference, p. 139. C.A.Villee, ed. The Josiah Macy Jnr. Foundation, New York.

HELLER H. (1952) The action and fate of vasopressin in newborn and infant rats. *J. Endocr.* **8**, 214.

HELLER H. & ZAIMIS E.J. (1949) The antidiuretic and oxytocic hormones in the posterior pituitary glands of newborn infants and adults. *J. Physiol.* **109**, 162.

HILAIRE G.S. (1836) *Traite de Tératologie*, Vol. II. Baillère, Paris.

HIRVONEN L. & LYBECK H. (1956) On the permeability of guinea-pig placenta for thyroxine. *Acta physiol. Scand.* **36**, 17.

HODGES R.E., EVANS I.C., BRADBURY J.T. & KEETTEL W.C. (1955) The accumulation of radioactive iodine by human foetal thyroids. *J. Clin. Endocr. Metab.* **15**, 661.

HODGES R.E., HAMILTON H.E. & KEETTAL W.C. (1952) Pregnancy in myxoedema. *Archs. intern. Med.* **90**, 863.

HOLLANDER W.F., GOWEN J.W. & STADLER J. (1956) A study of 25 gynandromorphic mice of the Bagg albino strain. *Anat. Rec.* **124**, 223.

HOSKINS F.M. & SNYDER F.F. (1928) Calcium content of maternal and foetal blood serum following injection of parathyroid extract in foetuses *in utero*. *Proc. Soc. Exp. Biol. Med.* **25**, 264.

HOUSE E.L., BURTON C., COOPER H. & ANDERSON E. (1958) The implantation of neonatal pancreas into the cheek pouch of the Alloxan diabetic hamster. *Endocrinology*, **63**, 389.

HSIANG, MEI LIU & POTTER E.L. (1962) Development of the human pancreas. *Archs. Path.* **74**, 439.

JACQUOT R. (1959) Recherches sur le contrôle endocrinien de l'accumulation de glycogène dans le foie chez le foetus de rat. *J. Physiol. (Paris)*, **51**, 655.

JACQUOT R. & KRETCHNER N. (1964) Effect of fetal decapitation on enzymes of glycogen metabolism. *J. Biol. Chem.* **239**, 1301.

JONES I.C., JARRETT J.G., VINSON G.P. & POTTER K. (1964) Adrenocorticosteroid production of foetal sheep near term. *J. Endocr.* **29**, 211.

JOSIMOVICH J.B. & ATWOOD B.L. (1964) Human placental lactogen, a trophoblastic hormone synergizing with chorionic gonadotrophin and potentiating the effects of pituitary growth hormone. *Am. J. Obst. & Gynec.* **88**, 867.

JOSIMOVICH J.B. & KNOBIL E. (1961) Placental transfer of I^{131} insulin in the rhesus monkey. *Am. J. Physiol.* **200**, 471.

JOSIMOVICH J.B. & MACLAREN J.A. (1962) Presence in the human placenta and term serum of a highly lactogenic substance immunologically related to pituitary growth hormone. *Endocrinology*, **71**, 209.

JOST A. (1948) Influence de la décapitation sur le developpement du tractus génital et des surrénales de l'embryon de Lapin. *C.r. Séanc. Soc. Biol.* **142**, 173.

JOST A. (1950) Dégénérescence des extrémités du foetus de rat sous l'action de certaines préparations hypophysaires. *C.r. Séanc. Soc. Biol.* **144**, 1324.

JOST A. (1951a) Sur le role de la vasopressine et de la corticostimuline (ACTH) dans la production expérimentale de lésions des extremités foetales (hémorragies, nécroses, amputations congénitales). *C.r. Séanc. Soc. Biol.* **145**, 1805.

JOST A. (1951b) Recherches sur la différenciation sexuelle de l'embryon de lapin. IV. Organogenèse sexuelle masculine apres décapitation du foetus. *Archs. Anat. microsc. Morph. exp.* **40**, 247.

JOST A. (1953a) Sur le developement de la thyroide chez le foetus de lapin décapité. *Archs. Anat. microsc. Morph. exp.* **42**, 168.

JOST A. (1953b) Problems of fetal endocrinology: The gonadal and hypophyseal hormones. *Recent Prog. Horm. Res.* **8**, 379.

JOST A. (1957) The secretory activities of foetal endocrine glands and their effects upon target organs. In *Gestation*, p. 129. C.Villee, ed. Josiah Macy, Jnr. Foundation.

JOST A. (1961a) The role of fetal hormones in prenatal development. In *The Harvey Lectures* 1959–60, p. 201. Academic Press, New York.

JOST A. (1961b) Physiologie des hormones thyroidiennes chez les foetus. In *Colquio Sobre le Tireoide*, p. 81. C.Chagas & L.C.Lobo, eds. Instituto de Biofisica, Rio de Janiero.

JOST A. & COHEN A. (1966) Signification de l'atrophie des surrénales foetales du rat provoquée par l'hypophysectomie (décapitation). *Develop. Biol.* **14**, 154.

JOST A. & DANYSZ P. (1952) Recherches histochimiques (réaction de MacManus) et expérimentales (décapitation) sur la physiologie de l'hypophyse foetale du Lapin. *C.r. Séanc. Soc. Biol.* **146**, 1062.

JOST A. & JACQUOT R. (1955) Recherches sur les facteurs endocriniens de la charge en glycogène du foie foetal chez le lapin (avec quelques indications sur le glycogène placentaire). *Annls. Endocr.* **16**, 849.

JOST A. & PICON L.O. (1958) Influence de la thyroidectomie du foetus de lapin sur la teneur de son corps en lipides et en azote. *C.r. hebd. Seanc. Acad. Sci. Paris*, **246**, 1281.

JOST A. & TAVERNIER R. (1956) Application de la methode à l'acide periodique–Schiff à l'etude de l'hypophyse foetale du rat. *C.r. hebd. Seanc. Acad. Sci. Paris*, **243**, 1353.

JOST A., MOREL F. & MAROIS M. (1949) Données préliminaires sur la fixation de radio-iode ^{131}I par la thyroide foetale du lapin. *C.r. Séanc. Soc. Biol.* **143**, 142.

JOST A., MOREL F. & MAROIS M. (1952) Nouvelles recherches à l'aide du radio-iode ^{131}I sur la physiologie thyroidienne du foetus de lapin décapité. *C.r. Seanc. Soc. Biol.* **146**, 1066.

JOST A., MOREAU G. & FOURNIER C. (1960) Date et ordre d'apparition des premiers centres d'ossification chez le foetus de rat normal ou soumis au propylthiouracile. *Archs. Anat. microsc. Morph. exp.* **49**, 431.

JOST A., JACQUOT R. & COHEN A. (1962) The pituitary control of the foetal adrenal cortex. In *The Human Adrenal Cortex*, p. 569. A.R.Currie, T.Symington & J.K. Grant, eds. Livingstone, Edinburgh.

JOST A., PIC P., MANIEY J. & LEGRAND C. (1963) Action du propylthiouracile donné à la ratte gestante sur les parathyroides et sur la calcemie des foetus. Remarques sur la physiologie des parathyroides. *Acta Endocr.* (*Kbh*), **43**, 618.

KAIJSER K. (1959) In *Physiologische entwicklung des Kindes*. F.Linneweh, ed. Springer, Berlin.

KIM J.M., RUNGE W., WELLS L.T. & LAZAROW A. (1960) Pancreatic islets and blood sugars in prenatal and postnatal offspring from diabetic rats; beta granulation and glycogen infiltration. *Anat. Rec.* **138** 239.

KITCHELL R.L. & WELLS L.T. (1952a) Reciprocal relation between hypophysis and adrenals in fetal rats: effects of unilateral adrenalectomy and of implanted cortisone, DOCA and sex hormones. *Endocrinology*, **50**, 83.

KITCHELL R.L. & WELLS L.T. (1952b) Functioning of the hypophysis and adrenals in fetal rats: effects of hypophysectomy, adrenalectomy, castration, injected ACTH and implanted sex hormones. *Anat. Rec.* **112**, 561.

KNOBIL E. & JOSIMOVICH J.B. (1959) Placental transfer of thyrotrophic hormone, thyroxine, tri-iodothyronine and insulin in the rat. *Ann. N.Y. Acad. Sci.* **75**, 895.

LAMPÉ L., KERTESZ J. & DZVONYAR J. (1964) Iodine storage in the thyroid of the human foetus. *Orv. Hetil.* **105**, 981.

LANMAN J.T. (1953) The fetal zone of the adrenal gland. Its developmental course, comparative anatomy and possible physiologic functions. *Medicine*, **32**, 389.

LANMAN J.T. (1961) The adrenal gland in the human foetus. An interpretation of its physiological and unusual developmental pattern. *Paediatrics, Springfield*, **27**, 140.

LANMAN J.T. (1962) An interpretation of human foetal adrenal structure and function. In *The Human Adrenal Cortex*, p. 547. A.R.Currie, T.Symington & J.K. Grant, eds. Livingstone, Edinburgh.

LARON Z., MANNHEIMER S. & GUTTMANN S. (1966) Lack of transplacental passage of growth hormone in rabbits. *Experentia* (*Basel*), **22**, 831.

LEGRAND J., KRIEGEL A. & JOST A. (1961) Déficience thyroidienne et maturation du cervelet chez le rat blanc. *Archs. Anat. microsc. Morph. exp.* **50**, 507.

LING W., MACNAUGHTON M.C., COUTTS J.R.T. & SOLOMON S. (1969) Metabolism of 17α hydroxyprogesterone in the human foeto-placental unit at mid term. In preparation.

LITTLE B., SHAW A. & PURDY R. (1963) The conversion of progesterone to 16α-hydroxy-pregn-4-ene-3,20-dione and androst-4-ene-3,17-dione by human placenta *in vitro*. *Acta Endocr.* (*Kbh*), **43**, 510.

MCCANCE R.A. & WIDDOWSON E.M. (1953) Renal function before birth. *Proc. Roy. Soc. B. Biol. Sc. Lond.* **141**, 488.

MANN E.B., PICKERING D.E., WALKER J. & COOKE R.E. (1952) Butanol-extractable iodine in the serum of infants. *Pediatrics, Springfield*, **9**, 32.

MARGOLIS F.L., ROFFI J. & JOST A. (1966) Norepinephrine methylation in foetal rat adrenals. *Science*, **154**, 275.

MÉGEVAND A., MATHIEU H. & ROYER P. (1961) *Anomalies Squelettiques et Troubles de Métabolisme du Calcium dans l'Insuffisance Thyroidienne de l'Enfant.* 18eme Congrès de l'Association des Pédiatres de Langue Francaise; le hypothyroides, p. 205. F.Bamatter & V.Megevand, eds. Genève 1.

MILNER R.D.G. & HALES C.N. (1965) Effect of intravenous glucose on concentration of insulin in maternal and umbilical cord plasma. *Br. Med. J.* i, 284.

MIZUSAWA S. (1966) Fetal thyrotropin. *Folia Endocr. Jap.* **42**, 69.

MOORE C.R. (1939) Modification of sexual development in the opossum by sex hormones. *Proc. Soc. Exp. Biol. Med.* **40**, 544.

MUNGER B.L. (1958) A light and electron microscope study of cellular differentiation in the pancreatic islets of the mouse. *Am. J. Anat.* **103**, 275.

MUSCHOLL E. & VOGT M. (1964) Secretory responses of extra medullary Chromaffin tissue. *Br. J. Pharmac. Chemother.* **22**, 193.

MYANT N.B. (1958) The passage of thyroxine and tri-iodo thyronine from mother to foetus in pregnant rabbits, with a note on the concentration of protein bound iodine in foetal serum. *J. Physiol.* **142**, 329.

MYANT N.B. & OSORIO C. (1959) Serum proteins, including thyroxine-binding proteins, in maternal and foetal rabbits. *J. Physiol.* **164**, 344.

NANANGAS J.C. (1925) A Comparison of the growth of the body dimensions of anencephalic human foetuses with normal foetal growth as determined by graphic analysis and empirical formulae. *Am. J. Anat.* **35**, 455.

NATAF B. & SFEZ M. (1961) Début du fonctionnement de la thyroide foetale du rat. *C.r. Seanc. Soc. Biol.* **155**, 1235.

NIEMINEVA K. (1950) Observations on the development of the hypophyseal-portal system. *Acta Paediat. Stockh.* **39**, 366.

NOUMURA T. (1959) Development of the hypophyseal-thyroidal system in the rat embryo and its relation to the maternal system. *Jap. J. Zool.* **12**, 301.

OBER W.B. & BERSTEIN J. (1955) Observations on the endometrium and ovary in the newborn. *Pediatrics*, **16**, 445.

ORTIZ E., PRICE D. & ZAAIJER J.J.P. (1966) Organ culture studies of hormone secretion in endocrine glands. II. Secretion of androgenic hormone in adrenals and testis during early stages of development. *Proc. Kon. Med. Akad. Wet. Ser. C.* **69**, 400.

OSLER M. (1960) Body water of newborn infants of diabetic mothers. *Acta Endocr. (Kbh)*, **34**, 261.

OSLER M. & PEDERSEN J. (1960) The body composition of newborn infants of diabetic mothers. *Pediatrics*, **26**, 985.

OSORIO C. & MYANT N.B. (1960a) The passage of thyroxine-binding substances between mother and foetus in pregnant rabbits. *J. Physiol.* **151**, 66.

OSORIO C. & MYANT N.B. (1960b) The passage of thyroid hormone from mother to foetus and its relation to foetal development. *Br. med. Bull.* **16**, 159.

PARKER M.L., UTIGER R.D. & DAUGHADAY W.H. (1962) Studies on human growth hormone. II. The physiological disposition and metabolic fate of human growth hormone in man. *J. Clin. Invest.* **41**, 262.

PASSMORE R. & SCHLOSSMANN H. (1938) The effect of large doses of insulin on the foetal sheep and goat. *J. Physiol.* **92**, 459.

PETERSON R.R. & YOUNG W.C. (1952) The problems of placental permeability for thyrotrophin, propylthiouracil and thyroxine in the guinea-pig. *Endocrinology*, **50**, 218.

PICKERING D.E., SETTERGREN K.F. & KONTAXIS N.E. (1961) Thyroid function in the foetus of the macaque monkey. *J. Endocr.* **23**, 261.

PICON L.O. (1957) Influence de l'hypophysectomie et de la surrénalectomie de la ratte gestante sur le poids des foetus. *C.R. Seanc. Soc. Biol.* **151**, 1314.

PICON L. & BOUHNIK J. (1966) Action de la cortico-surrénale sur la teneur du coeur en glycogène chez le foetus de rat et le rat nouveau-né. *C.R. Soc. Biol.* (*Paris*), **160**, 288.

PINKERTON J.H.M. (1959) Oestrogen production in the immature human ovary (observations based upon histochemical studies). *J. Obstet. Gyn. Brit. Emp.* **66**, 820.

PRICE D. (1957) Influence of hormones on sex differentiation in explanted fetal reproductive tracts. In *Gestation*. Transactions of the Third Conference, p. 173. C.A.Villee, ed. The Josiah Macy, Jnr. Foundation.

PRICE D. & PANNABECKER R. (1959) Comparative responsiveness of homologous sex ducts and accessory glands of foetal rats in culture. *Archs. Anat. microsc. Morph. exp.* 48bis. 223.

PURVIS H.D. (1964) Control of thyroid function. In *The Thyroid Gland*, Vol. 2, p. 1. R.Pitt Rivers & W.R.Trotter, eds. Butterworth, London.

RAYNAUD A. (1950) Recherches expérimentales sur le développement de l'appareil génital et le fonctionnement des glandes endocrines des foetus de souris et de mulot. *Archs. Anat. microsc. Morph. exp.* **39**, 518.

RAYNAUD A. & FRILLEY M. (1947) Destruction des glandes génitales de l'embryon de souris, par une irradiation au moyen des rayons X, à l'age de treize jours. *Annl. Endocr.* **8**, 400.

RAYNAUD A. & FRILLEY M. (1948) Procedé d'irradiation localisée au moyen des rayons X, des embryons de souris, dans l'uterus maternel et principaux resultats obtenus. *Bull. Soc. Zool.* (*Fr.*), **73**, 186.

ROBERTS J.D. & WARREN J.C. (1964) Steroid biosynthesis in the foetal ovary. *Endocrinology*, **74**, 846.

ROSA P. (1954) In *Endocrinologie Séxuelle du Foetus Féminin*. Masson et Cie, Paris.

RUMPH P. & SMITH P.E. (1926) The first occurrence of secretory products of a specific structural differentiation in the thyroid and anterior pituitary during the development of the pig foetus. *Anat. Rec.* **33**, 289.

RUNNEBAUM B. & ZANDER J. (1962) Progesterone, Δ^4-Pregnan-20α-ol-3-on, Δ^4-Pregnan-20β-ol-3-on and 17α-hydroxyprogesterone im Plasma der Nabelvene und der Nabelarterien. *Klin. Wschr.* **40**, 453.

SALHANICK (1959) Quoted by Grumbach M.M., Ducharme, J.R. & Moloshok R.E. 'On the fetal masculinising action of certain oral progestins'. *J. Clin. Endocr. Metab.* **19**, 1369.

SANTOS R.F., MCCANCE R.A. & RANDLE P.J. (1955) Insulin activity of cord plasma. *Nature, Lond.* **176**, 115.

SCHLOSSMANN H. (1933) *Der Stoffaustavsch Zwischen Mutter und Frucht durch die Plazenta*. J.F.Bergmann, Munchen.

SCHLOSSMANN H. (1938) Carbohydrate metabolism of foetal dog under influence of insulin. *J. Physiol.* **92**, 219.

SCOTHORNE R.J. (1964) Functional capacity of foetal parathyroid glands with reference to their clinical use as homografts. *Ann. N.Y. Acad. Sci.* **120**, 669.

SCOW R.O. (1964) Hormonal control of postnatal growth of skeletal muscle. *Proceedings of the Second International Congress of Endocrinology II*, p. 772.

SCOW R.O., BECKS H., SIMPSON M., ASLING C. & EVANS H. (1948) Skeletal changes in rats thyroidectomized on the day of birth and effects of growth hormone in such animals. *Anat. Rec.* **100**, 561.

SELLER M.J. (1964) The effect of glucose and insulin on the pregnant rat and foetus. *J. Physiol.* **172**, 353.

SHAH P.N., NAIK S.N., MAHAGAN D.K., DANE M.J. & PAYMASTER J.C. (1961) A new variant of human intersex with discussion on the developmental aspects. *Br. Med. J.* ii, 474.

SHEPHERD T.H., ANDERSEN H. & ANDERSEN H.J. (1964) Histochemical studies of the human fetal thyroid during the first half of fetal life. *Anat. Rec.* **149**, 363.

SMITH C.A. (1959) *The Physiology of the Newborn Infant*, p. 391. Charles C.Thomas, Illinois.

SMITH P.E. & DORTZBACH C. (1929) The first appearance in the anterior pituitary of the developing pig foetus of detectable amounts of the hormones stimulating ovarian maturity and general body growth. *Anat. Rec.* **43**, 277.

SNOECK J. (1958) In *Le Placenta Humain*, p. 375. Masson et Cie, Paris.

SOLOMON S., LANMAN J.T., LIND J. & LIEBERMAN S. (1958) The biosynthesis of androstenedione and 17α-hydroxyprogesterone by surviving human fetal adrenals. *J. Biol. Chem.* **233**, 1084.

SOLOMON S., BIRD C.E., WILSON R., WIQVIST N. & DICZFALUSY E. (1964) Progesterone metabolism in the fetal placental unit. *Proceedings of the Second International Congress of Endocrinology*, p. 721.

SPIVAK M. (1934) Polycystic ovaries in the newborn and early infancy and their relation to the structure of the endometrium. *Am. J. Obst. & Gynec.* **27**, 157.

STERN L., GREENBERG R.E. & LIND J. (1961) Catecholamine excretion in the newborn period: Effect of short periods of induced hypoxia. *Acta Paediat. Stockh.* **50**, 497.

SWEAT M.L., BERLINER D.L., BRYSON M.J., NABOSS C., HASKELL J. & HOLMSTROM E.G. (1960) The synthesis and metabolism of progesterone in the human and bovine ovary. *Biochem. Biophys. Acta*, **40**, 289.

TAYLOR N.R.W., LORAINE J.A. & ROBERTSON H.A. (1953) Estimation of ACTH in human pituitary tissue. *J. Endocr.* **9**, 334.

TILLINGER K.G., DICZFALUSY E. & WESTMAN A. (1957) Studies on oestrogen metabolism in newborn boys. *Acta Endocr.* (*Kbh*), Suppl. 31, p. 47.

TOBIN C.E. (1939) The influence of adrenal destruction on the prenatal development of the albino rat. *Am. J. Anat.* **65**, 151.

VILLEE D.B. & VILLEE C. (1964) Synthesis of cortocosteroids in the fetal placental unit. *Proceedings Second International Congress of Endocrinology, London*, p. 709.

VILLEE D.B., ENGEL L.L. & VILLEE C.A. (1959) Steroid hydroxylation in human fetal adrenals. *Endocrinology*, **65**, 465.

VILLEE D.B., ENGEL L.L., LORING J.M. & VILLEE C.A. (1961) Steroid hydroxylation in human fetal adrenals: formation of 16α-hydroxyprogesterone, 17α-hydroxyprogesterone and deoxycorticosterone. *Endocrinology*, **69**, 354.

WAGNER G., TRANSBOL I. & MELCHIOR J.C. (1964) Hyperparathyroidism and pregnancy. *Acta Endocr. (Kbh)*, **47**, 549.

WALTON R.L. (1954) Neonatal tetany in two siblings: Effect of maternal hyperparathyroidism. *Pediatrics, Springfield*, **13**, 227.

WATERMAN A.J. & GORBMAN A. (1956) Development of the thyroid gland of the rabbit. *J. Exp. Zool.* **132**, 509.

WEISS R.M. & NOBACK C.R. (1949) The effect of thyroxine and thiouracil on the time of appearance of ossification centers of rat fetuses. *Endocrinology*, **45**, 389.

WELLS L.J., CAVANAUGH M.W. & MAXWELL E.L. (1954) Genital abnormalities in castrated foetal rats and their prevention by means of testosterone propionate. *Anat. Rec.* **118**, 109.

WEST G.B. (1955) Comparative pharmacology of the suprarenal medulla. *Rev. Biol.* **30**, 116.

WEST G.B., SHEPHERD D.M., HUNTER R.B. & MACGREGOR A.R. (1953) The function of the organs of Zuckerkandl. *Clin. Sci.* **12**, 317.

WILKINS L. (1957) In *The Diagnosis and Treatment of Endocrine Disorders in Childhood and Adolescence*, 2nd ed. Charles C.Thomas, Springfield, Ill.

WILKINS L. (1960) Masculinisation of the female foetus due to the use of orally given progestins. *J. Am. med. Ass.* **172**, 1028.

WOOLF H. & JACKSON W.P.U. (1957) Maternal prediabetes and the foetal pancreas. *J. Path. Bact.* **74**, 223.

YAMAZAKI E., NOGUCHI A. & SLINGERLAND D.W. (1959) The development of hormonal biosynthesis in human fetal thyroid. *J. Clin. Endocr. Metab.* **19**, 1437.

YAMAZAKI E., NOGUCHI A. & SLINGERLAND D.W. (1961) Thyrotrophin in the serum of mother and fetus. *J. Clin. Endocr. Metab.* **21**, 1013.

ZAAIJER J.J.P., PRICE D. & ORTIZ E. (1966) Organ culture studies of hormone secretion in endocrine glands of foetal guinea-pigs. I. Androgenic secretion as demonstrated by a bioindicator method. *Proc. Kon. Med. Akad. Wet. Ser. C*, **69**, 389.

ZANDER J. (1961) Relationship between progesterone production in the human placenta and the foetus. Ciba Foundation Study Group 9, p. 32.

ZANDER J., THIJSSEN J. & VON MUNSTERMANN A. (1962) Isolation and identification of 16α-hydroxyprogesterone from human corpora lutea and placental blood. *J. Clin. Endocr. Metab.* **22**, 861.

ZETTERSTROM R. & ALBERG B. (1955) Infants of diabetic mothers. *Acta Paediat. Stockh.* **44**, 1.

ZONDEK H. (1940) On the problem of foetal function of the thyroid gland. *Acta med. Scand.* **103**, 251.

ZUCKERKANDL E. (1901) Uber Nebenorgane des Sympathicus in Retroperitoneum des Menschen. *Anat. Anz..* **15**, 97.

Author Index

Bold figures are bibliographical references

Subject Index